# Geriatric Nutrition

## *The Health Professional's Handbook*

### Second Edition

**Ronni Chernoff, PhD, RD, FADA**
Associate Director
GRECC for Education and Evaluation
Department of Veterans Affairs
John L. McClellan Memorial Veterans' Hospital
Little Rock, Arkansas

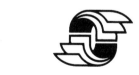

**AN ASPEN PUBLICATION®**
Aspen Publishers, Inc.
Gaithersburg, Maryland
1999

The authors have made every effort to ensure the accuracy of the information herein. However, appropriate information sources should be consulted, especially for new or unfamiliar procedures. It is the responsibility of every practitioner to evaluate the appropriateness of a particular opinion in the context of actual clinical situations and with due considerations to new developments. Authors, editors, and the publisher cannot be held responsible for any typographical or other errors found in this book.

Aspen Publishers , Inc., is not affiliated with the American Society of Parenteral and Enteral Nutrition.

Library of Congress Cataloging-in-Publication Data

Geriatric nutrition: the health professional's handbook/[edited by]
Ronni Chernoff—2nd ed.
p. cm.
Includes bibliographical references and index.
ISBN 0-8342-1082-7
1. Aged—Nutrition. I. Chernoff, Ronni.
[DNLM: 1. Aging—physiology. 2. Nutrition—Aged. QU 145 G3697 1999]
RC952.5.G44342 1999
613.2'084'6—dc21
DNLM/DLC
for Library of Congress
99-14492
CIP

Orders: (800) 638-8437
Customer Service: (800) 234-1660

**About Aspen Publishers** • For more than 35 years, Aspen has been a leading professional publisher in a variety of disciplines. Aspen's vast information resources are available in both print and electronic formats. We are committed to providing the highest quality information available in the most appropriate format for our customers. Visit Aspen's Internet site for more information resources, directories, articles, and a searchable version of Aspen's full catalog, including the most recent publications: **http://www.aspenpublishers.com**
**Aspen Publishers, Inc.** • The hallmark of quality in publishing
Member of the worldwide Wolters Kluwer group.

Editorial Services: Kathleen Ruby
Library of Congress Catalog Card Number: 99-14492
ISBN: 0-8342-1082-7

*Printed in the United States of America*

1  2  3  4  5

## Dedication

This book is dedicated to my mother Lynn—my number one fan;
very best friend; fun, loyal, and loving—to the end of time.
With love.

# Table of Contents

# Contributors

**Jeffrey Blumberg, PhD**
Associate Director and Professor
Chief, Antioxidants Research Laboratory
Jean Mayer USDA Human Nutrition
  Research Center on Aging
Tufts University
Boston, Massachusetts

**William J. Carter, MD**
Associate Chief of Staff, Geriatrics and
  Extended Care
Central Arkansas Veterans Healthcare
  System
Professor, Department of Geriatrics
University of Arkansas for Medical Sciences
Little Rock, Arkansas

**Gurkamal S. Chatta, MD**
Assistant Professor, Geriatrics and
  Oncology
Donald W. Reynolds Department of
  Geriatrics
University of Arkansas for Medical Sciences
Geriatric Research Education and Clinical
  Center
Central Arkansas Veterans Healthcare
  System
Little Rock, Arkansas

**Ronni Chernoff, PhD, RD, LD, FADA**
Associate Director for Education/Evaluation
Geriatric Research Education and Clinical
  Center
Central Arkansas Veterans Healthcare
  System
Professor, Nutrition and Dietetics
University of Arkansas for Medical Sciences
Little Rock, Arkansas

**Rebecca Couris, MS, PhD**
Assistant Professor of Pharmacy
Massachusetts College of Pharmacy and
  Allied Health Sciences
Boston, Massachusetts

**Jessica L. Dorey, BS**
Graduate Assistant
Department of Dietetics and Nutrition
University of Arkansas for Medical Sciences
Little Rock, Arkansas

**Valerie B. Duffy, PhD, RD**
Assistant Professor, Dietetics Program
School of Allied Health
University of Connecticut
Storrs, Connecticut

**Maria A. Fiatarone Singh, MD**
John Sutton Chair of Exercise and Sports
  Medicine
Professor of Medicine
University of Sydney
Sydney, Australia
Associate Professor
School of Nutrition Science and Policy
Jean Mayer USDA Human Nutrition
  Research Center on Aging
Tufts University
Boston Massachusetts

**Gary J. Fosmire, PhD**
Associate Professor of Nutrition Science
Department of Nutrition
Pennsylvania State University
University Park, Pennsylvania

**Jeanne P. Goldberg, PhD, RD**
Director, Center on Nutrition
  Communication
Tufts University School of Nutrition Science
  and Policy
Medford, Massachusetts

**Jennifer P. Hellwig, MS, RD**
Tufts University School of Nutrition Science
  and Policy
Medford, Massachusetts

**Manish Kohli, MD**
Fellow, Hematology/Oncology
Department of Medicine
University of Arkansas for Medical Sciences
Little Rock, Arkansas

**Elyse Levine, PhD, RD**
Research and Evaluation Specialist
Prospect Associates
Silver Spring, Maryland

**Robert D. Lindeman, MD**
Professor and Chief, Division of
  Gerontology
Department of Internal Medicine
University of New Mexico Health Sciences
  Center
Albuquerque, New Mexico

**David A. Lipschitz, MD, PhD**
Chairman, Department on Aging
Director, Donald W. Reynolds Center on
  Aging
University of Arkansas for Medical Sciences
Little Rock, Arkansas

**Robert Marcus, MD**
Professor of Medicine
Stanford University
Director, Aging Study Unit
Veterans Administration Medical Center
Palo Alto, California

**Wendy E. Martin, DDS, MPH**
Staff Gerondontist
St. Louis Veterans Administration Medical
  Center
Assistant Professor
Division of Geriatric Medicine
St. Louis University School of Medicine
St. Louis, Missouri

**Beverly J. McCabe, PhD, RD, LD**
Professor
Department of Dietetics and Nutrition
University of Arkansas for Medical Sciences
Little Rock, Arkansas

**Barbara E. Millen, DPH, RD**
Associate Dean for Research
Professor of Public Health and Medicine
Boston University School of Public Health
Boston University School of Medicine
Boston, MA 02118

**Carol O. Mitchell, PhD, RD**
Professor
Nutrition Graduate Program
Department of Consumer Science and
  Education
The University of Memphis
Memphis, Tennessee

**John E. Morley, MB, BCh**
Dammert Professor of Gerontology
Director, Division of Geriatric Medicine
Department of Internal Medicine
Saint Louis University Health Sciences
  Center
Director, Geriatric Research Education, and
  Clinical Center
St. Louis Veterans Administration Medical
  Center
St. Louis, Missouri

**John R. Saltzman, MD**
Assistant Professor of Medicine
Division of Digestive Disease and Nutrition
University of Massachusetts Medical Center
Worcestor, Massachusetts

**Paolo M. Suter, MD, MS**
Medical Policlinic
University Hospital
Zurich, Switzerland

# Preface

During the past decade, geriatric nutrition has become a burgeoning specialty. Aging is a compilation of complex interactions that occur among such variables as genetic inheritance, health habits, lifestyle, environmental factors, diet, and disease, to cite a few. Analysis of requirements for nutrients, nutrient utilization, nutritional risk, and related issues requires an integration of knowledge of physiologic aging, nutrition, and conditions of aging. There are so many uncontrollable variables that affect the human condition that it is difficult to isolate them and attribute any one of them to the development of a disabling condition. Assumptions must be made based on history, circumstances, population studies, and good clinical judgment.

Relationships between physiologic aging and nutrition, and nutrition and age-related conditions and diseases are getting clearer through research. The purpose of this book is to examine the present knowledge of nutrition in an aging population. The contributing authors are all experts in their field and provide the latest information and perspectives. All of the chapters have been updated and new chapters added for this second edition.

The first chapter addresses some of the issues facing our society that are related to shifting demographics and changes in the ethnic "melting pot" that is the United States. Because the American health care system is changing so rapidly and the population of elderly is about to increase dramatically as the baby boomers age, information about aging and nutrition commands attention. The beginning four chapters address present knowledge in nutrient requirements for macronutrients, vitamins, minerals, and trace metals.

The second group of eight chapters examines the impact of aging on organ systems. This review begins with oral health and a new chapter on taste and smell changes in older adults. This is a topic of great interest with little information readily available to clinicians. A completely revised chapter on the aging gastrointestinal tract follows. The cardiovascular, renal, hematopoietic, skeletal, and endocrine systems chapters are all updated with new information and recent research. These chapters contribute to a greater understanding of physiologic aging and the role that nutrition plays in the development and management of chronic illness. Interesting aspects of aging and nutrition are discussed in these chapters. Hopefully these chapters will contribute to a broader understanding of human aging and the various roles of nutrition in health and disease.

Polypharmacy, with related drug–drug and drug–nutrient interactions, is a problem that many chronically ill elderly experience. For this reason, an entire chapter is devoted to exploring this topic. It is known that elderly people use more prescription and over-the-counter drugs than do younger adults. The potential interactions and side effects of polypharmacy may have serious consequences on the health of elderly people.

A new chapter on exercise and aging is included in this edition. This is an area of great growth and a potential area for research. Exercise is key to the maintenance of health, functionality, and restoration of strength and mobility. Dr. Marie Fiatarone Singh, author of this chapter, was instrumental in bringing our attention to the importance of exercise as a maintenance and restorative therapy in the frail elderly.

The physiologic changes that are associated with advancing age make assessing nutritional status in the elderly challenging, even under the best of circumstances. The various components of a thorough and comprehensive nutritional assessment are discussed in the following chapter. A multidimensional picture of the patient being assessed must be drawn in order to make conclusions about nutritional status. Identifying risk factors and the signs of poor nutritional status is necessary so that appropriate and timely nutritional interventions can be instituted.

Nutritional interventions include diet modification, oral supplements, and enteral and parenterai nutrition. If appropriate choices are made, recommending and administering these interventions can minimize the effects of nutritional depletion by restoring nutritional status and correcting nutritional deficiencies. While many more older adults live at home than are institutionalized, a risk of poor nutrition still exists. This risk, once identified, can be addressed by ensuring access to needed services for older Americans. Revised chapters take a fresh look at nutritional interventions and nutrition services for the elderly.

The last chapter in this volume is a completely revised chapter on health promotion for the elderly. While this chapter focuses on elderly adults, the advice is applicable to all.

We are aware that this text is not perfect and that it is incomplete because of new knowledge discovered since these chapters were written, but we still believe that this book addresses geriatric nutrition in a thorough and rational way. Our hope is that the contents will contribute to a greater understanding of aging and nutrition, will contribute to the reader's successful aging, and will support any endeavor to enhance healthy aging in others.

*Ronni Chernoff, PhD, RD, FADA*

# CHAPTER 1

# Demographics of Aging

*Ronni Chernoff*

Aging is a process experienced by all living creatures as they approach the end of their predestined life spans. It has been described as "intrinsic, deleterious, universal, progressive and irreversible."[1] Most likely, it begins when growth and development cease, and it is a uniquely individual experience that is affected by many factors over which individuals have no control; even geriatrics experts do not possess the ability to predict how aging will occur in any particular individual.

Society and tradition have provided an arbitrary age—65 years—as a demarcation between middle age and old age that has no basis in the study of human aging processes. Biologic aging occurs on a continuum that varies among individuals. The arbitrary age of 65 years was established in the 1880s by Bismarck as the dividing line beyond which people became eligible for retirement pensions; this was an interesting decision considering that there was a shorter life expectancy.[1]

At the beginning of the 20th century, it was not common for people to live much beyond the age of 50 years; average life expectancy was approximately 42 years. Today, 95% of children born will live well past the age of 50. The advances in disease prevention and treatment that have been achieved during the last century have probably extended the human life span close to its predestined limits, but there is probably a limit to future extensions beyond several years.[2]

Factors that may affect individual aging include such diverse occurrences as genetic inheritance, food supply, social circumstances, political events, exposure to disease, climate and natural disasters, and other environmental events. The impacts of these factors and of other life events are impossible to quantify and are hard to interpret, especially since it is very difficult and expensive to conduct prospective aging studies for the entire life span of a large enough group of people to permit conclusions that make any sense. In fact, the premier study on aging that exists in the United States is the Baltimore Longitudinal Study of Aging, which has been going on prospectively since 1958. The most valuable information collected about human aging must be gathered prospectively so that events that occur throughout life can be linked to physiologic, physical, and psychologic changes experienced by aging individuals. It is certainly easier to conduct cross-sectional studies, in which groups of people of varying ages are examined and differences among them at one point in time are measured or described, but such studies tell us nothing about the events that preceded that point in time or which factors contributed to the differences measured.

This area of study is further complicated by the fact that humans are subject to an uncontrolled genetic pool; medical knowledge that changes from one generation to the next; advances in science that affect the quality of life, such as an improved food supply, refrigeration, transportation systems, availability of medicines, and environmental control; and the lack of biologic markers that indicate true physiologic age. Although this is an area that is demanding attention and research resources, little progress has been made in our ability to identify individual life expectancies or to quantify the impact of disease on life span. It is notable that the maximum human life span has been estimated at approximately 112 to 114 years and that this estimate has not changed in more than 200 years.

## DEMOGRAPHIC TRENDS

Until research provides us with a better definition of old age, people who have reached the age of 65 years or older will remain the reference group when the elderly population is discussed. Between 1950 and 1980, the population of those older than age 65 more than doubled so that one in every eight people fell into this age group. By 1996, there were 33.9 million people over age 65. Projections for the future indicate that by 2030 there will be about 70 million people over age 65 and that in 2050 one in every five people will be 65 years or older.[3]

What is truly significant about this increase is not the total size of this group but rather that the greatest increase occurs in the group older than 85 years. Between 1960 and 1980, the percentage of people older than 85 years increased by 281%[4] (Figure 1–1). In a 1996 Census Bureau report, there were 3.5 million people age 85 and older.[5] Projections are that the population of those 85 and older will double to 7 million by 2020 and then double again to 14 million by 2040 due to the aging

baby boomers, born between 1946 and 1964. If these projections prove accurate, by 2050, 1 out of 20 Americans will be age 85 or older compared to 1 in 100 at the end of the 20th century.[3]

Death rates have been declining or remaining constant throughout the 20th century; however, declines in mortality rates vary by age, race, and sex. Women have had a consistently greater decline in mortality rate, making the proportion of women larger, the older the age group. Actually, more boys than girls are born, but since there is a higher death rate for males and an improvement in mortality rate for women, this ratio changes quickly. In 1980, there were 44 males to every 100 females over age 85 years. In 1996, there were 20 million older women and 13.9 million older men. The ratio of males to females declines with advancing age; this ratio is expected to fall to 36 males for every 100 females by 2020.[4] The result will be an increasingly large group of women in the very old age group, and this is not expected to change (Figure 1–2).

The impact of this trend is yet to be seen. Women live longer, but they also have more disabilities than do elderly men. Disability in men is usually related to heart disease and stroke; in women, disability is related to osteoporosis and associated fractures, arthritis, and circulatory diseases. Women tend to live longer with disability than do men.[6]

There are differences in population demographics by race as well as by age and sex. By 2030, the elderly minority population will represent 25% of all older adults. At present, there are many more elderly white people than there are elderly African American people, despite a proportionately higher birth rate among African Americans. This discrepancy is due to a higher mortality rate at younger ages for African Americans as well as increased mortality from hypertension, less access to preventive health care services,

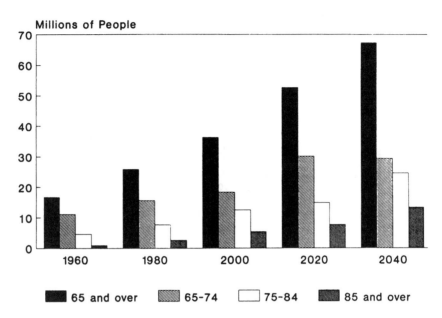

**Figure 1–1** Population projections for various age groups from 1960 to 2040, based on Social Security Administration data.

and a delay in seeing a physician until the terminal stages of disease.[7] Although the mortality rate for African Americans is expected to decrease, it is not projected to compensate for the gap between races in the near future. Between 1990 and 2030, the elderly African American population is expected to grow by 159%.

The ethnic diversity of the older population, as well as the working-age population, will increase due to the larger families and higher birth rates of both African Americans and Hispanic Americans.[3] The number of elderly Hispanic Americans grew 61% in the decade between 1970 and 1980 and is expected to increase by 570% between 1990 and 2030. Compared with elders in other groups, Hispanic American elders are 2.5 times more likely to live with incomes below the poverty line. However, they tend to spend a larger proportion of their disposable income on

health care, despite a lower likelihood of having health insurance than other groups of elderly people.[8] Health care tends to be through emergency departments, and admissions to the hospital are usually via this route. Along with the socioeconomic barriers to accessing health care, Hispanic American elderly also have cultural and language barriers to overcome. There appears to be a link between having English language skills and having a primary care provider. This may reflect a higher socioeconomic status or more successful acculturation among English speakers than among those who speak only Spanish.[8]

Asian and Pacific Islander elders have different cultural traditions than other minority groups. They tend to form a more cohesive family group that offers support for the elderly family members. Their cultural mores contribute to a unique approach to medical care, relying heavily on the customary view

## Population Growth by Age and Sex
### 1960-2040

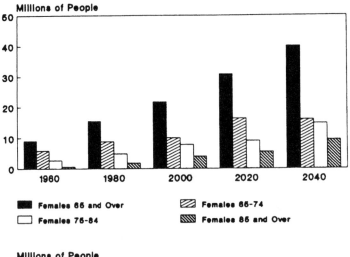

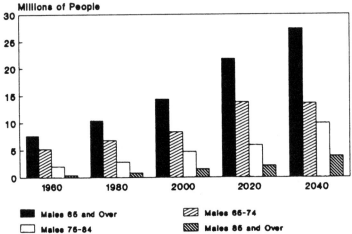

**Figure 1–2** Comparison of population growth by age and sex for men and women in the United States, based on Social Security Administration data.

of mind and body linkages and the use of traditional medicines. Although this group of older adults is a small proportion of the population, the number of elderly is expected to grow as the immigrants from the 1970s age.[9]

Life expectancy of Native Americans has increased dramatically during the past decade and is expected to increase by 294% by 2030. Data regarding the health status of elderly Native Americans are sparse, and their availability is highly variable among tribes. The Indian Health Service was elevated to agency status in the Public Health Service in 1988, and it can be anticipated that this will allow for greater awareness of the health needs of all Native Americans. It is known that heart disease, diabetes mellitus, cancer, oral health, and nutrition problems exist among Native

American groups.[10] Nutrition services and meals for Native Americans receiving care from the Indian Health Service are generally provided through Title III of the Older Americans Act.

The income of today's elderly populace is greater than that of similarly aged cohorts of previous generations. Social Security benefits represent the largest source of income for this group, followed by earnings and income from property, pensions, and investments. Although the current group of elderly people is less educated than are Americans of younger age groups, the gap between generations is closing and is expected to change by the end of the century. The next generation of elderly is much better educated and more affluent than the current age cohort.[11] This fact will have an impact on income levels of future groups of older people, most likely making them more sophisticated, with greater expectations of social care systems and medical care options,[4] and may thereby lead to greater expenditures for health care services. These factors will probably contribute to more of the elderly population's owning their own homes in the future and wanting to stay in them for as long as they can manage.

Demographic trends are affected by many factors, including migration, immigration, and "new elderly births." New elderly births are the number of people who are newly classified as "elderly" because they have passed their 60th birthday. This effect has shifted the elderly population in the United States faster than the total population growth. Elderly births are making a noticeable impact on African American, Hispanic, and Asian populations, where immigration occurred in large numbers in the years before World War II. The next significant force of this will occur in 2006, when the "baby boom" generation will start to turn 60. For the future, the impact of this phenomenon will continue to be greater than the effect of migration and immigration.[12]

Another demographic factor that distinguishes the present cohort of elderly people from future generations of older people is their mobility. Older people tend to move geographically less often, and less far, than do younger people; they tend to settle in the geographic region where they were born and raised or where they settled when they married.[4] This is likely to change as the next generation ages.

As population demographics shift, population projections by the Bureau of the Census predict significant differences in rates of change in different regions of the United States. The regions that are expected to grow the fastest are the South and the West, while the north central region of the country will lose population.[4] Immigration per se has a minimal effect on the demographics of this age group except in four states: Hawaii, California, Florida, and New York. Internal migration has a more noticeable impact on states that tend to be magnets for retirees, led by Nevada, Florida, and Arizona.[12] These factors will influence the need for, and accessibility to, health care resources in the future.

## IMPACT ON THE HEALTH CARE SYSTEM

One of the natural occurrences that accompanies aging is an increase in the prevalence of disabilities and diseases. The incidence of concurrent illnesses and multiple disabilities rises sharply with age and is greatest in the very old segment of the population, those older than 85 years.[4] When an acute episode occurs, the consumption of health care resources is greater in this group of patients because of the multiple chronic problems they may have that must be attended to along with their acute illnesses. Unfortunately, the health care system in the United States is becoming increasingly focused on the short-term delivery of acute health care, allowing expensive and limited technologies to be used for the maximal number of patients. Complex, frail, very old patients require these expensive, lifesaving technologies, but concurrently they also require extended periods of skilled care for adequate recuperation and rehabilitation. This increasingly large portion of the population will soon strain the resources of the existing health care system.

On the basis of relatively recent statistics, the population segment older than 65 years—approximately 12% of the total population—accounts for more than 38% of all hospital stays,[13] uses approximately 48% of the acute care hospital bed days,[14,15] buys 25% of all the prescription drugs, spends 30% of the health care dollars spent in the United States (about $53 billion), and accounts for more than 50% of the federal health budget (about $20 billion).[14] By 1993, the population older than 85 years represented 1.3% of the total population but accounted for 36% of all personal health expenditures, totaling approximately $162 billion.[13,16]

There is no doubt that health care managers must assess the growth of the older segment of the population carefully and plan accordingly. For example, although only 5% of elderly people are in nursing homes at any one time, 90% of those older than 65 years and 42% of those older than 85 years have experienced a nursing home admission, making the availability of nursing home beds and services an increasingly important part of planning for and allocating health care resources in the future.[16] The heaviest users of nursing home beds are women aged 85 and older (Figure 1–3).[17] It is projected that the nursing home population will increase from 1,511,000 in 1980 to 5,227,000 in 2040. There is an increased shift in resources toward home health care and community-based service providers, and this will be a factor in future policy making and planning.[16]

When the "baby boomers" come of elderly age, between 2020 and 2040, the largest demands for services will occur (Figure 1–2).[15] Other issues that will affect the utilization of services are that the next generation of elderly have a higher level of education, are more medically sophisticated, and have different expectations than their parents. Baby boomers want the health care system to keep them well, not just to take care of them when they are sick. They have had better childhood health and medical care and are generally healthier than previous generations. The next generation of older adults expects accessible, local, convenient, available, and cost-effective services.[11]

The issue of how health care services for the elderly will be paid for is a major policy problem to be addressed in the immediate future. As the "baby boomers" reach retirement age starting in 2006, there is expected to be a major stress on Social Security and Medicare benefits. Medicare pays for a notable percentage of the costs incurred by older adults; in 1987, Medicare expenditures for older people came to $72 billion.[17] Medicare Part A covers in-hospital costs. As health care costs rise, the likelihood that the funds paid in to Medicare will cover the projected health care demands is decreasing.[18]

Policy decisions to increase the retirement eligibility age will not address the problem with Medicare unless the eligibility age for Medicare changes too. One approach to saving Medicare Part A funds is to shift costs to Medicare Part B, which covers less costly outpatient services. Reducing acute care hospital lengths of stay and shifting health care

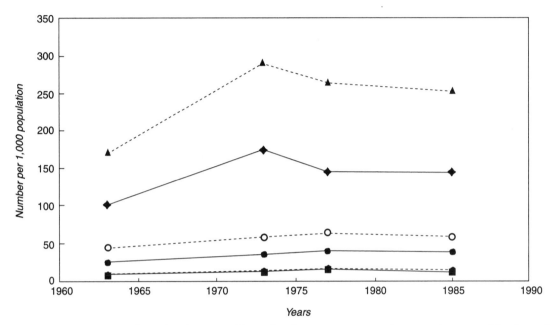

**Figure 1–3** Number of nursing home residents for three age groups of men and women. Number of residents per 1,000 persons for 1973–1974 and 1977 differs from that presented in the original source reports because the rates have been recomputed using revised census estimates for those years. For 1973–1974, data exclude residents in personal care domiciliary care homes. *Source:* Data from National Center for Health Statistics: *Health, United States, 1992,* National Nursing Home Survey.

delivery to outpatient clinics, day hospitals, and home-delivered services are potential options for saving money.[18]

Health care service utilization is a very complex issue. The major factor in this complicated matrix of resource utilization is health status, whether it is an individual perception or a medical diagnosis.[19] Utilization has been described using a supply/demand model with some secondary factors that have a major effect on both supply and demand. These secondary factors are demographic (e.g., age, gender, socioeconomics), socio-psychological (e.g., attitudes, personality, health beliefs), sociocultural (e.g., religion, norms and values, ethnicity), and financial-economic (e.g., health insurance, disposable income).[19] On the demand side are age, sex, household composition, education, income, housing, social support system, medical technologies, and attitudes. On the supply side are health insurance and health care policy decisions, productivity of providers, efficiency, efficacy and technological developments, and suppliers' cooperation in the provision of services.[17]

## QUALITY OF LIFE AND HEALTH STATUS

It is well known that older people have more health problems than do younger individuals. However, it is often overlooked that a large percentage of the population older than 65 years is relatively healthy and vigorous. Needless to say, good health status contributes to vitality and quality of life.

*Quality of life* is a difficult term to define well. Objective indicators of quality of life show only a weak relationship to individuals' perceptions of quality of life.[20] There are many subjective factors that contribute to quality of life, of which health status is only one. For example, general health and functional status represent one dimension of perceived quality of life, along with socioeconomic status, general life satisfaction, and self-esteem.[21] Of interest is that subjective estimates of health status by the individual do not correlate closely with objective assessment of health status as measured by laboratory tests and physical examination.[20] However, the dimension that appears to correlate better when perceptions are compared with objective measures is functional status. Functional status is defined as the ability to perform activities related to self-care and daily living and can be measured by several instruments.[22] Frequently, poor health status and physical disability have an impact on functional ability; it is difficult to separate the two dimensions.

Approximately 54% of all those older than age 65 report having at least one disability that limits their ability to carry out the activities of daily living, and 50% of those 85 years and older need assistance with the activities of daily living.[13] As the population ages, there will be an increased need for assistive services to supplement family support.[3]

*Quality of life* takes on different meanings when applied to institutionalized elderly people. Since their health status is questionable—or they would not need institutional care—factors that contribute to their perceptions of quality of life tend to relate to their immediate environment. The quality of their food; the ability to make choices and control some parts of their lives; participation in events in the institution, such as self-feeding or exercise programs; and the attitudes of the care providers and other residents all contribute to the quality of life for chronically ill, elderly people cared for in institutions.[23] Certainly, satisfaction with one's life and surroundings contributes to perception of the overall quality of life. A positive outlook can contribute to better cooperation and compliance with health care regimens and perhaps help to maintain health status for a greater part of the latter years of life. All of these factors contribute to successful aging.

## HEALTH CARE COSTS

As the elderly portion of the population expands, the consumption of health care resources may grow beyond their present availability. Efforts to curb expenditures have focused on acute care resources and have had an impact primarily on elderly, poor, and underprivileged patients. Many factors contribute to the large amounts of money spent on health care in the United States. Certainly, advances in medical technology, which result in the availability of expensive equipment needed to perform diagnostic tests and to provide technical treatment modalities, have contributed to rising costs. Another important contributing factor is that a large proportion of the population is living longer, since the management of chronic disease has become easier and since technologic advances have made the diagnosis and treatment of serious illnesses more effective.

Data from the National Center for Health Statistics support the proposal that one of the reasons the elderly segment of the population is getting larger is that their death rates are decreasing.[21] Because older people tend to have more disabilities and more chronic conditions, they require—and use—more health care resources. There is no doubt that people older than 65 years require more acute care hospital days than do younger people, and this need increases in even older groups: individuals older than 85 years use 8,300 days of acute care hospital resources per 1,000 persons[15]; for chronic care resources, individuals older than 85 years use 86,400 days per year per 1,000 persons.[15]

The need for health care services in the area of chronic care also requires an examination of the availability of appropriate providers. Models that analyze the requirements for physicians who are trained in geriatrics and are primary care providers indicate that there is probably not a compelling need for more physicians; rather, the kind of health care and services needed can, and should, be provided by midlevel providers such as physician assistants (PAs) and registered nurse practitioners (RNPs). It is estimated that if service delivery is shifted to ambulatory care practice with PAs and RNPs, the number of patient visits can be increased by 12% to 37%, improving physician efficiency.[24,25]

The need for quality long-term care and the complexity of the issue are attracting the attention of policy makers. There are few demographic data to describe residents of long-term care facilities because they are often missed or overlooked in censuses or household surveys. However, as the population of frail elderly people increases, interest in payment sources for their care becomes greater. Currently, public or private insurance to help defray the costs of long-term care is limited. Skilled nursing services are expensive, and it

is likely that in most cases public funds such as Medicare or Medicaid will not cover the costs of care. Proprietary nursing homes are reluctant to accept patients who require skilled care; facilities that accept this type of patient may have staff inadequately skilled to care for ill patients. This limitation often creates a difficult situation when services are needed but are not affordable or available.[3]

Alternatives to nursing home care are being explored through experimental or demonstration projects. Home health care services are one option that may prove to be a viable alternative to nursing home care. There are limitations to home care services, particularly the need for caregiver support required to make it work. In one model, a large portion of the care provided (about 72%) is delivered by family members, particularly if the patient's disabilities are not great. Costs for home services increase with the level of patient disability.[26]

Some physicians do not favor the home health care concept because they are concerned with malpractice issues, quality-of-care issues, loss of control over patient care, and loss of reimbursement, since the home health agencies take over managerial responsibilities.[26] Physicians have a limited role in the delivery of health care when the home care agencies become the primary providers. The physician is involved only in approving forms that allow home care professionals to be reimbursed or in providing telephone consultations to the primary care provider. To be paid for patients' home health care, physicians must see the patients in the office or visit them in their homes; these activities are very time-consuming and not very cost-effective.

Hospitals are becoming involved in developing home health services because they are a viable option for extending services and marketing other hospital programs. These have become prime objectives because hospital reimbursement systems have limited income in many facilities.[27] In fact, hospital-based home health care programs have grown much faster than independent home health care agencies.[28]

Other models of home care have been developed by the Department of Veterans Affairs. For frail but medically stable elderly individuals who have able caregivers, the hospital-based primary care (HBPC) program is a successful alternative. The hospital-based staff members make home visits within a 50-mile radius of their base, and skilled health care professionals (social workers, pharmacists, dietitians, nurses, and physicians) track patients on a regular schedule and assess their home situations. This program provides continuity of care, an important dimension of caring for frail elderly people. There is regular contact by telephone so that problems can be dealt with early and hospitalization arranged efficiently when needed.[29]

Another program alternative that may be a feasible solution to the problems of providing health care to elderly patients is adult day health care.[30] Access to appropriate adult day health care facilities may enable frail elderly people to remain in their home surroundings and maintain a relatively familiar lifestyle. There are different types of adult day care models. The most common model is the social model. Social day care programs are designed to meet the needs of clients who may be disabled but are medically stable. The primary purpose of these programs is to maintain social and physical capacities through recreational and other social programs and to prevent or delay institutionalization.[26]

Medical model day care programs are designed to provide rehabilitative and support services, with the goal being the restoration of physical and functional abilities. One type of medical model adult day care has been un-

der study through a multicenter health services research grant provided by the Department of Veterans Affairs.[26] In this program, elderly people can remain in their own homes yet receive health care through a day care center that provides therapeutic services. Family members, friends, or other support providers must arrange for transportation to the sites, or the program must provide transportation. Patients can be enrolled in the program if they require rehabilitative care, such as physical or occupational therapy, medical treatment, or respite care. Patients can attend the center as needed, but usually they visit two or three times per week. They are brought in early in the morning and are picked up in the late afternoon, making it possible for care providers, spouses, or adult children to continue to participate in other activities, such as work or household or child care responsibilities.

Although there may not be ready-made answers to the problems of providing health care to elderly people in the future, there are certainly options being explored.[25] It is obvious that something must be done to provide quality health care for this segment of the populace, but to develop the services and find the resources to pay for them, a great deal must be learned about aging, diseases that are common in old age, and the maintenance of health in aging people.

## CONCLUSION

There is no doubt that the expansion of the population segment older than 65 years will force health care providers to face problems associated with an aging society sooner than they might have liked. Many creative options have been proposed to provide appropriate quality health care to elderly people, but they need to be tested and evaluated before solutions can be found to the problems inherent in health care delivery to a large, distinct population of patients who have different income levels, unique medical problems, and diverse life experiences.

Within this context, health care providers must understand the role of nutrition in the maintenance of health, the management of chronic conditions, and the treatment of serious disease. The remainder of this text addresses the relationship among physiologic aging, nutrition, and disease. Comprehension of these important associations and the application of this knowledge will contribute to more effective health promotion, disease prevention, and disease management in elderly persons.

## REFERENCES

1. Haynes SG, Feinleib M. *Second Conference on the Epidemiology of Aging.* Washington, DC: US Public Health Service; 1980. US Dept of Health and Human Services publication NIH 80-969.

2. Olshansky SJ, Carnes BA, Grahn D. Confronting the boundaries of human longevity. *Am Scientist.* January/February 1998;86:52–61.

3. Waite LJ. The demographic face of America's elderly. *Inquiry.* 1996;33:220–224.

4. Gilford DM, ed. *The Aging Population in the Twenty-First Century: Statistics for Health Policy.* Washington, DC: National Academy Press; 1988.

5. *Census Report.* Government Printing Office, Washington, DC; 1996.

6. Manton KG. Demographic trends for the aging female population. *J Am Med Women's Assoc.* 1997;52(3):99–105.

7. Brangman SA. African-American elders: implications for health care providers. *Clin Geriatr Med.* 1995;11(1):15–23.

8. Pousada L. Hispanic American elders: implications for health-care providers. *Clin Geriatr Med.* 1995;11(1):39–52.

9. Douglas KC, Fujimoto D. Asian Pacific elders: implications for health care providers. *Clin Geriatr Med.* 1995;11(1):69–82.

10. Rousseau P. Native American elders: implications for health care providers. *Clin Geriatr Med.* 1995;11(1):83–95.

11. Chernoff R. Baby boomers come of age: nutrition in the 21st century. *J Am Diet Assoc.* 1995;95(6): 650–654.

12. Frey WH. Elderly demographic profiles of US states: impacts of "new elderly births," migration, and immigration. *Gerontologist.* 1995;35:761–770.

13. *A Profile of Older Americans: 1997.* Washington, DC: Program Resources Dept, American Association of Retired Persons and the Administration on Aging, Dept of Health and Human Services; 1998.

14. Hanson MJ. How we treat the elderly. *Hastings Center Rep.* 1994;24(5):4–6.

15. Pegels CC. *Health Care and the Older Citizen.* Gaithersburg, Md: Aspen Publishers, Inc; 1988.

16. Background materials. 1995 White House Conference on Aging; May 2–5, 1995; Washington, DC.

17. *Vital and Health Statistics: Trends in the Health of Older Americans: U.S. 1994.* Washington, DC: US Government Printing Office; 1995. Series 3, Analytic and Epidemiological Studies, No. 30.

18. Chen Y-P. "Equivalent retirement ages" and their implications for Social Security and Medicare Financing. *Gerontologist.* 1994;34:731–735.

19. van der Berg Jeths A, Thorslund M. Will resources for elders be scarce? *Hastings Center Rep.* 1994; 24(5):6–10.

20. Vinokur A, Cannell CF, Eraker SA, et al. *The Role of Survey Research in the Assessment of Health and the Quality-of-Life Outcomes of Pharmaceutical Interventions.* Ann Arbor, Mich: University of Michigan, Institute for Social Research; 1983. Cost-Effectiveness of Pharmaceuticals Report Series No. 6.

21. George L, Bearon L. *Quality of Life in Older Persons: Meaning and Measurement.* New York: Human Sciences Press; 1980.

22. Besdine RW. The data base of geriatric medicine. In: Rowe JW, Besdine RW, eds. *Health and Disease in Old Age.* Boston, Mass: Little, Brown & Co; 1982:1–14.

23. Institute of Medicine Committee on Nursing Home Regulations. *Improving the Quality of Care in Nursing Homes.* Washington, DC: National Academy Press; 1986.

24. Reuben DB, Bradley TB, Zwanziger J, Beck JC. Projecting the need for physicians to care for older persons: effects of changes of demography, utilization patterns, and physician productivity. *J Am Geriatr Soc.* 1983;41:1033–1038.

25. Beck C, Chumbler N. Planning for the future of long-term care: consumers, providers, and purchasers. *J Gerontol Nurs.* 1997;23(8):6–13.

26. Liu K, Manton KG, Liu BM. Home care expenses for the disabled elderly. *Health Care Financ Rev.* 1985;7(2):51–58.

27. Taeuber C. America in transition: an aging society. In: *Current Population Reports.* Washington, DC: Bureau of the Census; 1983. US Dept of Commerce Special Studies Series P-23, No. 128.

28. Weissert WG. One more battle lost to friendly fire—or if you spend too much it's hard to save money. *Med Care.* 1993;31(9):SS119–121.

29. Cummings J, Hughes S, Weaver F. Cost effectiveness of Veterans Administration hospital-based home care: a randomized clinical trial. *Arch Intern Med.* 1990;150:1274–1280.

30. Hedrick SC, Rothman ML, Chapko M, et al. Summary and discussion of methods and results of the Adult Day Health Care Evaluation Study. *Med Care.* 1993;31(9):SS94–SS103.

# CHAPTER 2

# Macronutrient Requirements for Elderly Persons

*William J. Carter*

## PROTEIN METABOLISM AND REQUIREMENT IN ELDERLY SUBJECTS

### Age-Related Changes in Body Protein Content, Distribution, and Turnover

Changes in body protein content, distribution, and turnover make consideration of protein intake particularly important in older persons. There is a decline in lean body mass with age that is manifested by a decrease in total body potassium, nitrogen, and water content.[1] Measurement of the components of lean body mass by neutron activation techniques indicates that a decline in muscle mass accounts for most of the age-related reduction in lean body mass.[2] In contrast, non-muscle lean tissue mass does not decrease substantially with age (Table 2–1). Direct measurement of muscle weight at autopsy demonstrates a substantial loss of muscle mass with age.[3] Skeletal muscle accounts for about 45% of body weight during young adulthood, but its contribution declines to about 27% at age 70.[3] Uauy and associates have shown that skeletal muscle makes a smaller contribution to total body protein metabolism with advancing age.[4] In young adulthood, skeletal muscle accounts for about 30% of whole-body protein turnover, but in old age it decreases to 20% or less. In addition to decreased strength, the decreased skeletal muscle reservoir may provide an inadequate supply of amino acids in response to illness or other stress.[4]

The diminishing muscle mass contributes greatly to the frailty of old age by causing loss of strength and declining functional reserve, which often leads to decreased mobility, postural instability, and falls. The age-related decline in muscle mass is a direct cause of the age-related decrease in muscle strength.[5] Furthermore, muscle strength is highly correlated with functional capacity in the very old. In one study, 40% of women 55 to 65 years of age, 45% of women aged 66 to 75, and 65% of women aged 76 to 85 could not lift 4.5 kg.[6] Similar percentages could not do heavy housework. Protein intake by older persons should be high enough to minimize the age-related loss of skeletal muscle. It is clear that an inadequate protein intake may accelerate this loss.

### Measurement of Dietary Protein Requirements

Most estimates of adult protein requirement have been made in young and middle-aged individuals. Two general methods have most often been used to estimate dietary pro-

**Table 2–1** Effects of Age on Body Composition in Normal Men

| Age (y) | Nonmuscle Mass (kg) | Muscle Mass (kg) | Total Body Fat (kg) |
|---------|---------------------|------------------|---------------------|
| 20–29 | 37 | 24 | 15 |
| 40–49 | 38 | 20 | 19 |
| 60–69 | 37 | 17 | 23 |
| 70–79 | 38 | 13 | 25 |

Source: Adapted with permission from S.H. Cohn et al., Effect of Age on Body Composition in Normal Men, *American Journal of Physiology*, Vol. 239, pp. E524, E526, and E527, © 1980, American Physiological Society.

tein requirement.[7] One method, the factorial method, measures all losses of nitrogen compounds in individuals adapted to a protein-free diet and assumes that the dietary protein requirement is equal to the amount of protein necessary to replace these losses. The second method determines directly the minimum amount of dietary protein needed for nitrogen equilibrium in adults and optimum growth in infants and children. On the basis of these methods, the adult requirement for protein of average quality appears to be approximately 0.8 g/kg per day.[7] Variation in energy intake reduces the accuracy of this estimate. At high energy intakes, less protein is required to achieve nitrogen balance than at low energy intakes.[7] In nitrogen balance studies, the energy intake has often been increased beyond basal requirement to prevent weight loss on low-protein diets.[7] This approach tends to produce estimates of protein requirement that are too low when applied to individuals with borderline or low energy intakes.

### Daily Protein Requirement for Elderly Persons

Although earlier studies suggested that the protein requirement of elderly subjects is less than that of young adults, more recent nitrogen balance studies indicate that protein requirement per kilogram of body weight increases with age.[1] A carefully performed nitrogen balance study showed that the current recommended daily allowance of 0.8 g of high-quality egg protein per kilogram of body weight per day did not maintain nitrogen balance in half of the elderly men and women studied for 30 days.[8] A recent balance study found that 1 g of protein per kilogram of body weight per day was required to maintain nitrogen equilibrium.[9] When protein requirements for nitrogen balance were calculated from the data of four previous studies using currently accepted formulas, the average value was 0.91 g/kg per day.[10] Allowing a safety factor to accommodate the needs of most individuals, the minimum recommended safe intake was 1 g/kg of body weight per day of high-quality protein.[10] This estimate applies to well elderly only. A number of stresses may increase the protein requirement well above this level, as indicated below. A dietary survey of 239 men and 452 women aged 60 to 95 suggested that 1 g of protein per kilogram of body weight is an adequate daily allowance.[11] Persons with debilitating diseases were excluded from this study, which focused on overtly healthy, free-living men and women in an urban environment. Nutrient intake was estimated from a diary listing all foods, beverages, and nutrient supplements consumed over a 3-day period. Protein intake was correlated with indices of protein nutrition including serum albumin, prealbumin, transferrin, ceruloplasmin, retinol-binding protein, and upper arm muscle mass.

On the other hand, leucine balance measured by short-term labeled leucine infusion at high and low protein intakes suggested that the protein requirement of healthy elderly subjects is similar to or less than that of young adults.[12] Five men and five women aged 68 to 91 were compared to five men and five women aged 21 to 31. The subjects received a 9-hour infusion of labeled leucine, beginning with 3 hours in the postabsorptive state (0–3 hours), followed by 3 hours during isoenergetic low-protein feeding (3–6 hours), and ending with 3 hours during isoenergetic high-protein feeding (6–9 hours). The metabolic demand for protein was assumed to be proportional to postabsorptive leucine oxidation, and the efficiency of postprandial protein utilization (PPU) was assumed to be proportional to the increase in leucine oxidation following feeding. The apparent protein requirement was calculated by dividing the metabolic demand by PPU. The apparent daily protein requirement was 0.99 g/kg for young adults, 0.66 g/kg for elderly men, and 0.84 g/kg for elderly women.

## Recommended Protein Allowance for Elderly Subjects

Since the studies examining protein requirements for elderly persons are few and inconsistent, a definitive recommendation is not possible.[13] Nevertheless, it appears prudent to use the more liberal recommendation derived from nitrogen balance studies until more information is available. On the basis of these studies, a daily intake of 1 g of high-quality protein per kilogram of body weight is recommended.[10] Since digestibility of dietary protein is about 90% and since mixed animal and plant protein is likely to be of lower quality (ie, reduced proportion of es-

sential amino acids) than egg protein, a 10% increase in this estimate provides an additional margin of safety. Since energy requirement declines with age, the dietary protein intake is likely to be a greater proportion of total energy intake (12–14%) as age advances.[1,11] When necessary, protein intake must be increased to satisfy the demand of specific diseases and to replete protein stores in malnourished subjects.

## Quality of Dietary Protein

An ideal protein provides all essential amino acids in optimum concentrations to meet requirements when fed in adequate amounts.[7] Although amino acid content is a useful means to describe the nutritional potential of dietary protein, it is not ideal. The ability of a test protein to support growth in infants and nitrogen balance in adults can be used as another index of protein quality.[7] Most animal proteins contain a satisfactory mixture of essential amino acids and can be considered to be high quality. On the other hand, many plant proteins have a lower nutritional value because they contain too little of one or more essential amino acids; this causes inefficient utilization and the need for a larger protein intake to maintain nitrogen equilibrium. Nevertheless, adequate protein nutrition can be obtained using predominantly or exclusively plant proteins provided that complementary groups of plant proteins (such as proteins of the cereal and legume families) are consumed during the course of a day in the same or separate meals.[1]

## Factors Affecting Protein Requirement in Elderly Subjects

Aging is accompanied by an increasing frequency of acute and chronic diseases. Enhanced protein catabolism in response to stresses such as surgery, infection, fractures, and other trauma can greatly increase protein requirement.[14] These catabolic responses are mediated by increased levels of cortisol, glucagon, and catecholamines and cause loss of lean body mass, especially muscle.[14] Although adequate protein intake during the first week following these stresses does not prevent increased proteolysis, it minimizes the negative nitrogen balance that ensues.[14] Protein intake should be increased 1.5 to 2-fold as soon as tolerated and continued until lean body mass is restored.[14] If the patient is malnourished at the onset of the illness or if enteral intake is delayed for more than 7 days, parenteral nutrition should be considered.[14]

Progressive resistance training (PRT), which is muscle contraction against a force that progressively increases as muscle strength increases, has increased muscle mass and strength in elderly subjects.[15] PRT has significant anabolic effects and has decreased nitrogen excretion by 10% to 15%.[15] This suggests that appropriate exercise may reduce the protein intake required to attain nitrogen balance.

### Effect of Protein Intake on the Age-Related Decline in Renal Function

Brenner and associates have suggested that the high and continuous protein intake common in current Western societies increases renal blood flow, glomerular filtration rate, and the transcapillary pressure gradient in the glomerulus.[16] They further suggest that these changes contribute to age-related glomerular sclerosis.[16] In support of this hypothesis, over half of the glomeruli are sclerotic in senescent rats fed a high-protein diet ad lib.[17] Development of these lesions is delayed by feeding a low-protein diet.[18] Although the 30% reduction in functioning glomeruli seen in humans between the fourth and eighth decades does not cause significant renal insufficiency by it-

self, it may be very important when combined with intrinsic renal disease.[16] However, recent studies do not support a relationship between protein intake and the age-related decrease in renal function.[19,20] When healthy individuals on a high protein intake were compared with vegetarians on a long-term low protein intake, no difference in the age-related deterioration in creatinine clearance was noted.[19] Furthermore, an analysis of male members of the Baltimore Longitudinal Study of Aging failed to show a relationship between high protein intake and impairment of creatinine clearance.[20] At present, there is little basis for reducing protein intake to spare renal function.

## AGE AND ENERGY REQUIREMENT

### Effect of Age on Energy Requirement

There is evidence that energy intake declines progressively with age. In a cross-sectional survey, the total energy intake of men enrolled in the Baltimore Longitudinal Study of Aging declined from 2700 kcal at age 30 to 2100 kcal at age 80.[21] About one third of this decrement was attributed to a declining basal metabolic rate (BMR) and the remainder to decreased physical activity.[21] A subsequent longitudinal analysis of this study population over 15 years confirmed the reduction in energy intake with age.[22] The decline in energy intake appeared to be a pure effect of age, with no confounding cohort or time effects. Reduced fat consumption by elderly subjects accounted for the decreased energy intake.[22] In addition, other cross-sectional studies such as the Framingham Study and the Health and Nutritional Examination Survey (HANES) have shown declining energy intake with age.[23,24] In HANES, energy intake in men decreased from 2700 kcal in the 23- to 34-year age group to 1800 kcal in the 65- to 74-year age group.[23] Although a declining BMR has been cited as contributing to the reduced energy requirement of older individuals,[21] Owen and associates found little effect of age on the resting metabolic rate (RMR) in healthy men.[25] In this study, RMR was measured by indirect calorimetry in 60 men, only 4 of whom were 65 years of age or older. Increasing age was associated with a small, statistically insignificant reduction in RMR. The small number of elderly subjects in this study reduces the impact of the authors' conclusion that age has an insignificant effect on RMR in healthy subjects.[25]

### Estimation of the Energy Requirement of Elderly Individuals

The BMR is determined by body size, body composition, and age.[26] Within a given sex and age range, weight is the most useful and practical index for predicting BMR.[26] The Food and Agriculture Organization (FAO)/ World Health Organization (WHO)/United Nations University (UNU) Expert Group has calculated regression equations relating BMR to body weight that can be used to estimate the BMR of adults.[26] The adult category has been divided into three age ranges: 18 to 30, 30 to 60, and older than 60 years. Regression equations have been presented in Table 2–2 for men and women in each age range.

Total energy requirement can be estimated by multiplying the BMR by factors covering the energy costs of physical activity, maintenance of muscle tone, and the thermic effect of food.[26] The energy costs of various levels of physical activity expressed as multiples of the BMR are presented in Table 2–3. The energy requirement per 24 hours can be estimated by summing the energy costs for different levels of activity that occur throughout the day.[26] The energy required for each level of activity is estimated by multiplying the rate of energy expenditure in kcal/h times the number of hours spent at that level of activity. Table 2–4 presents the daily energy require-

**Table 2–2** Estimate of BMR in kcal According to Age and Sex ($W$ = Body Weight in Kilograms)

| Age Range | Men | Women |
|---|---|---|
| 18–30 | $15.3W + 679$ | $14.7W + 496$ |
| 31–60 | $11.6W + 879$ | $8.7W + 829$ |
| 60+ | $13.5W + 487$ | $10.5W + 596$ |

*Source:* Adapted from: *Energy and protein requirements.* Report of a Joint FAO/WHO/UNU Expert Consultation. Geneva, World Health Organization, 1985 (WHO Technical Report Series, No. 724), Table 5.

ment of a healthy retiree, estimated as indicated above.[26]

Until recently, there was no way to directly measure total energy expenditure (TEE), so it was indirectly estimated by summing its principal components. This "factorial approach" may underestimate TEE because of difficulties in timing and accurately measuring activities not associated with specific tasks.[27] Recently, TEE has been directly estimated by measuring the metabolism of doubly labeled water.[27] Calorimetric validation studies have shown this to be an accurate and reasonably precise method. In 38 men ranging in age from 64 to 74 years with a mean age of 69,

**Table 2–3** Energy Costs of Physical Activity Expressed as Multiples of BMR

| Levels of Activity | Men | Women |
|---|---|---|
| Light work | 1.7 | 1.7 |
| Moderate work | 2.7 | 2.2 |
| Heavy work | 3.8 | 2.8 |
| Residual time (no activity, but awake) | 1.4 | 1.4 |
| Sleeping | 1.0 | 1.0 |

*Source:* Adapted from: *Energy and protein requirements.* Report of a Joint FAO/WHO/UNU Expert Consultation. Geneva, World Health Organization, 1985 (WHO Technical Report Series, No. 724), Table 8.

**Table 2–4** Estimated Energy Requirement of a Man Aged 75 Years, Weight 60 kg, with Estimated BMR of 54 kcal/h

| Level of Activity | Time at Level (h) | Energy Need (kcal) |
|---|---|---|
| In bed at 1.0 × BMR | 8.0 | 430 |
| Social activities at 3.3 × BMR | 2.0 | 355 |
| Household tasks at 2.7 × BMR | 1.0 | 145 |
| Cardiovascular fitness exercise at 3.8 × BMR | 0.3 | 70 |
| Residual time energy needs at 1.4 × BMR | 12.7 | 960 |
| Total | 24.0 | 1960 |

*Source:* Adapted from: *Energy and protein requirements.* Report of a Joint FAO/WHO/UNU Expert Consultation. Geneva, World Health Organization, 1985 (WHO Technical Report Series, No. 724), Table 8.

resting energy expenditure (REE) measured by doubly labeled water was 1514 kcal/d and TEE was 2478 kcal/d.[27] This value is slightly higher than the 2300-kcal intake previously recommended. In 36 women ranging in age from 64 to 74 years with a mean age of 70, REE was estimated at 1264 kcal/d and TEE at 2155.[27] Again, the value is slightly higher than the previously recommended intake of 1900 kcal/d. The ratio of TEE to REE was 1.66 when based on direct measurements, as compared to 1.51 when based on factorial estimation of TEE.[27]

### Recommended Daily Energy Intake for Elderly Persons

In 1996, an international panel of experts recommended that the equations used to estimate BMR (REE) be revised to include new data and to divide the older population into three age ranges of 65 to 75, 76 to 85, and 86 and older. The panel recommended that total energy needs be expressed as a multiple of REE and suggested that a healthy range was a 1.5 to 1.8 multiple of REE.[28] The greater the level of physical activity, the higher the ratio of total energy need to REE. The range of 1.5 to 1.8 was designed to provide enough energy for sufficient activity to prevent accelerated loss of muscle or bone.

### Effect of Progressive Resistance Exercise Training on Energy Requirements of Elderly Persons

PRT has significantly enhanced energy requirements and may become an important strategy to promote weight loss in obese persons.[29] In 12 subjects participating in upper and lower body resistance training 3 days a week in which eight muscle groups were exercised at an appropriate intensity at each session, an increase in energy intake of 15% was required to maintain body weight.[29] The increased energy expenditure was due to increases in BMR (REE) and the energy costs of the resistance exercise itself. This study has been replicated.[30] Therefore, PRT increases energy requirement, maintains metabolically active lean body mass, and has the potential to reduce body fat.

### WATER INTAKE IN ELDERLY INDIVIDUALS

Although required water intake is not substantially different in young and old adults, elderly individuals are prone to an inadequate water intake. In fact, dehydration is the most common fluid and electrolyte disturbance in the elderly.[31,32] In many instances, diseases that cause mental or physical incapacity also reduce the ability to recognize thirst, create an inability to express thirst, or decrease access to water.[33] In addition to the effects of acquired diseases, healthy elderly individuals appear to have reduced thirst in response to fluid deprivation.[31] Healthy elderly men (67–75 years old) and young men (20–31 years old) were deprived of all fluid intake for 24 hours followed by free access to water for 60 minutes. In spite of a higher serum osmolality in the elderly group following dehydration, they were less thirsty and consumed only half as much water during the 60-minute rehydration period as the young subjects.[31] Furthermore, young subjects fully corrected elevated serum osmolalities during the rehydration period, whereas elderly subjects did not.[31] In addition to reduced thirst, elderly subjects produced a moderately less concentrated urine following fluid deprivation.[31] Since elderly subjects had higher serum vasopressin levels in response to dehydration, the decreased capacity to concentrate the urine appears to be at the renal level.[31] As this study indicates, healthy as well as ill elderly subjects are less able to respond to dehydration.

### Detection of Dehydration

Three forms of dehydration can be distinguished: isotonic dehydration, resulting from a balanced loss of water and sodium; hypertonic dehydration, resulting from relatively greater water losses; and hypotonic dehydration, resulting from relatively greater sodium losses.[32] This discussion will focus on hypertonic dehydration, in which water losses exceed sodium losses. Although there is no absolute criterion for dehydration, a practical definition is the rapid loss of greater than 3% of body weight.[32] The serum sodium and osmolality values are often used to categorize dehydration. Since aging may affect skin turgor and cardiovascular responses to volume depletion, a general clinical evaluation with assessment of blood pressure, pulse, and blood values is the most useful means of detecting dehydration in elderly persons. A serum urea nitrogen/creatinine ratio of 25 or greater and a serum sodium of greater than 148 mmol/L are suggestive of dehydration.[32]

### Treatment of Dehydration

The free water deficit (FWD) can be estimated by the following formula[32]:

$$\text{FWD in liters} = \text{weight in kilograms} \times 0.45 - [(140/\text{measured serum sodium}) \times \text{weight in kilograms} \times 0.45]$$

*Weight* refers to the baseline before the onset of dehydration. In general, the estimated deficit should be replaced at the rate of 25% to 30% per day. If the patient is hemodynamically stable, water or 5% glucose may be used to replace losses. With hemodynamic instability, normal saline should be infused until stability is restored. Fluids may be replaced by mouth, supplementation of enteric feedings, or intravenous infusion. The fluid prescription should make provision for deficit replacement, maintenance needs, and extraordinary losses.[32]

### Prevention of Dehydration

Factors increasing the risk of dehydration include deterioration in cognitive status, immobility, swallowing problems, poor oral intake, enteral feedings, weight loss, diarrhea, fever, uncontrolled diabetes, diuretic use, and laxative abuse. Patients with these problems should be assessed for adequate fluid intake. Daily baseline water requirements range from 1500 to 2500 mL or approximately 30 mL/kg of body weight.[32,33] In cases of severe hypodipsia like that following strokes, fluid intake must be rigidly prescribed to prevent repeated episodes of dehydration.[33]

## DESIRABLE FAT INTAKE IN ELDERLY PERSONS

### Dietary Fat Requirement

The desirable fat intake for elderly individuals does not differ from that of younger adults.[34] Fats and carbohydrates are the major sources of dietary energy, providing 85% to 90% of the total intake. Fats are by far the most efficient energy source, with twice the energy content per gram as carbohydrate and protein. A minimum of 10% of the total energy intake should be fat to allow an adequate intake of fat-soluble vitamins and the essential fatty acids, linoleic and arachidonic acid.[34] Essential fatty acids are required for the synthesis of prostaglandins and cell membrane phospholipids.[35] It is widely believed that the fat content of the average American diet, approximately 40% of the total energy intake, is too high and contains a higher proportion of saturated fatty acids and cholesterol than is desirable for optimum health of adults.[36–38] To retard atherogenesis and combat obesity, the National Cholesterol Education Program (NCEP) recommends that total fat intake be limited to 30% or less of total calories, with saturated fatty acids providing 8% to 10%, polyunsaturated fatty acids up to 10%, and monounsaturated fatty acids up to 15% of total energy intake.[37] In addition, cholesterol intake should be limited to less than 300 mg/d and the total energy intake adjusted to achieve and maintain optimum body weight. In contrast to the great volume of evidence that high fat intake increases the risk of coronary disease,[36–38] a recent study suggests that decreased fat intake is associated with increased risk of ischemic stroke in middle-aged men.[39] In a 20-year follow-up of men in the Framingham Heart Study, the risk of ischemic stroke declined as intake of saturated and monounsaturated, but not polyunsatu-

rated, fat increased. This study raises the possibility that restriction of fat intake as recommended by the NCEP and others may not reduce and could possibly increase the incidence of ischemic strokes. Nevertheless, the authors of this study caution against premature recommendations to increase fat intake, since this might aggravate the coronary artery disease that is often associated with cerebrovascular disease. The significance of these findings and whether dietary recommendations should be changed are not clear.

In an alternative approach to prevention of coronary artery disease, the intake of saturated fat has been reduced and that of monounsaturated and polyunsaturated fat increased with little change in total fat intake.[40] In a secondary prevention trial, 289 experimental subjects with a prior myocardial infarction were given a Mediterranean-style diet with more bread, fruit, root and green vegetables, and fish but less beef, lamb, and pork.[41] Butter and cream were replaced by a rapeseed oil–based margarine, and oils used in food preparation were limited to rapeseed and olive oil. The 295 control subjects continued their usual diets. After an average follow-up of 2 years, total cardiac events and deaths were reduced in the experimental group. Although the experimental diet reduced total energy intake 10%, energy provided by total fat and saturated fat 6.7% and 29%, and cholesterol intake 32% and increased energy provided by unsaturated fat 9.1%, the total cholesterol (TC) and low-density lipoprotein-cholesterol (LDL-C) levels did not change.

### The Relationship of Serum Cholesterol and Coronary Heart Disease in Elderly Persons

Although TC is recognized as a powerful risk factor for coronary heart disease in middle-aged persons, its impact in elderly individuals is controversial.[42–44] A recent multisite study related TC level to risk of death from coronary heart disease in 4066 men and women older than 71 years who were followed for 5 years.[45] When this study population was characterized by TC level, the lowest 9.5% (values ≤160 mg/dL) had the highest incidence of preexisting cardiovascular disease, the highest risk factors for cardiovascular disease, and the highest indices of poor health. Crude coronary heart disease mortality was highest in this lowest TC group. When mortality rates were adjusted for age, preexisting cardiovascular disease, risk factors, and general health status, the highest risk of death from coronary artery disease shifted from the lowest TC group to the highest. With further exclusion of persons dying during the first year of follow-up, elevated TC levels predicted increased deaths from coronary disease in a pattern similar to that observed in middle-aged adults.[45] This study strongly suggests that the adverse effects of low TC levels result from comorbidity, frailty, and premorbid conditions. When these factors are accounted for, elevated TC levels remain risk factors for death from coronary artery disease in older persons. In addition, high-density lipoprotein-cholesterol (HDL-C) values less than 35 mg/dL predict coronary heart disease mortality and occurrence of new events in persons older than 70.[46]

## Dietary Treatment of Hypercholesterolemia

Diet may greatly influence TC and its atherogenic LDL-C component. TC and LDL-C are increased by excess intake of energy, saturated fats, and cholesterol.[47] They can be lowered by reduced intake of energy and total fat and substitution of unsaturated fats for saturated ones.[47] The great potential for dietary and lifestyle modification to reduce TC and LDL-C and prevent or even reverse coronary disease is suggested by the study of a stringent low-fat vegetarian diet combined with aerobic exercise, stress management, and smoking cessation.[48] Twenty-eight experimental subjects with an average age of 56 and coronary artery disease demonstrated by arteriography were placed on a diet restricting fat to 10% of total calories, cholesterol to 5 mg/d, and animal products to egg whites and one cup per day of nonfat milk or yogurt. Take-home meals were provided upon request. Moderate aerobic exercise was prescribed, and patients attended group support activities for 8 hours per week. Twenty-one control subjects with an average age of 60 and similar coronary artery lesions were not asked to make dietary or lifestyle changes but were free to do so. In the experimental group, the reduction in total fat intake from 32% of total calories to 7% and cholesterol intake from 213 mg/d to 12 mg was accompanied by a 24% reduction in TC and 37% reduction in LDL-C. After 1 year of treatment, repeat coronary arteriography showed that 82% of experimental subjects had a reduction in the extent of their lesions compared to 47% of controls.[48] Angina frequency and severity were also reduced in the experimental group.[48] However, reductions in dietary fat intake of this magnitude are not practical in large-scale outpatient settings and may not be desirable in view of recent evidence showing an inverse relationship between fat intake and ischemic stroke.[39] In a meta-analysis of the effectiveness of dietary advice in reducing fat intake and TC levels in more usual outpatient settings, TC levels were reduced approximately 3.7% in five trials lasting 9 to 18 months.[49] Even modest reductions in TC levels are likely to produce significant benefits. In a meta-analysis of 28 trials, each 10% reduction in TC in men 55 to 64 years of age produced a 20% reduction in coronary events after 2 to 5 years.[50] Furthermore, a lifetime 10% reduction in serum cholesterol was estimated to reduce the incidence of coronary events by 54% at age 40, 27% at age 60, and 20% at age 70.[50] Limited data for women indicated a similar benefit.

## Recommendations for Dietary Control of Hypercholesterolemia in the Elderly

Although large numbers of subjects older than age 70 have not been included in trials of cholesterol lowering in the primary and secondary prevention of atherosclerosis, the NCEP recommends aggressive attempts at cholesterol lowering in elderly persons with a reasonable outlook for several years of active, healthy life.[37] Extrapolating the beneficial effects of cholesterol lowering observed in middle-aged subjects to elderly ones is supported by observations that cholesterol levels respond as well to dietary and drug treatment in elderly subjects as in younger ones. Furthermore, treatment of hypertension, another major risk factor for vascular disease, has reduced coronary heart disease events and strokes in patients in their 70s and 80s.[51] On the other hand, the American College of Physicians Guidelines take a less aggressive stance by concluding that there is insufficient evidence to encourage or discourage cholesterol screening for primary prevention in persons 65 to 75 years of age and by not recommending screening for primary prevention in persons older than 75 years.[52] Aggressive attempts at cholesterol lowering are not indicated in elderly individuals who are severely incapacitated or who have their life span greatly limited by irreversible, life-threatening diseases.

The NCEP recommends dietary modification and lifestyle change (increased exercise and weight control) as the initial steps in cholesterol lowering.[37] Dietary modification is accomplished in two steps. The Step I diet limits total fat to 30% or less of total calories, with saturated fatty acids providing 8% to 10%, polyunsaturated fatty acids 10% or less, and monounsaturated fatty acids 15% or less. Carbohydrates provide about 55% of total calories and protein about 15%. The cholesterol intake is limited to 300 mg/d or less. This diet is suitable for the population at large. If the Step I diet is not sufficient, the Step II diet further reduces saturated fat to less than 7% of total calories and cholesterol intake to less than 200 mg/d. Threshold cholesterol levels for initiating and monitoring dietary therapy are listed in Table 2–5. The target of dietary therapy in primary prevention of atherosclerotic vascular disease is reduction of LDL-C below 160 mg/dL in patients with fewer than two risk factors and below 130 in individuals with two or more risk factors.[37] In patients with preexisting atherosclerotic vascular disease, the target is reduction of LDL-C below 100 mg/dL.[37] Risk factors to be considered in this algorithm include age greater than 45 in men and 55 in women, family history of premature vascular disease, cigarette smoking, hypertension, HDL-C less than 35 mg/dL, diabetes mellitus, obesity, and inactivity. In contrast, an HDL-C level greater than 60 mg/dL is protective and allows subtraction of one risk factor. If the individual is on the Step I diet at the outset or if it proves ineffective in 6 to 12 weeks, the Step II diet should be implemented. If dietary and lifestyle modification is not sufficient to reach LDL-C goals, drug therapy will be required, especially in persons with preexisting vascular disease.[53] Since measurement of the LDL-C level requires fasting and measurement of TC does not, it may be convenient to use TC as a substitute measurement. TC levels of 200 and 240 mg/dL are approximately equivalent to LDL cholesterol levels of 130 and 160. Once target TC levels are reached, a confirmatory lipoprotein analysis including LDL-C measurement should be obtained. Similarly, decisions to investigate and treat lipoprotein abnormalities can be based on TC and HDL-C levels as follows: a TC of 200 mg/dL or less with an HDL-C greater than 35 mg/dL requires no further study, with a recheck in 5 years; a TC of 200 mg/dL or less with an HDL-C less than 35 mg/dL requires lipoprotein analysis; a TC of 200 to 239 mg/dL with an HDL-C greater than 35 mg/dL and fewer than two risk factors requires no further study, with a recheck in 1 to 5 years; a TC of 200 to 239 mg/dL with an HDL less than 35 mg/dL or presence of two or more other risk factors requires lipoprotein analysis; and a TC greater than 240 mg/dL requires lipoprotein analysis.

## DESIRABLE CARBOHYDRATE AND FIBER INTAKE IN ELDERLY PERSONS

### Dietary Carbohydrate Requirement

The major function of dietary carbohydrate is to provide energy. Glucose can be utilized by all body tissues and is required for energy production in the brain and red blood cells.[54]

In the absence of dietary carbohydrate, fatty acids are incompletely oxidized, leading to ketosis, which may cause lethargy and depression.[40] To prevent ketosis, a minimum of 50 g of dietary glucose or complex carbohydrate equivalent is required per day.[54] Although sufficient carbohydrate (at least 100 g) to prevent ketosis is the minimum desirable intake, no ideal level of consumption has been defined. When the protein requirement and desirable fat intake have been defined, the remaining dietary energy needs should be met by prescribing the appropriate amount of carbohydrate. If the protein requirement is 15% of dietary energy and the desirable fat intake is 30% or less, as indicated above,[37] the carbohydrate intake should be 55% to 60% of dietary energy.

### Benefits of Dietary Fiber in Elderly Persons

Excessive refining of foods with removal of indigestible dietary fiber may contribute to disorders that are particularly prevalent in the elderly, such as constipation, diverticular disease of the colon, diabetes, and hyperlipidemia.[55] Dietary fiber is derived from structural components of plant cell walls and consists of plant polysaccharides and lignin,

**Table 2–5** Initiation and Target Cholesterol Levels for Dietary Therapy

|  | LDL Cholesterol | | Total Cholesterol |
|---|---|---|---|
|  | Initiation | Target | Monitoring Goal |
| Without CHD and <2 risk factors | ≥160 mg/dL | <160 mg/dL | <240 mg/dL |
| Without CHD and ≥2 risk factors | ≥130 mg/dL | <130 mg/dL | <200 mg/dL |
| With CHD | >100 mg/dL | ≤100 mg/dL | ≤160 mg/dL |

*Note:* CHD, coronary heart disease; LDL, low-density lipoprotein.

*Source:* Reprinted from the Report of the National Cholesterol Education Program.

which are resistant to digestive enzymes in people.[55] Water-holding particulate fiber with high pentosan content, like wheat bran, increases fecal bulk and decreases gut transit time and intraluminal pressure within the colon.[56] These effects are helpful in reducing constipation and the formation of colonic diverticula. On the other hand, soluble fibers such as gums and pectins increase the viscosity of intestinal contents, increase gut transit time, and decrease the rate of small intestinal absorption.[55] Increased consumption of fibers such as guar, pectin, and tragacanth reduced insulin secretion following a test meal in normal subjects and increased carbohydrate tolerance in diabetics.[57,58] The mechanism of the beneficial effect appears to be delayed gastric emptying and reduced rate of absorption of carbohydrate in the small intestine. As a consequence of these effects, the American, Canadian, and British Diabetes Associations have recommended increased consumption

of high-fiber carbohydrate–containing foods.[55] Although it is less well established, purified fibers such as guar, pectin, and oat bran and high-fiber foods such as cereals, starchy vegetables, and beans have been reported to lower serum lipids.[59] Decreases in TC, LDL-C, and triglycerides without change in HDL-C were observed.[59] Again, the mechanism appears to be delayed gastric emptying and reduced intestinal absorption of cholesterol and triglyceride.

**Desirable Fiber Intake**

For the above reasons, a fiber intake of 25 to 35 g/d appears prudent. Fiber from a variety of sources such as fresh fruits, vegetables, legumes, and whole-grain products is recommended, with two or more servings of fruits, three or more servings of vegetables, and six or more servings of grain products per day.[60]

---

**REFERENCES**

1. Fukagawa NK, Young VR. Protein and amino acid metabolism and requirements in older persons. *Clin Geriatr Med.* 1987;3:329–341.

2. Cohn SH, Vartsky D, Yasumura S, et al. Compartmental body composition based on the body nitrogen, potassium and calcium. *Am J Physiol.* 1980;239:E192–E200.

3. Korenchevsky V. In: Bourne GH, ed. *Physiological and Pathological Aging.* New York, NY: Hafner; 1961:514.

4. Uauy R, Winterer JC, Bilmazes C, et al. The changing pattern of whole body protein metabolism in aging humans. *J Gerontol.* 1978;33:663–671.

5. Frontera WR, Hughes VA, Evans WJ. A cross-sectional study of upper and lower extremity muscle strength in 45–78 year old men and women. *J Appl Physiol.* 1991;71:644–650.

6. Jette AM, Branch LG. The Framingham Disability Study: II. Physical disability among the aging. *Am J Public Health.* 1981;71:1211–1216.

7. Munro HN, Crim MC. In: Shils ME, Young VR, eds. *Modern Nutrition in Health and Disease.* 7th ed. Philadelphia, Pa: Lea & Febiger; 1988:25.

8. Gersovitz M, Motil K, Munro HN, et al. Human protein requirements: assessment of the adequacy of the current recommended allowance for dietary protein in elderly men and women. *Am J Clin Nutr.* 1982;35:6–14.

9. Campbell WW, Crim MC, Dallal GE, et al. Increased protein requirements in elderly people: new data and retrospective reassessments. *Am J Clin Nutr.* 1994;60:501–509.

10. Campbell WW, Evans WJ. Protein requirements of elderly people. *Eur J Clin Nutr.* 1996;50(suppl 1):S180–S185.

11. Munro HN, McGandy RB, Hartz SC, Russell RM, Jacob RA, Otradovec CL. Protein nutriture of a group of free-living elderly. *Am J Clin Nutr.* 1987;46:586–592.

12. Fereday A, Gibson NR, Cox M, Pacy PJ, Millward DJ. Protein requirements and ageing: metabolic demands and efficiency of utilization. *Br J Nutr.* 1997;77:685–702.

13. Clugston G et al. Report on the working group on protein and amino acid requirements. *Eur J Clin Nutr.* 1996;50(suppl 1):S193–S195.

14. Souba WW, Wilmore DW. In: Shils ME, Young VR, eds. *Modern Nutrition in Health and Disease.* 7th ed. Philadelphia, Pa: Lea & Febiger; 1988:1306.

15. Evans WJ. Effects of aging and exercise on nutrition needs of the elderly. *Nutr Rev.* 1996;54:S35–S39.

16. Brenner BM, Meyer TW, Hostetter TH. Dietary protein intake and the progressive nature of the kidney disease: the role of hemodynamically mediated glomerular injury in the pathogenesis of progressive glomerular sclerosis in aging, renal ablation, and intrinsic renal disease. *N Engl J Med.* 1982;307:652–659.

17. Elema JD, Arends A. Focal and segmental glomerular hyalinosis and sclerosis in the rat. *Lab Invest.* 1975;33:554–561.

18. Yu BP, Masoro EJ, Murata I, Bertrand AA, Lynd FT. Life span study of SPF Fischer 344 male rats fed ad libitum or restricted diets: longevity, growth, lean body mass and disease. *J Gerontol.* 1982; 37:130–141.

19. Blum M, Averbach M, Wolman Y, Aviram A. Protein intake and kidney function in humans: its effect on "normal aging." *Arch Intern Med.* 1989; 149:211–212.

20. Tobin J. Nutrition and organ function in a cohort of aging men. In: Hutchinson M, Munro HN, eds. *Nutrition and Aging: 5th Annual Bristol-Meyers Symposium on Nutritional Research.* New York, NY: Academic Press; 1986:23.

21. McGandy RB, Barrows CH, Spanias A, Meredith A, Stone JL, Norris AH. Nutrient intakes and energy expenditure in men of different ages. *J Gerontol.* 1966;21:581–587.

22. Elahi VK, Elahi D, Andres R, Tobin JD, Butler MG, Norris AH. A longitudinal study of nutritional intake in men. *J Gerontol.* 1983;38:162–180.

23. *Health and Nutrition Examination Survey No. 2.* Hyattsville, Md: US Public Health Service, Division of Health Statistics; 1981.

24. Kannel WB, Gordon T. *The Framingham Diet Study. An Epidemiological Investigation of Cardiovascular Disease.* Washington, DC: US Dept of Health, Education and Welfare, Public Health Service; 1970.

25. Owen OE, Holup JL, D'Alessio DA, et al. A reappraisal of the caloric requirements of men. *Am J Clin Nutr.* 1987;46:875–885.

26. Food and Agriculture Organization, World Health Organization, United Nations University. *Energy and Protein Requirements.* Geneva, Switzerland: World Health Organization; 1985. Technical Report Series No. 724.

27. Roberts SB. Energy requirements of older individuals. *Eur J Clin Nutr.* 1996;50(suppl 1):S112–S118.

28. Dupont JL, Durnin JVGA, Ferro-Luzzi A, et al. Report of the working group on energy requirements of older individuals. *Eur J Clin Nutr.* 1996;50(suppl 1):S192.

29. Campbell WW, Crim MC, Young VR, et al. Increased energy requirements and body composition changes with resistance training in older adults. *Am J Clin Nutr.* 1994;60:167–175.

30. Pratley R, Nicklas B, Rubin M, et al. Strength training increases resting metabolic rate and norepinephrine levels in healthy 50- to 65-yr-old men. *J Appl Physiol.* 1994;76:133–137.

31. Phillips PA, Rolls BJ, Ledingham JGG, et al. Reduced thirst after water deprivation in healthy elderly men. *N Engl J Med.* 1984;311:753–759.

32. Weinberg AD, Minaker KL, Council on Scientific Affairs, American Medical Association. Dehydration: evaluation and management in older adults. *JAMA.* 1995;274:1552–1556.

33. Miller PD, Krebs RA, Neal BJ, McIntyre DO. Hypodipsia in geriatric patients. *Am J Med.* 1982;73:354–356.

34. Lowenstein FW. Nutritional requirements of the elderly. In: Young EA, ed. *Nutrition, Aging and Health.* New York, NY: Alan R Liss; 1986:61.

35. Linscheer WG, Vergroesen AJ. In: Shils ME, Young VR, eds. *Modern Nutrition in Health and Disease.* 7th ed. Philadelphia, Pa: Lea & Febiger; 1988:72.

36. Kannel WB. Cholesterol and risk of coronary heart disease and mortality in men. *Clin Chem.* 1988;34:B53–B59.

37. National Cholesterol Education Program. Second report of the expert panel on detection, evaluation, and treatment of high blood cholesterol in adults. *Circulation.* 1994;89:1333–1432.

38. Caggiula AW, Mustad VA. Effects of dietary fat and fatty acids on coronary artery disease risk and total and lipoprotein cholesterol concentrations: epidemiologic studies. *Am J Clin Nutr*. 1997; 65(suppl):1597S–1610S.

39. Gillman MW, Cupples LA, Millen BE, Ellison RC, Wolf PA. Inverse association of dietary fat with development of ischemic stroke in men. *JAMA*. 1997;278:2145–2150.

40. Oliver MF. It is more important to increase the intake of unsaturated fats than to decrease the intake of saturated fats: evidence from clinical trials relating to ischemic heart disease. *Am J Clin Nutr*. 1997;66(suppl):980S–986S.

41. de Lorgeril M, Renaud S, Mamelle N, et al. Mediterranean alpha-linolenic acid-rich diet in secondary prevention of coronary heart disease. *Lancet*. 1994;343:1454–1459.

42. Garber AM, Sox HC Jr, Littenberg B. Screening asymptomatic adults for cardiac risk factors: the serum cholesterol level. *Ann Intern Med*. 1989; 110:622–639.

43. Kannel WB. Nutritional contributors to cardiovascular disease in the elderly. *J Am Geriatr Soc*. 1986;34:27–36.

44. Mariotti S, Capocuccia R, Farchi G, Menotti A, Verdecchia A, Keys A. Age, period, cohort and geographical area effects on the relationship between risk factors and coronary disease mortality. *J Chron Dis*. 1986;39:229–242.

45. Corti MC, Guralnik JM, Salive ME, et al. Clarifying the direct relation between total cholesterol levels and death from coronary heart disease in older persons. *Ann Intern Med*. 1997;126:753–760.

46. Corti MC, Guralnik JM, Salive ME, et al. HDL cholesterol predicts coronary heart disease mortality in older persons. *JAMA*. 1995;274:539–544.

47. Grundy SM. Cholesterol and coronary heart disease. *JAMA*. 1986;256:2849–2858.

48. Ornish D, Brown SE, Scherwitz LW, et al. Can lifestyle changes reverse coronary heart disease? *Lancet*. 1990;336:129–133.

49. Brunner E, White E, Thorogood M, Bristow A, Curle D, Marmot M. Can dietary interventions change diet and cardiovascular risk factors? A meta-analysis of randomized controlled trials. *Am J Public Health*. 1997;87:1415–1422.

50. Law MR, Wald NJ, Thompson SC. By how much and how quickly does reduction in serum cholesterol concentration lower risk of ischemic heart disease? *Br Med J*. 1994;308:367–372.

51. Applegate WB. Managing the older patient with hypertension. *Am J Hypertens*. 1993;6:277S–282S.

52. American College of Physicians. Guidelines for using serum cholesterol, high-density lipoprotein cholesterol, and triglyceride levels as screening tests for preventing coronary heart disease in adults. *Ann Intern Med*. 1996;124:515–517.

53. Gotto AM. Cholesterol management in theory and practice. *Circulation*. 1997;96:4424–4430.

54. MacDonald I. Carbohydrates. In: Shils ME, Young VR, eds. *Modern Nutrition in Health and Disease*. 8th ed. Philadelphia, Pa: Lea & Febiger; 1994:36–46.

55. Schneeman BO, Tietgen J. Dietary fiber. In: Shils ME, Young VR, eds. *Modern Nutrition in Health and Disease*. 8th ed. Philadelphia, Pa: Lea & Febiger; 1994:89–100.

56. Cummings JH, Branch W, Jenkins DJA, Southgate DAT, Houston H, James WPT. Colonic response to dietary fibre from carrot, cabbage, apple, bran and guar gum. *Lancet*. 1978;1:5–9.

57. Jenkins DJA, Wolever TMS, Leeds AR, et al. Dietary fibres, fibre analogues, and glucose tolerance: importance of viscosity. *Br Med J*. 1978;1:1392–1394.

58. Vinik AI, Jenkins DJA. Dietary fiber in management of diabetes. *Diabetes Care*. 1988;11:160–173.

59. Jenkins DJA, Reynolds D, Slavin B, Leeds AR, Jenkins AL, Jepson EM. Dietary fiber and blood lipids: treatment of hypercholesterolemia with guar crispbread. *Am J Clin Nutr*. 1980;33:575–581.

60. US Dept of Agriculture, US Dept of Health and Human Services. *Dietary Guidelines for Americans*. Washington, DC: US Government Printing Office; 1990. No. 232.

# CHAPTER 3

# Vitamin Status and Requirements of the Elderly

*Paolo M. Suter*

In the United States and worldwide, the elderly segment of the population is rapidly increasing in age and numbers. Those older than 60 years constitute the fastest growing group in most Western countries and will soon also be the fastest growing group in many other countries (such as the People's Republic of China). Many of these elderly are enjoying good health, but for a large segment, aging is associated with continuing impairment of health and well-being. Chronic conditions affect all age groups, but in view of the declining mortality rates, the number of people with one or more chronic conditions will increase continuously.[1]

In recent years, new important roles of certain vitamins in reducing disease risk have been more closely described (eg, a relationship among folic acid, homocysteine, and the risk of atherosclerosis).[2] In view of the increasing aging of our society, the maintenance of adequate intake of all essential nutrients, and especially of the vitamins, becomes more important than ever. Selected new aspects of the vitamin metabolism will be discussed in relation to the aging process and diseases.

The aim of any medical strategy in relation to aging should be not only that more people live longer but also that they live well. This is a function not only of vitamin nutrition, but

of overall nutrition and other lifestyle factors that are not directly related to nutrition (such as exercise, smoking, and psychological factors). Nevertheless, in formulating recommendations for the nutriture of the elderly, it should be remembered that a 60-year-old is very different from a 90-year-old. The whole elderly population represents an extremely heterogeneous group as compared to younger population groups. This heterogeneity has important consequences for medical therapy and especially for recommendations regarding vitamin nutriture. The elderly also share several factors putting them at an increased risk of malnutrition. The prevention of the chronic diseases of aging by dietary means will have a central role in any future health system.[3]

An adequate intake of the different vitamins is not only of importance for the prevention of the development of deficiency. During the last few years, new functions and health effects of vitamins have been identified.[4-6] Some of these will be discussed in the following sections.

## VITAMIN A

The importance of vitamin A and vitamin A precursors in the form of carotenoids was recognized a long time ago, and the classical deficiency signs were described long ago.[7] Vitamin A (retinol) plays an important role in growth and cell differentiation, vision, and maintenance of immune function. The discovery of many new functions of vitamin A, especially its role in the regulation of gene expression in the nuclear retinoid receptors, constitutes what has been called a "retinoid revolution."[8]

The present recommended dietary allowance (RDA) for the age group of those older than 51 years is, as in earlier editions of the recommendations,[9] 1000 μg of retinol equivalents (RE) for men and 800 μg for women.[10] Others, however, have recommended a lower intake of 700 μg and 600 μg RE for men and women, respectively.[11] Epidemiological studies would support the lower figures of intake recommendations, since the vitamin A intake of many elderly is below the recommendations but their vitamin A levels remain well within the limits of normality.[12-20] In the follow-up analysis of the Euronut Survey in Europe on Nutrition and the Elderly, a Concerted Action (SENECA) study, the regulation of gene expression in the nuclear retinoid receptors, retinol levels decreased over the period of 4 to 5 years, but the prevalence of biochemical vitamin A deficiency was zero.[21] Vitamin A intakes vary widely, and up to 70% of elderly people, depending on their income, sex, and race, have been shown to have vitamin A intakes less than two thirds of the RDA. These data must be interpreted with caution, since the vitamin A content of food varies considerably and since there are technical difficulties in analyzing the vitamin A content of food. Some elderly populations, however, may consume more than the recommendations.[17] Institutionalization is associated with an overall impairment of nutritional status, including lower vitamin A intakes than in free-living elderly.[18]

Some studies describe a sex difference in plasma retinol levels and beta carotene levels that is in part attributable to differences in the plasma lipid levels as well as changes in the concentration of retinol-binding protein.[17,22]

Plasma carotenoids are a very heterogeneous group of chemical substances, including lycopene, beta carotene, alpha carotene, zeaxanthin, lutein, and beta cryptoxanthin.[23] The importance of these carotenoids varies considerably, but they may be of great importance in the pathogenesis of different age-related chronic conditions such as cardiovascular disease or age-related macular degeneration and cataract.[23] A recent study reported a direct association between lycopene status and functional capacity (including dependence in self-care) in women aged 77 to 98 years.[24] Whether this described relationship between functional parameters and lycopene is causal remains unclear. Low-density lipoprotein (LDL) cholesterol is the major carrier of lycopene in the blood.

The protective effects of antioxidants in different disease processes are well known.[6,25,26] The increased intake of carotenoids from fruits and vegetables was found to be associated with a decreased cardiovascular mortality in an elderly population of Massachusetts residents.[27] Others described a similar finding but reported only a small effect of carotenoid supplementation on the reduction of cardiovascular risk.[28] The lower mortality in subjects with plasma carotenoids above the median in the latter study is probably caused not only by improved carotenoid status but probably also by other nutrients and phytochemicals. A colinearity of different antioxidative vitamins has been described in the elderly. The colinearity of nutrients is very important and must be considered in any interpretation of the association between a single nutrient and a specific disease. An increase of vitamin C, vitamin E, or carotenoids is usually associated with a greater plasma concentration of one or both other vitamins.[29]

Vitamin A may have considerable toxicity.[11] In view of the widespread vitamin A supplement use by the elderly, it has been suggested that the increased absorption of vitamin A with age could contribute to toxicity in elderly individuals who have high vitamin A intakes from supplements.[30-33] There are two forms of hypervitaminosis A: chronic and acute. Acute hypervitaminosis A is rare in elderly people, but chronic toxicity can be seen in this group.[34] Chronic diseases of old age may influence vitamin A nutriture at the level of intake, absorption, recycling, tissue utilization, and storage. Of special importance in the elderly are chronic liver diseases, often related to the chronic ingestion of alcohol, which impairs the storage of vitamin A in the liver as well as the ability of the liver to synthesize retinol-binding proteins.[35-38] In normal aging, defined as aging in the absence of any relevant disease, the liver hardly senesces, and constitutive liver functions are maintained, suggesting no alterations in vitamin A metabolism. In view of the widespread intake of drugs in the elderly, it must be remembered that several drugs (including ethanol and barbiturates) are capable of affecting the metabolism of vitamin A by accelerating hepatic retinol breakdown. Chronic toxicity is mainly due to the intake of vitamin A supplements and is hardly due to excessive intakes of vitamin A from diet alone. Due to the availability of over-the-counter vitamin A capsules containing up to 20,000 IU of vitamin A, the risk of toxicity may be high. Recently it was shown that supplemental intake of vitamin A may be associated with greater levels of circulating retinyl esters in fasting blood. These high retinyl esters may be an indicator of vitamin A toxicity and liver damage.[34]

In a recent study using the relative dose response (RDR) for assessing vitamin A intake in the elderly, the maximum plasma retinol response occurred in elderly subjects 60 to 120 minutes later than in younger subjects.[39] Therefore, the procedures of the RDR should be modified when used with the elderly. Unlike young people or children, the elderly should have their fasting vitamin A levels measured for correct assessment of vitamin A intake.[40]

The effects of vitamin A deficiency on the immune functions in children are well known. In recent years, the effects of vitamin A and carotenoids on the immune function of the elderly have been evaluated in several studies. The effects of this vitamin are of special interest, since the immune system plays a crucial role in health maintenance and potentially also the aging process per se.

Santos and colleagues evaluated the effect of beta carotene on natural killer cell activity in a small sample of young old (aged 51 to 64 years) and older old (age range 65 to 86 years) participants of the Physician's Health Study. In this placebo-controlled study, the subjects received 50 mg of beta carotene every second day. With increasing age, natural killer cell activity declined only in the placebo group. In the younger subjects, however, beta carotene had no effect on natural killer cell activity.[41] Other nutrients such as vitamins C and E have also been shown to have the potential to modulate immune function in aging. In this context, the effect of vitamin A on pulmonary function in patients with chronic obstructive pulmonary disease (COPD) is interesting. This disease is becoming more prevalent with age, and it is estimated that up to 20% of the elderly are afflicted to some degree with COPD. Several epidemiologic studies have shown an inverse association between COPD and vitamin A nutriture. Lower plasma vitamin A levels have been described in subjects with COPD, and supplementation with vitamin A may result in improved lung function tests.[42] Future studies will show whether this association is of clinical relevance. Functional abnormalities due to COPD are often complicated by miscellaneous nutritional deficiencies, since breathing is impaired, especially during food intake, leading to higher energy requirements and reduced food intake to avoid breathing difficulties during eating. A recent study in younger subjects accumulated evidence suggesting that the different antioxidants may play an important role in bronchial reactivity and thus the prevalence and incidence of asthma and other allergic diseases.[43] Vitamin A deficiency results in an impairment of the response to viral and bacterial infection at several stages of the immune response.[44]

The safety of beta carotene supplements is at present a matter of dispute. In view of current knowledge, a recommendation of beta carotene supplements is warranted only after a careful evaluation of the clinical constellation of a patient. Several large trials reported a higher mortality in subjects receiving beta carotene.[45–47] The exact mechanisms of the excess mortality are not yet known. New data from the Finnish study and the Carotene and Retinol Efficiency Test (CARET) trial suggest an association with alcohol intake.[45,48] The negative beta carotene effects became stronger in subjects consuming more than 11 g of alcohol per day. In view of this, the intake of fruits and vegetables should be increasingly promoted, particularly in the elderly. The promotion of supplements for everyone should be reconsidered critically.

Healthy elderly persons are able to maintain adequate body stores of vitamin A and normal vitamin A plasma/serum levels despite intakes below the actual RDA. It can be concluded that the vitamin A status of healthy elderly individuals does not require special attention and that the present recommendations are adequate.

## VITAMIN D

Vitamin D and the vitamin D endocrine system are involved not only in the regulation of bone mass and bone mineral metabolism but also in the modulation of several fundamental cellular processes. The current RDA for vitamin D in elderly subjects (ie, older than 51 years) is 200 IU (5 μg) of cholecalciferol per day.[10] This is half of the recommended intake for subjects during the growth period. Vitamin D can be obtained either from dietary sources or by synthesis in the skin upon exposure to the sun; however, it is controversial which of the two possible sources is more important for maintaining adequate vitamin D nutriture in elderly people. Due to the importance of vitamin D in bone health and osteoporosis, the literature is expanding very rapidly.

The vitamin D nutriture depends on the cutaneous synthesis of the vitamin and the diet. Food is, however, a rather bad source for vitamin D, except for certain selected foods such as deep sea fish and vitamin D–fortified food products. Thus, up to 75% of the elderly consume less than two thirds of the present RDA.[32,49–52] McKenna[53] reviewed the vitamin D intakes in 31 studies. In many studies, there was no difference in the vitamin D intake of young and elderly subjects.[53] In the northern countries of Europe, the intake of vitamin D in the elderly is a little higher due to the ingestion of more oily deep sea fish. The intake of vitamin D from supplements varies according to the geographic region. The prevalence of elderly subjects taking supplements is higher in the northern European countries and North America than in other parts of Europe. There are hardly any elderly ingesting more than 5 μg of vitamin D per day. In view of the low vitamin D content of natural food products, this is not surprising. The assessment of nutritional vitamin D status is defined by the amount of circulating 25(OH) vitamin D.[54] Plasma and serum levels of 25-hydroxyvitamin $D_3$ (25(OH)$D_3$), the marker for vitamin D nutriture, decline with age.[16,49,53,55–57]

Plasma vitamin D levels in the elderly are more than 50% lower than those of younger controls. Blood levels of 25(OH)$D_3$ below 10 ng/mL have been reported in up to 50% of the free-living elderly.[58–60] In institutionalized elderly, this proportion may be as high as 90%.[61–64] Besides the low intakes, other mechanisms may contribute to the lower and decreasing plasma 25(OH)$D_3$ levels with aging (Table 3–1). Some evidence exists that even higher intake of vitamin D does not ensure an adequate biochemical vitamin D status.[65,66] Decreased plasma levels of 1-25(OH)$_2$ vitamin D, the most active form of vitamin D, may parallel the decreased levels of the precursor (ie, 25(OH)$D_3$). This decrease is caused not only by a lack of the precursor molecule (ie, 25(OH)$D_3$) but by an age-related decline in 1-α-hydroxylase activity.[67,68] Even at the level of the bone itself, an age-related decline of 1-25(OH)$_2D_3$ levels has been found.[69]

Vitamin D absorption and the hydroxylation in the liver are probably not affected during the normal aging process.[70] The capacity to hydroxylate the vitamin D molecule in the 21-position is, however, decreased due to age-specific changes.[71,72] The exact mecha-

nisms of the latter phenomenon are not known, but parathormone resistance may be of causal importance. Specific age-related effects at the level of the end organs (intestine and bone) may lead to a resistance to the effects of the activated form of the vitamin (ie, 1,25(OH)$_2$D).[73,74] The decline in estrogen levels with age may also play a central role in the modulation of end-organ responsiveness,[75] along with alterations of locally synthesized estrogens as a function of differences of the expression of vitamin D receptors.[76] Recently, particular steroid hormone receptors for vitamin D have been identified and studied intensively. At present it is controversial whether polymorphisms of vitamin D receptors may account for the genetic variations in bone mass or are also part of the age-related decline of bone mass.[77]

Casual sun exposure covers the vitamin D requirements of elderly people.[78] Many different factors can influence the synthesis of vitamin D in the skin. Geographical latitude may contribute to a large seasonal variation in the capacity of the skin to synthesize vitamin D. At high latitudes, there may be no vitamin D synthesis in the skin for up to 6 months of the year.[79,80] Sunlight exposure may cover most vitamin D requirements, but the capacity to synthesize vitamin D in the skin upon sunlight exposure decreases with age. Elderly individuals do show a decline in the precursor for the vitamin D synthesis, 7-dehydrocholesterol, in the skin, and the conversion of the provitamin after exposure to ultraviolet light decreases in the skin of elderly people, leading to suboptimal endogenous vitamin D synthesis.[79] This is also reflected in less markedly expressed seasonal variations in 25(OH)$D_3$ plasma levels in the elderly compared to younger adults. Living in the South with a potential for much more sun exposure does not ensure adequate vitamin D nutriture. In the Euronut SENECA study, eld-

---

**Table 3–1** Age-Related Changes in the Vitamin D Endocrine System

Low vitamin D intake
Decreased synthesis in the skin
Decreased 1-hydroxylation in the kidney
Decreased plasma-binding capacity for different vitamin D metabolites
Decreased sunlight exposure
Increased risk for vitamin D drug interactions

erly from southern European countries had the lowest mean plasma 25(OH)-vitamin D concentrations.[58] This study shows that sun exposure per se is not enough and that the factors of intensity and duration of sun exposure should also be accounted for. The elderly should expose themselves regularly to sunlight, especially during the summer months. Exposure of suberythemal duration seems to be "safe" also from the dermatologist's point of view regarding the development of skin cancer.[81]

Dietary fortification and enrichment of food and the ingestion of vitamin D supplements have a high potential for improving vitamin D status as well as preventing bone loss and associated fracture risk. Also in the elderly, the ingestion of vitamin D supplements will lead to an increase in the plasma/serum concentration of 25(OH) vitamin D. The change in 25(OH)-vitamin D levels may eventually be accompanied by changes in the plasma concentration of other calcium-regulating hormones such as parathormone (PTH) or 1-25(OH)$_2$ vitamin D.[82] Despite many studies, the ideal amount of vitamin D intake to maintain adequate vitamin D nutriture is still a matter of controversy. Krall and colleagues[83] reported that at least 5.5 µg of vitamin D per day was needed to maintain stable (25)OH-vitamin D serum levels and normal PTH concentrations. According to these authors, the recommended vitamin intake should therefore be at least in this range. As discussed above, hardly any elderly are receiving this amount of vitamin D from their diet. Several studies have reported a reduction of bone loss in elderly subjects due to the ingestion of vitamin D supplementation alone or in combination with calcium supplements.[84–86] Vitamin D supplementation is not necessarily associated with an increase in 1-25(OH)$_2$-vitamin D levels,[87] but other biochemical parameters of bone formation and resorption may be changed favorably. Osteocalcin, a bone matrix protein, is increased in vitamin D–deficient elderly but can be lowered upon vitamin D supplementation.[88,89]

Thus, many changes in vitamin D nutriture and metabolism would suggest that the present intake recommendations for the elderly are too low to maintain bone health. Increased sun exposure during the summer months as well as the consumption of vitamin D–fortified food may help to improve overall vitamin D nutriture. Elderly people with a low degree of sun exposure may qualify for low-dose vitamin D supplementation in the range of 10 µg/d (400 IU), alone or in combination with calcium supplements.

## VITAMIN E

Antioxidants, especially vitamin E, seem to be of special importance in the modulation of certain age-related phenomena. Many different theories of aging have been formulated, but most of them lack universality regarding different organ systems and functions.[6,26,90] Age-related changes due to oxidation are found in most organ systems and are therefore rather universally applicable.

The 1989 RDAs for vitamin E in the elderly are identical to the RDAs from 1980: 10 mg of α-tocopherol (α-TE) equivalents for men and 8 mg of α-tocopherol equivalents for women.[9,10] In an animal study with rats using intestinal perfusion with $^3$H-methyl-α-tocopherol, it was reported that animals 24 months old had an increase in vitamin E absorption up to 35% as compared to young controls (aged 4 months).[91] Many different factors may influence the bioavailability of vitamin E, including not only intraluminal events but also the dosage and the form of vitamin E.[92] Further, there is some confusion whether the absorptive phenomena differ from species to species; therefore, it remains open whether vitamin E bioavailability is increased in humans as they age. Most studies of the elderly have reported plasma/serum vitamin E levels well within the normal range. In a cross-sectional study of 206 institutionalized elderly (mean age for men and women 68.8 ± 15 and 76.4 ± 13.2 years, respectively), only 2 subjects had low α-tocopherol plasma levels by the Euronut SENECA criteria.[12] In a group of over 200 institutionalized elderly in Wülflingen, Switzerland, we found an adequate vitamin E status in all patients. The mean plasma vitamin E concentration was 27.3 ± 6.97 µmol/L; only one patient had a plasma vitamin E level below 15 µmol/L (Morell R, Suter PM, Haller J, et al. Unpublished data, 1993). Our data are in agreement with those of other studies reporting in most elderly an adequate plasma/serum vitamin E content.[21,22,93–99] Schmuck et al[100] reported a low intake of most antioxidants in a hospitalized geriatric population. Some studies report a decline in vitamin E levels with aging. This can be explained by a decline in the LDL cholesterol levels with increasing age (especially in the very old), since the LDL molecule is the major carrier of vitamin E in the blood.

The maintenance of adequate blood vitamin E levels suggests an adequate intake in most elderly. Illness associated with low food intake is one of the major determinants of vitamin E nutriture. Data regarding changes in tissue levels of vitamin E with age are inconsistent. Low platelet vitamin E levels have been described in a small group of old subjects (aged 78–94 years) as compared to young controls (aged 25–35 years).[101] These authors concluded that the increased platelet aggregation in aging may be caused by this decreased vitamin E concentration at the level of the platelets. A group of elderly on low intakes of eicosapentaenoic acid platelets showed a higher vitamin E concentration as compared to a control group.[102] Several animal studies analyzing vitamin E tissue levels in the central nervous system in different age groups have been performed recently. Meydani and colleagues[103] reported a selective decrease in the tocopherol concentration in the cerebellum of the brainstem. This decline was especially due to a decrease in α-tocopherol content. The authors concluded that these changes may be caused by a higher vitamin E turnover in these brain areas and that these brain areas require more vitamin E to maintain an adequate concentration of α-tocopherol. Supporting this conclusion were marked differences in the response upon supplementation in old versus young animals as assessed by the measurement of lipid peroxidation products.[104] A similar study measuring the effect of vitamin E deficiency in aging animals on the accumulation of age pigments in neuronal structures was performed by Koistinaho et al.[105] Recent animal studies, however, have reported that dietary vitamin E could affect lipofuscin accumulation only up to middle age, but not in old age.[106]

In a Swedish study, human adipose tissue tocopherol concentrations showed large variability depending on the serum tocopherol content ($r = 0.24–0.31$), but there was (contrary to other studies) no age-associated increase in the adipose tissue tocopherol content.[107] These controversial data need to be clarified in future studies. At present it is not known whether changes in vitamin E metabolism with age in certain selected tissues are representative of other tissues and organs or even overall requirements. From these studies, no conclusions regarding the requirements of vitamin E in aging can be drawn.

In the present context, the potential importance of vitamin E and other antioxidants in the pathogenesis of atherosclerosis must be discussed briefly.[26,90] LDL cholesterol plays a central role in the induction and progression of atherosclerosis. Evidence suggests that oxidatively modified LDL-cholesterol molecules bear a much higher pathophysiologic potential than native nonmodified LDL molecules, since these particles do show functional changes leading to improved recognition by the scavenger receptor.[108] Antioxidants may interfere basically at all pathophysiological steps of atherogenesis. Thus, the lipoproteins and the different structures of the vessel wall have to be protected from oxidative attack. The antioxidant hypothesis of atherosclerosis is very attractive, but causality needs to be proven. The development of atherosclerosis is probably a chronic lifelong process, so an adequate supply of antioxidants should be ensured during all periods of life.

In view of the antioxidative effects of vitamin E and its membrane-stabilizing properties, the effects of vitamin E on many chronic diseases of aging have been studied. Epidemiological and experimental studies suggest a potential role of this vitamin in the prevention of atherosclerosis, cancer, cataracts, central nervous system disorders such as Alzheimer's disease and Parkinson's disease, immune function, impaired glucose tolerance, and many more conditions.[26,90,109–113] These are all interesting associations, but despite fascinating pathophysiological phenomena, they do not imply causality. Ongoing trials may eventually clarify the controversy of causality for many different clinical conditions. In view of the available evidence, the present RDA for vitamin E seems to be adequate for the elderly population. To resolve the controversy around the importance of vitamin E, the results of some large-scale prospective studies are awaited. Further, it should be noted that the control of oxidative stress includes not only the supply of adequate amounts of antioxidants, but the control of any pro-oxidative metabolic conditions.

## VITAMIN K

During the past few years, new functions of vitamin K have been elucidated that may be of special importance for the elderly. One of the most important roles of vitamin K is to support the post-translational carboxylation of glutamate residues, which are involved in the formation of the modified amino acid γ-carboxyglutamate.[114]

Despite the new discoveries concerning the function of vitamin K and its metabolites, only incomplete information is available on the vitamin K requirements of the elderly. Reasons for this lack of knowledge are the limited knowledge of the amount of vitamin K in food sources as well as the difficulties in assessing biochemical vitamin K status correctly. It was in 1989 that an RDA for vitamin K was formulated for the first time. On the basis of a few studies, it is assumed that a dietary intake of 1 μg/kg of body weight per day should be sufficient to maintain normal blood clotting in adults.[10] The RDA for vitamin K is currently 80 μg (176 nmol) for adult men and 65 μg (143 nmol) for adult women. These recommendations are based on the maintenance and function of normal clotting mechanisms, but it is not known whether more vitamin K is needed for optimal functioning of other vitamin K–dependent proteins containing γ-carboxyglutamyl residues. Not only the diet but also the bacterial flora in the jejunum and the ileum contribute to the maintenance of the vitamin K status.[115] The relative contribution of the intestinal source of vitamin K depends on many factors, mainly the composition and the amount of the gut microflora. New evidence based upon the induction of vitamin K deficiency in normal healthy subjects by dietary restriction alone argues against the nutritional relevance of the intestinal bacteria as an important vitamin K source.[116]

There are hardly any data available on vitamin K nutriture in the elderly. It is estimated that the average U.S. diet provides a daily intake of about 150 to 500 μg vitamin K.[10] In view of newer data from the FDA Total Diet Study (TDS), these data seem to be overestimated. In the oldest groups of the TDS (ie, aged 60 years and older), the highest mean dietary intakes of vitamin $K_1$ from the whole population were reported. The estimated vitamin $K_1$ intake in this age category ranged from 76 to 80 μg/d, which is well above the present recommendation.[117] In the latter study, gender differences in the dietary sources of vitamin $K_1$ were identified. For adult women, green vegetables represented a more important source than they did for men. Nevertheless, green vegetables represent the major source of vitamin K in elderly men and women, followed by grain products, meat, and fats (in the form of dressings). This interesting study revealed that the addition of fat and oils to mixed meals and desserts represents an important modifier of vitamin K intake. In view of the trend of low-fat meals and different weight control strategies, this observation gains importance for the elderly. With increasing age, the contribution of vitamin $K_1$ from mixed meals declined, especially in women.[117] In agreement with the TDS, a cross-sectional study of 402 healthy postmenopausal women showed the mean total dietary intake of phylloquinone to be 89 μg/d.[118] In this study, there was a significant relationship ($r = 0.13$, $P = 0.01$) between the dietary intake of phylloquinones and the plasma levels. These apparently adequate intakes in the elderly would be in agreement with the observation that the elderly had higher vitamin K plasma levels than younger subjects.[116] The higher plasma levels in the elderly may, however, only represent higher vitamin K hepatic stores (as in the case of vitamin A). The reported mean plasma phylloquinone levels in the elderly are in the range of 1.05 to 1.15 nmol/L.[116,118,119]

Whether vitamin K absorption changes with age is not known. Alcohol consumption was associated with decreased fasting levels of vitamin $K_1$.[119] It seems that vitamin K–dependent proteins could be used to assess vitamin K nutriture.[120,121] Several studies have reported a relationship between osteocalcin and vitamin K nutriture.[122,123] Osteocalcin is less carboxylated when vitamin K status is impaired. In a recent biochemical study of 263 subjects (age range 18–85 years), the urinary γ-carboxyglutamic acid (Gla)–to-creatinine excretion ratios increased significantly with age in both genders ($r = 0.63$ and $0.68$, $P < 0.001$, for females and males, respectively).[120] In the same study, increased levels of total, carboxylated, and undercarboxylated osteocalcin levels with aging were reported.

The measurement of blood-clotting factors can be used to assess vitamin K nutriture. Newer methods (direct measurements of vitamin K and its metabolites, gla-proteins) are used today to assess vitamin K nutriture. Nevertheless, some older studies using measurements of clotting factors may reveal alterations in the vitamin K metabolism of the elderly. It was shown, with a test depending on all four vitamin K–dependent clotting factors, that 50% of a group of randomly selected elderly (age range 56–100 years) had an impairment suggestive of a vitamin K deficiency.[124] The subjects in this study were afflicted with various diseases and thus were not representative of the normal healthy aging process. In animal experiments, experimental vitamin K deficiency is more easily induced in older animals than in younger.[125] Further, despite the absence of significant age-related changes in warfarin pharmacokinetics, healthy elderly persons do have an increased sensitivity to warfarin.[126]

Despite the increased interest in vitamin K metabolism due to new analytical methods for the determination of the vitamin's levels and the new roles of vitamin K in bone health, no statement regarding the adequacy of the present recommendations for vitamin K in the elderly can be made. It seems that the lack of knowledge of the metabolism of this vitamin may be inversely related to its importance in health maintenance, especially regarding issues of age and aging.

## VITAMIN C

The vitamin C (ascorbic acid) deficiency disease of scurvy is rare in Western societies, but due to an increasing knowledge of new metabolic properties of vitamin C, an adequate supply of this vitamin remains the cornerstone for health maintenance, especially in the elderly. For the prevention of the development of scurvy, a daily intake of approximately 10 mg of ascorbic acid is needed; nevertheless, scurvy may still be found in our society in subjects consuming an inadequate diet.[127] The 1989 RDA for elderly males and females is 60 mg/d, which is identical to the RDA for the younger adults.[10] Olson and Hodges recommended lower RDAs: for men, 40 mg/d, and for women, 30 mg/d.[128] Despite the wide distribution of vitamin C in food, vitamin C intakes in elderly people vary widely, and up to 60% of the elderly may have intakes below 30 mg/d.[16,32,129–133] Dietary vitamin C intakes vary mainly as a function of the presence of illness associated with overall poor nutrient intake, institutionalization, and age.[134] The variability in intakes is nicely illustrated in two recent studies. In the Boston survey, the median vitamin C intakes for free-living elderly men and women were 132 mg and 128 mg, respectively.[135] In an Italian population of free-living elderly aged 70 to 75 years, 45% of the subjects had dietary intakes below 40 mg/d.[130] Similarly, a free-living population of elderly people on the Greek island of Crete had vitamin C intakes well above the U.S. RDA.[136] During the last decade, the intake of different supplements, especially vitamin C supplements, has increased widely and contributes considerably to the nutrient intake of large segments of the elderly population.

With increasing age, there is a decrease in ascorbic acid levels in whole blood, serum/plasma, and leucocytes.[137,138] Since the vitamin C plasma/serum levels depend mainly on vitamin C intake, there is a very wide variability in plasma/serum vitamin C levels. Between 1% and 60% of the free-living elderly may have low vitamin C levels (ie, <11.4 μmol/L).[129,139–143] Up to 80% of the institutionalized elderly may show low vitamin C levels in the blood. In the 155 institutionalized elderly of the Wülflingen study in Switzerland, the mean plasma ascorbic acid concentration was 25.8 ± 19.6 μmol/L. The lowest plasma concentration was 5.7 μmol/L, and 72% of the men and 42% of the women had plasma levels below 20 μmol/L (Morell R, Suter PM, Haller J, et al. Unpublished data, 1993). Institutionalization, hospitalization, and illness lead to a sharp decrease of vitamin C intakes[63,100] and thus low plasma levels. Most studies show lower ascorbic acid levels in elderly men than in elderly women; it has been suggested that the sex difference in plasma ascorbic acid concentration may be caused by a lower tubular reabsorption of the vitamin in elderly men.

Despite the high prevalence of low intakes and a low biochemical status in elderly subjects, the pharmacokinetic properties of a large dose of vitamin C (500 mg per os) were not affected by age.[144] In a depletion/repletion study of elderly subjects (aged 66–74 years) as compared to young controls (aged 21–28 years), no age-related difference in the response pattern was found.[145] In this study, 10 mg of ascorbic acid was given per day over a prolonged time period, and there was no difference in the half-life during the depletion period. In a metabolic study, elderly persons (aged >65 years) needed a larger dose of vitamin C to maintain a plasma concentration at which the ascorbic acid body pools were saturated (in this study, 56.7 µmol/L).[146] To maintain saturated ascorbic acid pools, the elderly men had to ingest approximately 150 mg/d and the elderly women approximately 80 mg/d, an intake considerably higher than the present RDA. Interestingly, at an ascorbic acid intake of 60 mg/d, some elderly men were not able to achieve an adequate plasma ascorbic acid concentration (ie, above 22.7 µmol/L). These data suggest that at least certain subsets of the elderly may indeed need higher vitamin C intakes to maintain adequate vitamin C nutriture. Whether tissue vitamin C levels do change with age is controversial.[147] Pinto et al,[148] using a vitamin C–loading test, reported a small increase of the plasma vitamin C levels in elderly subjects, suggestive of low tissue levels.

Low levels of vitamin C in the blood of healthy elderly people can be corrected easily by the administration of oral ascorbic acid supplements,[149] but upon withdrawal, a rapid decrease of the blood levels is seen. This supports the hypothesis that the low blood levels seen in the elderly are mainly attributable to low intakes and not to an age-related physiologic alteration at the level of absorption and/or other metabolic steps. Elderly persons with low vitamin C levels do not necessarily show clinical symptoms, so it has been concluded that there is no real need to raise the ascorbic acid levels in the blood through supplementation. In view of the functions of vitamin C, this conclusion may be wrong, since the health consequences of marginal vitamin C deficiency and its pathophysiologic role in the development of different diseases are not yet exactly known.

Ascorbic acid may be of importance in the pathogenesis of most chronic diseases of aging.[150] Ascorbic acid has been found to be potentially of importance in the prevention of atherosclerosis, cancer, senile cataract, lung diseases, cognitive function, and degenerative diseases of miscellaneous organs.[149–158] Further, ascorbic acid may be of great importance in immunomodulation in the elderly.[150] It is controversial which of the different antioxidative vitamins is of major importance. Present evidence suggests that an adequate supply of all the different antioxidatively active vitamins is needed and that it may be wrong to stress the importance of one single vitamin. The relative importance of the miscellaneous vitamins depends upon many different factors, such as body compartment, type of tissue or organ, and biochemical function. In a recent study by Sahyoun et al[159] looking at the association between mortality and different antioxidants (carotenoids, vitamin E, and vitamin C) in 747 free-living elderly subjects, only high intakes of vitamin C and frequent consumption of vegetables were significantly protective against early mortality. These findings would suggest a special importance of vitamin C, but adequacy of all nutrients is central for health maintenance, and the adequate intake of vitamin C may be a proxy for a more protective overall diet. Similar results were reported in other studies.[160,161]

Coronary artery disease and atherosclerosis are the leading causes of morbidity and mortality. The antioxidant hypothesis of atherosclerosis (see the section "Vitamin E") seems very attractive, but the effects of vitamin E on oxidative processes at the level of the LDL-cholesterol molecule have drawn more attention than the effects of ascorbic acid. It must be noted that vitamin C may decrease the oxidation of LDL and play an important role in the regeneration of vitamin E.[162] It also must be considered that a large fraction of the free radicals develop in the water phase of the different body compartments, where vitamin C is the major antioxidant. In addition, vitamin C may elicit a direct lipid-modifying effect.[163] And it may play a role in the pathogenesis of essential hypertension; several studies have reported an inverse relationship between vitamin C nutriture and blood pressure.[164,165]

Several modifiable factors, such as stress and smoking, influence vitamin C requirements. Vitamin C requirements of smokers may be up to 60 mg higher than those of nonsmokers.[154] Low levels in smokers can be corrected by a higher dietary or supplemental intake of vitamin C, but the maintenance of high plasma levels cannot counteract and counterbalance the negative health effects of smoking. Smoking cessation without an additional nutritional intervention leads rapidly to an improvement of vitamin C status as reflected in higher plasma levels.[166] The intake of vitamin C supplements seems to be fairly safe, but there is as yet no convincing evidence to advocate the intake of vitamin C supplements.

Present evidence suggests the absence of any specific age-related change in the metabolism of ascorbic acid. The present RDA of 60 mg of ascorbic acid per day seems to be adequate for the elderly, although some evidence suggests that for some individuals, needs may be higher. Nevertheless, intake should be optimized in certain substrata of the elderly (the institutionalized, the ill, and those of lower socioeconomic strata), especially during the winter months.

## VITAMIN B$_1$

The classical vitamin B$_1$ (thiamine hydrochloride) deficiency disease of beri-beri is hardly seen in Western populations, except in alcoholics. Vitamin B$_1$ plays an important role in carbohydrate metabolism, so the RDA of this vitamin depends on the total carbohydrate and overall energy intake. The present RDAs for thiamine are 1.2 mg/d for men and 1.0 mg/d for women.[10] The suggested minimal requirement appears to be between 0.20 and 0.23 mg/1000 kcal. To be on the safe side, an intake of 0.5 mg/1000 kcal is recommended. For elderly people, an intake of 1 mg/d is recommended, even if their energy consumption is below 2000 kcal/d.[10] These recommendations are the subject of some debate, since in young subjects with an intake of 0.3 mg/1000 kcal no biochemical deficiency could be detected.[167,168] As mentioned earlier, data from young subjects could not necessarily be extrapolated to the elderly, who represent a very heterogeneous population.

Up to 70% of the elderly, depending on income, race, and socioeconomic status, have been shown to have low thiamine intakes.[13,129,130,139,169–175] For thiamine, institutionalization, socioeconomic level, and illness are the major determinants of vitamin status.[130,169] Physical activity stimulates overall energy intake, which is also associated with improved overall nutriture, including better thiamine status. In the Wülflingen study, on the basis of the measurement of the thiamine transketolase activity, 82% of the elderly men and 74% of the women did show a thiamine deficiency. When the α-erythrocyte transketolase activity coefficient (ETKAC) was used, 14% of the elderly revealed a deficiency and 34% had a marginal status; about 50% had an adequate thiamine nutriture by this index (Morell R, Suter PM, Haller J, et al. Unpublished data, 1993). These data are in agreement with data from other studies.[175] However, there is, as for most water-soluble vitamins, a very wide variability in thiamine nutriture in the elderly: in an Irish study, up to 70% of elderly women showed a marginal and/or deficient thiamine status based upon the ETKAC,[174] whereas in other studies (as cited above) only about 10% showed a vitamin $B_1$ deficiency. This variability of intakes has been also reported in the Euronut SENECA study, where the median daily intakes of this vitamin ranged from 0.84 mg/d (Yverdon, Switzerland) to 1.59 mg/d (North Ireland).[139] In the same study, the longitudinal data revealed a median decline in the intakes of this vitamin during a 4- to 5-year period in the range of 0.00 to 0.20 mg/d. In looking at these data, it must be remembered that the assessment of nutrient intakes is a very difficult task, due not only to the incompleteness of the food tables but also to the inadequacy of the reports of intake by the subjects. In a study by Nichols and Basu,[171] the average thiamine intake was 0.4 mg/1000 kcal, which is well above the recommendation, but up to 50% of the subjects had a thiamine pyrophosphate activity coefficient above 14%, suggestive of a deficiency. This finding may be caused by either an inadequate dietary assessment or age-related changes in thiamine metabolism. Up to now, no specific age-related alterations in the metabolism of this vitamin have been identified.

Elderly subjects admitted for a medical or psychiatric hospitalization very often show a thiamine deficiency.[176–178] Aside from the latter factors, excessive alcohol intake is the most important factor in impaired thiamine status in the elderly.[179] Alcohol interferes with thiamine nutriture at basically all levels of metabolism. Since alcohol (even in small to moderate quantities) blocks active thiamine absorption, this may become clinically relevant, especially in elderly persons with low thiamine intakes who depend on the active mechanisms of the vitamin's uptake.[180] Patients with cardiac failure may represent a high-risk population for thiamine deficiency due to the chronic ingestion of diuretics.[181] In the latter study, thiamine nutriture worsened as a function of the New York Heart Association (NYHA) functional class. Some evidence suggests that chronic diuretic treatment leads to increased thiamine losses in urine[182]; supplementation with thiamine has further been shown to improve left ventricular function.[183] These data are very suggestive that especially elderly patients with a chronic diuretic therapy may be at higher risk for a thiamine deficiency and that low-dose thiamine supplementation (e.g., 50 mg/d) may be helpful in these patients. Oral supplementation with thiamine has been reported to improve cognitive function and overall well-being in the elderly.[174]

In summary, there are no specific changes in thiamine nutriture due to aging alone. The high prevalence of thiamine deficiency in some groups of the elderly is caused by poor intakes only.

## VITAMIN B₂

Vitamin $B_2$ (riboflavin) acts with its coenzymes flavin mononucleotide (FMN) and flavin adenin dinucleotide (FAD) in many electron transfer reactions. The present RDA for this vitamin is 1.4 mg/d for men and 1.2 mg/d for women.[10] For practical reasons, the riboflavin allowance in the 1989 RDA has been computed as 0.6 mg/1000 kcal for people of all ages, and 0.5 mg/1000 kcal has been considered to be the minimal requirement for adults.

Depending on race, income, gender, age, and health status, up to 70% of the elderly ingest less than two thirds of the present RDA.[13,129,136,169,173,184–191] Intake is the major determinant of riboflavin status. The intake of dairy products is, for the elderly, one of the most important sources of riboflavin. The latter relationship is nicely reflected in the different populations within the Euronut SENECA study, where the median riboflavin intake in the Danish population was 2.0 mg/d,[13] whereas at study sites with a lower consumption level of milk products the riboflavin intake was found to be well below the lowest European intake recommendation of 1.0 mg/d. Nevertheless, the median intake in the latter study ranged from 1.24 mg/d (Hamme, Belgium) to 2.19 mg/d (North Ireland).[139] In a carefully performed study in Guatemala, the rather high prevalence of riboflavin deficiency was mainly caused by an inadequate intake of dairy products.[188] In the same study, it was also found that a lower fat-to-carbohydrate ratio in the diet can be associated with *decreased* dietary needs for riboflavin.[192] Although the riboflavin content of alcoholic beverages varies widely, wine was identified as an important riboflavin source in a sample of elderly in Italy (aged >60 years)[184]; in contrast, in a survey of free-living elderly in the Boston area, high alcohol consumers were found to have the lowest blood levels of riboflavin and also vitamin $B_{12}$.[193]

Assessments of riboflavin nutriture by the erythrocyte glutathione reductase activity coefficient (EGRAC) have reported a similarly high prevalence of suboptimal or even deficient nutriture. In the Wülflingen study, in which milk products were daily consumed by a group of institutionalized elderly, low levels of EGR activity (ie, <30 μkatal/L) were found only in 10% of the men and 2% of the elderly women. The lowest EGR was 20.1 μkatal/L. When the EGRAC was used, only

8% of the subjects were found to be deficient; when the reference range of 1.2 to 1.3 was used to define a marginal status, 19% of these elderly subjects were identified to have marginal riboflavin nutriture (Morell R, Suter PM, Haller J, et al. Unpublished data, 1993). A similarly low prevalence of impaired riboflavin status was found in other studies from Italy[173] and in the Boston survey.[189] In a poor group of elderly (aged >60 years) in Hong Kong, an EGRAC greater than 1.3 was found in about 70% of the surveyed population.[128] Recent data suggest that riboflavin deficiency is especially widespread in the elderly in developing countries.[194,195] Riboflavin absorption seems to be unaffected by age, and there are probably no specific changes in vitamin $B_2$ tissue levels with age.[196,197]

Recent evidence suggests a role for riboflavin in the pathogenesis of age-related cataract, since this vitamin may be important as a photosensitizing agent.[198] Biochemical analysis of human lens capsules and epithelium revealed a high prevalence (over 20%) of severe glutathione reductase deficiency, suggestive of a dietary riboflavin deficiency.[199] Others have reported a decrease of glutathione reductase in red blood cells with advancing age independent of riboflavin nutriture.[200] Although these data are contradictory, they may point to possible age-related changes in the glutathione redox system at the tissue level.

A recent depletion study in elderly subjects suggests that the elderly may have higher riboflavin requirements. This study was performed in a healthy elderly population aged 60 years or older in Guatemala, eating a Western-type diet. Using urinary excretion of riboflavin, it found the requirement for this vitamin to be in the range of 1.1 to 1.3 mg/d.[192] These new data are in agreement with older data in different younger age groups using similar techniques for the assessment of riboflavin nutriture.[201–205] Since these rather old data are in good agreement with the new data from Boisvert et al,[192] aging per se apparently does not affect riboflavin requirements. Therefore, these data are very suggestive of higher riboflavin requirements in the elderly subjects than the current RDA.

In summary, at present there is no evidence suggesting age-related changes in the metabolism of riboflavin. The high variability of riboflavin nutriture in healthy elderly people is mainly due to low intakes and thus is easily corrected. Nevertheless, several lines of evidence show that the requirements for this vitamin do not change with age and seem to be similarly high in elderly and younger subjects. These data imply that an increase in $B_2$ intake of the elderly to the same levels as in younger subjects would be desirable.

## NIACIN

Niacin plays an important role as a coenzyme in nicotinamide adenine dinucleotide (NAD) and nicotinamide adenine dinucleotide phosphate (NADP). Since the amino acid tryptophan can be converted to niacin, niacin requirements are expressed as niacin equivalents (NE). Accordingly, the 1989 RDA is 15 mg NE per day for men and 13 mg NE per day for women.[10] The niacin deficiency disease pellagra is uncommon in Western societies, except in association with chronic alcoholism.[179]

The analytical procedures for the measurement of the niacin content of food as well as the biochemical assessment of niacin nutriture are uncertain and very incomplete and therefore of only limited practical value. Accordingly, the data about the niacin nutriture in the elderly are very limited. There is still much controversy regarding the ideal method for the assessment of niacin nutriture.

Niacin intake in the elderly varies widely as a function of socioeconomic background, race, age, health status, and institutionalization. In the Boston survey, around 25% of the elderly consumed less than the RDA.[135] In the Health and Nutrition Examination Survey I (HANES I), 53% of the surveyed black elderly with incomes below the poverty level had intakes below two thirds of the RDA.[133] However, only 54% of healthy free-living, middle-income elderly surveyed by Garry et al[32] in New Mexico had intakes of less than three fourths of the RDA. As in the case of most other nutrients, nutritional intake of niacin is related to the mortality of the elderly.[206] When urinary excretion of *N*-methyl nicotinamide is used as a measure, 1% to 50% of the elderly are shown to be niacin deficient.[207–209] Different factors affect the bioavailability of this vitamin, but on the basis of the present data, aging per se does not affect absorption.[210,211]

Niacin may be obtained from the conversion of tryptophan to this vitamin. Many different factors (such as hormonal factors, amino acids, or certain nutrients) may influence the conversion of tryptophan to niacin.[212–214] At present it is not known whether there are age-related changes in the conversion of tryptophan to niacin. Age-related changes in hormonal balance or in vitamin nutriture may affect the conversion. Animal data suggest that the conversion rate may depend highly on the adequacy of the vitamin $B_6$ status.[215] Since aging is associated with a high prevalence of an impairment of vitamin $B_6$ nutriture (see the section "Vitamin $B_6$"), this relationship may become important. Due to the lack of data, no conclusion can be drawn about the adequacy of the present intake recommendations of this vitamin.

## VITAMIN $B_6$

Vitamin $B_6$ is of major importance as a cofactor in many reactions of intermediary metabolism. Compared to the 1980 RDAs, the 1989 RDAs have been lowered—for the age group of men aged 51 years or older, by 0.2 mg to 2.0 mg/d, and for women, by 0.4 mg to 1.6 mg/d.[10] High protein intakes are associated with a higher requirement of this vitamin, and an intake of 0.016 mg of vitamin $B_6$ per gram of protein eaten is recommended. The intake of vitamin $B_6$ varies widely among the elderly as a function of absolute age, socioeconomic level, and state of health. Intakes below the RDA have been reported in up to 50% or even 90% of elderly populations.[12,21,130,133,135,139,169,216–224] Even in the healthy, free-living, upper–middle-class elderly surveyed by Garry et al,[32] 61% of the women consumed less than 1 mg of vitamin $B_6$ per day, and 54% of the elderly men consumed less than 1.1 mg (corresponding to 55% of the 1989 RDA). In the Euronut SENECA study, all populations in the different study centers had a median vitamin $B_6$ intake below the present U.S. RDA. When pyridoxal levels for the biochemical assessment of vitamin $B_6$ nutriture and a cutoff of 20 nmol/L are used, close to 25% of the subjects must be classified as deficient.[12] In the Boston survey of free-living elderly, 56% of the subjects had a low dietary intake, but only 5% showed a biochemical deficiency by the index of aspartate aminotransferase activity coefficients (AST-AC).[135] A similarly low prevalence of deficiency (9%) by the same index was found in a nationwide survey in the Netherlands, in which the surveyed elderly (aged 65–79 years) consumed around 0.016 mg of vitamin $B_6$ per gram of protein ingested.[223] On the basis of their data, the latter authors concluded that a normal AST-AC could be achieved with vitamin $B_6$ intakes of at least 0.020 mg/g of protein. The discrepancy between a high prevalence of low intakes and a rather low prevalence of deficiency in some of the cited studies may be caused in part by the use of only incomplete dietary databases for vitamin $B_6$.

The prevalence of diagnosed deficiency depends on the biochemical methods used for the assessment of the $B_6$ status. In the Wülflingen study of institutionalized elderly in Switzerland, we observed a deficiency in about 33% of the elderly when the erythrocyte aspartate aminotransferase activity (AST; former EGOT) was used as an index. Using the AST-AC with a cutoff of less than 1.8 to define deficiency, we found 85% of the subjects to be deficient. On the basis of pyridoxal-5-phosphate levels, 93% were found to be deficient (Morell R, Suter PM, Haller J, et al. Unpublished data, 1993). Also, in other studies, socioeconomic level, institutionalization, and health status were the major determinants of the vitamin $B_6$ status.

Serum and plasma vitamin $B_6$ levels are subject to large variations, depending mainly on recent food intake, and thus do not reflect long-term vitamin $B_6$ nutritional status. Several studies have shown a decline in serum and plasma levels of pyridoxal phosphate (PLP, which represents the most active form of the vitamin) with age.[225–227] The reported decrease of plasma PLP was approximately 0.90 ng/mL and was associated with an increased prevalence of low plasma PLP levels (ie, <5 ng/mL) from around 3% in healthy younger subjects (aged <40 years) to about 12% in individuals aged 80 years or older. It has been suggested that the age-related increase of the activity of the alkaline phosphatase, which is considered to be of major importance in the degradation of PLP, and low intakes are the major causes of the age-related decline in plasma PLP levels with aging.[228]

Animal data suggest, however, an impairment of the formation of PLP in different tissues.[229] It is not established whether the capacity to phosphorylate this vitamin changes with age. Little evidence for an alteration in pyridoxine phosphorylation with age comes from a few clinical case reports of primary sideroachrestic anemias responsive solely to the administration of pyridoxal phosphate and not to pyridoxine.[230] Using the tryptophan-loading test and an index of vitamin $B_6$ nutriture, several older studies found an age-related increase in abnormal loading tests.[225,227] These abnormalities of vitamin $B_6$ nutriture can be corrected by the ingestion of vitamin $B_6$ supplements in most elderly persons.[207,231–233] However, a few studies report the inability of some elderly (up to 20%) to correct their biochemical vitamin $B_6$ status upon supplement intakes.[234–236] The latter observations are very suggestive of age-related changes in vitamin $B_6$ requirements of the elderly. Nevertheless, effects of diseases and unknown comorbidities in these studies could not be ruled out as a cause of this nonresponsiveness to supplements.

Functional or dynamic tests may be a better means to study potential age-related changes in the metabolism of most vitamins. Despite the possibility of age-related changes in vitamin $B_6$ metabolism (as outlined above), Kant et al[237] were unable to detect a change of the urinary 4-pyridoxic acid excretion after an oral vitamin $B_6$ load as a function of age. However, it is not exactly known whether these excretion tests can reliably detect any age-related changes. Therefore, it has been recommended that more than one biochemical index be used for the optimal assessment of vitamin $B_6$ nutriture.

Interesting and important data about the vitamin $B_6$ requirements of the elderly were obtained in a recent depletion/repletion study of elderly subjects (>60 years) in a metabolic unit.[221] This study consisted of several experimental periods with well-defined amounts of vitamin $B_6$ ranging from 0.003 up to 0.03375 mg/kg of body weight per day. After the initial depletion, the subjects were repleted in a stepwise fashion; the tryptophan-loading test (ie, the measurement of urinary xanthurenic acid excretion) was used to assess $B_6$ nutriture. The major result of this study was that in elderly subjects consuming the RDA or 1.5 times the RDA for protein, the estimated vitamin $B_6$ requirements are about 1.96 mg for elderly men and 1.90 mg for elderly women. These data from Ribaya-Mercado et al[221] strongly suggest that the RDA for this vitamin should be higher, since at present the RDA is based on a ratio of 0.016 mg of vitamin $B_6$ per gram of protein, which seems, in view of these data, to be inadequate. Furthermore, in this study, the repletion was done with a highly bioavailable pyridoxine hydrochloride supplement. The bioavailability of vitamin $B_6$ from food is much lower, so the RDA based upon the intake of the vitamin from food sources may be even higher than that actually recommended.

Vitamin $B_6$ deficiency or suboptimal status may result in an enhancement of the pathogenesis of different diseases and/or impairment of specific organ functions. The depletion of vitamin $B_6$ in studies by Meydani et al resulted in an impairment of the immune function in these elderly.[238,239] Vitamin $B_6$ plays an important function as a cofactor for the cystathionine synthase, and a lack of this vitamin may result in high homocysteine levels in the blood. Recent evidence suggests that elevated plasma homocysteine levels should be regarded as an independent cardiovascular risk factor.[240–243] Several nutrients (folate, vitamin $B_6$, and vitamin $B_{12}$) are important modulators of the plasma homocysteine levels.[240] Retrospective and prospective studies have described a relationship between the risk of coronary artery disease and myocardial infarction and the intake of vitamin $B_6$.[233,244–246] This relationship is, however, strongest for folic acid.[240] The relationship between the different vitamins and the risk of atherosclerosis, especially coronary artery disease, has a high potential to be of great pathophysiologic and public health importance but needs to be proven in more prospective interventional studies. The importance of homocysteine and the potential relationship between nutrition and the pathogenesis of atherosclerosis will be discussed in the next section. Vitamin $B_6$ plays an important role in the synthesis of neurotransmitters and neural function in general. Accordingly, it is not surprising that vitamin $B_6$ supplementation in the elderly may be associated with an improvement of memory and mental performance.[247]

The prevalence of impaired vitamin $B_6$ nutriture in elderly people is variable compared to that of other vitamins but is rather high, is consistently found in different populations, and is mainly caused by low dietary intakes. Further, vitamin $B_6$ metabolism may be affected by aging. In view of the present evidence, especially from metabolic studies, the present RDA should be reevaluated carefully. Data strongly suggest a higher requirement than is currently recommended.

## FOLATE

One of the main functions of folate is the transport of single carbon atoms in intermediary metabolic processes. The 1989 folate RDAs are the same for elderly as for well young adults: 200 μg for men and 180 μg for women.[10] This recommendation was lower than the 1980 RDA.

Folate intakes in the elderly may vary considerably, but most elderly people ingest amounts close to the RDA. The prevalence of low intakes varies between 0% and 50%[32,49,139,248,249] and is influenced mainly by institutionalization and health status.[63,250] In the Wülflingen study, 27% of the men and 14% of the women had folate plasma levels below 10 nmol/L. The lowest value was 7.5 nmol/L, so none of these surveyed elderly were below the level of 6.8 nmol/L, which is regarded as the threshold level for deficiency. Nevertheless, about 50% of these institutionalized elderly had a marginal biochemical status (ie, plasma levels between 6.8 and 13.4 nmol/L) (Morell R, Suter PM, Haller J, et al. Unpublished data, 1993). This marginal status may be of pathophysiological relevance regarding the relationship with the metabolism of homocysteine. Other studies reported a similarly low prevalence of biochemical deficiency in the elderly. The median dietary folate intake in the Boston survey was 254 μg/d for the men and 216 μg/d for the women.[135] In agreement with these intakes, only 2.5% of this group of elderly showed plasma concentrations below 7 nmol/L.[135] A similarly low rate of deficiency was reported in a study from New York City and a town in New Zealand.[251,252] As in the Wülflingen study and the SENECA study, no elderly subjects had plasma folate levels below 6.8 nmol/L.[12] In some studies, despite low intakes, hardly any elderly had low plasma folate levels[32]; this discrepancy may in part be caused by an underestimation of folate intakes due to the incompleteness of the food tables used.

Folate is widely distributed in food, where it is found mainly in the form of polyglutamates. Before absorption, polyglutamates must be deconjugated by an intestinal folate conjugase (pteroylpolyglutamyl hydrolase) present in the brush border and intracellular fraction of the jejunal mucosa.[253] Whether the activity of this enzyme is subject to age-related alterations is controversial; however, present evidence suggests that folic acid absorption is not influenced by age alone.[132,254] The activity of the folate conjugase, and thus folate absorption per se, is highly pH dependent. Russell and colleagues[254] reported a diminished folic acid absorption in elderly subjects with atrophic gastritis, which is characterized by diminished gastric acid output and thus a higher proximal small intestinal pH, leading to bacterial overgrowth in the upper gastrointestinal tract. This malabsorption may be due to a high intraluminal pH that negatively influences the pH-sensitive active uptake of folic acid by small intestinal epithelial cells. In this study, the folic acid malabsorption in subjects with atrophic gastritis was completely corrected (ie, normalized) by the oral administration of 0.1 N of hydrochloric acid.

Despite this folate malabsorption in atrophic gastritis, these individuals had normal serum folate levels, which might have been due to folate synthesis by the bacteria that were overgrowing the upper intestinal tract.[254] Different modifiable factors may affect folate absorption. A high intake of alcohol alone or in combination with an inadequate diet is one of the most important factors contributing to a clinical folate deficiency.[179] Alcohol has the potential to block several metabolic pathways of folic acid. Animal experiments using rats chronically fed a low-folate diet suggest changes in methyl group metabolism with aging, independent of the amount of folate in the diet.[255]

In the elderly, the combination of low folate intakes and elevated plasma homocysteine levels represents a rather prevalent clinical situation. In the original Framingham Study cohort of subjects aged 67 to 96 years, 29% showed high plasma homocysteine levels (hyperhomocysteinemia, defined as >14 µmol/L).[240] These elevated levels of plasma homocysteine are mainly attributable to an impairment of folate, vitamin $B_6$, and/or vitamin $B_{12}$ nutriture. But in most people, folic acid seems to be the major determinant of plasma homocysteine levels.[2,240]

Several lines of evidence suggest that homocysteine may be a risk factor for coronary artery disease and atherosclerosis.[243,256–258] In view of the potential importance of folate as a modulator of the plasma homocysteine levels and therefore potentially also of cardiovascular risk, folate nutriture should be optimized in all age groups, and theoretical considerations suggest that a folic acid fortification of the food supply may be beneficial for the elderly.[2] In this context, it should be mentioned that food fortification with folic acid alone should be considered only very carefully, since vitamin $B_{12}$ deficiency is also rather prevalent in the elderly. To clarify the therapeutic potential of lowering homocysteine by the administration of folate, large prospective placebo-controlled trials are urgently needed.

Besides its role in atherosclerosis, folic acid may have great importance in the maintenance of many different organ functions in the aged, especially cognitive function. In a recent study of the noninstitutionalized elderly, a relationship between the Mini-Mental Test and biochemical folate status was described.[259] Further, it is possible that folic acid status may be of crucial importance in the pathogenesis and/or management of depression and other neuropsychiatric disturbances in the elderly.[260–262]

Despite the rather strong evidence of the role of folate in the development of diseases and/or the potential to modulate different metabolic functions, present evidence does not yet support strongly enough an increase of the present RDA. Nevertheless, adequate intakes based on present guidelines should be more strongly encouraged.

## VITAMIN $B_{12}$

The 1989 RDA for vitamin $B_{12}$ is 2.0 µg/d for men and 1.6 µg/d for women.[10] The primary dietary sources of this vitamin are animal products. Vitamin $B_{12}$ intake in free-living elderly varies widely, and approximately

0% to 50% of the elderly have been reported to have intakes below the present recommendation.[32,49,131,263,264] In the study by Garry et al[264] of middle-class elderly subjects in New Mexico, 24% of the men and 39% of the women had intakes below the present RDA; up to 15% had intakes below 75% of the RDA. The male elderly surveyed in the Boston study had a median vitamin $B_{12}$ dietary intake of 3.1 µg/d, and for the female elderly it was 2.6 µg/d.[135] Only 3% of the elderly men but 12% of the elderly women had intakes below two thirds of the present recommendation. The prevalence of low blood vitamin $B_{12}$ levels varies between 0% and 30% of the surveyed elderly.[251,252,265–274] In the Wülflingen study, only 3.8% of the surveyed institutionalized elderly had plasma vitamin $B_{12}$ levels below 100 pmol/L. Despite this low prevalence of biochemical deficiency, 28.3% of the elderly had plasma levels below 200 pmol/L, and most of the elderly (ie, 85.3%) had levels below 400 pmol/L. The lowest detected value was 14 pmol/L, and 86% of the elderly had levels above 147 pmol/L. Using the Euronut criteria, 6.3% have to be judged as deficient (Morell R, Suter PM, Haller J, et al. Unpublished data, 1993). In the Euronut SENECA study, only 2.7% of the subjects had vitamin $B_{12}$ levels below 111 pmol/L.[12] These data are further in good agreement with the Boston survey, in which only 5% of the elderly were found to have vitamin $B_{12}$ values below 74 pmol/L.[135]

Several studies have reported a gradual decline in the plasma vitamin $B_{12}$ levels with age; however, despite this decline, the values remain within the limits of normality in most studies. The cutoff value of the limit of normality is, however, controversial. In a longitudinal study by Nilsson-Ehle et al,[275] an annual decline of the serum vitamin $B_{12}$ levels of 3.4 pmol/L for men and 3.2 pmol/L for women was observed. In agreement with this decline, the prevalence of low vitamin $B_{12}$ levels increases with age in most studies. It has been suggested that this age-related decline in plasma/serum vitamin $B_{12}$ levels might be related to the increased occurrence of atrophic gastritis with increasing age.[263,276]

The prevalence of atrophic gastritis increases with age to almost 40% to 50% in those aged 80 years or older. It has been shown that atrophic gastritis decreases the bioavailability of dietary vitamin $B_{12}$ (ie, protein-bound vitamin $B_{12}$).[277–279] In natural food sources, vitamin $B_{12}$ is bound to food proteins and must be released from protein binding before the absorptive process can be initiated. Several mechanisms may lead to the malabsorption of protein-bound vitamin $B_{12}$ in atrophic gastritis. Because of diminished or completely lacking gastric acid production, protein digestion is impaired, and vitamin $B_{12}$ cannot be released from its protein binding. Additionally, bacteria that overgrow the upper gastrointestinal tract may bind vitamin $B_{12}$ and/or convert it to vitamin $B_{12}$ analogues, rendering the vitamin $B_{12}$ unavailable. Some of the analogues may even inhibit vitamin $B_{12}$ malabsorption.

The decreased output of intrinsic factor in atrophic gastritis is probably of no clinical significance because usually the degree of parietal cell destruction is only partial. In a recent study, it was shown that the malabsorption of the protein-bound vitamin $B_{12}$ in subjects with atrophic gastritis could be reversed by an antibiotic treatment with tetracycline.[279] In this study, the bacterial counts in the upper gastrointestinal tract could have been reduced, and this decrease was associated with a normalization of the absorption of the protein-bound vitamin $B_{12}$, suggesting that the malabsorption was mainly due to bacterial overgrowth. In this context, it should be mentioned that the absorption of crystalline vitamin $B_{12}$ is not impaired in atrophic gastritis. This possibility (ie, normal crystalline vitamin $B_{12}$ absorption) should be accounted for in the selection of the type of vitamin $B_{12}$ absorption test (crystalline or protein bound) used in clinical practice. Age per se (ie, in the absence of atrophic gastritis) does not affect the absorption of vitamin $B_{12}$. Therefore, it must be remembered that a normal absorption of crystalline vitamin $B_{12}$ is not equal to a normal absorption of protein-bound vitamin $B_{12}$.[280]

It is controversial whether adequate plasma vitamin $B_{12}$ levels always reflect adequacy of vitamin $B_{12}$ status correctly. Recently it has been shown that vitamin $B_{12}$ deficiency, diagnosed by the measurements of serum methylmalonic acid and total homocysteine, might be present even in the absence of hematologic abnormalities, a normal Schilling test, and normal or only minimally depressed serum/plasma cobalamin levels.[281] This suggests that vitamin $B_{12}$ deficiency could be a major undetected problem in apparently healthy elderly.[270] In view of the importance of vitamin $B_{12}$ in intermediary metabolism as a cofactor for the L-methylmalonyl-CoA mutase and the methionine synthase, the measurement of serum metabolites in the diagnosis of cobalamin deficiency may be indicated in certain cases.[282,283] Some evidence even suggests that the measurement of serum cobalamin to detect deficiency is a rather insensitive tool.[266] This should be remembered in any discussion of the implementation of generous folate fortification and/or supplementation for the control of plasma homocysteine levels. Measurement of plasma homocysteine and methylmalonic acid levels may be helpful in the evaluation of the adequacy of vitamin $B_{12}$ nutriture. But besides vitamin nutriture, other factors, especially kidney function, may represent an important modulator of plasma homocysteine levels. These factors have to be considered in the formulation of "normal values," and the definition of reference intervals should be adjusted for different age groups separately.[284] The controversy regarding the lower limit of normal plasma levels of vitamin $B_{12}$ continues so elderly subjects with low plasma levels of vitamin $B_{12}$ should be monitored more closely, and in view of the potential benefit, even a parenteral supplementation of this vitamin may be indicated in certain patients.

Because of the primary importance of folate for the regulation of plasma homocysteine levels, fortification of food and/or folate supplementation has been recommended. In view of the high prevalence of abnormalities in vitamin $B_{12}$ metabolism, supplementation with folate alone may be associated with some risk; therefore, only combined supplementation/fortification with folate *and* vitamin $B_{12}$ should be considered.[2,284]

Evidence suggests that elderly individuals, even with plasma vitamin $B_{12}$ levels within the lower limit of normality, may show metabolic disturbances indicative of a "subclinical" vitamin $B_{12}$ deficiency. Consequently, the reduction of vitamin $B_{12}$ intake recommendations in the last edition of the RDA seems unwarranted and may even present some risk for certain subgroups of the elderly.

## BIOTIN

Biotin deficiency seems to occur rarely but has been reported in persons who have been on long-term total parenteral nutrition, who have ingested raw eggs excessively, or who have an inborn error of metabolism. There is no RDA for biotin; in view of the incomplete data, an intake of 30 to 100 µg/d is provisionally recommended for adults.[10] There are hardly any data available on biotin nutriture in the aged. One study reported lower biotin plasma levels in a small group of elderly as compared with young athletes, but others have reported no change in these levels with age.[285–288] In the Wülflingen study, only 20 patients (9.7%) had plasma biotin levels below 1 nmol/L; 21 patients (10.2%) showed a marginal biotin status (defined as plasma biotin levels between 0.5 and 1.0 nmol/L). The lowest biotin plasma level was 0.61 nmol/L. If deficiency is defined as a plasma biotin level below 0.5 nmol/L, none of our subjects were deficient. The present evidence, although scarce, suggests that biotin nutriture is not a major concern for the elderly.

## PANTOTHENIC ACID

There is no RDA for pantothenic acid, but the estimated safe and adequate daily intake is 4 to 7 mg for both men and women. In a study in a nursing home, the daily pantothenic acid intake was 3.75 mg/d or 2.22 mg/1000 kcal, which is less than the recommended allowance for the elderly.[289] In humans as well as in animals, a decrease in protein-bound pantothenic acid in blood has been reported; however, some investigators have failed to find an age-related decline in blood levels of this vitamin. Using urinary excretion as an index of pantothenic acid nutriture in elderly people is not conclusive and is contradictory.[290,291] On the basis of the present evidence, no statement about the adequacy of pantothenic acid nutriture in the elderly or the recommended allowance can be made.

## CONCLUSION AND RECOMMENDATIONS

In this chapter, selected aspects of the vitamin nutriture of the elderly have been reviewed. The elderly are a very heterogeneous population group, so they vary widely in their vitamin status in general. The evidence suggests that the present recommendations for vitamin D, vitamin $B_6$, and probably vitamin $B_{12}$ may be too low for the elderly. For these vitamins, age-related changes in metabolism may account in part for the deficiency. For riboflavin, some evidence suggests that the recommendations may be too low, but increasing intake of milk products can improve riboflavin status immediately. The intake recommendations for vitamin A seem to be too high for the elderly, but a large fraction of vitamin A can be obtained by intake of the vitamin A precursor beta carotene, and due to the potentially important health effects of carotenoids, lowering the vitamin A RDA may be counterproductive. For vitamin K, niacin, biotin, and pantothenic acid, no statement about vitamin status and metabolism in the elderly can be formulated due to lack of data. All other vitamins show no age-related changes in metabolism; a deficiency is usually caused by poor intakes and is therefore correctable with increased food intake.

When discussing vitamin metabolism in the elderly, modifiable effects on the basic requirements of the different vitamins should be mentioned. Vitamins may play an important role in primary and secondary aging processes[4] (Table 3–2 and Figure 3–1). The effect of overall lifestyle, including nutrition, on the aging process and homeostatic competence (ie, the potential to develop diseases) is illustrated in Figure 3–2. However, as illustrated, many immediately modifiable factors influence both vitamin and overall nutriture, as well as the rate of aging. These factors have to be controlled for in the elderly. They include smoking, excessive ethanol consumption, energy overconsumption, and physical inactivity. In the presence of these factors, an apparently adequate nutrient intake becomes inadequate, resulting in de-

**Table 3–2** The Role of Vitamins in Modulating the Primary and the Secondary Aging Processes

*Secondary Aging Processes*

Modulation of comorbidity—the pathogenesis of the chronic diseases of aging:

Cell differentiation
Tissue differentiation
Atherogenesis
Cancer
Osteoporosis
Immune function
Brain function (cognitive function)
Degenerative diseases
Diabetes
Intermediary metabolism
Drug metabolism
Detoxification

*Primary Aging Process(es)*

Interaction with the primary "rate" of aging:

Free-radical theory of aging
Genetic determination
Cross-linking theory
Metabolic theory
Immunological theory
Programmed senescence
Dysdifferentiation theory
Collagen theory

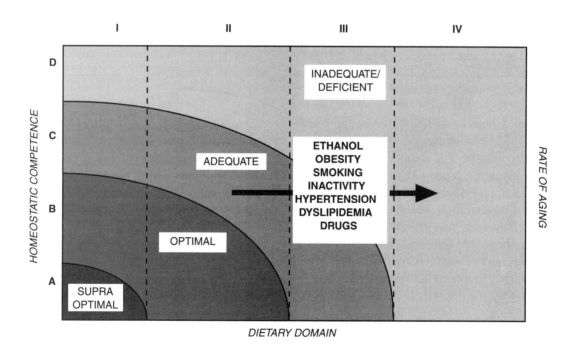

**Figure 3–1** Relationship among nutrient intake, rate of aging, and homeostatic competence. Control of risk factors modulating the nutrient requirements may be of primary importance in daily life.

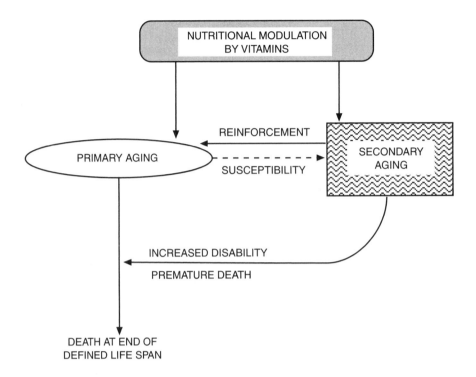

**Figure 3–2** Relationship between nutritional status and the primary and secondary aging processes.

creased functional homeostasis and an increased rate of aging and eventually deterioration of nutritional status. As discussed, the primary aging process does not significantly affect the metabolism of most vitamins (except for vitamin D and, eventually, vitamin $B_6$). However, many secondary aging phenomena (ie, the different chronic diseases of aging) may directly and indirectly affect nutrient requirements and especially nutrient status by the modification of food intake. Therefore, the maintenance of optimal vitamin nutriture includes also the minimization of any secondary aging phenomena (ie, chronic disease risk) by the control of the well-known modifiable risk factors (Figures 3–1 and 3–2).

As mentioned in this review, there is still much controversy regarding vitamin nurture and vitamin requirements in the elderly. The maintenance of an adequate supply of single vitamins remains essential for the assurance of an adequate status. Nutrient supplements may be indicated on an individual basis, however, rather than for all elderly. The question "Who can profit from supplemental vitamin intake?" is still unsolved and controversial. Nevertheless, the vitamin nutrition for the elderly does not start when someone has reached retirement age; the optimization of daily nutrient supply at a young age probably remains the cornerstone for optimal vitamin nutriture at older ages.

## REFERENCES

1. Hoffman C, Rice D, Sung HY. Persons with chronic conditions: their prevalence and costs. *JAMA*. 1996;276:1473–1479.

2. Tucker KL, Mahnken B, Wilson PWF, Jacques P, Selhub J. Folic acid fortification of the food supply: potential benefits and risks for the elderly. *JAMA*. 1996;276:1879–1885.

3. *Diet, Nutrition, and the Prevention of Chronic Diseases*. Geneva, Switzerland: World Health Organization; 1990.

4. Suter PM, Vetter W. The role of vitamins in ageing and the ageing process. *Age Nutr*. 1996;7:86–95.

5. Sauberlich HE, Machlin LJ. Beyond deficiency: new views on the function and health effects of vitamins. *Ann NY Acad Sci*. 1992;669:1–398.

6. Cutler RG, Packer L, Bertram J, Mori A, eds. *Oxidative Stress and Aging*. Basel, Switzerland: Birkhäuser Verlag; 1995.

7. Wolf G. A history of vitamin A. *FASEB J*. 1996;10:1102–1107.

8. Bollag W. The retinoid revolution. *FASEB J*. 1996;10:938–939.

9. National Research Council. *Recommended Dietary Allowances*. Washington, DC: National Academy of Sciences; 1980.

10. National Research Council. *Recommended Dietary Allowances*. Washington, DC: National Academy Press; 1989.

11. Olson JA. Recommended dietary intakes (RDI) of vitamin A in humans. *Am J Clin Nutr*. 1987;45:704–716.

12. Euronut SENECA Investigators. Nutritional status: blood vitamins A, E, $B_6$, $B_{12}$, folic acid and carotene. *Eur J Clin Nutr*. 1991;45(suppl 3):63–82.

13. Euronut SENECA Investigators. Intake of vitamins and minerals. *Eur J Clin Nutr*. 1991;45(suppl 3):121–138.

14. Johnson EJ, Russell RM. Vitamin A. In: Hartz SC, Rosenberg IH, Russell RM, eds. *Nutrition in the Elderly: The Boston Nutritional Status Survey*. London, England: Smith-Gordon & Co Ltd; 1992:87–101.

15. Saito M, Itoh R. Nutritional status of vitamin A in a healthy elderly population in Japan. *Int J Vitam Nutr Res*. 1991;61:105–109.

16. Russell RM, Suter PM. Vitamin requirements of the elderly: an update. *Am J Clin Nutr*. 1993;58:4–11.

17. Mino M, Tamai H, Tanabe T, et al. Nutritional status of antioxidant vitamins (A, E, and beta-carotene) in elderly Japanese. *J Nutr Sci Vitaminol (Tokyo)*. 1993;39(suppl):S67–S74.

18. Lipski PS, Torrance A, Kelly PJ, James OF. A study of nutritional deficits of long-stay geriatric patients. *Age Ageing*. 1994;22:244–255.

19. Haller J, Lowik MR, Ferry M, Ferro-Luzzi A. Nutritional status: blood vitamin A, E, $B_6$, folic acid and carotene. Euronut SENECA investigators. *Eur J Clin Nutr*. 1991;45(suppl 3):63–82.

20. Monget AL, Galan P, Preziosi P, et al. Micronutrient status in elderly people. *Int J Vitam Nutr Res*. 1996;66:71–76.

21. Haller J, Weggemans RM, Lammi-Keefe CJ, Ferry M. Changes in the vitamin status of elderly Europeans: plasma vitamins A, E, B-6, B-12, folic acid and carotenoids. *Eur J Clin Nutr*. 1996;50(suppl 2):S32–S46.

22. Morinobu T, Tamai H, Tanabe T, et al. Plasma alpha-tocopherol, beta-carotene, and retinol levels in the institutionalized elderly individuals and in young adults. *Int J Vitam Nutr Res*. 1994;64:104–108.

23. Mayne ST. Beta-carotene, carotenoids, and disease prevention in humans. *FASEB J*. 1996;10:690–701.

24. Snowdon DA, Gross MD, Butler SM. Antioxidants and reduced functional capacity in the elderly: findings from the Nun Study. *J Gerontol A Biol Sci Med Sci*. 1996;51:M10–M16.

25. Pryor WA. The antioxidant nutrients and disease prevention: what do we know and what do we need to find out? *Am J Clin Nutr*. 1991;53:391–393.

26. Packer L, Fuchs J, eds. *Vitamin E in Health and Disease*. New York, NY: Marcel Dekker Inc; 1993.

27. Gaziano JM, Manson JE, Branch LG, Colditz GA, Willett WC, Buring JE. A prospective study of consumption of carotenoids in fruits and vegetables and decreased mortality in the elderly. *Ann Epidemiol*. 1995;5:255–260.

28. Greenberg ER, Baron JA, Karagas MR, et al. Mortality associated with low plasma concentration of beta carotene and the effect of oral supplements. *JAMA*. 1996;275:699–703.

29. Jacques PF, Halpner AD, Blumberg JB. Influence of combined antioxidant nutrient intakes on their plasma concentration in an elderly population. *Am J Clin Nutr.* 1995;62:1228–1233.

30. Processing of dietary retinoids is slowed in the elderly. *Nutr Rev.* 1991;49:116–118.

31. Chevalier S, Ferland G, Tuchweber B. Lymphatic absorption of retinol in young, mature, and old rats: influence of dietary restriction. *FASEB J.* 1996; 10:1085–1090.

32. Garry PJ, Goodwin JS, Hunt WC, Hooper EM, Leonard AG. Nutritional status in a healthy elderly population: dietary and supplemental intakes. *Am J Clin Nutr.* 1982;36:319–331.

33. Garry PJ, Hunt WC, Bandrofchak JL, VanderJagt D, Goodwin JS. Vitamin A intake and plasma retinol in healthy men and women. *Am J Clin Nutr.* 1987;46:989–994.

34. Krasinski SD, Russell RM, Otradovec CL, et al. Relationship of vitamin A and vitamin E intake to fasting plasma retinol, retinol binding protein, retinyl esters, carotene, alpha-tocopherol, and cholesterol among elderly people and young adults: increased plasma retinyl esters among vitamin A supplement users. *Am J Clin Nutr.* 1989;49:112–120.

35. Leo MA, Lieber CS. Hepatic vitamin A depletion in alcoholic liver injury. *N Engl J Med.* 1982; 307:597–601.

36. Leo MA, Lieber CS. Hypervitaminosis A: a liver's lover lament. *Hepatology.* 1988;8:412–417.

37. Sato M, Lieber CS. Hepatic vitamin A depletion after chronic ethanol consumption. *J Nutr.* 1981; 111:2015–2023.

38. Mobarhan S, Seitz HK, Russell RM, et al. Age related effects of chronic ethanol intake on vitamin A status in Fisher 344 rats. *J Nutr.* 1991;121:510–517.

39. Bulux J, Carranza E, Castaneda C, et al. Studies on the application of the relative dose response test for assessing vitamin A status in older adults. *Am J Clin Nutr.* 1992;56:543–547.

40. Rasmussen HM, Dallal GE, Phelan E, Russell RM. Serum concentrations of retinol and retinyl esters in adults in response to mixed vitamin A and carotenoid containing meals. *J Am Coll Nutr.* 1991; 10:460–465.

41. Santos MS, Meydani SN, Leka L, et al. Natural killer cell activity in elderly men is enhanced by β-carotene supplementation. *Am J Clin Nutr.* 1996; 64:772–777.

42. Paiva SAR, Godoy I, Vannucchi H, Favaro RMD, Geraldo RRC, Campana AO. Assessment of vitamin A status in chronic pulmonary disease patients and healthy smokers. *Am J Clin Nutr.* 1996;64:928–934.

43. Soutar A, Seaton A, Brown K. Bronchial reactivity and dietary antioxidants. *Thorax.* 1997;52:166–170.

44. Ross AC, Stephensen CB. Vitamin A and retinoids in antiviral responses. *FASEB J.* 1996;10:979–985.

45. Omenn GS, Goodman GE, Thornquist MD, et al. Risk factors for lung cancer and for intervention effects in CARET, the beta-carotene and retinol efficacy trial. *J Natl Cancer Inst.* 1996;88:1550–1559.

46. Omenn GS, Goodman GE, Thornquist MD, et al. Effects of a combination of beta carotene and vitamin A on lung cancer and cardiovascular disease. *N Engl J Med.* 1996;334:1150–1155.

47. Alpha-tocopherol b-cP: the effect of vitamin E and beta-carotene on the incidence of lung cancer and other cancers in male smokers. *N Engl J Med.* 1994;330:1029–1035.

48. Albanes D, Heinonen OP, Taylor PR, et al. α-Tocopherol and β-carotene supplements and lung cancer incidence in the Alpha-Tocopherol, Beta-Carotene Cancer Prevention Study: effects of baseline characteristics and study compliance. *J Natl Cancer Inst.* 1996;88:1560–1570.

49. Suter PM, Russell RM. Vitamin nutriture and requirements of the elderly. In: Munro HN, Danford DE, eds. *Nutrition, Aging and the Elderly.* New York, NY: Plenum Press; 1989:245–291.

50. Delvin EE, Imbach A, Copti M. Vitamin D nutritional status and related biochemical indices in an autonomous elderly population. *Am J Clin Nutr.* 1988;48:373–378.

51. Keane EM, Healy M, Coakley D, Walsh JB. Hypovitaminosis D in the elderly. *Br J Clin Pract.* 1995;49:301–303.

52. Guggenheim K, Kravitz M, Tal R, Kaufmann NA. Biochemical parameters of vitamin D nutriture in old people in Jerusalem. *Nutr Metab.* 1979; 23:172–178.

53. McKenna MJ. Differences in vitamin D status between countries in young adults and the elderly. *Am J Med.* 1992;93:69–77.

54. Hollis BW. Assessment of vitamin D nutritional and hormonal status: what to measure and how to do it. *Calcif Tissue Int.* 1996;4–5.

55. Baker MR, Peacock M, Nordin BEC. The decline in vitamin D status with age. *Age Ageing.* 1980; 9:249–252.

56. Boonen S, Aerssens J, Dequeker J. Age-related endocrine deficiencies and fractures of the proximal femur. II. Implications of vitamin D deficiency in the elderly. *J Endocrinol.* 1996;149:13–17.

57. Gallagher JC. Vitamin D metabolism and therapy in elderly subjects. *South Med J.* 1992;85:2S43–2S47.

58. van der Wielen RP, Löwik MRH, van den Berg H, et al. Serum vitamin D concentrations among elderly people in Europe. *Lancet.* 1995;346:207–210.

59. Mäenpää P, Pirhonen A, Pirskanen A, et al. Biochemical indicators related to antioxidant status and bone metabolic activity in Finnish elderly men. *Int J Vitam Nutr Res.* 1989;59:14–19.

60. Villareal DT, Civitelli R, Chines A, Avioli LV. Subclinical vitamin D deficiency in postmenopausal women with low vertebral bone mass. *J Clin Endocrinol Metab.* 1991;72:628–634.

61. Gloth FM, Gundberg CM, Hollis BW, Haddad JG, Tobin JD. Vitamin D deficiency in homebound elderly persons. *JAMA.* 1995;274:1683–1686.

62. Goldray D, Mizrahi-Sasson E, Merdler C, et al. Vitamin D deficiency in elderly patients in a general hospital. *J Am Geriatr Soc.* 1989;37:589–592.

63. Löwik MRH, van den Berg H, Schrijver J, Odink J, Wedel M, van Houten P. Marginal nutritional status among institutionalized elderly women as compared to those living more independently (Dutch Nutrition Surveillance System). *J Am Coll Nutr.* 1992;11:673–681.

64. Sem SW, Sjoen RJ, Trygg K, Pedersen JI. Vitamin D status of two groups of elderly in Oslo: living in old people's homes and living in own homes. *Compr Gerontol A.* 1987;1:126–130.

65. Gloth FM, Tobin JD, Sherman SS, Hollis BW. Is the recommended daily allowance for vitamin D too low for homebound elderly? *J Am Geriatr Soc.* 1991;39:137–141.

66. Aksnes L, Rodland O, Aarskog D. Serum levels of vitamin $D_3$ and 25-hydroxyvitamin $D_3$ in elderly and young adults. *Bone Miner.* 1988;3:351–357.

67. Slovik DM, Adams JS, Neer RM, Holick MF, Potts JT. Deficient production of 1-25-dihydroxyvitamin D in the elderly. *N Engl J Med.* 1981;13:372–374.

68. Quesada J, Coopmans W, Ruiz R, Aljama P, Jans I, Bouillon R. Influence of vitamin D on parathyroid function in the elderly. *J Clin Endocrinol Metab.* 1992;75:494–501.

69. Sagiv P, Hallel T, Edelstein S. Decrease in bone level of 1-25-dihydroxyvitamin D in women over 45 years old. *Calcif Tissue Int.* 1992;51:24–26.

70. Clemens TL, Zhou XY, Myles M, Endres D, Lindsay R. Serum vitamin $D_2$ and vitamin $D_3$ metabolite concentrations and absorption of vitamin $D_2$ in elderly subjects. *J Clin Endocrinol Metab.* 1986; 63:656–660.

71. Silverberg SJ, Shane E, de la Cruz L, Segre GV, Clemens TL, Bilezikian JP. Abnormalities in parathyroid hormone secretion and 1,25-dihydroxyvitamin $D_3$ formation in women with osteoporosis. *N Engl J Med.* 1989;320:277–281.

72. Dandona P, Menon RK, Shenoy R, Houlder S, Thomas M, Mallinson WJW. Low 1,25-dihydroxyvitamin D, secondary hyperparathyroidism, and normal osteocalcin in elderly subjects. *J Clin Endocrinol Metab.* 1986;63:459–462.

73. Eastell R, Yergey AL, Vieira NE, Cedel SL, Kumar R, Riggs BL. Interrelationship among vitamin D metabolism, true calcium absorption, parathyroid function, and age in women: evidence of an age-related intestinal resistance to 1-25-dihydroxyvitamin D action. *J Bone Miner Res.* 1991;6:125–132.

74. Wood RJ, Fleet JC, Cashman K, Bruns ME, DeLuca HF. Intestinal calcium absorption in the aged rat: evidence of intestinal resistance to 1, 25 $(OH)_2$ vitamin D. *Endocrinology.* 1998;139:3843–3848.

75. Gennari C, Agnusdei D, Nardi P, Civitelli R. Estrogen preserves a normal intestinal responsiveness to 1,25-hydroxyvitamin $D_3$ in oophorectomized women. *J Clin Endocrinol Metab.* 1990;71:1288–1293.

76. Tanaka S, Haji M, Takayanagi R, Tanaka S, Sugioka Y, Nawata H. 1,25-Dihydroxyvitamin $D_3$ enhances the enzymatic activity and expression of the messenger ribonucleic acid for aromatase cytochrom P450 synergistically with dexamethasone depending on the vitamin D receptor level in cultured human osteoblasts. *Endocrinology.* 1996;137:1860–1869.

77. Houston LA, Grant SF, Reid DM, Ralston SH. Vitamin D receptor polymorphism, bone mineral density, and osteoporotic vertebral fracture: studies in a UK population. *Bone.* 1996;18:249–259.

78. Holick MF. McCollum Award Lecture 1994: vitamin D: new horizons for the 21st century. *Am J Clin Nutr.* 1994;60:619–630.

79. Webb AR, Holick MF. The role of sunlight in the cutaneous production of vitamin $D_3$. *Annu Rev Nutr.* 1988;8:75–99.

80. Webb AR, Pilbeam C, Hanafin N, Holick MF. An evaluation of the relative contributions of exposure to sunlight and of diet to the circulating concentrations of 25-hydroxyvitamin D in an elderly nursing home population in Boston. *Am J Clin Nutr.* 1990;51:1075–1081.

81. Prystowsky JH. Photoprotection and the vitamin D status of the elderly. *Arch Dermatol.* 1988; 124:1844–1848.

82. Brazier M, Kamel S, Maamer M, et al. Markers of bone remodeling in the elderly subject: effects of vitamin D insufficiency and its correction. *J Bone Miner Res.* 1996;10:1753–1761.

83. Krall EA, Sahyoun N, Tannenbaum S, Dallal GE, Dawson-Hughes B. Effect of vitamin D intake on seasonal variations in parathyroid hormone secretion in postmenopausal women. *N Engl J Med.* 1989;321:1777–1783.

84. Chevalley T, Rizzoli R, Nydegger V, et al. Effects of calcium supplements on femoral bone mineral density and vertebral fracture rate in vitamin-D-replete elderly patients. *Osteoporos Int.* 1994; 4:245–252.

85. Ooms ME, Roos JC, Bezemer PD, van der Vijgh WJ, Bouter LM, Lips P. Prevention of bone loss by vitamin D supplementation in elderly women: a randomized double blind trial. *J Clin Endocrinol Metab.* 1995;80:1052–1058.

86. Dawson-Hughes B, Dallal GE, Krall EA, Harris S, Sokoll LJ, Falconer G. Effect of vitamin D supplementation on wintertime and overall bone loss in healthy postmenopausal women. *Ann Intern Med.* 1991;115:505–512.

87. Himmelstein S, Clemens TL, Rubin A, Lindsay R. Vitamin D supplementation in elderly nursing home residents increases 25(OH)D but not 1,25(OH)$_2$D. *Am J Clin Nutr.* 1990;52:701–706.

88. Douglas AS, Robins SP, Hutchison JD, Porter RW, Stewart A, Reid DM. Carboxylation of osteocalcin in post-menopausal women following vitamin K and D supplementation. *Bone.* 1995; 17:15–20.

89. Pietschmann P, Woloszczuk W, Pietschmann H. Increased serum osteocalcin levels in elderly females with vitamin D deficiency. *Exp Clin Endocrinol.* 1990;95:275–278.

90. Reznick AZ, Rappaport B, Landvik SV, Simon-Schnass I, Packer L. Vitamin E and the aging process. In: Packer L, Fuchs J, eds. *Vitamin E in Health and Disease.* New York, NY: Marcel Dekker Inc; 1993:435–454.

91. Hollander D, Dadufalza V. Lymphatic and portal absorption of vitamin E in aging rats. *Dig Dis Sci.* 1989;34:768–772.

92. Traber MG, Cohn W, Muller DPR. Absorption, transport and delivery to tissues. In: Packer L, Fuchs J, eds. *Vitamin E in Health and Disease.* New York, NY: Marcel Dekker Inc; 1993:35–51.

93. Birlouez-Aragon I, Girard F, Ravelontseheno L, Bourgeois C, Belliot JP, Abitbol G. Comparison of two levels of vitamin C supplementation on antioxidant vitamin status in elderly institutionalized subjects. *Int J Vitam Nutr Res.* 1995;65:261–266.

94. Hallfrisch J, Muller DC, Singh VN. Vitamin A and E intakes and plasma concentrations of retinol, beta-carotene and alpha-tocopherol in men and women of the Baltimore longitudinal study of aging. *Am J Clin Nutr.* 1994;60:176–182.

95. Heseker H, Schneider R. Requirement and supply of vitamin C, vitamin E and beta-carotene for elderly men and women. *Eur J Clin Nutr.* 1994; 48:118–127.

96. Vandewoude MFJ, Vandewoude MG. Vitamin E status in a normal population: the influence of age. *J Am Coll Nutr.* 1987;6:307–311.

97. Campbell D, Bunker VW, Thomas AJ, Clayton BE. Selenium and vitamin E status of healthy institutionalized elderly subjects: an analysis of plasma, erythrocytes and platelets. *Br J Nutr.* 1989;62:221–227.

98. Pokorn D, Accetto B, Prevorcnik A. Vitamin E status in men and women aged 60-90 years. *Acta Med Iugosl.* 1990;44:223–232.

99. Meydani M, Blumberg JB. Vitamin E. In: Hartz SC, Rosenberg IH, Russell RM, eds. *Nutrition in the Elderly. The Boston Nutrition Status Survey.* London: Smith-Gordon & Co Ltd; 1992:103–109.

100. Schmuck A, Ravel A, Coudray C, Alary J, Franco A, Roussel AM. Antioxidant vitamins in hospitalized elderly patients: analysed dietary intakes and biochemical status. *Eur J Clin Nutr.* 1996;50:473–478.

101. Vericel E, Croset M, Sedivy P, Courpron P, Dechavanne M, Lagarde M. Platelets and aging, I-aggregation, arachidonate metabolism and antioxidant status. *Thromb Res.* 1988;49:331–342.

102. Croset M, Vericel E, Rigaud M, et al. Functions and tocopherol content of blood platelets from elderly people after low intake of purified eicosapentaenoic acid. *Thromb Res.* 1990;57:1–12.

103. Meydani M, Macauley JB, Blumberg J. Influence of dietary vitamin E, selenium, and age on regional distribution of α-tocopherol in the rat brain. *Lipids.* 1989;21:786–791.

104. Meydani M, Verdon CP, Blumberg JB. Effect of vitamin E, selenium and age on lipid peroxidation events in rat cerebrum. *Nutr Res.* 1985;5:1227–1236.

105. Koistinaho J, Alho H, Hervonen A. Effect of vitamin E and selenium supplement on aging peripheral neurons of the Sprague-Dawley rat. *Mech Ageing Dev.* 1990;51:63–72.

106. Monji A, Morimoto N, Okuyama I, Yamashita N, Tashiro N. Effect of dietary vitamin E on lipofuscin accumulation with age in the rat brain. *Brain Res.* 1994;634:62–68.

107. Ohrvall M, Tengblad S, Vessby B. Tocopherol concentration in adipose tissue: relationships of tocopherol concentrations and fatty acid composition in serum in a reference population of Swedish men and women. *Eur J Clin Nutr.* 1994;48:212–218.

108. Luc G, Fruchart JC. Lipoprotein oxidation and atherosclerosis. In: Packer L, Fuchs J, eds. *Vitamin E in Health and Disease.* New York, NY: Marcel Dekker Inc; 1993:635–648.

109. Bogden JD, Bendich A, Kemp FW, et al. Daily micronutrient supplements enhance delayed-hypersensitivity skin test responses in older people. *Am J Clin Nutr.* 1994;60:437–447.

110. Paolisso G, Dimaro G, Galzerano D, et al. Pharmacological doses of vitamin E and insulin action in elderly subjects. *Am J Clin Nutr.* 1994; 59:1291–1296.

111. Steinberg D. Antioxidant vitamins and coronary heart disease. *N Engl J Med.* 1993;328:1487–1489.

112. Taylor A. Cataract: relationships between nutrition and oxidation. *J Am Coll Nutr.* 1993;12:138–146.

113. Knekt P, Aromaa A, Maatela J, et al. Vitamin E and cancer prevention. *Am J Clin Nutr.* 1991; 53:283S–286S.

114. Hauschka PV, Lian JB, Cole DE, Gundberg CM. Osteocalcin and matrix gla protein: vitamin K-dependent proteins in bone. *Physiol Rev.* 1989; 69:990–1047.

115. Conly JM, Stein RT. The production of manaquinones (Vitamin $K_2$) by intestinal bacteria and their role in maintaining coagulation homeostasis. *Prog Food Nutr Sci.* 1992;16:307–343.

116. Ferland G, Sadowski JA, O'Brien ME. Dietary induced vitamin K deficiency in normal human subjects. *J Clin Invest.* 1993;91:1761–1768.

117. Booth SL, Pennington JAT, Sadowski JA. Food sources and dietary intakes of vitamin K-1 (phylloquinone) in the American diet: data from the FDA Total Diet Study. *J Am Diet Assoc.* 1996; 96:149–154.

118. Booth SL, Sokoll LJ, O'Brien ME, Dawson-Hughes B, Sadowski JA. Assessment of dietary phylloquinone intake and vitamin K status in postmenopausal women. *Eur J Clin Nutr.* 1995; 49:832–841.

119. Sadowski JA, Hood SJ, Dallal GE, Garry PJ. Phylloquinone in plasma from elderly and young adults: factors influencing its concentration. *Am J Clin Nutr.* 1989;50:100–108.

120. Sokoll LJ, Sadowski JA. Comparison of biochemical indexes for assessing vitamin K nutritional status in a healthy adult population. *Am J Clin Nutr.* 1996;63:566–573.

121. Suttie JW. Synthesis of vitamin K-dependent proteins. *FASEB J.* 1993;7:445–452.

122. Koshihara Y, Hoshi K, Ishibashi H, Shiraki M. Vitamin $K_2$ promotes 1α-25(OH)$_2$ vitamin $D_3$-induced mineralization in human periosteal osteoblasts. *Calcif Tissue Int.* 1996;59:466–473.

123. Jie KSG, Bots ML, Witteman JCM, Grobbee DE. Vitamin K status and bone mass in women with and without aortic atherosclerosis: a population based study. *Calcif Tissue Int.* 1996;59:352–356.

124. Hazell K, Baloch KH. Vitamin K deficiency in the elderly. *Gerontol Clin.* 1970;12:10–17.

125. Doisy EA. Nutritional hypoprothrombinemia and metabolism of vitamin K. *Fed Proc.* 1961; 20:989–994.

126. Shepherd AM, Hewick DS, Moreland TA, Stevenson IH. Age as a determinant of sensitivity to warfarin. *Br J Clin Pharmacol.* 1977;4:315–320.

127. Connelly TJ, Becker DOA, McDonald JW. Bachelor scurvy. *Int J Dermatol.* 1982;21:209–211.

128. Olson JA, Hodges RE. Recommended dietary intakes (RDI) of vitamin C in humans. *Am J Clin Nutr.* 1987;45:693–703.

129. Woo J, Ho SC, Mak YT, et al. Nutritional status of the water-soluble vitamins in an active Chinese elderly population in Hong Kong. *Eur J Clin Nutr.* 1988;42:415–424.

130. Bianchetti A, Rozzini R, Carabellese C, Zanetti O, Trabucchi M. Nutritional intake, socioeconomic conditions, and health status in a large elderly population. *J Am Geriatr Soc.* 1990;38:521–526.

131. Suter PM, Russell RM. Vitamin requirements of the elderly. *Am J Clin Nutr.* 1987;45:501–512.

132. Yearik ES, Wang MSL, Pisias SJ. Nutritional status of the elderly: dietary and biochemical findings. *J Gerontol.* 1980;5:663–671.

133. Bowmann BB, Rosenberg IH. Assessment of the nutritional status of the elderly. *Am J Clin Nutr.* 1982;35:1142–1451.

134. Lowik MR, Hulshof KF, Schneijder P, Schrijver J, Colen AA, van-Houten P. Vitamin C status in elderly women: a comparison between women living in a nursing home and women living independently. *J Am Diet Assoc.* 1993;93:167–172.

135. Sahyoun N. Nutrient intake by the NSS elderly population. In: Hartz SC, Rosenberg IH, Russell RM, eds. *Nutrition in the Elderly: The Boston Nutritional Status Survey.* London, England: Smith-Gordon & Co Ltd; 1992:31–44.

136. Kafatos A, Diacatou A, Labadarios D, et al. Nutrition status of elderly in Anogia, Crete, Greece. *J Am Coll Nutr.* 1993;12:685–692.

137. Loh HS. The relationship between dietary ascorbic acid intake and buffy coat and plasma ascorbic acid concentration at different ages. *Int J Vitam Nutr Res.* 1972;42:80–85.

138. Kirk JE, Chieffi M. Vitamin studies in middle-aged and old individuals. XI. The concentration of total ascorbic acid in whole blood. *J Gerontol.* 1953;8:301–304.

139. Cruz JAA, Moreiras O, Brzozowska A. Longitudinal changes in the intake of vitamins and minerals of elderly Europeans. *Eur J Clin Nutr.* 1996;50(suppl 2):S77–S85.

140. Porrini M, Simonetti P, Ciappellano S, Testolin G. Vitamin A, E and C nutriture of elderly people in North Italy. *Int J Vitam Nutr Res.* 1987;57:349–355.

141. Mandal SK, Ray AK. Vitamin C status of elderly patients on admission into an assessment geriatric ward. *J Int Med Res.* 1987;15:96–98.

142. Marazzi MC, Mancinelli S, Palombi L, et al. Vitamin C and nutritional status of institutionalized and noninstitutionalized elderly women in Rome. *Int J Vitam Nutr Res.* 1990;60:351–359.

143. Chavance M, Herbeth B, Fournier C, Janot C, Vernhes G. Vitamin status, immunity and infections in an elderly population. *Eur J Clin Nutr.* 1989;43:827–835.

144. Blanchard J, Conrad KA, Mead RA, Garry PJ. Vitamin C disposition in young and elderly men. *Am J Clin Nutr.* 1990;51:837–845.

145. Blanchard J. Depletion and repletion kinetics of vitamin C in humans. *J Nutr.* 1991;121:170–176.

146. VanderJagt DJ, Garry PJ, Bhagavan HN. Ascorbic acid intake and plasma levels in healthy elderly people. *Am J Clin Nutr.* 1987;46:290–294.

147. Schaus R. The ascorbic acid content of pituitary, cerebral cortex, heart and skeletal muscle and its relation to age. *Am J Clin Nutr.* 1957;5:39–42.

148. Pinto RM, Unamuno MDR, Rodrigues MM, dos-Santos JE, Marchini JS, de-Oliveira JE. Vitamin C load test in elderly subjects. *Arch Latinoam Nutr.* 1993;43:20–22.

149. Bendich A, Langseth L. Health effects of vitamin C supplementation: a review. *J Am Coll Nutr.* 1995;14:124–136.

150. Brown LAS, Jones DP. The biology of ascorbic acid. In: *Handbook of Antioxidants.* Cadenas E, Packer L, eds. New York, NY: Marcel Dekker Inc; 1996:117–154.

151. Gale CR, Martyn CN, Cooper C. Cognitive impairment and mortality in a cohort of elderly people. *Br Med J.* 1996;312:608–611.

152. Jha P, Flather M, Lonn E, Farkouh M, Yusuf S. The antioxidant vitamins and cardiovascular disease: a critical review of epidemiologic and clinical trials. *Ann Intern Med.* 1995;123:860–872.

153. Flagg EW, Coates RJ, Greenberg RS. Epidemiologic studies of antioxidants and cancer in humans. *J Am Coll Nutr.* 1995;14:419–427.

154. Weber P, Bendich A, Schalch W. Vitamin C and human health: a review of recent data relevant to human health. *Int J Vitam Nutr Res.* 1996;66:19–30.

155. Jialal I, Vega GL, Grundy SM. Physiologic levels of ascorbate inhibit the oxidative modification of

low density lipoprotein. *Atherosclerosis*. 1990; 82:185–191.

156. Jacques PF, Hartz SC, Chylack LT, McGandy RB, Sadowski JA. Nutritional status in persons with and without senile cataract: blood vitamin and mineral levels. *Am J Clin Nutr*. 1988;48:152–158.

157. Jacques PF, Chylack LT, McGandy RB, Hartz SC. Antioxidant status in persons with and without senile cataract. *Arch Ophthalmol*. 1988;106:337–340.

158. Frei B. Ascorbic acid protects lipids in human plasma and low-density lipoprotein against oxidative damage. *Am J Clin Nutr*. 1991;54:1113S–1118S.

159. Sahyoun NR, Jacques PF, Russell RM. Carotenoids, vitamin C and E, and mortality in an elderly population. *Am J Epidemiol*. 1996;144:501–511.

160. Gale CR, Martyn CN, Winter PD, Cooper C. Vitamin C and risk of death from stroke and coronary artery disease in a cohort of elderly people. *Br Med J*. 1995;310:1563–1566.

161. Losonczy KG, Harris TB, Havlik RJ. Vitamin E and vitamin C supplement use and risk of all-cause and coronary heart disease mortality in older persons: the Established Populations for Epidemiologic Studies of the Elderly. *Am J Clin Nutr*. 1996;64:190–196.

162. Jialal I, Fuller CJ. Effect of vitamin E, vitamin C and beta-carotene on LDL oxidation and atherosclerosis. *Can J Cardiol*. 1995;11(suppl G):97G–103G.

163. Howard PA, Meyers DG. Effect of vitamin C on plasma lipids. *Ann Pharmacother*. 1995;29:1129–1136.

164. Jacques PF. A cross-sectional study of vitamin C intake and blood pressure in the elderly. *Int J Vitam Nutr Res*. 1992;62:252–255.

165. Ness AR, Khaw KT, Bingham S, Day NE. Vitamin C status and blood pressure. *J Hypertens*. 1996;14:503–508.

166. Lykkesfeldt J, Priemé H, Loft S, Poulsen HE. Effect of smoking cessation on plasma ascorbic acid concentration. *Br Med J*. 1996;313:91.

167. Rosenberg IH. Nutritional needs of the elderly. In: Bianchi L, Holt P, James OFW eds. *Aging in Liver and Gastrointestinal Tract*. Lancaster, England: MTP Press; 1988.

168. Iber FL, Blass JP, Brin M, Leevy CM. Thiamin in the elderly: relation to alcoholism and to neurological degenerative disease. *Am J Clin Nutr*. 1982;36:1067–1082.

169. van der Wielen RP, de Wild GM, de Groot LC, Hoefnagels WH, van Staveren WA. Dietary intakes of energy and water soluble vitamins in different categories of aging. *J Gerontol A Biol Sci Med Sci*. 1996;51:B100–B107.

170. Ben-Hur T, Wolff E, River Y. Thiamin deficiency is common in Israel. *Harefuah*. 1992;123:382–384.

171. Nichols HK, Basu TK. Thiamine status of the elderly: dietary intake and thiamin pyrophosphate response. *J Am Coll Nutr*. 1994;13:57–61.

172. Chapman KM, Ham JO, Perlman RA. Longitudinal assessment of the nutritional status of veterans. *J Gerontol A Biol Sci Med Sci*. 1996;51:B261–B269.

173. Porrini M, Testolin G, Simonetti P, Moneta A, Rovati P, Aguzzi F. Nutritional status of non-institutionalized elderly people in North Italy. *Int J Vitam Nutr Res*. 1987;57:203–216.

174. Smidt LJ, Cremin FM, Grivetti LE, Clifford AJ. Influence of thiamin supplementation on the health and general well-being of an elderly Irish population with marginal thiamin deficiency. *J Gerontol*. 1991;46:M16–M22.

175. Sokoll LJ, Morrow FD. Thiamin. In: Hartz SC, Rosenberg IH, Russell RM, eds. *Nutrition in the Elderly: The Boston Nutritional Status Survey*. London, England: Smith-Gordon & Co Ltd; 1992:111–117.

176. Sumner AD, Simons RJ. Delirium in the hospitalized elderly. *Cleve Clin Med J*. 1994;61:258–262.

177. Kwok T, Falconer-Smith JF, Potter JF, Ives DR. Thiamine status of elderly patients with cardiac failure. *Age Ageing*. 1992;21:67–71.

178. Mookhoek EJ, Colon EJ. Nutritional status of elderly patients at admission to a general psychiatric hospital. An inventory. *Tijdschr Gerontol Geriatr*. 1992;23:127–131.

179. Seitz HK, Suter PM. Ethanol toxicity and the nutritional status. In: Kotsonis FM, Mackey M, Hjelle J, eds. *Nutritional Toxicology*. New York, NY: Raven Press; 1994:95–116.

180. Baum RA, Iber FL. Thiamin: the interaction of aging, alcoholism and malabsorption in various

populations. *World Rev Nutr Diet*. 1984;44:85–116.

181. Pfitzenmeyer P, Guilland JC, d'Athis P, Petit-Marnier C, Gaudet M. Thiamine status of elderly patients with cardiac failure including the effects of supplementation. *Int J Vitam Nutr Res*. 1994;64:113–118.

182. Brady JA, Rock CL, Horneffer MR. Thiamine status, diuretic medications, and the management of congestive heart failure. *J Am Diet Assoc*. 1995;95:541–544.

183. Seligmann H, Halkin H, Rauchfleisch S, et al. Thiamine deficiency in patients with congestive heart failure receiving long-term furosemide therapy: pilot study. *Am J Med*. 1991;91:151–155.

184. Krogh V, Freudenheim JL, D'Amicis A, et al. Food sources of nutrients of the diet of elderly Italians: II. Micronutrients. *Int J Epidemiol*. 1993;22:869–877.

185. Toh SY, Thompson GW, Basu TK. Riboflavin status of the elderly: dietary intake and FAD-stimulating effect on erythrocyte glutathione reductase coefficients. *Eur J Clin Nutr*. 1994; 48:654–659.

186. Lowik MR, van den Berg H, Kistemaker C, Brants HA, Brussaard JH. Interrelationships between riboflavin and vitamin $B_6$ among elderly people (Dutch Nutrition Surveillance System). *Int J Vitam Nutr Res*. 1994;64:198–203.

187. Mares-Perlman JA, Klein BE, Klein R, Ritter LL, Freudenheim JL, Luby MH. Nutrient supplements contribute to the dietary intake of middle- and older-aged adult residents of Beaver Dam, Wisconsin. *J Nutr*. 1993;123:176–188.

188. Boisvert WA, Castaneda C, Mendoza J, et al. Prevalence of riboflavin deficiency among Guatemalan elderly people and its relationship to milk intake. *Am J Clin Nutr*. 1993;85:85–90.

189. Sadowski JA. Riboflavin. In: Hartz SC, Rosenberg IH, Russell RM, eds. *Nutrition in the Elderly: The Boston Nutritional Status Survey*. London, England: Smith-Gordon & Co Ltd; 1992:119–125.

190. Garry PJ, Goodwin JS, Hunt WC. Nutritional status in a healthy elderly population: riboflavin. *Am J Clin Nutr*. 1982;36:902–909.

191. Beauchenne RE, Davis TA. The nutritional status of the aged in the USA. *Age*. 1979;2:23–28.

192. Boisvert WA, Mendoza J, Castaneda C, et al. Riboflavin requirement of healthy elderly and its relationship to macronutrient composition of the diet. *J Nutr*. 1993;123:915–925.

193. Tucker KL, Dallal GE, Rush D. Dietary pattern of elderly Boston-area residents defined by cluster analysis. *J Am Diet Assoc*. 1992;92:1487–1491.

194. Pongpaew P, Tungtrongchitr R, Lertchavanakul A, et al. Anthropometry, lipid- and vitamin status of 215 health-conscious Thai elderly. *Int J Vitam Nutr Res*. 1991;61:215–223.

195. Bates CJ, Powers HJ, Downes R, Brubacher D, Sutcliffe V, Thurnhill A. Riboflavin status of adolescent vs elderly Gambian subjects before and during supplementation. *Am J Clin Nutr*. 1989; 50:825–829.

196. Schaus R, Kirk JE. The riboflavin concentration of brain, heart, and skeletal muscle in individuals of various ages. *J Gerontol*. 1957;11:147–150.

197. Said HM, Hollander D. Does aging affect the intestinal transport of riboflavin? *Life Sci*. 1985; 36:69–73.

198. Ugarte R, Edwards AM, Diez MS, Valenzuela A, Silva E. Riboflavin-photosensitized anaerobic modification of rat lens proteins: a correlation with age-related changes. *J Photochem Photobiol B*. 1992;13:161–168.

199. Straatsma BR, Lightfood DO, Barke RM, Horwitz J. Lens capsule and epithelium in age-related cataract. *Am J Ophthalmol*. 1991;112:283–296.

200. Matsubara LS, Machado PE. Age-related changes of glutathione content, glutathione reductase and glutathione peroxidase activity of human erythrocytes. *Braz J Med Biol Res*. 1991;24:449–454.

201. Williams RD, Mason HL, Cusick PL, Wilder RM. Observations on induced riboflavin deficiency and the riboflavin requirement of man. *J Nutr*. 1943;25:361–377.

202. Keys A, Heuschel AF, Mickelson O, Brozek JM, Crawford JH. Physiological and biochemical functions in normal young men on a diet restricted in riboflavin. *J Nutr*. 1944;27:165–178.

203. Friedmann TE, Ivy AC, Jung FT, Sheft BB, Kinney VM. Utilization of thiamin and riboflavin at low and high dietary intake. *Q Bull Northwest School (Chicago)*. 1949;23:177–189.

204. Davis MV, Oldham HG, Roberts LJ. Riboflavin excretions of young women on diets containing

various levels of the B vitamins. *J Nutr.* 1946; 32:143–161.

205. Horwitt MK, Harvey CC, Hill OW, Liebert E. Correlation of urinary excretion with dietary intake and symptoms of ariboflavinosis. *J Nutr.* 1950;41:247–264.

206. Magni E, Bianchetti A, Rozzini R, Trabucchi M. Influence of nutritional intake on 6-year mortality in an Italian elderly population. *J Nutr Elder.* 1994;13:25–34.

207. Harrill I, Cervone V. Vitamin status of older women. *Am J Clin Nutr.* 1977;30:431–440.

208. Bonati B, Nani S, Rancati GB. Eliminazione urinaria di vitamine del complesso B nei vecchi. *Acta Vitaminol.* 1956;10:241–244.

209. Morgan AG, Kelleher J, Walker BE, et al. A nutritional survey in the elderly: blood and urine vitamin levels. *Int J Vitam Nutr Res.* 1975;45:448–462.

210. Fleming BB, Barrows CH. The influence of aging on intestinal absorption of vitamin $B_{12}$ and niacin in rats. *Exp Gerontol.* 1982;17:121–126.

211. Rose RC. Intestinal absorption of water-soluble vitamins. *Proc Soc Exp Biol Med.* 1996;212:191–198.

212. Peters JC. Tryptophan nutrition and metabolism: an overview. *Adv Exp Med Biol.* 1991;294:345–358.

213. Oduho GW, Han Y, Baker DH. Iron deficiency reduces the efficacy of tryptophan as a niacin precursor. *J Nutr.* 1994;124:444–450.

214. Shibata K. Effects of adrenalin on the conversion ratio of tryptophan to niacin in rats. *Biosci Biotechnol Biochem.* 1995;59:2127–2129.

215. Shibata K, Mushiage M, Kondo T, Hayakawa T, Tsuge H. Effects of vitamin $B_6$ deficiency on the conversion ratio of tryptophan to niacin. *Biosci Biotechnol Biochem.* 1995;59:2060–2063.

216. Driskel JA. The vitamin $B_6$ status of the elderly. In: National Academy of Sciences, eds. *Human Vitamin $B_6$ Requirements.* Washington, DC: National Academy of Sciences; 1978.

217. Osler M, Schroll M. A dietary study of elderly in the city of Roskilde 1988/1989 (II): a nutritional risk assessment. *Dan Med Bull.* 1991;38:410–413.

218. Mantero-Atienza E, Beach RS, Sotomayor MG, Christakis G, Baum MK. Nutritional status of institutionalized elderly in south Florida. *Arch Latinam Nutr.* 1992;42:242–249.

219. Ortega RM, Andres P, Redondo MR, Zamora MJ, Lopez-Sobaler AM, Encinas-Sotillos A. Dietary assessment of a group of elderly Spanish people. *Int J Food Sci Nutr.* 1995;46:137–144.

220. Ribaya-Mercado JD. Vitamin $B_6$. In: Hartz SC, Rosenberg IH, Russell RM, eds. *Nutrition in the Elderly: The Boston Nutritional Status Survey.* London, England: Smith-Gordon & Co Ltd; 1992:127–134.

221. Ribaya-Mercado JD, Russell RM, Sahyoun N, Morrow FD, Gershoff SN. Vitamin B-6 requirements of elderly men and women. *J Nutr.* 1991;121:1062–1074.

222. Manore MM, Vaughan LA, Carroll SS, Leklem JE. Plasma pyridoxal 5'-phosphate concentration and dietary vitamin B-6 intake in free-living, low-income elderly people. *Am J Clin Nutr.* 1989; 50:339–345.

223. Löwik MRH, vandenBerg H, Westenbrink S, Wedel M, Schrijver J, Ockhuizen T. Dose-response relationships regarding vitamin B-6 in elderly people: a nationwide nutritional survey (Dutch Nutritional Surveillance System). *Am J Clin Nutr.* 1989;50:391–399.

224. Kant AK, Block G. Dietary vitamin B-6 intake and food sources in the US population: NHANES II, 1976-1980. *Am J Clin Nutr.* 1990;52:707–716.

225. Hamfelt A. Age variation of vitamin $B_6$ metabolism in men. *Clin Chim Acta.* 1964;10:48–54.

226. Rose CS, Gyorgy P, Butler M, et al. Age difference in vitamin $B_6$ status of 617 men. *Am J Clin Nutr.* 1976;29:847–853.

227. Driskell JA. Vitamin $B_6$. In: Machlin LJ, ed. *Handbook of Vitamins. Nutritional, Biochemical, and Clinical Aspects.* New York, NY: Marcel Dekker, Inc; 1984:379–401.

228. Reynolds RD, Moser-Veilon PB, Kant AK. Effect of age on status and metabolism of vitamin $B_6$ in man. In: Leklem JE, Reynolds RE, eds. *Current Topics in Nutrition and Disease: Clinical and Physiological Applications of Vitamin $B_6$.* New York, NY: Alan R Liss Inc; 1988:19–30.

229. Fonda ML, Eggers DK. Vitamin $B_6$ metabolism in the blood of young adult and senescent mice. *Exp Gerontol.* 1980;15:465–472.

230. Mason DY, Emerson PM. Primary acquired sideroblastic anemia: response to treatment with pyridoxal-5-phosphate. *Br Med J.* 1973;1:389–390.

231. Darnton-Hill I, Sriskandarajah N, Stewart PM, Craig G, Truswell AS. Vitamin supplementation and nutritional status in homeless men. *Aust J Public Health*. 1993;17:246–251.

232. Woo J, Ho SC, Mak YT, Law LK, Cheung A. Nutritional status of elderly patients during recovery from chest infection and the role of nutritional supplementation assessed by a prospective randomized single blind trial. *Age Ageing*. 1994; 23:40–48.

233. Naurath HJ, Joosten E, Riezler R, Stabler SP, Allen RH, Lindenbaum J. Effects of vitamin $B_{12}$, folate, and vitamin $B_6$ supplements in elderly people with normal vitamin concentrations. *Lancet*. 1995;346:85–89.

234. Hoorn RKJ, Flikweert JP, Westerink D. Vitamin $B_1$, $B_2$, and $B_6$ deficiencies in geriatric patients, measured by coenzyme stimulation of enzyme activities. *Clin Chim Acta*. 1975;61:151–162.

235. Vir SC, Love AHG. Vitamin $B_6$ status of hospitalized aged. *Am J Clin Nutr*. 1978;31:1383–1391.

236. Vir SC, Love AHG. Vitamin $B_6$ status of institutionalized aged. *Int J Vitam Nutr Res*. 1977; 47:364–372.

237. Kant AK, Moser-Veillon PB, Reynolds RD. Effect of age on changes in plasma, erythrocyte, and urinary B-6 vitamins after an oral vitamin B-6 load. *Am J Clin Nutr*. 1988;48:1284–1290.

238. Meydani SN, Ribaya-Mercado JD, Russell RM, Sahyoun N, Morrow FD, Gershoff SN. The effect of vitamin $B_6$ on immune response of healthy elderly. *Ann NY Acad Sci*. 1990;587:303–306.

239. Meydani SN, Ribaya-Mercado JD, Russell RM, Sahyoun N, Morrow FD, Gershoff SN. Vitamin B-6 deficiency impairs interleukin 2 production and lymphocyte proliferation in elderly adults. *Am J Clin Nutr*. 1991;53:1275–1280.

240. Selhub J, Jacques PF, Wilson PW, Rush D, Rosenberg IH. Vitamin status and intake as primary determinants of homocysteinemia in an elderly population. *JAMA*. 1993;270:2693–2698.

241. Mudd SH, Skovby F, Levy HL, et al. The natural history of homocystinuria due to cystathionine beta-synthase deficiency. *Am J Hum Genet*. 1985;37:1–31.

242. Serfontein WJ, Ubbink JB, De-Villiers LS, Rapley CH, Becker PJ. Plasma pyridoxal-5-phosphate level as risk index for coronary artery disease. *Atherosclerosis*. 1985;55:357–361.

243. McCully KS. Homocysteine and vascular disease. *Nat Med*. 1996;2:386–389.

244. Robinson K, Meyer E, Miller DP, et al. Hyperhomocysteinemia and low pyridoxal phosphate: common and independent reversible risk factors for coronary artery disease. *Circulation*. 1995; 92:2825–2830.

245. Ellis JM, McCully KS. Prevention of myocardial infarction by vitamin $B_6$. *Res Commun Mol Pathol Pharmacol*. 1995;89:208–220.

246. Chasan-Taber L, Selhub J, Rosenberg IH, et al. A prospective study of folate and vitamin $B_6$ and risk of myocardial infarction in US physicians. *J Am Coll Nutr*. 1996;15:136–143.

247. Deijen JB, van der Beek BJ, Orlebeke JF, van den Berg H. Vitamin B-6 supplementation in elderly men: effects on mood, memory, performance and mental effort. *Psychopharmacology (Berl)*. 1992;109:489–496.

248. Rosenberg IH, Bowman BB, Cooper BA, et al. Folate nutrition in the elderly. *Am J Clin Nutr*. 1982;36:1060–1066.

249. Rosenberg IH. Folate. In: Hartz SC, Rosenberg IH, Russell RM, eds. *Nutrition in the Elderly: The Boston Nutritional Status Survey*. London, England: Smith-Gordon & Co Ltd; 1992:135–139.

250. Infante-Rivard C, Krieger M, Gascon-Barre M, Rivard GE. Folate deficiency among institutionalized elderly. *J Am Geriatr Soc*. 1986;34:211–214.

251. Hanger HC, Sainsbury R, Gilchrist NL, Beard MEJ, Duncan JM. A community study of vitamin $B_{12}$ and folate levels in the elderly. *J Am Geriatr Soc*. 1991;39:1155–1159.

252. Grinblat J, Marcus DL, Hernandez F, Freedman ML. Folate and vitamin $B_{12}$ levels in an urban elderly population with chronic diseases: assessment of two laboratory folate assays: microbiologic and radioassay. *J Am Geriatr Soc*. 1986;34:627–632.

253. Davis RE, Nichol DJ. Folic acid. *Int J Biochem*. 1988;20:133–139.

254. Russell RM, Krasinski SD, Samloff IM, Jacob RA, Hartz SC, Brovender SR. Folic acid malabsorption in atrophic gastritis: compensation by bacterial folate synthesis. *Gastroenterology*. 1986;91:1476–1482.

255. Varela-Moreiras G, Perez-Olleros L, Garcia-Cuevas M, Ruiz-Roso B. Effects of ageing on folate metabolism in rats fed a long term folate

deficient diet. *Int J Vitam Nutr Res*. 1994;64:294–299.

256. Selhub J, Jacques PF, Bostom AG, et al. Association between plasma homocysteine concentrations and extracranial carotid artery stenosis. *N Engl J Med*. 1995;332:286–291.

257. Stabler SP, Marcell PD, Podell ER, Allen RH, Savage DG, Lindenbaum J. Elevation of total homocysteine in the serum of patients with cobalamin or folate deficiency detected by capillary gas chromatography-mass spectrometry. *J Clin Invest*. 1988;81:466–474.

258. Kang SS, Wong PWK, Cook HY, Norusis M, Messer JV. Protein-bound homocyst(e)ine: a possible risk factor for coronary artery disease. *J Clin Invest*. 1986;77:1482–1486.

259. Ortega RM, Manas LR, Andres P, et al. Functional and psychic deterioration in elderly people may be aggravated by folate deficiency. *J Nutr*. 1996;126:1992–1999.

260. Nilsson K, Gustafson L, Faldt R, Andersson A, Hultberg B. Plasma homocysteine in relation to serum cobalamin and blood folate in a psychiatric population. *Eur J Clin Invest*. 1994;24:600–606.

261. Santhosh-Kumar CR, Hassell KL, Deutsch JC, Kolhouse JF. Are neuropsychiatric manifestations of folate, cobalamin and pyridoxine deficiency mediated through imbalances in excitatory sulfur amino acids? *Med Hypotheses*. 1994;43:239–244.

262. Guaraldi G, Fava M, Mazzi F, et al. An open trial of methyltetrahydrofolate (MTHF) in elderly depressed patients. *Ann Clin Psychiat*. 1993;5:101–106.

263. Prothro J, Mickles M, Tolbert B. Nutritional status of a population sample in Macon County, Alabama. *Am J Clin Nutr*. 1976;29:94–104.

264. Garry PJ, Goodwin JS, Hunt WC. Folate and vitamin $B_{12}$ status in a healthy elderly population. *J Am Geriatr Soc*. 1984;32:719–726.

265. Meuleman JR, Hoffman NB, Conlin MM, Lowenthal DT, Delafuente JC, Graves JE. Health status of the aged: medical profile of a group of functional elderly. *South Med J*. 1992;85:464–468.

266. Pennypacker LC, Allen RH, Kelly JP, et al. High prevalence of cobalamin deficiency in elderly outpatients. *J Am Geriatr Soc*. 1992;40:1197–1204.

267. Basu TK, Donald EA, Hargreaves JA, et al. Vitamin $B_{12}$ and folate status of a selected group of free living older persons. *J Nutr Elder*. 1992;11:5–19.

268. Crystal HA, Ortof E, Frishman WH, Gruber A, Hershman D, Aronson M. Serum vitamin $B_{12}$ levels and incidence of dementia in a healthy elderly population: a report from the Bronx Longitudinal Aging Study. *J Am Geriatr Soc*. 1994;42:933–936.

269. Cals MJ, Bories PN, Devanlay M, et al. Extensive laboratory assessment of nutritional status in fit, health-conscious, elderly people living in the Paris area (Research Group on Aging). *J Am Coll Nutr*. 1994;13:646–657.

270. Matthews JH. Cobalamin and folate deficiency in the elderly. *Baillieres Clin Haematol*. 1995;8:679–697.

271. Quinn K, Basu TK. Folate and vitamin $B_{12}$ status of the elderly. *Eur J Clin Nutr*. 1996;50:340–342.

272. Bunting RW, Bitzer AM, Kenney RM, Ellman L. Prevalence of intrinsic factor antibodies and vitamin $B_{12}$ malabsorption in older patients admitted to a rehabilitation hospital. *J Am Geriatr Soc*. 1990;38:743–747.

273. Marcus DL, Shadick N, Crantz J, Gray M, Hernandez F, Freedman ML. Low serum $B_{12}$ levels in a hematologically normal elderly subpopulation. *J Am Geriatr Soc*. 1987;35:635–638.

274. Nilsson-Ehle H, Jagenburg R, Landahl S, Lindstedt G, Swolin B, Westin J. Cyanocobalamin absorption in the elderly: results for healthy subjects and for subjects with low serum cobalamin concentration. *Clin Chem*. 1986;32:1368–1371.

275. Nilsson-Ehle H, Jagenburg R, Landahl S, Lindstedt S, Svanborg A, Westin J. Serum cobalamins in the elderly: a longitudinal study of a representative population sample from age 70 to 81. *Eur J Haematol*. 1991;47:10–16.

276. Tauber S, Goodhart RS, Hsu JM, et al. Vitamin $B_{12}$ deficiency in the aged. *Geriatrics*. 1957;12:368–374.

277. King CE, Leibach J, Toskes PP. Clinically significant vitamin $B_{12}$ deficiency secondary to malabsorption of protein-bound vitamin $B_{12}$. *Dig Dis Sci*. 1979;24:397–402.

278. Doscherholmen A, Ripley D, Chang S, et al. Influence of age and stomach function on serum vitamin $B_{12}$ concentration. *Scand J Gastroenterol*. 1977;12:313–319.

279. Suter PM, Golner BB, Goldin BR, Morrow FD, Russell RM. Reversal of protein-bound vitamin $B_{12}$ malabsorption with antibiotics in atrophic gastritis. *Gastroenterology.* 1991;101:1039–1045.

280. Lucas MH, Elgazzar AH. Detection of protein bound vitamin $B_{12}$ malabsorption: a case report and review of the literature. *Clin Nucl Med.* 1994;19:1001–1003.

281. Lindenbaum J, Healton EB, Savage DG, et al. Neuropsychiatric disorders caused by cobalamin deficiency in the absence of anemia or macrocytosis. *N Engl J Med.* 1988;318:1720–1728.

282. Joosten E, Pelemans W, Devos P, et al. Cobalamin absorption and serum homocysteine and methylmalonic acid in elderly subjects with low serum cobalamin. *Eur J Haematol.* 1993;51:25–30.

283. Allen RH, Stabler SP, Savage DG, Lindenbaum J. Metabolic abnormalities in cobalamin (vitamin $B_{12}$) and folate deficiency. *FASEB J.* 1993; 7:1344–1353.

284. Joosten E, Lesaffre E, Riezler R. Are different reference intervals for methylmalonic acid and total homocysteine necessary in the elderly people? *Eur J Haematol.* 1996;57:222–226.

285. Dickinson CJ. Does folic acid harm people with vitamin $B_{12}$ deficiency? *Q J Med.* 1995;88:357–364.

286. Markkanen T, Mustakallio E. Absorption and excretion of biotin after feeding minced liver in achlorhydria and after partial gastrectomy. *Scand J Clin Lab Invest.* 1963;15:57–61.

287. Bonjour JP. Biotin in man's nutrition and therapy: a review. *Int J Vitam Nutr Res.* 1977;47:107–118.

288. Bonjour JP. Biotin. In: Machlin LJ, ed. *Handbook of Vitamins: Nutritional, Biochemical and Clinical Aspects.* New York, NY: Marcel Dekker Inc; 1984.

289. Walsh JH, Wyse BW, Hansen RG. Pantothenic acid content of a nursing home diet. *Ann Nutr Metab.* 1981;25:178–181.

290. Sugarman B, Munroe HN. [C-14]-Pantothenate accumulation by isolated adipocytes from adult rats of different age. *J Nutr.* 1980;110:2297–2301.

291. Ishiguro K. Aging effect of blood pantothenic acid content in females. *Tohoku J Exp Med.* 1972; 107:367–372.

# CHAPTER 4

# Mineral Requirements

*Robert D. Lindeman*

Establishing requirements for minerals in humans is difficult, and although most of them are known to be essential to human life, specific recommendations regarding necessary intake are not available. There are no recommended dietary allowances (RDAs) for sodium or potassium, although they are required for physiologic function; there are recommendations for calcium and magnesium. However, with the development of accurate, inexpensive techniques for quantifying sodium, potassium, calcium, and magnesium concentrations in biologic fluids, a vast literature has been generated documenting that deficits and excesses of these minerals create many clinical challenges for practitioners. The ability of elderly people to maintain concentrations within normal ranges is often impaired by the frequently observed decrease in renal function (Chapter 10) and by aberrations in other homeostatic mechanisms designed to conserve or excrete excess minerals. Certainly for some of the minerals, specifically calcium and magnesium, what is of concern is the failure to consume amounts adequate to meet known nutritional needs.

## SODIUM       135-145

Sodium is an essential component in human nutrition and in the maintenance of fluid and electrolyte homeostasis. Serum sodium concentration is an accurate, precise, routinely performed laboratory measure that is useful in classifying sodium balance into hyponatremic, hypernatremic, and normal categories. Water balance status is judged by the clinical assessment of extracellular fluid volume (ECFV), which is much more subjective than the measurement of serum sodium concentration. Figure 4–1 demonstrates the relationships of sodium and water in various deficit or excess states.

*Dehydration* means a decrease in total body water, but the pathophysiology of its development may focus on either primary water loss or salt loss with obligated water. Water depletion, which occurs when there is water loss without proportionate sodium loss, is reflected by an increased serum sodium concentration—that is, hypernatremia. Normally, with free access to water, normal thirst mechanisms ensure that the individual maintains an adequate fluid intake, but in elderly individuals, especially those with cerebral disease such as strokes, thirst may become impaired. Patients who have primary salt depletion become volume depleted (dehydrated), and they maintain normal serum sodium concentrations and osmolalities until the volume depletion becomes sufficient to stimulate release of antidiuretic hormone (ADH). If fluid then is replaced, water is retained, and hyponatremia begins to develop.

## SALT and WATER IMBALANCES

| SERUM SODIUM CONCENTRATION | | | | |
|---|---|---|---|---|
| | **LOW** | **DEHYDRATION** (Primary Salt Loss)<br><br>$Na^+$ Loss > $H_2O$ Loss | **REDISTRIBUTION** Hyperglycemia **DISPLACEMENT** Hyperlipemia Hyperproteinemia **SYNDROME OF INAPPROPRIATE ADH WATER INTOXICATION** | **DILUTIONAL HYPONATREMIA**<br><br>$H_2O$ Retention > . $Na^+$ Retention |
| | **NORMAL** | **DEHYDRATION**<br><br>$Na^+$ Loss = $H_2O$ Loss | **NORMAL** | **UNCOMPLICATED EDEMA**<br><br>$H_2O$ Retention = $Na^+$ Retention |
| | **HIGH** | **DEHYDRATION** (Primary Water Loss)<br><br>$H_2O$ Loss > $Na^+$ Loss | **HYPERALDOSTERONISM HYPERCORTISONISM** | **STEROID EXCESS SALT INTOXICATION**<br><br>$Na^+$ Retention > $H_2O$ Retention |
| | | **LOW** | **NORMAL** | **HIGH** |
| | | **EXTRACELLULAR FLUID VOLUME** | | |

**Figure 4–1** Salt and water imbalances. ADH, antidiuretic hormone.

The excessive retention of body fluids (overhydration) may result from primary salt retention with its osmotically obligated water (simple edema) or from retention of water in excess of salt (dilutional hyponatremia). Simple edema may be local or generalized. Generalized edema occurs with increasing frequency as one ages because those disease states, specifically congestive heart failure, renal insufficiency, cirrhosis, nephrotic syndrome, and hypoalbuminemia, that are associated with edema are more common in elderly people.

### Hyponatremia

A low serum sodium concentration may result from (1) a loss of sodium in excess of osmotically obligated water (primary salt depletion), (2) a retention of water in excess of sodium (dilutional hyponatremia), or (3) a combination of both (syndrome of inappropriate ADH, or SIADH) (Table 4–1). Hyponatremia also may result from a displacement of plasma water with large–molecular weight solute (eg, protein, lipids) or from the addition of an uncharged solute (eg, glucose) to the ECFV.

A reduction in serum sodium concentration to less than 125 mmol/L, regardless of etiology, may produce symptoms ranging from mild, nonspecific complaints, such as malaise, irritability, muscle weakness, and change in personality, to marked functional central nervous system impairment. Serious central nervous system impairment occurs when the shift of fluid from the hypoosmotic extracellular fluid into isotonic brain cells increases brain volume and intracranial pressure significantly. Depending on the severity

**Table 4–1** Hyponatremic Syndromes

I. Hyponatremia with contracted ECFV
   A. Urinary sodium <10 mmol/L
      1. Inadequate intake
      2. Excessive sweating
      3. Excessive gastrointestinal loss
         (a) Diarrhea
         (b) Fistulous tracts (bowel, biliary)
   B. Urinary sodium >10 mmol/L
      1. Severe metabolic alkalosis due to vomiting (bicarbonaturia)
      2. Excessive urinary losses
         (a) Adrenal insufficiency (Addison disease, hypoaldosteronism)
         (b) Renal salt wasting (renal tubular acidosis, interstitial nephritis, end-stage renal disease)
         (c) Diuretic induced
II. Hyponatremia with normal ECFV
   A. Displacement syndromes
      1. Hyperglycemia
      2. Hyperlipemia
      3. Hyperglobulinemia
   B. SIADH
      1. Malignancies (eg, lung, pancreas)
      2. Pulmonary diseases, including treatment with positive pressure breathing
      3. Cerebral conditions (eg, trauma, infection, tumor, cerebrovascular accident)
      4. Drugs (eg, sulfonylureas, thiazides, antitumor agents, psychotropics, antidepressants)
      5. Myxedema
      6. Porphyria
      7. Idiopathic
   C. Water intoxication (schizophrenia)
III. Hyponatremia with expanded ECFV
   A. Dilutional hyponatremia (low solute excretion)
      1. Congestive heart failure
      2. Cirrhosis
      3. Nephrotic syndrome
      4. Renal failure
      5. Hypoalbuminemia

of hyponatremia and the state of hydration, a spectrum of alterations of consciousness, ranging from confusion to coma, may appear. Seizures are also frequent manifestations of these conditions.

### Hyponatremia with Contracted ECFV (Primary Salt Depletion)

Early in primary salt depletion, salt and water are lost at comparable rates, so that serum sodium concentrations and osmolality remain normal. After volume depletion becomes evident, ADH release is stimulated, resulting in water retention while salt loss continues. If the urinary sodium concentration is less than 10 mmol/L, suspected etiologies include decreased salt intake, excessive sweating with only water provided to replace losses, or gastrointestinal salt losses. If urinary sodium concentration is greater than 10 mmol/L, inappropriate renal losses of sodium and water may be due to excessive use of diuretics, adrenal or pituitary insufficiency, or intrinsic renal disease (ie, salt-losing nephritis, renal insufficiency, or renal tubular acidosis). In severe vomiting with metabolic alkalosis and bicarbonate wasting, urinary sodium concentrations also may be elevated despite hypovolemia and hyponatremia. Elderly subjects may be more prone to hyponatremia while developing these disorders. Epstein and Hollenberg[1] have shown that there is a modest reduction in the capacity of the kidney to conserve sodium in normal elderly subjects when subjected to salt depletion (Chapter 10). Treatment generally is accomplished with isotonic saline, although in severe cases hypertonic saline may be used initially. When it remains unclear whether the etiology is primary salt depletion or SIADH, one can place a central venous pressure (CVP) catheter and infuse normal saline until the CVP climbs, unless the patient has left ventricular failure or pulmonary hypertension and thus requires a Swan-Ganz catheter. An important clue to making the differential diagnosis may be the blood urea nitrogen concentration, as this is elevated in primary salt depletion and is usually subnormal in SIADH.

## Hyponatremia with Expanded ECFV (Dilutional Hyponatremia)

Impairment in water excretion occurs commonly in conditions in which salt excretion also is severely impaired. Patients with advanced cardiac, hepatic, and renal disease and generalized edema often are placed on diets that sharply restrict salt intake without placing limitations on fluid intake. Once hyponatremia begins to develop, restriction of water intake may become necessary. Although total ECFV in such patients often is increased, the blood volume in the arterial vascular system tends to be decreased, stimulating baroreceptors in the arterial system to initiate retention of salt and water. A decrease in glomerular filtration rate or an increase in sodium reabsorption in the proximal tubule limits water excretion by decreasing delivery of tubular salt and water to the distal diluting segment of the nephron. If little salt and water reach the distal nephron, the individual becomes unable to dilute his or her urine much below isotonic levels. Since normally the relative intakes of salt and water constitute a hypotonic solution, this results in the development of hyponatremia. Decreases in intra-arterial or left atrial pressure or volume, which are potent stimuli to ADH release, also have a role in the pathogenesis of hyponatremia. Treatment consists of diuretic administration and fluid restriction in addition to treatment of the underlying etiology. Diuretics active in the loop of Henle, such as furosemide, that promote excretion of hypotonic to isotonic urine even in the presence of ADH, are the diuretics of choice.

## Hyponatremia with Normal ECFV (SIADH)

A diagnosis of SIADH can be made only when other causes of hyponatremia have been excluded. The following criteria must be met: (1) the extracellular fluid osmolality and sodium concentration must be decreased; (2) the urine must be hypertonic to serum; (3) urinary sodium excretion must exceed 10 mmol/L; (4) adrenal, renal, cardiac, and hepatic functions must be normal; and (5) the hyponatremia must be able to be corrected by water restriction. Persistence of circulating ADH is considered inappropriate when neither serum hyperosmolality nor volume depletion is present. Inability to excrete water normally leads to volume expansion, which, by several mechanisms, promotes urinary salt loss. SIADH is seen most frequently in patients with pulmonary neoplasm, most notably oat cell carcinomas, but it may also be seen in numerous other conditions, as listed in Table 4–1. Often the etiology for SIADH is impaired blood flow through the pulmonary circulation, resulting in impaired filling of the left atrium, which stimulates ADH release. Any person treated with positive pressure breathing has the potential for a similar consequence.  *BuN closer to NL.*

### Hyponatremia in the Elderly

Surveys of older persons in both acute and chronic care facilities show a high prevalence of hyponatremia. Kleinfeld and colleagues[2] reported that 36 of 160 chronically ill patients (23%) had serum sodium concentrations below 132 mmol/L (mean 120 mmol/L). In most patients, low serum sodium concentrations were not readily explained except by the presence of debilitating diseases and old age.

In another nursing home study,[3] over half the patients had been hyponatremic on at least one occasion over the preceding year (serum sodium concentrations measured monthly; hyponatremia defined as a serum sodium less than 135 mmol/L). Water loading (20 cc of $H_2O$ per kilogram of body weight) resulted in an impaired response in the hyponatremic residents, as they excreted only 56% as much water as comparable elderly with normal sodium concentrations and achieved only a minimum urine osmolality of 195 mOsm/kg of $H_2O$ compared to 84 mOsm/kg of $H_2O$ in normonatremic resi-

dents. In a study of an ambulatory geriatric population,[4] using a similar definition for hyponatremia, 11% had hyponatremia, with SIADH being the apparent cause in nearly 60% of the hyponatremic individuals. In a quarter of these individuals (seven subjects) with SIADH-like hyponatremia, there was no apparent underlying etiology other than age.

Anderson and colleagues[5] prospectively evaluated the prevalence, cause, and outcome of hyponatremia in an acute care facility. The prevalence was 2.5%, with two thirds being iatrogenic. The mean age of these subjects was nearly 60 years. The most frequent cause was SIADH (normovolemic hyponatremia), accounting for 34% of cases; hypovolemia, hypervolemia, and hyperglycemia each accounted for 16% to 19% of cases; and renal failure (overhydration) and error accounted for the remainder. The authors demonstrated that nonosmotic (baroreceptor) stimulation of vasopressin release was a major factor in this electrolyte disorder, regardless of cause. Other evidence suggests that elderly persons may be more susceptible to the development of hyponatremia similar to that seen in patients with SIADH than are their younger counterparts. Antidiuresis and hyponatremia have been observed postoperatively, primarily in elderly patients. Sulfonylureas create SIADH almost exclusively in older persons. Diuretic-induced hyponatremia is an entity occurring primarily in older patients.

Observations reported by Helderman and associates[6] may help to explain the increased susceptibility of older patients to the development of hyponatremia. In older subjects, serum arginine vasopressin (AVP) concentrations showed a greater increase (twofold) after a standardized hypertonic saline infusion designed to raise serum osmolality to 306 mmol/L than did those of younger subjects, despite comparable baseline AVP concentrations. In contrast, ethanol infusion, known to inhibit ADH secretion, produced a more prolonged depression in serum AVP concentrations in young than in old subjects. These two observations suggest an increasing osmoreceptor sensitivity with age, with a greater release of AVP and therefore more water retention in response to any given stimulus or balance state.

Rowe and associates[7] subsequently reported studies designed to determine whether this phenomenon represented a consistent, age-related increase in vasopressin responsiveness or whether it was specific for osmotic stimuli. Older subjects, after 8 minutes of quiet standing, failed to increase their serum AVP concentrations as much as did younger subjects. Furthermore, Rowe and associates could divide their subjects into those who released AVP (responders) and those who failed to release AVP (nonresponders) in response to orthostasis. Whereas less than 10% of the young subjects were nonresponders, nearly half of the older subjects failed to release AVP in response to orthostasis. Because these subjects had an intact norepinephrine response to orthostasis, the authors felt that the age-related defect was distal to the vasomotor center in the afferent limb of the baroreceptor reflex arc. They further suggested that the altered vasopressin response to osmolar and volume-pressure stimuli in some elderly subjects might be related primarily to impaired baroreceptor input to the supraoptic nucleus. Secondarily, there would be an impaired responsiveness to osmotic stimuli. Subsequent studies have provided some supporting and some conflicting evidence as to whether AVP responses to a variety of stimuli really are different in elderly compared to younger subjects. These studies are nicely summarized in a recent review by Epstein.[8]

It is very difficult for a normal person to ingest sufficient water to become symptomatically hyponatremic. Some patients with schizophrenic illnesses, however, have been reported to be capable of ingesting sufficient fluids without vomiting to become symptomatically hyponatremic.

A decrease in serum sodium concentration does not always indicate a decrease in the osmolality of body fluids. With hyperglycemia, the cause of hyponatremia is the glucose-related increase in the osmolality of extracellular fluid, which results in a movement of water from the intracellular to extracellular fluid compartments. Expansion of the extracellular fluid space triggers a diuresis of excess fluid along with sodium.

The serum sodium concentration in hyperlipemia and hyperproteinemia is decreased because of the volume occupied by lipids or proteins, respectively. If lipids or proteins are removed from the plasma, the sodium concentration in the remaining plasma water is normal.

## Hypernatremia

An increase in serum sodium concentration is a result of loss of body water in excess of salt loss, although it also can result from ingestion or administration of salt without sufficient water to provide an isotonic solution. Among elderly patients, hypernatremia is most common in those who are bedfast and are not provided sufficient water to satisfy their thirst, or in those whose thirst sensation is diminished by impaired central nervous system function. A net deficit of water also can be associated with vomiting and diarrhea, diabetes insipidus, an osmotic diuresis such as is seen with hyperosmolar nonketotic diabetic acidosis, and hyperpyrexia (excessive sweating).

In general, older patients appear to be predisposed to the development of hypernatremia. Snyder and associates[9] reported that more than 1% of their hospital admissions were patients older than 60 years who developed hypernatremia (serum sodium concentration >148 mmol/L). Over half of these patients developed hypernatremia while in the hospital. Surgery, febrile illnesses, infirmity, and diabetes mellitus accounted for two thirds of the diagnoses of these cases. Hypernatremia is a marker for severe associated illness, and the mortality rate in this group of patients was 42%. In these patients, rapid fluid replacement contributed to increased mortality rates.

Lavizzo-Mourey and colleagues,[10] in a systematic evaluation of the factors leading to dehydration in hospitalized nursing home residents, found a constellation of important risk factors that included advanced age, female sex, several chronic diseases, number of medications (especially laxatives), and decreased functional status. Alterations in thirst perception in healthy young and old persons were studied by Phillips and colleagues.[11] All subjects were deprived of water for 24 hours, after which free access to water was allowed. The older individuals drank less water even though they lost more fluid during the period of water deprivation and ended with higher plasma sodium concentrations and osmolalities, suggesting an impaired thirst responsiveness in older subjects. Furthermore, the decline in renal concentrating ability commonly observed with age (Chapter 10) might increase the potential for hypernatremia by augmenting urinary losses of water.

Hypernatremia reflects an increase in serum osmolality, which results in a shift of water from the intracellular to extracellular spaces. One consequence of this phenomenon is a shrinkage of brain cells, causing intracranial injury to blood vessels, which may lead to hemorrhage, venous thrombosis, or infarction.

The earliest manifestation of hypernatremia is thirst, followed by confusion and lethargy and, ultimately, delirium, stupor, and coma. Because intravascular volume is preserved at the expense of cell water, changes in blood pressure, pulse rate, and skin turgor are not prominent features of hypernatremia.

Once life-threatening hypernatremia has occurred, parenteral restoration of fluid and electrolyte balance usually is necessary. The amount of water (or dextrose and water, when given parenterally) needed can be estimated by multiplying the percentage increase in sodium concentration over normal by the total body water (60% of body weight). To prevent a recurrence, a fluid prescription establishing the quantity of fluid to be ingested daily may be an important part of treatment.

## POTASSIUM

3.5-5.0 mEq/L

Potassium is the primary intracellular cation, with less than 2% of total body potassium contained in the extracellular fluid compartment. Therefore, the serum concentration of potassium may not reflect accurately total body potassium stores. A potassium flux into the cells occurs with cell growth, intracellular nitrogen and glycogen deposition, and increases in extracellular pH; potassium leaves the cell with cell destruction, glucose utilization, and decreases in extracellular pH. When one is interpreting serum potassium concentrations, those factors that affect the ratio of intracellular to extracellular concentration must be considered, since normally a steep concentration gradient is maintained. For example, the patient with diabetic ketoacidosis has a high serum potassium concentration, but rehydration, correction of the acidosis with bicarbonates, and treatment of the hyperglycemia with insulin combine to produce a dramatic decrease in plasma potassium concentration as the cation moves intracellularly. Age alone does not appear to affect the ability to maintain this concentration gradient. Isotopic dilution studies and muscle biopsies, however, have been used to demonstrate that intracellular stores of potassium can be decreased in a variety of clinical conditions commonly seen in elderly patients, such as metabolic and respiratory acidosis, congestive heart failure, cirrhosis, and uremia, with serum potassium concentrations remaining within normal limits.

## Hypokalemia

The causes of hypokalemia are listed in Table 4–2. The most frequent cause of hypokalemia in elderly people is diuretic therapy used for treatment of edematous and hypertensive conditions. Probably the most frequently overlooked cause of hypokalemia in elderly people is excessive use of enemas and purgatives, behavior that should be suspected whenever unexplained hypokalemic alkalosis occurs in older persons.

Multiple pathophysiologic mechanisms occur in many, if not most, cases to explain the development of hypokalemia. For example, the patient who vomits not only has a reduction in potassium intake and some loss of potassium in the vomitus but loses hydrogen ions, producing a metabolic alkalosis that in turn shifts potassium intracellularly and augments urinary potassium losses. The contracted intravascular volume increases proximal tubular sodium and bicarbonate reabsorption, which further enhances the metabolic alkalosis and induces a secondary hyperaldosteronism that increases urinary potassium losses.

Although the normal kidney is not as effective in conserving potassium as it is in conserving sodium, it can reduce excretions below 15 mmol/d even in the presence of acidosis or alkalosis. Since little potassium normally is lost through the gastrointestinal tract, it takes 2 to 3 weeks on a virtually potassium-free intake for a person to reduce his or her potassium concentration to 3.0 mmol/L, provided that all organ systems are functioning normally. A reasonable criterion for establishing a diagnosis of potassium wasting when the serum potassium concentration falls below 3.5 mmol/L would be the daily excretion of more than 20 mmol of potassium per day. The etiologies of excessive urinary loss have been separated into four categories: (1) pituitary-adrenal disturbances, (2) renal defects, (3) drug-induced losses, and (4) idiopathic and miscellaneous causes.

The structural and functional defects associated with potassium deficiency are shown in Table 4–3. These involve the kidney, the myocardium and cardiovascular system, the neuromuscular and central nervous system, and the gastrointestinal tract. Potassium deficiency also contributes to an impairment in carbohydrate metabolism and protein synthesis.

Since alkalosis (chloride depletion) usually accompanies hypokalemia, replacement therapy should be instituted with potassium chloride rather than with the alkaline salts of potassium. Foods rich in potassium (citrus and tomato juices, bananas, meats, and vegetables) provide the safest way to administer potassium. When additional oral replacement is needed, most commercial liquid preparations contain 20 mmol/15mL; this amount can be given one to three times daily in a glass of water. Preparations also are available in tablet form and single-dose packets (20 mmol). Slow-release formulations have been designed to reduce the incidence of gastrointestinal side effects. Intravenous potassium repletion may be necessary but can be hazardous, especially if infusion rates exceed 20 mmol/h or if concentrations of infusate exceed 40 mmol/L. Adequate urine output should be demonstrated, and electrocardiographic monitoring should be a requirement before potassium infusions are pushed above these levels.

The need for replacement potassium therapy in edematous and hypertensive pa-

**Table 4–2** Causes of Hypokalemia

I. Inadequate intake

II. Excessive sweating

III. Dilution of extracellular fluid volume

IV. Shift of potassium intracellularly
   A. Increase in blood pH (alkalosis)
   B. Glucose and insulin
   C. Familial hypokalemic periodic paralysis ·

V. Excessive gastrointestinal losses
   A. Vomiting
   B. Biliary, pancreatic, and intestinal drainage from fistulas and ostomies
   C. Diarrhea
      1. Chronic infections and inflammatory lesions
      2. Malabsorption
      3. Villous adenomas of colon and rectum
      4. Catechol-secreting neural tumors
      5. Abdominal lymphomas
      6. Non-alpha, non-beta islet cell tumors of pancreas
      7. Excessive use of enemas and purgatives
   D. Ureterosigmoidostomy

VI. Increased urinary losses
   A. Pituitary-adrenal disturbances
      1. Primary aldosteronism
      2. Secondary aldosteronism (renal artery stenosis, accelerated hypertension, volume depletion)
      3. Cushing syndrome (adrenal adenomas, carcinomas, and hyperplasia, pituitary corticotropin hypersecretion, ectopic corticotropin secretion secondary to tumor)
   B. Renal disorders
      1. Distal or proximal renal tubular acidosis
      2. Renin-secreting renal tumor
      3. Salt-losing nephritis
      4. Diuretic phase of acute tubular necrosis
      5. Postobstructive diuresis
   C. Drug induced
      1. Diuretics (thiazides, loop diuretics)
      2. Licorice extracts (glycyrrhizic acid)
      3. Large, nonabsorbable anions (eg, carbenicillin)
      4. Cisplatin, aminoglycosides, amphotericin B
      5. Acetylsalicylic acid (respiratory alkalosis)
   D. Idiopathic and other pathologies
      1. Bartter's and Gitelman's syndromes
      2. Hypomagnesemia
      3. Leukemia (lysozymuria)
      4. Idiopathic or familial

**Table 4–3** Manifestations of Hypokalemia

I. Myocardial and cardiovascular
   A. Focal myocardial necrosis
   B. Electrocardiographic changes (Figure 4–2)
      1. Depressed ST segment, inversion of T waves
      2. Accentuated U waves
   C. Arrhythmias
   D. Potentiation of digitalis toxicity
   E. Salt retention
   F. Hypotension
II. Neuromuscular and psychiatric
   A. Muscle weakness to flaccid paralysis
   B. Muscle pain and tenderness secondary to muscle necrosis (rhabdomyolosis)
   C. Depressive reaction (anorexia, constipation, weakness, lethargy, apathy, fatigue, depressed mood)
   D. Acute brain syndrome (memory impairment, disorientation, confusion)
III. Renal
   A. Defect in urine concentrating ability with polyuria
   B. Paradoxical aciduria
   C. Sodium retention
IV. Gastrointestinal
   A. Decreased motility and propulsive activity of intestine
   B. Paralytic ileus
V. Metabolic
   A. Carbohydrate intolerance (delayed release of insulin)
   B. Growth failure due to impaired protein synthesis

---

tients receiving diuretic therapy is questionable. In hypokalemic patients receiving diuretics, intracellular potassium concentrations are decreased more in patients with edematous or acidotic conditions than in hypertensive patients, making it appear necessary to give supplements to patients with edema and acidosis more often than to hypertensive patients. In fact, several studies have shown that hypertensive patients receiving diuretics, even though they may develop mild hypokalemia, maintain normal intracellular potassium concentrations; supplements do little to change these levels.

A great deal of concern and discussion has been generated suggesting that hypokalemia may precipitate cardiac arrhythmias and sudden death in patients made hypokalemic with diuretics, especially patients receiving digitalis for cardiac disorders or patients with acute myocardial infarctions. Controlled trials with patients either receiving supplements or not receiving supplements suggest that treatment with potassium supplementation fails to affect outcome.[12] A significant incidence of life-threatening hyperkalemia in patients receiving supplements suggests that the potential benefits of supplemental therapy be weighed against the risks.

**Hyperkalemia**

The causes of hyperkalemia are outlined in Table 4–4. Most cases of hyperkalemia are

**Table 4–4**  Causes of Hyperkalemia

I. Hyperkalemia caused by
   A. Decreased urinary excretion of potassium
   B. Increased exogenous or endogenous potassium
   C. Both

II. Decreased urinary excretion
   A. Renal insufficiency
   B. Potassium-retaining diuretics (spironolactone, triamterene)
   C. ACE inhibitors, NSAIDs, β-adrenergic antagonists
   D. Adrenal hypofunction (Addison disease, hyporeninemic hypoaldosteronism)

III. Increased exogenous or endogenous load
   A. Supplemental potassium (with diuretics)
   B. Potassium-containing drugs (eg, penicillin)
   C. Tissue catabolism (starvation, crush injury)
   D. Metabolic acidosis

---

observed in patients with impaired renal function. However, most patients with chronic renal failure who maintain good flow rates do not develop significant hyperkalemia until the azotemia becomes life threatening. Because the distal nephron has such a large capacity for secreting potassium, even in advanced renal failure, hyperkalemia develops only when there is some associated factor, such as (1) oliguria (eg, acute renal failure), (2) excessive potassium load (tissue catabolism, potassium supplementation, or administration of excess potassium in some other form, such as potassium penicillin G), (3) severe acidosis, (4) spironolactone or triamterene diuretic therapy, (5) a deficiency of endogenous steroid (aldosterone, cortisol), or (6) administration of a drug that inhibits potassium secretion in the distal nephron (eg, an angiotensin-converting enzyme [ACE] inhibitor or a nonsteroidal anti-inflammatory drug [NSAID]).

Poorly monitored potassium supplementation in patients receiving diuretic therapy leads to potentially lethal hyperkalemia with frightening frequency, especially in older patients who have some level of renal impairment. In the Boston Collaborative Drug Surveillance Program,[13] more than 16,000 consecutive patients were monitored for adverse reactions to medications they were taking. In this group, 31% received potassium chloride as a supplement for diuretic therapy. There were 7 deaths directly attributable to hyperkalemia and 21 lives threatened by significant hyperkalemia. Two significant risk factors were identified. Azotemia as a risk factor was predictable, but the second risk factor, age, was not. Only 0.8% of 1404 patients under age 50 years who received potassium supplements developed hyperkalemia. In contrast, the frequency of hyperkalemia in groups over age 50 years increased from 4.2% to 6.0% with advancing age. To explain this observation, reports have shown that elderly subjects on both restricted and unrestricted salt intakes, both upright and supine, have much lower plasma renin activities and urinary aldosterone excretions than do comparable young subjects.[14,15] This failure of the renin-aldosterone system in older patients produces an appearance of type IV renal tubular acidosis in the more severe cases.

The clinical manifestations of hyperkalemia often are subtle and may occur only shortly before death occurs from cardiac arrhythmia. Anxiety, restlessness, apprehension, weakness, stupor, and hyporeflexia should alert the clinician to the potential existence of this imbalance in patients at risk. Characteristic electrocardiographic changes are peaking of T waves followed by widening and then loss of P waves, and widening of the QRS complex (Figure 4–2).

Therapy should be started when the serum potassium concentration exceeds 5.5 mmol/L; a true medical emergency exists when it exceeds 7.0 mmol/L. Acute treatment is with glucose, insulin, and sodium bicarbonate to shift potassium intracellularly, and with calcium and sodium salts, which act as physiologic antagonists. Sodium polystyrene sulfonate (Kayexalate) resins are used to remove excess potassium from the body and can be given orally or in enema form. To avoid constipation and fecal impaction with oral administration of these resins, sorbitol can be given as necessary, titrating the dose. When hyperkalemia is due to a mineralocorticoid deficiency, 9-fluorohydrocortisone (Florinef) can be given. If all else fails, hemodialysis can be used to remove excess potassium.

One last observation that deserves further investigation is that in hypertensive laboratory animals, a high potassium intake protects against the development of cerebrovascular accidents. In the only study in humans,[16] a cohort of southern Californians followed for 10 years showed a 40% decrease in the risk of stroke mortality for every 10 mmol/d increase in potassium intake. Although the consensus seems to be now that supplemental

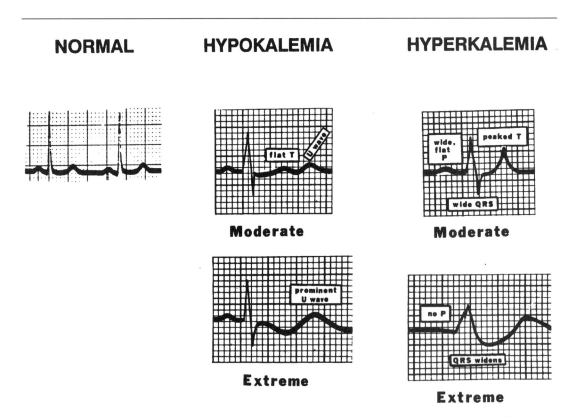

**NORMAL**     **HYPOKALEMIA**     **HYPERKALEMIA**

**Figure 4–2** Impact of moderate and severe hypokalemia and hyperkalemia on the electrocardiogram.

potassium lowers blood pressure and potassium depletion raises blood pressure,[17] the protection afforded by potassium supplementation is not totally explained by its effect on blood pressure. If these observations can be corroborated by further study, supplemental potassium may become a rational prophylactic therapy in high-risk persons.

## CALCIUM

A finely tuned endocrine system exists to maintain serum ionized calcium concentrations within a narrow normal range by controlling intestinal absorption, bone exchange, and renal excretion of calcium (Chapter 12). Whenever serum ionized calcium concentrations decrease, parathyroid hormone (PTH) secretion increases, resulting in mobilization of calcium from bone, decreased renal tubular phosphate resorption with resultant decreased serum phosphate concentration (this facilitates bone resorption of calcium), increased renal tubular calcium resorption, and increased intestinal calcium absorption, either directly or by enhancing the effect of vitamin D. Vitamin D is converted by the liver to the carrier metabolite 25-hydroxycholecalciferol ($25(OH)D_3$) and by the kidney to the active metabolite 1,25-dihydroxycholecalciferol ($1,25(OH)_2D_3$). The conversion in the kidney acts primarily to increase calcium absorption in the intestine, but it also increases bone resorption of calcium and decreases urinary calcium and phosphate excretion. PTH appears to produce its effects on the intestine by accelerating the conversion of $25(OH)D_3$ to $1,25(OH)_2D_3$. When serum calcium concentrations increase, serum thyrocalcitonin concentrations increase, producing effects counter to those of PTH.

Serum calcium exists in both the ionized and bound states, but only ionized calcium is physiologically active. The un-ionized calcium is either bound to serum proteins, primarily albumin, or bound in a complex with various anions, such as citrate. The binding is dependent on the concentration of serum protein (albumin) and the blood pH, with calcium binding increasing as the pH increases. Since most laboratories report only serum total calcium concentrations, these factors must be recognized in evaluating a specific serum calcium concentration.

Both hypocalcemia and hypercalcemia occur with increasing frequency in elderly individuals, primarily because specific disease entities causing these imbalances are more common in elderly persons. Of more importance in the elderly, however, is the inevitable age-related loss of bone calcium that occurs in both sexes but is more severe in women; this loss leads to the development of osteoporosis, with increased risk of fractures (Chapter 12). Since this entity is also discussed elsewhere, this narrative covers primarily the problems encountered in evaluating severity and progression or improvement of osteoporosis and the calcium requirement known to prevent its development and progression.

### Osteoporosis

Riggs and Melton[18] have postulated that at least two distinct clinical entities exist, specifically, type I (postmenopausal osteoporosis) and type II (senile osteoporosis). The distinctions between these two types of osteoporosis are based on different clinical features, densitometric and hormonal changes, and relation of disease patterns to menopause and age. In women, the impact may be additive. Among the different mechanisms involved in bone losses, dietary factors appear to play an important role in both entities. In older persons, calcium intake is generally low and is associated with reduced calcium absorption.[19,20] In addition, hypovitaminosis D is frequently associated with increased age through mechanisms of avoidance of dairy products, intestinal malabsorption of fat-soluble vitamin D, decreased exposure to sunlight, and a decreased ability of the skin to produce provitamin D[20–22] (Chapter 3). As vitamin D is a major regulator of calcium absorption, the cumulative response of a deficit of calcium intake and an inadequate intake of vitamin D is a negative calcium balance, which stimulates parathyroid hormone secretion. This secondary hyperparathyroidism increases bone calcium resorption and the risk of fractures, with its subsequent morbidity and mortality.[18]

The requirement for calcium, especially in older persons, continues to be a controversial subject. Calcium deficiency is difficult to define and hard to measure, and uncertainty remains about its impact. These problems arise from the slow turnover of bone tissue, which makes the monitoring of both breakdown and repair a long-term procedure, since bone status monitoring techniques are still relatively crude.

The requirements and RDAs of most nutrients are derived from experimental and clinical evidence of the effects of a deficiency and the amount of nutrient that is needed to prevent these effects from occurring. After the deficiency syndrome is characterized, the amount of the nutrient required to prevent or cure it is determined, and an allowance is decided on. With most nutrients, the deficiency develops relatively rapidly, and the effect of the intervention also is manifested rapidly. Calcium differs from most other minerals in that the plasma calcium concentration is not a guide to the individual's calcium nutriture. The regulation of plasma calcium levels is so fine that intraindividual variation is not much greater than the technical error in its measurement, and interindividual variation is not much larger. This fine regulation is mediated

by the parathyroid glands. Because there are 1200 g of calcium in the skeleton and only 1 g in extracellular fluid, serum calcium concentration does not reflect calcium economy in the body. Calcium deficiency has been shown to lower the plasma calcium concentration by 0.15 mg/dL when large numbers of subjects are studied by paired observations.[23] It is not possible to discriminate between individuals in positive and negative calcium balance by means of serum calcium concentration alone.

Since serum calcium concentrations cannot be used to gauge calcium balance, measurement of the blood level of PTH, which increases in response to calcium deficiency, and the plasma $1,25(OH)_2D_3$ level, which also increases in response to calcium deprivation, might be used as indicators of calcium nutritional status. However, the assay for PTH is still too imprecise, and there are many other regulators of plasma $1,25(OH)_2D_3$ levels (eg, phosphorus intake, growth hormone, prolactin), precluding its use as a reliable indicator of calcium nutriture.

The quantification of bone density itself also might provide a criterion of nutritional calcium status. However, the wide individual variation in bone density ($\pm10\%$) and the many hormonal and other factors that affect bone density, along with the relatively severe depletion that must occur before bone deficiency can be detected, preclude this end point, even if it were agreed that osteoporosis was the clinical end point of calcium deficiency. When everything is considered, the only practical definition of calcium requirement is the amount of calcium required to maintain calcium balance, and the only way to determine it is by balance techniques. If calcium requirement is defined as the amount required to maintain calcium balance, then it can be determined by calculating from calcium balances the mean intake at which intake and output are equal. In healthy young adults, this is estimated to be around 500 mg/d.[24] From available data, an RDA of 800 mg/d was proposed for the United States, with the recognition that pregnant and lactating women and postmenopausal women have higher requirements. These recommendations were not changed in the 1989 revisions made by the Food and Nutrition Board of the National Academy of Sciences and the National Research Council.[25] Nordin et al[26] and Heaney et al[27] found that the requirements in postmenopausal women were 900 and 1500 mg/d, respectively. Older persons generally do not attain these levels of intake. One study[28] reported that 62% of the subjects studied had an intake less than 500 mg/d and that 21% had less than 300 mg/d.

There is no evidence of bone loss in premenopausal women on a normal diet; bone loss starts abruptly at menopause. Women 1 year after the start of menopause have significantly higher serum concentrations and urinary excretions of calcium, serum alkaline phosphatase activity (evidence of new bone formation or osteoblastic activity), and urinary hydroxyproline excretions (evidence of bone resorption or osteoclastic activity)[29] (Table 4–5) (Chapter 12). Several theories have been proposed to define the pathophysiology of the change at menopause. First, the loss of estrogen activity may cause a small increase in plasma calcium concentration (perhaps due to a change in the PTH set point), which increases urinary calcium excretion, bone resorption, and bone re-formation. The other possibility is that increased bone resorption is the primary event, resulting in an increase in plasma and urine calcium levels. Under normal circumstances, the efficiency of intestinal calcium absorption is regulated to meet the body's need for calcium. In elderly persons, the adaptive response to a low calcium intake is reduced. The negative calcium balance is due not only to a low intake but also to the reduced vitamin D level, which impairs intestinal absorption. Vitamin D status is influenced significantly by length of exposure to sunlight. Ambulatory elderly persons had much higher plasma $25(OH)D_3$ levels than did long-term hospitalized patients who did not go outdoors.[28] The same risk exists for institutionalized elderly patients. Supplements of calcium (1000 mg/d) and ergocalciferol (20 mg/d) induced a significant increase in serum calcium and $25(OH)D_3$ concentrations and a decrease in serum PTH concentrations in 65 elderly patients.[26] These data provide evidence that bone resorption can be retarded by adequate intakes of calcium and vitamin D.

**Table 4–5** Immediate Biochemical Effects of Menopause

| Variable | Premenopausal Women | Women 1 y after Menopause | P |
|---|---|---|---|
| Plasma calcium (mmol/L) | 2.38 ± 0.016 | 2.42 ± 0.015 | <.05 |
| Urinary calcium:creatinine (mmol/mmol) | 0.18 ± 0.026 | 0.26 ± 0.033 | <.05 |
| Plasma alkaline phosphatase (U/L) | 62.1 ± 3.0 | 77.6 ± 4.3 | <.005 |
| Urinary hydroxyproline:creatinine (mmol/μmol) | 14.2 ± 0.83 | 22.0 ± 1.7 | <.001 |

*Note:* Mean values ± standard error; *N* = 22.
*Source:* reference 29.

## Hypocalcemia

The causes of hypocalcemia are listed in Table 4–6. In patients with unexplained hypocalcemia or hypokalemia, or both, clinicians should be aware that hypomagnesemia may be the underlying etiology; hypomagnesemia causes a peripheral resistance to PTH and decreases the release of PTH in response to the hypocalcemic stimulus.

The symptomatology associated with hypocalcemia is primarily related to increased neuromuscular excitability, as manifested by tetany. Long-term manifestations include cataracts; abnormalities of the nails, skin, and teeth; and mental and growth retardation.

Acute correction of symptomatic hypocalcemia can be accomplished with parenteral calcium gluconate. Oral calcium salts (carbonate, gluconate, or lactate) can be used to treat mild or latent hypocalcemia. Vitamin D and its metabolites increase serum calcium concentration by increasing intestinal absorption and bone resorption of calcium.

---

**Table 4–6** Causes of Hypocalcemia

   I.  Malignancies, especially with osteoblastic metastases (prostate)
   II. Renal insufficiency
  III. Hypoparathyroidism; pseudohypoparathyroidism
  IV. Gastrointestinal disorders (malabsorption)
   V. Vitamin deficiency or resistance
  VI. Acute pancreatitis
 VII. Calcitonin-producing tumors (medullary carcinoma of thyroid)
VIII. Hypomagnesemia or hyperphosphatemia, or both

*Note:* Patients in categories II and III have high serum phosphorus concentrations; phosphorus concentrations tend to be normal in others.

## Hypercalcemia

The two most common causes of hypercalcemia are malignancy and hyperparathyroidism, which together are responsible for 80% to 90% of all cases.[30] Malignancy-associated hypercalcemia is the most common paraneoplastic syndrome, occurring in up to 10% of all patients with cancer, and is most frequently observed in patients with breast, renal cell, and lung cancers, squamous cell carcinomas of the head and neck, and multiple myeloma. Rarely, instances of ectopic production of true PTH, documented by radioimmunoassay, have been reported. In most cases reported, however, a humoral factor with many, but not all, of the physiologic characteristics of PTH (stimulates osteoclastic bone reabsorption, activates renal adenylate cyclase, and suppresses tubular phosphate reabsorption) has been identified as the mediator of hypercalcemia of malignancy.[31] This factor does not have the radioimmunoassay characteristics of PTH, however. Other causes of hypercalcemia are listed in Table 4–7. Early symptoms are vague and nonspecific and include anorexia, nausea, vomiting, constipation, fatigue, somnolence, muscle weakness, pruritus, and psychiatric disturbances. Ultimately, polyuria with dehydration and azotemia with cardiac arrhythmias, especially in digitalized patients, are likely to occur. Nephrolithiasis and nephrocalcinosis are manifestations of chronic hypercalcemia.

The initial therapy for patients with hypercalcemia is rehydration with normal saline. This decreases the serum calcium concentration by hemodilution and increases urinary calcium excretion. Loop diuretics (furosemide) also greatly increase urinary calcium excretion, whereas thiazide diuretics decrease urinary calcium excretion and may potentiate hypercalcemia. Prednisone in high

**Table 4–7** Causes of Hypercalcemia

I. Malignancies
   A. With osteolytic metastases (enhanced bone resorption)
   B. Without osteolytic metastases
      1. Ectopic hyperparathyroidism (rare)
      2. Humoral PTH-like peptide
      3. Osteolytic activating factor (myeloma, lymphoma)
II. Hyperparathyroidism
III. Thiazide administration
IV. Immobilization
V. Miscellaneous (vitamin A or D intoxication, tuberculosis, sarcoidosis, hyperthyroidism, Addison disease, milk alkali syndrome, acute renal failure)

doses is effective when the mechanism of the hypercalcemia is increased vitamin D–mediated calcium absorption from the intestine (sarcoid, multiple myeloma, vitamin D intoxication) but is less effective in malignancies with metastatic bone disease and hyperparathyroidism. Mithramycin is another option available for treating the hypercalcemia associated with malignancy. This antitumor agent acts by inhibiting bone resorption and blocking vitamin D action. Its application is limited by the necessity of intravenous administration. Transient nausea and vomiting and bone marrow suppression are the major adverse effects. Injections of calcitonin decrease the skeletal release of calcium, phosphorus, and hydroxyproline. The most impressive results are seen in conditions in which a high rate of bone turnover occurs, such as in immobilization, thyrotoxicosis, and vitamin D intoxication. NSAIDs may be helpful in reducing the hypercalcemia in some malignancies, such as renal cell carcinoma, in which prostaglandin E appears to be the mediator of excessive bone breakdown without evidence of bony metastases. The biphosphonates are an important group of drugs in the treatment of hypercalcemia regardless of cause.[32] The use of etidronate, the first biphosphonate available, has largely been supplanted by newer, more potent biphosphonates. A single-dose infusion of pamidronate (60–90 mg) can be delivered in a liter of normal saline over 24 hours or over multiple shorter periods of time if given as outpatient therapy. The drug is highly effective and can maintain normocalcemia for 1 to 2 weeks after each infusion; it can safely be used repeatedly to maintain normocalcemia. Oral agents have been developed but are not yet approved in the United States. Another agent available for treating cancer-induced hypercalcemia is gallium nitrate, which also acts by blocking bone reabsorption. If all else fails, hemodialysis is effective in acutely lowering serum calcium concentrations.

## PHOSPHORUS

Selective phosphorus deficiency induced in normal subjects by an inadequate diet or by ingestion of large quantities of phosphate-binding antacids leads to a distinctive clinical syndrome characterized by anorexia, weakness, and bone pain.[33] Symptoms appear primarily when the serum phosphorus concentration falls below 0.32 mmol/L, and clinical improvement occurs rapidly when dietary phosphorus is restored. Severe hypophosphatemia has been documented in association with alcohol withdrawal, diabetes mellitus, excessive antacid ingestion, recovery from burns, unsupplemented hyperalimentation, nutritional recovery syndrome, and severe respiratory alkalosis. Patients with severe hypophosphatemia may develop a metabolic encephalopathy (irritability, muscle weakness, hypoesthesias and paresthesias, dysarthria, confusion, seizures, and coma), rhabdomyolysis, hemolysis, leukocyte dysfunction (abnormal phagocytic, chemotactic, and bacteriocidal activities of granulocytes), and platelet dysfunction. Milk is the best dietary source of phosphorus; oral or intravenous phosphorous salts can be used as a supplement in individuals with severe deficits.

The 1989 RDA for adults is 800 mg/d; 1200 mg/d is recommended during pregnancy and lactation. A one-to-one ratio of calcium to phosphorus provides sufficient phosphorus, and since there is more phosphorus than calcium in most diets, phosphorus deficiency generally does not occur until calcium intake also is deficient.[25]

## MAGNESIUM

Magnesium is the second most important intracellular cation; about 60% of body magnesium is located in bone, 40% is in the intracellular space (half of this in skeletal muscle), and only 1% exists extracellularly. The normal serum magnesium concentration is remarkably constant (0.7–1.1 mmol/L) and correlates poorly with intracellular magnesium. About 30% of serum magnesium is protein bound, with most of the remainder in ionized form, making it ultrafilterable through the kidney. Most of the intracellular magnesium is bound to protein and energy-rich phosphates. Magnesium is important in over 300 different enzyme systems, being indispensable to the metabolism of adenosine triphosphate. Therefore it affects glucose utilization; synthesis of fat, protein, and nucleic acids; muscle contraction; and several membrane transport systems.

The National Research Council, utilizing available balance data, has established an RDA of 350 mg/d for adult men and 280 mg/d for adult women, with slightly higher values for pregnant and lactating women.[24] These recommendations were not changed in the 1989 revisions made by the Food and Nutrition Board of the National Academy of Sciences and the National Research Council.[25] Studies by Pao and Mickle[34] on 37,000 healthy adults showed that the mean intakes for men and women were 266 and 228 mg/d, respectively. For elderly persons with chronic conditions that might affect gastrointestinal absorption or urinary excretion of magnesium, a deficiency of magnesium becomes a very real concern.

### Magnesium Deficiency

The causes of magnesium deficiency are listed in Table 4–8; the first two entities are the most commonly encountered. Hypomagnesemia produces neuromuscular and psychiatric disturbances, including neuromuscular hyperirritability, tetany, hyperacusis, seizures, muscle weakness, vertigo, gross tremors, and mental changes (eg, irritability and aggressiveness). Individuals with hypomagnesemia also may develop polyuria and other electrolyte disturbances (hypocalcemia, hypokalemia, hypophosphatemia).

There is no evidence that older patients have a higher incidence of magnesium depletion than do younger people, and no decrease in serum magnesium concentration is observed with advancing age. Significant depletion of intracellular magnesium can occur, however, before the serum magnesium concentration falls below the normal range.[35] The concern then arises of how best to measure

**Table 4–8** Causes of Hypomagnesemia

I. Gastrointestinal disorders with malabsorption and/or diarrhea
II. Chronic alcoholism and diabetes mellitus
III. Endocrine disorders
   A. Hyperaldosteronism
   B. Hyperparathyroidism
   C. Diabetic ketoacidosis
IV. Acute pancreatitis
V. Renal magnesium loss
   A. Diuretic therapy
   B. SIADH
   C. Sodium, calcium, and/or magnesium wasting (interstitial nephropathy)
   D. Renal tubular acidosis
   E. Other drugs (cisplatin, aminoglycoside antibiotics, pentamadine, cyclosporine)
VI. Protein-calorie malnutrition

intracellular magnesium; most methods are invasive, requiring tissue (muscle) biopsy, which is not practical for human studies. One method for quantifying a magnesium deficit is to determine the amount of magnesium retained, or excreted, in a 24-hour urine sample after infusion of a standardized quantity of magnesium.[36] This procedure has been useful in patients with suspected symptomatology of magnesium depletion despite normal serum magnesium concentrations, but it has not been used specifically in comparing young and old subjects. Whether magnesium supplementation is warranted in conditions such as hypokalemia associated with diuretic therapy in elderly people remains speculative.

**Hypermagnesemia**

The earliest manifestations of hypermagnesemia are somnolence and hypotension, and an electrocardiogram may show prolongation of the PR interval and QRS duration with peaking of the T waves. Later, respiratory depression or paralysis and cardiac arrest

can be terminal events. Such hypermagnesemia is usually seen only in patients with renal insufficiency who also are taking magnesium-containing antacids or cathartics.

**CONCLUSION**

Elderly patients are more susceptible to the development of both hyponatremia and hypernatremia. There appears to be an increasing osmoreceptor responsiveness and a decreasing baroreceptor responsiveness in elderly people, which make them prone to the development of SIADH. Elderly individuals also develop a defect in their thirst mechanisms, especially when they have cerebral disease, making them more prone to develop hypernatremia resulting from dehydration secondary to primary water depletion.

Hypokalemia and hyperkalemia are more common in elderly people. Hypokalemia frequently occurs in the elderly because of their increased use of medications (eg, diuretics, purgatives, and enemas). Hyperkalemia is related to the lower renin-aldosterone levels seen in older persons under comparable conditions, making it more difficult to clear any excess potassium via the kidneys.

Osteoporosis is a major problem in elderly individuals, but a finely tuned endocrine system tends to ensure that serum calcium concentrations are maintained within a narrow normal range. Calcium and vitamin D intakes often are inadequate to prevent a negative calcium balance and bone demineralization.

Hypercalcemia occurs more frequently in elderly persons, primarily because the malignancies that cause hypercalcemia are more frequent.

Disorders of magnesium balance, even though they are not more common in elderly subjects, may be overlooked because serum magnesium concentrations are not routinely measured.

### REFERENCES

1. Epstein M, Hollenberg N. Age as a determinant of renal sodium conservation in normal man. *J Lab Clin Med.* 1976;87:411–417.

2. Kleinfeld M, Casimir M, Borra S. Hyponatremia as observed in a chronic disease facility. *J Am Geriatr Soc.* 1979;27:156–161.

3. Miller M, Morley JE, Rubenstein LZ. Hyponatremia in a nursing home population. *J Am Geriatr Soc.* 1995;43:1410–1413.

4. Miller M, Hecker MS, Friedlander DA, et al. Apparent idiopathic hyponatremia in an ambulatory geriatric population. *J Am Geriatr Soc.* 1996;44:404–408.

5. Anderson RJ, Chung HM, Kluge R, et al. Hyponatremia: a prospective analysis of its epidemiology and the pathogenetic role of vasopressin. *Ann Intern Med.* 1985;102:164–168.

6. Helderman JH, Vestal RE, Rowe JW, et al. The response of arginine vasopressin to intravenous ethanol in man: the impact of aging. *J Gerontol.* 1978;33:39–47.

7. Rowe JW, Minaker KL, Sparrow D, et al. Age related failure of volume-pressure mediated vasopressin release. *J Clin Endocrinol Metab.* 1982;54:661–664.

8. Epstein M. Aging and the kidney. *J Am Soc Nephrol.* 1996;7:1106–1122.

9. Snyder NA, Feigal DW, Arieff AI. Hypernatremia in elderly patients: a heterogeneous, morbid, and iatrogenic entity. *Ann Intern Med.* 1987;107:309–319.

10. Lavizzo-Mourey R, Johnson J, Stolley P. Risk factors for dehydration among elderly nursing home residents. *J Am Geriatr Soc.* 1988;36:213–218.

11. Phillips PA, Rolls BJ, Ledingham JG, et al. Reduced thirst after water deprivation in healthy elderly men. *N Engl J Med.* 1984;311:753–759.

12. Fries ED. Diuretic induced hypokalemia: the debate over its relationship to cardiac arrhythmias. *Postgrad Med.* 1987;81:123–129.

13. Lawson DH. Adverse reactions to potassium chloride. *Q J Med.* 1974;171:433–440.

14. Weideman P, DeMyttenaeu-Bursztein S, Maxwell MH, et al. Effect of aging on plasma renin and aldosterone in normal man. *Kidney Int.* 1975;8:325–333.

15. Crane MG, Harris JJ. Effect of aging on renin activity and aldosterone excretion. *J Lab Clin Med.* 1976;87:947–959.

16. Khaw KT, Barrett-Conner E. Dietary potassium and stroke associated mortality. *N Engl J Med.* 1987;316:235–240.

17. Barri YM, Wingo CS. The effects of potassium depletion and supplementation on blood pressure: a clinical review. *Am J Med Sci.* 1997;314:37–40.

18. Riggs BL, Melton LJ III. Involutional osteoporosis. *N Engl J Med.* 1986;314:1676–1684.

19. Bullamore JR, Gallagher JC, Wilkinson R, et al. Effect of age on calcium absorption. *Lancet.* 1970;2:535–537.

20. Gallagher JC, Riggs BL, Eisman J, et al. Intestinal calcium absorption and serum vitamin D metabolites in normal subjects and osteoporotic patients: effect of age and dietary calcium. *J Clin Invest.* 1979;64:729–736.

21. Tsai KS, Heath H III, Kumar R, et al. Impaired vitamin D metabolism with aging in women: possible role in pathogenesis of senile osteoporosis. *J Clin Invest.* 1984;73:1668–1672.

22. MacLaughlin J, Holick MF. Aging decreases the capacity of skin to produce vitamin $D_3$. *J Clin Invest.* 1985;76:1536–1538.

23. McFadyen IM, Nordin BEC, Smith DA, et al. Effect of variation in dietary calcium. *Br Med J.* 1985;1:161–164.

24. Food and Nutrition Board, National Research Council. *Recommended Dietary Allowances.* 8th ed. Washington, DC: National Academy Press; 1980.

25. Food and Nutrition Board, National Research Council. *Recommended Dietary Allowances.* 10th ed. Washington, DC: National Academy Press; 1989.

26. Nordin BEC, Horsman A, Marshall DM, et al. Calcium requirement and calcium therapy. *Clin Orthop.* 1979;140:216–246.

27. Heaney RP, Recker RR, Saville P. Menopausal changes in calcium balance performance. *J Lab Clin Med.* 1978;94:953–963.

28. Chapuy MC, Chapuy P, Meunier PJ. Calcium and vitamin D supplements: effects of calcium metabolism in elderly people. *Am J Clin Nutr.* 1987;46:324–328.

29. Nordin BEC, Pollen KJ, Need AG, et al. The problem of calcium transport. *Am J Clin Nutr.* 1987;45:1296–1304.

30. Lafferty FW. Differential diagnosis of hypercalcemia. *J Bone Miner Res.* 1991;6:S51–S59.

31. Broadus AE, Mangin M, Ikeda K, et al. Humoral hypercalcemia of cancer: identification of a novel parathyroid hormone-like peptide. *N Engl J Med.* 1988;319:556–563.

32. Bilezikian JP. Clinical review: management of hypercalcemia. *J Clin Endocrinol Metab.* 1993; 77:1445–1449.

33. Knochel JP. The pathophysiology and clinical characteristics of severe hypophosphatemia. *Arch Intern Med.* 1977;137:203–220.

34. Pao EM, Mickle SJ. Problem nutrients in the United States. *Food Technol.* 1981;35:58–69.

35. Reinhart RA. Magnesium metabolism: a review with special reference to the relationship between intracellular content and serum levels. *Arch Intern Med.* 1988;148:2415–2420.

36. Al-Ghandi SMG, Cameron EC, Sutton RAL. Magnesium deficiency: pathophysiologic and clinical overview. *Am J Kidney Dis.* 1994;24:737–752.

# CHAPTER 5

# Trace Metal Requirements

*Gary J. Fosmire*

There is growing concern about the nutritional needs of the elderly, with increasing attention focused on various trace metals. Studies of dietary intake and status, both generally and in association with various disease states, have revealed that elderly people may be particularly vulnerable to developing deficiencies, or in some cases toxicities, of one or more of the trace metals. Reasons for this increased vulnerability include decreased energy intake without an increased density of trace metals in the diet; changes in food intake patterns; age-related physiologic changes that impair absorption, retention, or excretion; and various chronic and acute diseases experienced by the elderly and the medications used to treat them.

Several physiologic changes associated with aging[1] might be expected to affect the metabolism of most trace minerals. Changes in body composition, including a decline in lean body mass and a relative increase in body fat, can be expected to alter body pool sizes of, or requirements for, most of the trace metals, as they tend to be associated primarily with nonadipose tissues. The decline in basal metabolic rate associated with advancing age is usually accompanied by a decrease in energy intake, exacerbating problems of insufficient density of trace minerals in the diet. The impairment in kidney function observed with aging may result in less efficient elimination, with a concomitant retention of certain minerals, or less efficient reabsorption with resultant increased losses (Chapter 10). The relative hypochlorhydria associated with aging adversely affects the solubility of the minerals and results in a decreased bioavailability or decreased absorption of various trace metals. The senescent changes in the intestine (Chapter 8) include a decreased mucosal surface area and decreased motility, potentially contributing to an impaired absorption of trace metals; such impairment with aging has not been a consistent finding, however, suggesting that in the absence of disease there is sufficient capacity for appropriate absorption.[2] The greater prevalence of disease states among the elderly may adversely affect nutritional status as a direct result of the disease processes or through drug-nutrient interactions (Chapter 14).

Dietary choices may also influence trace metal status. In an obvious way, selection of foods that do not contain substantial quantities of a particular trace mineral can result in a deficient state, but other dietary choices such as the incorporation of large amounts of fiber or foods containing phytate (myo-inositolhexaphosphate), found in whole grains and legumes, can decrease the absorption or retention of various minerals.[3] The complexing of minerals by the fiber or phytate could impair absorption of exogenous sources as well as complex with those minerals, such as zinc, that are secreted into the intestine, thereby preventing their reabsorption. Although it is difficult to generalize, many elderly may restrict energy intake or have other restrictive dietary practices that would predispose them to developing deficiencies.[4]

## ZINC

Zinc has been known to be an essential trace metal since the 1930s, and its importance to human health has been recognized for the last 40 years. Zinc is a component of more than 80 metalloenzymes and proteins, where it may have catalytic, structural, or regulatory roles. It has important but as yet not clearly understood roles in the structure and function of biomembranes. Zinc is reported to help stabilize the structures of RNA, DNA, and ribosomes and is involved in gene regulation by its role in zinc fingers and twists.[5] At a more physiologic level, zinc is essential for growth, cell division, reproduction, taste acuity, wound healing, and normal immune function. Given the important physiologic roles that zinc plays and the likelihood that these may be disrupted in some fashion by a deficient state, it is important to consider the dietary adequacy of zinc and other factors that may affect zinc status.

Among the factors affecting zinc status is the amount in the diet. The recommended dietary allowances (RDAs) for men and women 51 years of age and older have been set at 15 mg and 12 mg, respectively[6]; there are no more specific recommendations for intakes for older individuals. A review of 10 studies of elderly people revealed that mean intakes were between 7 mg and 10 mg/d.[7–9] In a recent commentary on dietary intakes of minerals, Pennington reported that zinc intakes were only 72% of the RDA for women 60 to 65 years of age and 85% of the RDA for men[10] and that dietary adequacy of zinc is of concern for a number of age and gender groups. These lower levels of dietary intakes are, in part, a reflection of the density of zinc in the diet and the diminished energy intake associated with aging. If one uses the concept of "critical nutrient density," defined by Solomons[11] as the amount of a given micronutrient contained in 1000 kcal of diet that will supply the RDA when energy intake is minimally adequate for maintenance of health, the critical nutrient density is 8.2 mg/1000 kcal for men aged 51 to 74 years and is 7.9 mg/1000 kcal for women of the same age range, as based on RDAs for energy intake and the RDA for zinc.[6] It is recognized that recommended energy intakes for those older than 74 years should be less and thus that the density of zinc in the diet should increase at older ages. Actual densities of zinc in the diets of elderly individuals are less than those calculated for critical nutrient density. Usual densities of zinc range between 4.0 and 6.0 mg/1000 kcal. For example, Fosmire and colleagues[9] found the density of zinc in the diet of a rural elderly population to be 6.0 mg/1000 kcal for men and 5.8 mg/1000 kcal for women. Other studies using younger populations have reported densities of 4.7[12] and 4.2 mg/1000 kcal.[13] It is evident that unless people are particularly careful to choose foods rich in zinc, it is unlikely that their RDA will be met. If elderly people consume proportionately less of the foods that are richer in zinc (ie, meats, fish, and poultry), the density of zinc in their diets will decline further, exacerbating problems of obtaining sufficient zinc from dietary sources. The zinc content of selected foods is given in Table 5–1. In addition, differences in the bioavail-

**Table 5–1** Zinc Content of Selected Foods

| Food, Portion Size | Zinc Content (mg) |
|---|---|
| *Beverages* | |
| Carbonated, nonalcoholic, 12 fl oz | (0.2–0.4g) |
| Coffee, 1 cup | Trace |
| Tea, 1 cup | 0.1 |
| Wine, 4 fl oz | 0.1 |
| Beer, 12 fl oz | 0.1 |
| *Bread, 1 slice* | |
| White | 0.2 |
| Mixed grain | 0.5 |
| Rye | 0.4 |
| Whole wheat | 0.6 |
| *Dairy products* | |
| Milk, 1 cup | 0.9–1.0 |
| Cheese, 1 oz | 0.9 |
| Cottage cheese, 1 cup | 0.7–1.0 |
| *Eggs, 1 each* | 0.6 |
| *Fish, 3½ oz* | |
| Bass | 0.5 |
| Cod | 0.8 |
| Swordfish | 1.1 |
| Tuna | 0.9 |
| *Fruits, fresh, 1 each* | |
| Apple | Trace |
| Peach | 0.1 |
| Pear | 0.2 |
| Plum | 0.1 |
| Orange | 0.1 |
| *Legumes, 1 cup cooked* | |
| Kidney beans | 2.0 |
| Soybeans | 2.1 |
| Black-eyed peas | 1.3 |
| Dried peas | 1.9 |
| *Meat* | |
| Beef, cooked, 3 oz | 5.1 |
| Pork roast, 3 oz | 2.2 |
| Chicken, 1 cup | 2.9 |
| Beef liver, 3 oz | 5.2 |
| Chicken liver, 3 oz | 3.6 |
| *Nuts, 1 cup* | |
| Almonds | 4.2 |
| Cashews | 7.7 |
| Filberts | 2.8 |
| Peanuts | 4.8 |

| Food, Portion Size | Zinc Content (mg) |
|---|---|
| Pecans | 6.5 |
| Walnuts | 3.3 |
| *Shellfish* | |
| Oysters, eastern, 3½ oz | 62.0 |
| Oysters, western, 3½ oz | 48.0 |
| Clams, 3½ oz | 2.7 |
| *Vegetables* | |
| Green beans, 1 cup | 0.5 |
| Beets, ½ cup | 0.2 |
| Carrots, 1 each | 0.1 |
| Corn, 1 ear | 0.4 |
| Green peas, 1 cup | 1.8 |
| Potato, baked without skin, 1 each | 0.5 |
| Cabbage, raw, 1 cup | 0.1 |

*Source:* Values from *Nutrition for Living* (pp A12–A37) by JL Christian and JL Greger, Benjamin Cummings Publishing Company, 1988.

ability of zinc from various dietary sources may influence dietary adequacy. It is clear from a number of studies that zinc is generally less available for absorption from foods of vegetable origin than is the zinc from foods of animal origin.[3]

A great deal of research has been directed toward elucidating the mechanisms of zinc absorption and maintenance of zinc homeostasis.[14] Zinc absorption by the small intestine occurs by two processes, a saturable process that is stimulated by zinc depletion and a nonsaturable process that is not affected by zinc status. At lower levels of intake, absorption is primarily via a carrier-mediated (saturable) process. Secretion of endogenous zinc into the gastrointestinal tract is a part of the maintenance of zinc homeostasis. Such secretion may occur by desquamation of intestinal cells and by secretion via the pancreatic fluids, bile, and the succus entericus. Zinc homeostasis is accomplished primarily by modulation of the rate of absorption and the rate of endogenous secretions; conditions that interfere with these processes can adversely affect maintenance of appropriate levels of zinc in the body. Several studies have shown that the efficiency of zinc absorption is less in elderly than in younger subjects.[15,16] Another study by Bales et al[17] showed that elderly subjects failed to absorb as much zinc after a 25-mg zinc load as did younger subjects. Others have failed to observe such a decrease in efficiency of absorption with aging,[18] and a study by Turnlund et al[16] found that the elderly could absorb zinc as well as young subjects when presented with a very low-zinc diet. Reasons for the discrepancy in findings are not readily apparent. It has been reported[16] that the elderly can maintain zinc balance as well as younger subjects. Further studies will be required to establish whether aging results in a loss of efficiency of absorption of zinc and to assess whether older women follow patterns similar to men's.

In addition to the amount of zinc in the diet, a number of other factors, called "conditioning factors" by Sandstead and colleagues,[8] that impair the absorption or increase the excretion (or both) of zinc from endogenous pools may influence requirements or lead to a deficient state. Chronic malabsorption syndromes, such as gluten-sensitive enteropathy or Crohn's disease, can result in decreased zinc absorption and an impaired ability to control zinc homeostasis, as the gut is the apparent major point of control. Any physiologic stress that results in substantially increased zinc losses into the urine will increase requirements. Examples of such stresses would include physical trauma, wounds (including surgery), thermal burns, and muscle-wasting diseases, all of which result in dramatic increases in urinary zinc losses. The consumption of alcohol results in increased urinary losses of zinc due to alcohol consumption per se. If consumption has been prolonged enough to cause alcohol-induced cirrhosis, urinary losses of zinc will be high, and the zinc content of the liver will be abnormally low. Many of the medications (both those sold over the counter and those sold by prescription) used by the elderly can affect zinc status. Diuretics, chelating agents, antacids, laxatives, and iron supplements may decrease absorption or increase excretion from the body.

Given the poor intakes reported for the elderly and the likelihood of having one or more of the conditioning factors, it is reasonable to suppose that zinc deficiency would be prevalent in the elderly. The data that can be used to estimate prevalence rates for zinc deficiency are meager and clearly insufficient to allow confident estimates of such rates among the elderly as a whole. Data from a number of studies using relatively small subject population groups have been reviewed by Greger,[7] and data from several other studies[9,19–24] have been used to evaluate zinc nutriture among the elderly. Prevalence of deficient status, defined somewhat arbitrarily as plasma or serum zinc concentrations below 10.7 μmol/L or 70 μg/dL, ranged between 0% and 61%. As the studies examined populations varying in age, socioeconomic class, and health status, such variability in prevalence is not unexpected. Studies that have examined larger population groups, such as a subset of the population sampled by the Health and Nutrition Examination Survey II (HANES II), showed that about 12% of both men and women had zinc plasma or serum values below 10.1 μmol/L.[25] These findings would suggest that a considerable number of elderly people have biochemical evidence of zinc deficiency; prevalence rates appear strikingly higher among those with poor health or low socioeconomic status.

Consequences of zinc deficiency may be serious and varied, depending in part on the severity of the deficiency. Manifestations of the deficiency have been reviewed by Prasad[26] and may include growth retardation, impaired sexual development and performance, various manifestations of dermatitis, delayed wound healing, anorexia, altered taste acuity, and impaired immune function. A number of these symptoms arise as a result of a severely deficient state, but even moderate or mild deficiency may adversely affect the health of an individual. A number of these deficiency symptoms resemble problems commonly observed in elderly individuals, and attempts have been made to relate zinc status to the occurrence of several of these symptoms. Most attention has focused on taste acuity, wound healing, dermatitis, and immune function.

Taste acuity has been reported to decline with aging,[27] but it is unclear to what extent this can be attributed to zinc deficiency. It has been clearly shown that severe zinc deficiency will result in hypogeusia[28]; it is less clear that a less severely deficient state will result in diminished taste. Several studies have examined the interaction between zinc and taste acuity. Most studies of elderly subjects who did not have medical conditions that led to a severely deficient state have failed to observe such a relationship or to see a positive change—that is, lower thresholds for the different tastes in response to zinc supplementation.[17,29–31] It is of note, however, that a recent study by Prasad et al[32] reported that zinc supplementation (30 mg of zinc for 6 months) improved taste acuity among elderly subjects who had normal plasma zinc values but depressed values for granulocytes and lymphocytes on entry into the study. For patients rendered severely zinc deficient due to medical conditions, zinc supplementation

has been clearly shown to improve taste acuity.[33,34]

An essential role for zinc in wound healing is now well established.[35] It is apparent, however, that the increased rate of wound healing in response to zinc supplementation will occur only if the individual is in suboptimal zinc status; that is, there is no additional benefit obtained by supplementation once the deficiency has been corrected.[36] Initial poor status, due to insufficient intake and/or losses associated with surgery or physical trauma, could limit the amount of zinc available for tissue repair and diminish the effectiveness of the healing process.

Zinc deficiency in experimental and domestic farm animals results in parakeratotic skin lesions.[14] Severe zinc deficiency in humans may manifest as bullous pustular dermatitis of the extremities and in the oral, anal, and genital areas. The hypothesis that a portion of the dermatitis seen in the elderly is due to zinc deficiency has not been tested extensively. Weismann and colleagues[37] identified a number of individuals in an institution for elderly people who had skin problems similar to those described in zinc deficiency. A number of these subjects had subnormal plasma zinc concentrations; supplementation with zinc for 4 weeks did not result in improvement in their skin lesions, however.

The hypothesis that zinc nutriture is related to the immune response in elderly people has attracted considerable attention. Elderly individuals are more susceptible to some infectious diseases, and the consequences of such infections may be more severe.[38] Data in humans indicate that the defect associated with aging is in the delayed immune mechanisms, expressed as deficits in delayed dermal hypersensitivity and a failure of T lymphocytes to respond to stimulation.[39] It is known that severe zinc deficiency markedly impairs cellular immunity,[40–42] but the effects of a less severely deficient state are not as well documented. Two studies have reported beneficial effects of zinc supplementation on cellular immunity in elderly subjects,[43,44] although neither study was conducted with a double-blind research design and the number of individuals examined was small. A double-blind zinc intervention trial by Bogden and colleagues[24] was begun in 1987. Baseline data revealed that responses to seven skin test antigens were significantly associated with plasma zinc concentrations and that in vitro lymphocyte proliferative responses to various mitogens were related to various measures of cellular zinc levels. Although subsequent findings by this group[45] reported a decrease in delayed dermal hypersensitivity in response to supplementation with 15 mg of zinc per day, a further study by this group found that zinc supplementation did improve immune status[46]; reasons for the differences in findings are not readily apparent. Others have reported that zinc supplementation for the elderly resulted in improvement in various measures of immunity.[32,47]

Given that dietary intakes are generally less than the RDA and that there are potential beneficial effects of normalizing suboptimal zinc status, it seems prudent to recommend that all elderly people routinely take a small supplement of zinc. It should be pointed out, however, that excessive use of zinc supplements can result in alterations in copper balance and may affect lipoprotein profiles by reducing high-density cholesterol levels. Use of pharmacologic dosages of zinc for prolonged periods can result in frank copper deficiency and impaired immune responses.[48]

## COPPER

Of the various trace minerals, copper was one of the first to be recognized as an essential nutrient. The concentration of copper in milk is very low.[49] Feeding a milk-based diet to rats resulted in a severe hypochromic, microcytic anemia that was unresponsive to iron but that was cured by copper administration.[50] Further research has identified many of the biological roles of copper, which are primarily as a component of various copper-containing enzymes. As reviewed by Linder,[51] important roles for copper-containing enzymes include the production of free energy (adenosine triphosphate [ATP]) by the electron transport chain of oxidative phosphorylation in the mitochondria (cytochrome c oxidase) and the maintenance of antioxidant defenses (superoxide dismutases, both intracellular and extracellular, ceruloplasmin, and intracellular copper thioneins). Other important functions associated with copper-containing enzymes include the molecular oxygen-requiring reactions that lead to cross-linking of amino acids such as the lysyl oxidase of connective tissue, needed for proper maturation of collagen, and elastin, essential for wound healing and the maintenance of the integrity of blood vessels. In addition, the production of the melanin important to protect the skin from ultraviolet light and the pigmentation of hair are accomplished by a copper-containing enzyme (tyrosinase).

Copper deficiency has been produced experimentally in a number of species and has been observed in livestock and occasionally in humans. Symptoms of the deficient state are somewhat species specific but are usually manifest in humans as a hypochromic, microcytic anemia; a deficiency of white blood cells (leukopenia), especially of the neutrophilic leukocytes; decreases in ceruloplasmin and erythrocyte superoxide dismutase; hypercholesterolemia; increased turnover of red blood cells; and development of abnormal electrocardiographic patterns.[51] These manifestations of the deficiency can be largely explained by decreased activity of the various copper-containing enzymes or proteins.

Although copper has been known to be an essential trace metal for more than 60 years, there is substantial uncertainty about the requirements for humans.[52] Copper deficiency has been observed in humans and its essentiality thus proven, but RDAs are not available. Instead, the Committee on Dietary Allowances of the Food and Nutrition Board lists copper in the Estimated Safe and Adequate Daily Dietary Intake (SADDI) category; for adults, this value is 1.5 to 3.0 mg/d.[6] Evaluation of various diets for copper content showed that many provided less than 2.0 mg/d and that intakes of less than 1 mg/d were not uncommon.[7,53] Actual intakes of copper by adults on self-selected diets have been estimated to be slightly more than 1 mg/d on average but vary considerably (0.6–1.6 mg/d).[54]

Although the exact amount of copper required is not firmly established and is known to be affected by other dietary variables such as protein and zinc intakes, the requirement for young men seems to be in the range of 1.0 to 2.0 mg/d.[53,55] There are relatively few studies of copper requirements of elderly people. With mean intakes of 3.2 mg/d, copper balance was close to zero for elderly men in two studies conducted by Turnlund and colleagues.[56,57] Burke and colleagues found that 8 of 10 elderly subjects were in positive copper balance at 2.33 mg/d.[58] Healthy elderly subjects studied by Bunker and colleagues were not able to maintain balance at intakes of 1.28 mg/d.[21] For house-bound elderly, intakes of 0.87 mg/d resulted in substantial negative copper balance.[21] When these observations are combined with those of Turnlund and colleagues that younger individuals could maintain balance at intakes as low as 0.8 mg/d[59] and perhaps lower if sufficient periods of adaptation were allowed,[60] it appears that the elderly have a higher requirement for copper to maintain balance than do younger individuals and that the requirement is probably within the range of the SADDI of 1.5 to 3.0 mg/d.

Relatively few studies have been designed to assess copper intakes of elderly people directly. Gibson and colleagues[61] reported that the mean copper intake of vegetarian women (mean age of 69 years) was 2.1 mg/d. More recently, Gibson and colleagues,[19] using duplicate diet analyses, reported that mean intake for elderly Canadian women was 1.2 mg/d. This value was similar to that of 1.28 mg/d obtained for healthy elderly people in England.[20] For house-bound elderly people, copper intake was determined to be 0.87 mg/d.[20] Even lower intakes (mean of 0.67 with a range from 0.23 to 1.15 mg/d) were reported for hospitalized elderly women ranging in age from 76 to 99 years.[62] A recent nationwide survey of individuals in the United States aged 60 to 65 years showed mean daily intakes of 0.86 mg for women and 1.18 mg for men.[63] These data indicate that many or most elderly do not consume sufficient copper to meet the SADDI of 1.5 to 3.0 mg/d and that for a subset of the elderly, copper consumption is clearly inadequate to meet required needs.

The density of copper in the diet affects an individual's ability to meet physiological needs. Solomons[64] has estimated the critical nutrient density for copper to be 1.2 mg/1000 kcal for elderly men and 1.7 mg/1000 kcal for elderly women. In examining diets of house-bound elderly people, Bunker and colleagues[21] obtained values of 0.63 mg/1000 kcal for men and 0.70 mg/1000 kcal for women. These values are similar to values for healthy elderly subjects in an earlier study by the same group.[20] Nutrient densities that are approximately the same (0.75 mg/1000 kcal) can be estimated from the study conducted by Gibson and colleagues.[19] Thus, given the energy intake of elderly people, it would seem unlikely that they could choose diets that would meet their needs for copper without inclusion of some very concentrated sources of copper. Copper content of foods can vary more than 100-fold, and examples of the content of copper in various foods are given in Table 5–2.

In addition to food choices that influence nutrient density, several factors may affect the adequacy of copper in the diet. Among these are dietary components that may affect the absorption of copper. Absorption is regulated, in part, by the copper status of the individual but can also be influenced by a substantial number of factors affecting bioavailability.[65] Among those factors that increase copper absorption are citric acid, L-amino acids, phosphate, and gluconic acid. Factors that decrease copper utilization include zinc, iron, cadmium, phytate, fiber, unabsorbed fat, and vitamin C. Individuals who supplement their diets with large quantities of zinc, iron, or vitamin C have added risk of copper deficiency.

The essentiality of copper is well established. Severe deficiencies have been reported in premature infants, in children with severe malnutrition, in patients with severe malabsorption syndromes, and among individuals receiving total parenteral nutrition without adequate copper supplementation. The deficiency is usually manifested by severe anemia, neutropenia, and osteoporosis and, if untreated, may result in death. Such severe copper deficiency is relatively rare and does not usually occur in the absence of other medical problems that impair absorption or storage of copper or that increase the rate of copper lost from the body. The more common state, although the prevalence rate cannot be

**Table 5–2** Copper Content of Common Food

| Food | Amount of Copper/ Portion (mg) |
|---|---|
| Oysters, 3 oz | 3.7 |
| Crab, 3 oz | 1.0 |
| Almonds, 1 oz | 0.3 |
| Peanuts, 1 oz | 0.2 |
| Rye flour, 1 cup | 0.96 |
| Beans, black, 1 cup | 0.5 |
| Codfish, 3 oz | 0.03 |
| Broccoli, 1/2 cup | 0.03 |
| Beef, ground, 3.5 oz | 0.07 |
| Milk, 8 fl oz | 0.02 |

*Source:* Data from J. Pennington, *Bowes and Church's Food Values of Portions Commonly Used*, 17th ed., pp. 3–319, © 1998, Lippincott.

accurately established at present, is that of a mild, chronic copper deficiency. The question of whether mild copper deficiency is a significant nutritional problem in humans was recently addressed by Danks.[66] Possible features of chronic copper deficiency proposed by Danks are anemia and neutropenia refractory to other treatments, osteoporosis, arthritis, arterial and myocardial disease, loss of pigmentation, and neurological effects.

Although none of the above features are proven consequences of a mild, chronic copper deficiency, each has a biochemical or observational rationale that supports its inclusion in this list of suspected outcomes. For example, the anemia seen in copper deficiency has been related to decreased levels of ceruloplasmin, a copper-containing protein in plasma with ferroxidase activity. Ceruloplasmin oxidizes iron from a ferrous to a ferric state, a valence change required in order for the iron released from the intestinal mucosa or parenchymal cells in the liver to bind to transferrin for transport to the erythropoietic cells for the formation of hemoglobin.

Copper's role in bone metabolism and in the prevention of skeletal abnormalities is primarily related to the activity of lysyl oxidase. This copper-containing enzyme is required for establishing cross-linkages in collagen that are essential for the structural integrity of bone. There is a long history of empirical observations consistent with an anti-inflammatory role for copper, perhaps related to its moderating effects in autoimmune diseases such as some forms of arthritis. The role of copper in arterial and myocardial disease is partially related to its function in lysyl oxidase. The formation of cross-linkages of desmosine and isodesmosine in elastin requires lysyl oxidase. Failure to form these cross-linkages results in less elasticity and a weakening of the major blood vessels. Copper deficiency has also been shown to result in hypercholesterolemia, hypertriglyceridemia, glucose intolerance, and hypertension—all risk factors for cardiovascular disease.

Since many of the problems observed with substantial frequency in the elderly are similar to those listed as possible features of chronic copper deficiency, it seems important to obtain better estimates of the prevalence of suboptimal copper intake and status in this group. This is made more difficult by the absence of an unambiguous indicator of copper status and by the lack of clear dietary recommendations or requirements for copper for this age group. Older individuals might be encouraged to include some of the richer sources of copper in their diet; legumes, mushrooms, chocolate, seeds, nuts, crab, peanut butter, liver, and oysters are among those foods having the highest concentration of copper.[52]

## CHROMIUM

The essentiality of chromium for mammals was discovered in 1959 by Schwarz and Mertz,[67] who observed an impaired glucose tolerance in rats fed purified diets that could be corrected by chromium supplementation. Observations with other species, including humans, have confirmed this alteration in glucose tolerance in chromium deficiency, an alteration that can be normalized by provision of adequate chromium.[68] Despite its acceptance as an essential trace mineral, information about the exact biologic function of chromium is limited, in part due to the many technologic difficulties in chromium analysis and uncertainty about the validity of much of the earlier work.[69] It is clear, however, that chromium deficiency manifests with many of the symptoms of diabetes, especially those of impaired glucose tolerance, altered plasma lipid profile, and peripheral neuropathy.[70]

It has been difficult to accurately estimate dietary intake due to the problems associated with the analysis of this mineral. Recent analyses of dietary intake by elderly subjects[71,72] that have used appropriate techniques have reported intakes that are well below the SADDI range of 50 to 200 μg.[6] Offenbacher[73] has also reported intakes for elderly subjects that are well below the SADDI range. It is, however, not clear that the SADDI range is appropriate for it was established using data obtained by older methods of chromium analysis that gave falsely elevated values. Currently available data suggest that a lower SADDI range might be appropriate.[68]

A number of factors can affect the chromium status of an individual. One of these is the amount of chromium in the diet. An evaluation is made difficult by the uncertainty about the requirement or recommended intake against which to gauge intake, as noted above. A second problem is the paucity of data about chromium concentrations with foods—data made more difficult to obtain by the need to use methodology that is available only in a very limited number of laboratories. One of those laboratories is that of Anderson et al,[74] who have recently published values for chromium intakes for various foods. Some values from this reference are given in Table 5–3.

Examination of the values presented in Table 5–3 indicates that there are no clearly rich sources of chromium, with the possible exception of broccoli, which has a concentration of 22 µg/cup. Previous research has also indicated that rich sources of chromium are mushrooms, brewer's yeast, prunes, raisins, nuts, asparagus, and wine.[70] Given the usual density of chromium in the diet, it has been suggested that individuals would need to consume in excess of 3000 kcal/d to meet the minimal recommended intake of 50 µg—intakes of energy greater than usual intakes among the elderly[75] and greater than recommendations of the RDAs.[6] While these data may be taken to imply that individuals do not require as much as 50 µg/d, the elderly are also likely to be more vulnerable to developing a chromium-deficient state because their energy intake is so low. In addition to dietary intakes, chromium status may be affected by other dietary choices. For example, the consumption of high-sugar diets (35% of total calories from simple sugars) was reported to increase urinary chromium excretion when compared with excretion where diets contained only 15% of total calories from simple sugars.[76]

The lack of an accurate method for assessing chromium status has made it difficult to estimate prevalence of chromium deficiency in any population. An inference of a chromium-deficient state has been made by several investigators on the basis of a positive response in some indicator (usually glucose tolerance) to chromium supplementation.

**Table 5–3** Chromium Content of Selected Foods (µg/Serving)

| | |
|---|---|
| Whole milk, 1 cup | <0.12 |
| Eggs, 1 egg | 0.20 |
| Beef cubes, 3 oz | 2.0 |
| Haddock, 3 oz | 0.60 |
| Whole wheat bread, 1 slice | 0.98 |
| Dinner roll, 1 roll | 0.62 |
| Spaghetti, 1 cup | 0.28 |
| Rice, white, 1 cup | 1.2 |
| Apple, peeled, 1 med | 0.40 |
| Orange, peeled, 1 med | 0.39 |
| Juice, orange, 1 cup | 2.2 |
| Green beans, 1 cup | 2.2 |
| Carrots, raw, 1 carrot | 0.29 |
| Broccoli, 1 cup | 22.0 |
| Orange sherbet, 1 cup | 1.4 |
| Peanut butter, 1 tbsp | 0.61 |

*Source:* Reprinted with permission from R. Anderson et al., Dietary Chromium Intake: Freely Chosen Diets, Institutional Diets, and Individual Foods, *Biological Trace Element Research*, Vol. 32, pp. 117–121, © 1992, Humana Press, Inc.

Among those studies using elderly subjects, Urberg and Zemel[77] observed improved glucose tolerance with supplementation of 200 µg of chromium per day as chromium chloride, and a study by Martinez and colleagues[78] found that about half of their elderly subjects showed improved glucose tolerance with chromium supplementation. Abraham and colleagues[79] did not report lower fasting glucose concentrations among subjects given chromium supplements but did find an improvement in lipid profiles. Although the lack of a method for clearly assessing status makes determination of a deficient state difficult, it seems reasonable to infer that subjects who are chromium deficient will be those who will respond to normalization of chromium status and that the removal of a deficient state should be reflected in an improved glucose tolerance and improvement in lipid profile measures.

## SELENIUM

Selenium is known to be an essential nutrient for a number of species, including humans.[80] A number of diseases are caused by simultaneous deficiencies of selenium and vitamin E. For example, liver necrosis in rats, exudative diathesis in chicks, mulberry heart in swine, and some forms of muscular dystrophy in lambs and calves can be prevented or cured by supplementation with either selenium or vitamin E. These examples demonstrate the known biochemical roles for selenium as a component of glutathione peroxidase and for vitamin E as an antioxidant, both providing protection against the peroxides and free radicals that have their most damaging effects on cell membranes in blood, liver, and other tissues.

Roles for selenium independent of vitamin E status have also been demonstrated. Pancreatic degeneration occurs in chicks, even if vitamin E intake is adequate. Pure selenium deficiency in experimental animals resulted in growth retardation, cataract formation, sparse hair coats, and reproductive failure.[81] For humans, selenium deficiency is clearly a causative factor in Keshan disease (a cardiomyopathy primarily affecting children in the Keshan region of China) and is related to Kashin-Beck disease (an osteoarthropathy with disturbances of endochondral ossification and deformity of the affected joints, observed in people living in some regions of China where there are low levels of selenium in the soil). In addition, cardiomyopathy and skeletal muscle weakness have been associated with the use of total parenteral nutrition without adequate levels of selenium.[82] All of these conditions respond to selenium supplementation.

A role for selenium as an anticancer agent seems well established in animal experiments,[83] although the levels of selenium required to provide protection are relatively high.[84] Epidemiological studies have linked lower selenium intakes with higher incidences of cancers of the colon, rectum, prostate, breast, and leukocytes.[85] Several studies of humans suggest that selenium status does play a protective role in the development of several cancers,[86,87] particularly if the levels of other antioxidants (ie, vitamin E and carotenoids) are low.[88] These studies suggest that selenium, through its function as an antioxidant, has a role in cancer prevention, although definitive proof of this in humans is still not available. It has also been suggested that selenium may have a role, again as a component of glutathione peroxidase acting as an antioxidant, in slowing some of the changes seen as part of the aging process. This is most evident in reductions in the levels of lipofuscein pigments and peroxidative damage to cellular membranes and subcellular components.[89]

Mean selenium intake in the United States as assessed by nationwide food surveys is 108 µg/d,[90] and thus a well-balanced diet will provide adequate selenium to satisfy the newly established RDAs of 70 µg for men and 55 µg for women.[6] Studies reporting selenium intakes and status in elderly populations are quite limited. For healthy elderly, selenium intake and status do not appear to be low,[91] and intakes do not differ between healthy young and healthy elderly individuals. Other studies have shown selenium intakes of 77.6 ± 44.5 µg for a population of elderly Canadian women; 21% of these had intakes of less than 50 µg/d.[19] These values were similar to those reported for adults aged 60 years and older in the United States[92] and a bit lower than values (94 ± 43 µg) reported by

Lane and colleagues[93] for elderly adults. Lower selenium status has been reported for elderly house-bound individuals and could be related to lower selenium intakes,[94] and Schmuck and colleagues[62] reported very low intakes of selenium and lower levels of glutathione peroxidase activities, indicating selenium deficiency, among elderly women who were hospitalized.

When levels of intake were near the RDAs, most elderly subjects had biochemical indications of sufficient status as assessed by serum selenium concentration (0.115 ± 0.03 µg/mL)[19] in comparison with a reference value of 0.096 µg/mL.[95] The selenium content of food varies widely, as does its relative bioavailability. In general, organ meats and seafoods contain 0.4 to 1.5 µg/g, muscle meats 0.1 to 0.4 µg/g, cereals and grains less than 0.1 to greater than 0.8 µg/g, dairy products less than 0.1 to 0.3 µg/g, and fruits and vegetables less than 0.1 µg/g.[82]

Although the role of selenium in the antioxidant defenses of an organism is well recognized, there is little evidence of clear clinical disorders that can be directly related to suboptimal selenium intakes or marginal levels of selenium deficiency. Nor is there any evidence that provision of selenium at levels in excess of the current RDAs would provide beneficial effects in preventing chronic diseases such as cancer or cardiovascular disease.[96] Any use of selenium supplementation in excess of the RDAs would need to be considered in light of the known toxic effects of this essential trace metal. An estimate of an intake that would be safe is 5 µg/kg of body weight per day, or 350 µg of total intake for a 70-kg man.[97] Symptoms associated with selenium toxicity include nausea, vomiting, hair loss, nail changes, irritability, fatigue, and peripheral neuropathy.[82]

## ALUMINUM

Aluminum is not known to be required for any natural metabolic process and therefore is not thought to be an essential nutrient.[98] Although aluminum-containing compounds were considered to be essentially nonhazardous for many years, concerns about the potentially toxic effects of aluminum as it accumulates in tissues have been increasing during the last two decades.[99] This concern has prompted examinations of dietary intakes of aluminum, of response to pharmaceutical-based exposure, and of manifestations of toxicity.

Dietary exposure to aluminum includes that which is present naturally and that which comes from aluminum-containing food additives; other exposure arises from contact with aluminum used in food containers, cookware, utensils, and food wrapping. Most foods and beverages contain low concentrations of aluminum naturally; exceptions are tea, herbs, and spices.[100] Of the three factors affecting the aluminum content of foods, the aluminum-containing food additives have the greatest effects in increasing aluminum levels. For example, processed cheese contains 0.3 mg of aluminum per gram, whereas cheddar cheese contains 0.002 mg; white bread contains 0.003 mg/g, whereas baking powder biscuits contain 0.016 mg/g due to the inclusion of baking powder, which contains 2.3 mg/g.[101] The major food sources of aluminum in daily diets are grain products with aluminum additives, along with processed cheese, tea, herbs, spices, and salt with aluminum additives. Little aluminum is contributed to the diet by meat, poultry, fish, fruit, vegetables, fats and oils, or sugar and sweeteners. A distribution of aluminum intakes among various food groups has been calculated for a mixed diet containing 2541 kcal (Table 5–4).

**Table 5–4** Aluminum Intake in a Diet of 2541 kcal/d

| Foods | Aluminum Intake | |
| --- | --- | --- |
| | mg/d | % |
| Milk, yogurt, cheese | 3.69 | 27.0 |
| Meat, poultry, fish | 0.41 | 3.0 |
| Grains and grain products | 4.98 | 36.5 |
| Vegetables | 0.52 | 3.8 |
| Fruits | 0.02 | 0.1 |
| Mixed dishes | 0.69 | 5.1 |
| Fats, sweets, condiments | 0.23 | 1.7 |
| Beverages | 0.83 | 6.1 |
| Desserts | 2.26 | 16.6 |
| Nuts and seeds | 0.02 | 0.1 |
| Total | 13.65 | 100.0 |

*Source:* Values from *Journal of American Dietetic Association* (1989;89:659–664).

Aluminum can be transferred from aluminum food preparation equipment, particularly if the foods are acidic or exposure is prolonged. For example, the aluminum in tomato sauce increased from 0.1 mg/kg (net weight) to 57.1 mg/kg after the sauce was cooked in an aluminum pan.[102] This route is not, however, a major or consistent source of dietary aluminum. Total intakes of aluminum are variable, primarily depending on the inclusion of aluminum-containing food additives in the diet, but they are estimated to be about 9 mg/d for adult women and 12 to 14 mg/d for adult men.[100] Intakes in this range currently are not thought to pose a health risk.

The quantities of aluminum consumed in food and beverages are small when compared with those that can be ingested in pharmaceutical products such as antacids, buffered analgesics, antidiarrheal medications, and certain antiulcer drugs. Lione[103] estimated that daily intakes of aluminum could be 800 to 5000 mg from antacids and 126 to 728 mg from buffered analgesics. Such high levels of intake may have adverse consequences, particularly when there is a preexisting medical condition such as uremia.

Consequences of aluminum toxicity have been reported for several clinical conditions. Uremic patients undergoing dialysis and receiving dialysate fluids contaminated with aluminum and patients receiving aluminum-containing parenteral fluids have manifested aluminum toxicity.[104] Clinical signs of toxicity generally include osteodystrophy, encephalopathy, and anemia.[105] The osteodystrophy may be expressed as bone pain, an increased incidence of fractures, and a histological manifestation with aluminum-containing osteomalacic components. The symptoms of encephalopathy include dementia, speech difficulties, and motor abnormalities. The anemia is of the normochromic, normocytic type, most likely related to disturbances in heme synthesis and porphyrin metabolism, although the exact mechanism involved has yet to be identified. These symptoms are sometimes seen in uremic patients, especially children, who have not been exposed to aluminum-contaminated dialysis or intravenous fluids; the source of aluminum in these cases appears to be the aluminum-containing binder used to treat hyperphosphatemia.[106]

Most interest in aluminum toxicity as it relates to elderly people who are not on dialysis or parenteral feeding regimens is related to the putative connection between deposition of aluminum in the brain and the development of various senile dementias, including Alzheimer's disease.[107] It has been reported that individuals with Alzheimer's disease and with amyotrophic lateral sclerosis (Lou Gehrig disease) with Parkinsonism dementia had increased levels of aluminum in regions of the brain that also contain the neurofibrillary tangles associated with these dementias.[108] *Dementia* refers here to a progressive loss of cognitive function commonly involving memory, orientation, abstract thinking, and the ability to learn new tasks. The hypothesis that aluminum is part of the etiology of various dementias remains controversial. However, it is clear from experimental studies using animal models and in those humans who have had severe exposure to aluminum that if aluminum does gain access to the central nervous system, it acts as a potent neurotoxin.[109]

Under normal physiologic conditions, relatively little aluminum is absorbed by the gastrointestinal system after oral exposure, and, of the portion absorbed, only a much smaller amount is deposited in the central nervous system. It is therefore likely that under normal conditions, these natural barriers keep virtually all of the aluminum out of the central nervous system. However, Perl[108] has suggested that under conditions of advancing age, genetic predisposition, or possibly viral damage, these barriers may become impaired, allowing the element to gain access to the central nervous system, possibly inducing the neurofibrillary tangles. Supporting this hypothesis are reports that aluminum tends to accumulate in the brain with age.[110,111] The body's ability to remove the aluminum that has been absorbed may be diminished in the older individual. The decline in renal function observed with aging,[112] and the fact that the major excretory route for aluminum absorbed into the body is via the urine,[113] suggests that aging might promote accumulation of aluminum in the body. There has been very little research on the effects of aging on aluminum metabolism; therefore, much of the concern about the potential hazards of aluminum exposure for older individuals remains unresolved.

## MOLYBDENUM

The essentiality of molybdenum has been established for a number of species, including humans.[114] Molybdenum participates in a variety of enzymatic reactions as an essential cofactor termed *molybdopterin*, an alkylphosphate-substituted pterin to which molybdenum is coordinated through two sulfur atoms.[115] These molybdenum-containing enzymes are involved in the metabolism of purine, pyrimidines, pteridines, and aldehydes and in the oxidation of sulfite.[116] Demonstration of essentiality for humans has been based largely on studies of inborn errors of metabolism involving deficiencies in one or more of the molybdenum-containing enzymes. Affected individuals experience seizures, severe mental retardation, dislocation of the ocular lenses, and eventually death.[117] There is one report of a nutritional deficiency of molybdenum in a patient undergoing total parenteral nutrition.[118] Clinical symptoms included mental disturbances that progressed to coma, tachycardia, tachypnea, and night blindness; symptoms were eliminated by supplementation with 300 µg of ammonium molybdate per day. Changes were attributed to a loss of sulfite oxidase activity.

Molybdenum is widely distributed in soils, plants, and animal tissues. The richest sources of the element include legumes, cereal grains (and hence bread and baked products), leafy vegetables, milk, liver, and kidney. Fruits, stem and root vegetables, and muscle meats are among the poorest sources.[117] By chemical analysis of common foods, Tsongas and colleagues[119] have determined that the average intake in the United States is 0.18 mg/d. Intakes were lower for older individuals (men aged 65 to 74 years, 0.16 mg; men aged 75+ years, 0.14 mg; women aged 65 to 74 years, 0.12 mg; women aged 75+ years, 0.12 mg). These data are consistent with more recently obtained data by Pennington and Jones,[120] but it should be noted that many diets provided intakes of 50 to 100 µg/d, values less than the SADDI of 75 to 250 µg/d set by the Committee on Dietary Allowances.[6] With intakes of 0.1 to 0.2 mg of molybdenum per day, there are no reports of molybdenum deficiency in human populations. American diets appear to provide such levels of molybdenum intake easily. The use of molybdenum supplements is not advised. In animals, excessive molybdenum intake results in copper deficiency and other deleterious effects unrelated to impaired copper status; in humans, there is some suggestion that elevated levels of molybdenum intake may increase the incidence of gout.[116] Humans exposed to 10 to 15 mg of molybdenum per day displayed abnormally high serum uric acid levels and tissue xanthine oxidase activities, with symptoms of recurrent pain in the knees, interphalangeal joints of the hands, and metatarsalphalangeal joints of the feet, associated with erythema, edema, and joint deformity.[119]

## MANGANESE

Manganese is an essential element for many species, including humans. Among various animal species, the main manifestations of manganese deficiency include impaired growth, skeletal abnormalities, disturbed or depressed reproductive function, ataxia of the newborn, and defects in lipid and carbohydrate metabolism.[121] For a single human subject inadvertently rendered manganese deficient during an experimental study, the manifestations included hypocholesterolemia, weight loss, transient dermatitis, occasional nausea and vomiting, changes in hair and beard color, and slow growth of beard and hair.[122] A recent study by Friedman and colleagues[123] that fed a manganese-deficient diet to young men observed a dermatitis and reported changes in plasma calcium, phosphorus, and alkaline phosphatase concentrations consistent with alterations in bone remodeling that have been proposed by Strause and colleagues[124] as a manifestation of manganese deficiency.

Manganese can function in the body both as an enzyme activator and as a constituent of metalloenzymes. Arginase, the cytosolic enzyme responsible for urea synthesis; pyruvate carboxylase, a key enzyme in gluconeogenesis required for the synthesis of oxaloacetate from pyruvate; and mitochondrial manganese-superoxide dismutase, which catalyzes the disproportionation of superoxide to hydrogen peroxide and oxygen, are examples of manganese metalloenzymes. Defects in carbohydrate metabolism and increased lipid peroxidation, especially after exposure to hyperbaric oxygen, ozone, or ethanol, may be related to loss of enzymatic activity subsequent to development of manganese deficiency. Manganese can also activate various enzymes. Of particular importance is the manganese-specific activation of glycosyltransferases.[125] It is believed that the skeletal deformities and neonatal ataxia seen in manganese deficiency are due to impairment of cartilage synthesis as a result of decreased activity of the glycosyltransferases.

Common foods in human diets are highly variable in manganese concentration. In general, the highest manganese levels occur in nuts and whole-grain cereals; variable amounts are found in vegetables, and low concentrations are found in meat, fish, and dairy products. Tea and coffee are exceptionally rich in manganese.[126] Only a few studies have evaluated the manganese intake of older persons. A study of Canadian women by Gibson and colleagues[61] revealed that vegetarians (mean age 69 years) had greater dietary intakes (4.4 mg/d) than did nonvegetarian women (mean age 60 years; intakes of 2.6 mg/d); among the nonvegetarians, 43% had dietary intakes less than the lower value of 2.5 to 5.0 mg/d of the SADDI.[6] In a subsequent study of Canadian women ranging in age from 58 to 89 years with a mean age of 66 years, average intake was 3.8 mg/d; 27% had intakes less than 2.5 mg/d.[127] In the United States, Pennington and colleagues[63] reported intakes of 2.2 mg/d for women aged 60 to 65 years and 2.6 mg/d for men aged 60 to 65 years.

The SADDI for manganese of 2.5 to 5.0 mg/d[6] is based on data obtained from a relatively small number of subjects and from studies using a very limited range of intakes. More recent studies have reported that 3.5 mg/d is required to maintain balance in young men,[128] that intakes of 2.43 mg/d resulted in negative balance in postmenopausal women,[129] and that recalculation of data derived from a number of manganese balance studies in the literature suggests a recommended range of intakes of 3.5 to 7.0 mg/d.[130] Reports that a number of dietary components such as fiber and phytate,[131,132] calcium,[133] iron,[134] and sugar[129] have detrimental effects on either the absorption or the retention of manganese would seem to indicate that the needs for manganese might be greater than values set in the SADDI.

It is not clear why the apparently insufficient dietary intakes of manganese (based on both the published SADDI and the more recent estimates of requirements to maintain balance) are not reflected in recognized manganese-deficient states. It may be that more

marginal levels of deficiency are not easily recognized. Clearly, there is insufficient information or research about which manifestations of manganese deficiency might be observed if the deficiency were less severe. However, the use of balance experiments, although these are the most commonly used techniques to determine manganese requirements, may not be entirely appropriate. Results from a factorial design experiment (one designed to determine obligatory losses) indicate that the minimal requirement is 0.74 mg/d.[123] Reconciliation of these vastly different estimates of manganese requirements requires further work. Particular concerns that older individuals may have for how their bodies handle manganese, whether there are additional needs or larger requirements for this essential element, and whether some of the consequences of aging can be related to insufficient manganese status remain to be addressed.

## NICKEL

Nickel is probably an essential nutrient for humans, although this has not been definitely proven on the basis of the development of a deficient state, the presence of consistent deficiency symptoms, or the prevention or cure of a deficient state by provision of physiologic levels of this element. Nickel deficiencies, however, have been produced in a number of animal models (chicks, cows, goats, minipigs, rats, and sheep); the most prominent and consistent symptoms are reduced hematopoiesis, depressed growth, and various metabolic alterations.[135] Despite the recognition of these deficiency signs in animals, there is no firmly established biologic function for nickel in humans or animals. It is thought that nickel functions as a cofactor or structural component in specific metalloenzymes (as is the case for enzymes from a number of plants and microorganisms).[114]

The great effort that must be made to minimize dietary and environmental contamination in order to generate nickel deficiency in animals and the failure to observe the deficiency in humans suggest that the requirement for nickel is quite low and easily met by the diets consumed or, in some cases, even by environmental pollution with nickel-containing dust.[135] Inhalation and ingestion constitute the major routes of nickel intake in humans. Total dietary intakes vary greatly in the amounts and proportions of foods with varying nickel content. Foods that contain generally high concentrations of nickel (more than 0.3 μg/g) include nuts, leguminous seeds, shellfish, cacao products, and hydrogenated shortenings; grains, cured meats, and vegetables are generally intermediate in concentration (0.1 to 0.3 μg/g); and fish, milk, and eggs are generally low (less than 0.1 μg/g).[136] Nickel intake is probably in the range of 150 to 700 μg/d.[135] Such intakes easily meet the needs of the individual. The use of nickel supplements is not advisable. Oral nickel, in not particularly high doses, can adversely affect human health. Nickel dermatitis has been estimated to occur at a prevalence rate of between 3% and 13%. For sensitive individuals, an oral dose of as little as 0.6 mg has been shown to be sufficient to produce a positive reaction.[136]

## IODINE

Iodine is an integral part of the thyroid hormones thyroxine and triiodothyronine and as such is an essential nutrient for all animal species. A deficiency in iodine can result in endemic goiter and cretinism. Severe deficiencies of iodine remain a serious public health problem, particularly in less economi-cally developed regions of the world. For more industrialized regions of the world, iodine exposure is more than adequate to meet metabolic demands.

Iodine occurs in the food supply from endogenous sources and from the use of iodized salt. In addition, several adventitious sources of iodine contribute to total intake. Iodates are used as dough-conditioning agents in the continuous-vacuum/mix process for making bread and in iodine-containing disinfectants and iodine-containing additives in animal feeds. Milk and dairy products, as well as bread and bakery products, are the largest sources of iodine in human foods.[137]

The RDA for iodine for both men and women is set at 150 μg/d.[6] It is unlikely that individual intake would fall below this amount. Intakes for persons aged 60 to 65 years recently have been determined to be 270 μg for women and 360 μg for men; these intakes were averaged over the years 1982 to 1986.[63] There has been a decline in the intake of iodine over the last few years, resulting in intakes nearer the recommended allowance. Intakes of up to 2.0 mg/d are not thought to present a hazard to adults, although higher levels of intake have been associated with an increased incidence of thyrotoxicosis. It is thought that the present iodine intake in the United States is safe and decreasing toward recommended levels.[6]

## CONCLUSION

It is clear that we do not know enough about the requirements for various trace minerals, particularly about the needs of older individuals. Many of the physiologic changes that accompany aging probably interfere with optimal absorption, utilization, or retention of these minerals. Changes in dietary practices, both the decrease in food consumption that typically accompanies aging and changes in dietary choices, can be expected to adversely affect the trace mineral adequacy of the diet. When these changes are coupled with the effects of various disease processes and the medications used to treat these conditions, the potential for deficiency states is increased substantially. Evidence has been presented to indicate that the adequacies of zinc, copper, chromium, and manganese are of greatest concern. Intakes of selenium, molybdenum,

nickel, and iodine are unlikely to be deficient in other than very unusual circumstances. Aluminum is of concern only as a toxic mineral; minimization of exposure is appropriate. It is clear that most of the trace minerals discussed are essential for normal health and well-being, and it is very important that optimal status be maintained; however, the theory that some of the deleterious effects of aging can be related to deficiencies in one or more of these essential nutrients remains to be proven.

### REFERENCES

1. Timiras PS. *Physiological Basis of Geriatrics*. New York, NY: Macmillan Publishing Co; 1988.

2. Mertz W. Trace elements and the needs of the elderly. In: Hutchinson M, Munro H, eds. *Nutrition and Aging*. Orlando, Fla: Academic Press, Inc; 1986.

3. Solomons N. Biological availability of zinc in humans. *Am J Clin Nutr*. 1982;35:1046–1075.

4. Smiciklas-Wright H. Aging. In: Brown M, ed. *Present Knowledge in Nutrition*. 6th ed. Washington, DC: International Life Sciences Institute-Nutrition Foundation; 1990.

5. Vallee B, Auld D. Zinc metallochemistry in biochemistry. In: Jolles P, Jornvall H, eds. *Interface between Chemistry and Biochemistry*. Basel, Switzerland: Birkhauser Verlag; 1995.

6. Food and Nutrition Board, National Research Council. *Recommended Dietary Allowances*. 10th ed. Washington, DC: National Academy Press; 1989.

7. Greger J. Trace minerals. In: Chen L, ed. *Nutritional Aspects of Aging*. Boca Raton, Fla: CRC Press; 1986.

8. Sandstead H, Henrikson L, Greger J, et al. Zinc nutriture in the elderly in relation to taste acuity, immune response, and wound healing. *Am J Clin Nutr*. 1982;36:1046–1059.

9. Fosmire G, Manuel P, Smiciklas-Wright H. Dietary intakes and zinc status of an elderly rural population. *J Nutr Elder*. 1984;4:19–30.

10. Pennington J. Intakes of minerals from diets and foods: is there a need for concern? *J Nutr*. 1996;126:2304S–2308S.

11. Solomons N. Trace elements in nutrition of the elderly, 1: established RDAs for iron, zinc, and iodine. *Postgrad Med*. 1986;79:231–242.

12. Harland B, Johnson R, Blenderman E, et al. Calcium, phosphorus, iron, iodine, and zinc in the "total diet." *J Am Diet Assoc*. 1980;77:16–20.

13. Holden J, Wolf W, Mertz W. Zinc and copper in self-selected diets. *J Am Diet Assoc*. 1979;75:23–28.

14. Cousins R. Zinc. In: Ziegler EL, Filer L Jr, eds. *Present Knowledge in Nutrition*. 7th ed. Washington, DC: ILSI Press; 1996.

15. August D, Janghorbani M, Young V. Determination of zinc and copper absorption at three dietary Zn-Cu ratios by using stable isotope methods in young adult and elderly subjects. *Am J Clin Nutr*. 1989;50:1457–1463.

16. Turnlund J, Durkin N, Costa F, Margen S. Stable isotope studies of zinc absorption and retention in young and elderly men. *J Nutr*. 1986;116:1239–1247.

17. Bales C, Steinman L, Freeland-Graves J, et al. The effect of age on plasma zinc, uptake, and taste acuity. *Am J Clin Nutr*. 1986;44:664–669.

18. Couzy F, Kastenmayer P, Mansourian R, et al. Zinc absorption in healthy elderly humans and the effect of diet. *Am J Clin Nutr*. 1993;58:690–694.

19. Gibson R, Martinez O, MacDonald A. The zinc, copper, and selenium status of a selected sample of Canadian elderly women. *J Gerontol.* 1985; 40:296–302.

20. Bunker V, Hinks L, Lawson M, et al. Assessment of zinc and copper status of healthy elderly people using metabolic balance studies and measurement of leukocyte zinc concentrations. *Am J Clin Nutr.* 1984;40:1096–1102.

21. Bunker V, Hinks L, Stansfield M, et al. Metabolic balance studies for zinc and copper in housebound elderly people and the relationship between zinc balance and leukocyte zinc concentrations. *Am J Clin Nutr.* 1987;46:353–359.

22. Patterson P, Lee E, Christensen D, et al. Zinc levels of hospitalized elderly. *J Am Diet Assoc.* 1985;85:186–191.

23. Sahyoun N, Otradovic C, Hartz S, et al. Dietary intakes and biochemical indicators of nutritional status in an elderly, institutionalized population. *Am J Clin Nutr.* 1988;47:524–533.

24. Bogden I, Olesky I, Munves E, et al. Zinc and immunocompetence in the elderly: baseline data on zinc nutriture and immunity in unsupplemented subjects. *Am J Clin Nutr.* 1987;46:524–533.

25. Fulwood R, Johnson C, Bryner I, et al. *Hematological and Nutritional Biochemistry Reference Data for Persons 6 Months–74 Years of Age: United States 1976–1980.* Washington, DC: Public Health Service; 1982. US Dept of Health and Human Services publication PHS 83-1628.

26. Prasad A. Clinical spectrum and diagnostic aspects of zinc deficiency. In: Prasad A, ed. *Essential and Toxic Trace Elements in Human Health and Disease.* New York, NY: Alan R Liss, Inc; 1988.

27. Weiffenbach I, Baum B, Burghauser R. Taste thresholds: quality specific variation with human aging. *J Gerontol.* 1982;37:372–377.

28. Henkin R, Patten B, Re P, et al. Syndrome of acute zinc loss. *Arch Neurol.* 1975;32:745–751.

29. Greger J, Geissler A. Effect of zinc supplementation on taste acuity of the aged. *Am J Clin Nutr.* 1978;31:633–637.

30. Hutton C, Hayes-Davis R. Assessment of the zinc nutritional status of selected elderly subjects. *J Am Diet Assoc.* 1983;82:148–153.

31. Greger J. Dietary intake and nutritional status in regard to zinc of institutionalized aged. *J Gerontol.* 1977;32:549–553.

32. Prasad A, Fitzgerald J, Hess J, et al. Zinc deficiency in elderly patients. *Nutrition.* 1993;9:218–224.

33. Atkin-Thor E, Goddard B, O'Nion J, et al. Hypogeusia and zinc depletion in chronic dialysis patients. *Am J Clin Nutr.* 1978;31:1948–1951.

34. Mahajan S, Prasad A, Lambujon J, et al. Improvement of uremic hypogeusia by zinc: a double blind study. *Am J Clin Nutr.* 1980;33:1517–1521.

35. Wacker W. Biochemistry of zinc: role in wound healing. In: Hambidge K, Nichols B, eds. *Zinc and Copper in Clinical Medicine.* New York, NY: Spectrum Publications; 1978.

36. Hallbook T, Hedelin H. Zinc metabolism and surgical trauma. *Br J Surg.* 1977;64:271–273.

37. Weismann K, Wanscher B, Krakaver R. Oral zinc therapy in geriatric patients with selected skin manifestations and a low plasma zinc level. *Acta Dermatol (Stockholm).* 1978;58:157.

38. Carder I. The effect of aging on susceptibility to infection. *Rev Infect Dis.* 1980;2:801–810.

39. Fernandes G, West A, Good R. Nutrition, immunity and cancer: a review, III: effects of diet on the diseases of aging. *Clin Biol.* 1979;9:91–106.

40. Allen J, Kay N, McClain C. Severe zinc deficiency in humans: association with a reversible T-lymphocyte dysfunction. *Ann Intern Med.* 1981;95:154–157.

41. Oleski J, Westphal M, Shore S, et al. Zinc therapy of depressed cellular immunity in acrodermatitis enteropathica. *Am J Dis Child.* 1979;133:915–918.

42. Pekarek R, Sandstead H, Jacob R, et al. Abnormal cellular immune responses during acquired zinc deficiency. *Am J Clin Nutr.* 1979;32:1466–1471.

43. Duchateau J, Delepresse G, Vrigens R, et al. Beneficial effects of oral zinc supplementation on the immune response of old people. *Am J Med.* 1981;70:1001–1004.

44. Wagner P, Jernigan J, Bailey L, et al. Zinc nutriture and cell-mediated immunity in the aged. *Int J Vitam Nutr Res.* 1983;53:94–101.

45. Bogden J, Oleske J, Lavenhar M, et al. Effects of one year of supplementation with zinc and other micronutrients on cellular immunity in the elderly. *J Am Coll Nutr.* 1990;51:214–225.

46. Bogden J, Bendich A, Kemp F, et al. Daily micronutrient supplements enhance delayed-type hypersensitivity skin test responses in older people. *Am J Clin Nutr.* 1994;60:437–447.

47. Boukaiba N, Flament C, Archer S, et al. A physiological amount of zinc supplementation: effects on nutritional, lipid, and thymic status in an elderly population. *Am J Clin Nutr*. 1993;57:566–572.

48. Fosmire G. Zinc toxicity. *Am J Clin Nutr*. 1990;51:225–227.

49. Pennington J. *Bowes and Church's Food Values of Portions Commonly Used*. 17th ed. Philadelphia, Pa: JB Lippincott; 1998.

50. Hart E, Steenbock H, Waddell J, et al. Iron in nutrition, VII: copper as a supplement to iron for hemoglobin building in the rat. *J Biol Chem*. 1928;77:797–812.

51. Linder M. Copper. In: Ziegler E, Filer L Jr, eds. *Present Knowledge in Nutrition*. 7th ed. Washington, DC: ILSI Press; 1996.

52. Klevay L, Medeiros D. Deliberations and evaluations of the approaches, endpoints and paradigms for dietary recommendations about copper. *J Nutr*. 1996;126:2419S–2426S.

53. Sandstead H. Copper bioavailability and requirements. *Am J Clin Nutr*. 1982;35:809–814.

54. Linder M. *The Biochemistry of Copper*. New York, NY: Plenum Press; 1991.

55. Sandstead H. Are estimates of trace element requirements meeting the needs of the user? In: Mills C, Bremner I, Chesters J, eds. *Trace Elements in Man and Animals-TEMA 5*. Farnham Royal, England: Commonwealth Agricultural Bureaux; 1985.

56. Turnlund J, Costa B, Margen S. Zinc, copper, and iron balance in elderly men. *Am J Clin Nutr*. 1981;34:2641–2647.

57. Turnlund J, Reager R, Costa F. Iron and copper absorption in young and elderly men. *Nutr Res*. 1988;8:333–343.

58. Burke D, DeMicco F, Taper L, et al. Copper and zinc utilization in elderly adults. *J Gerontol*. 1981;36:558–563.

59. Turnlund J, Keen C, Smith R. Copper status and urinary and salivary copper in young men at three levels of dietary copper. *Am J Clin Nutr*. 1990;51:658–664.

60. Turnlund J. Human whole-body copper metabolism. *Am J Clin Nutr*. 1998;67:960S–964S.

61. Gibson R, Anderson B, Sabry J. The trace metal status of a group of post-menopausal vegetarians. *J Am Diet Assoc*. 1983;82:246–250.

62. Schmuck A, Roussel A-M, Arnaud J, et al. Analyzed dietary intakes, plasma concentrations of zinc, copper, selenium, and related antioxidant enzyme activities in hospitalized elderly women. *J Am Coll Nutr*. 1996;15:462–468.

63. Pennington J, Young B, Wilson D. Nutritional elements in U.S. diets: results from the total diet study, 1982 to 1986. *J Am Diet Assoc*. 1989;89:659–664.

64. Solomons N. Trace elements in nutrition of the elderly, 2: SADDIs for copper, manganese, selenium, chromium, molybdenum, and fluoride. *Postgrad Med*. 1986;79:251–263.

65. Cousins R. Absorption, transport, and hepatic metabolism of copper and zinc: special reference to metallothionein and ceruloplasmin. *Physiol Rev*. 1985;65:238–309.

66. Danks D. Copper deficiency in humans. *Annu Rev Nutr*. 1988;8:235–257.

67. Schwarz K, Mertz W. Chromium (III) and the glucose tolerance factor. *Arch Biochem Biophys*. 1959;85:292–295.

68. Stocker B. Chromium. In: Ziegler E, Filer L Jr, eds. *Present Knowledge in Nutrition*. 7th ed. Washington, DC: ILSI Press; 1996.

69. Offenbacher E, Pi-Sunyer F. Chromium in human nutrition. *Annu Rev Nutr*. 1980;8:543–563.

70. Anderson R. Chromium requirements and needs of the elderly. In: Watson R, ed. *Handbook of Nutrition in the Aged*. Boca Raton, Fla: CRC Press; 1985.

71. Bunker V, Lawson M, Delves H, et al. The uptake and excretion of chromium by the elderly. *Am J Clin Nutr*. 1984;39:797–802.

72. Gibson R, Scythes C. Chromium, selenium, and other trace element intakes of a selected sample of Canadian premenopausal women. *Biol Trace Elem Res*. 1984;6:105–116.

73. Offenbacher E. Chromium in the elderly. *Biol Trace Elem Res*. 1992;32:123–131.

74. Anderson R, Bryden N, Polansky M. Dietary chromium intake: freely chosen diets, institutional diets, and individual foods. *Biol Trace Elem Res*. 1992;32:117–121.

75. Hartz SC, Rosenberg IH, Russell RM, eds. *Nutrition in the Elderly: The Boston Nutritional Status Survey*. London, England: Smith-Gordon & Co Ltd; 1992.

76. Kozlovsky A, Moser P, Reiser S, et al. Effects of diets high in simple sugars on urinary chromium losses. *Metabolism*. 1986;35:515–518.

77. Urberg M, Zemel M. Evidence for synergism between chromium and nicotinic acid in the control of glucose tolerance in elderly humans. *Metabolism*. 1987;36:896–899.

78. Martinez O, MacDonald A, Gibson R, et al. Dietary chromium and effect of chromium supplementation on glucose tolerance of elderly Canadian women. *Nutr Res.* 1985;5:609–620.

79. Abraham A, Brooks B, Eylath U. The effect of chromium supplementation on serum glucose and lipids in patients with and without non-insulin dependent diabetes. *Metabolism.* 1992;41:768–771.

80. Combs G Jr, Levander D, Spallholz I, et al. *Selenium in Biology and Medicine, Parts A and B.* New York, NY: Van Nostrand Reinhold Co; 1987.

81. McCoy K, Weswig P. Some selenium responses in the rat not related to vitamin E. *Euro J Nutr.* 1969;98:383–389.

82. Levander O, Burk R. Selenium. In: Ziegler E, Filer L Jr, eds. *Present Knowledge in Nutrition.* 7th ed. Washington, DC: ILSI Press; 1996.

83. Milner J. The effects of selenium on virally induced and transplantable tumor models. *Fed Proc.* 1985;44:2568–2572.

84. Combs G Jr, Combs S. *The Role of Selenium in Nutrition.* Orlando, Fla: Academic Press; 1986.

85. Schrauzer G, White D, Schneider C. Cancer mortality correlation studies, III: statistical associations with dietary selenium intakes. *Bioinorg Chem.* 1977;7:23–24.

86. Lewko W, McConnell U. Observations on selenium in human breast cancer. In: Combs G Jr, Levander O, Spallholz I, et al, eds. *Selenium in Biology and Medicine, Parts A and B.* New York, NY: Van Nostrand Reinhold Co; 1987.

87. Saito K, Saito T, Hosokawa T, et al. Blood selenium level and the interaction of copper, zinc, and manganese in stomach cancer. In: Combs G Jr, Levander O, Spallholz I, et al, eds. *Selenium in Biology and Medicine, Parts A and B.* New York, NY: Van Nostrand Reinhold Co; 1987.

88. Clark L, Turnbull B, Graham G, et al. Nonmelanoma skin cancer and plasma selenium: a prospective cohort study. In: Combs G Jr, Levander O, Spallholz I, et al, eds. *Selenium in Biology and Medicine, Parts A and B.* New York, NY: Van Nostrand Reinhold Co; 1987.

89. Yuncie A, Hsu I. Role of selenium in aging. In: Combs G Jr, Levander O, Spallholz I, et al, eds. *Selenium in Biology and Medicine, Parts A and B.* New York, NY: Van Nostrand Reinhold Co; 1987.

90. Pennington J, Wilson D, Newell R, et al. Selected minerals in food surveys, 1974–1981/82. *J Am Diet Assoc.* 1984;84:771–780.

91. Abdulla M, Behbehani A, Dashti H. Dietary intake and bioavailability of trace elements. *Biol Trace Elem Res.* 1989;21:173–178.

92. Thimaya S, Ganapathy S. Selenium in human hair in relation to age, diet, pathological condition, and serum levels. *Sci Total Environ.* 1982;24:41–49.

93. Lane A, Warran D, Taylor B, et al. Blood selenium and glutathione peroxidase levels and dietary selenium of free-living and institutionalized elderly subjects. *Proc Soc Exp Biol Med.* 1983; 173:87–95.

94. Lowik M, van den Berg H, Schrijver J, et al. Marginal nutritional status among institutionalized elderly women as compared to those living more independently (Dutch Nutrition Surveillance System). *J Am Coll Nutr.* 1992;11:673–681.

95. Iyengar V, Woittiez J. Trace elements in human clinical specimens: evaluations of literature data to identify reference values. *Clin Chem.* 1988; 34:474–481.

96. Levander O. A global view of human selenium nutrition. *Annu Rev Nutr.* 1987;7:227–250.

97. Abernathy C, Cantilli R, Du J, et al. Essentiality versus toxicity: some considerations in the risk assessment of essential trace elements. In: Saxena J, ed. *Hazard Assessment of Chemicals.* Vol. 8. Washington, DC: Taylor & Francis; 1993.

98. Underwood E. *Trace Elements in Human and Animal Nutrition.* 4th ed. New York, NY: Academic Press; 1977.

99. Greger J. Aluminum and tin. *World Rev Nutr Diet.* 1987;54:255–285.

100. Pennington J. Aluminum content of foods and diets. *Food Addit Contam.* 1988;5:161–232.

101. Greger J. Dietary and other sources of aluminum intake. In: Chadwick D, Whelan J, eds. *Aluminum in Biology and Medicine.* Chichester, England: Wiley and Sons Ltd; 1992.

102. Greger J. Aluminum in the diet and mineral metabolism. In: Sigel H, ed. *Metal Ions in Biological Systems.* New York, NY: Marcel Dekker; 1988.

103. Lione A. Aluminum intake from non-prescription drugs and sucralfate. *Gen Pharmacol.* 1985; 16:223–228.

104. Greger J. Potential for trace mineral deficiencies and toxicities in the elderly. In: Bales C, ed. *Min-*

*eral Homeostasis in the Elderly.* New York, NY: Alan R Liss Inc; 1989.

105. Wills M, Savory J. Aluminum toxicity and chronic renal failure. In: Sigel H, ed. *Metal Ions in Biological Systems.* New York, NY: Marcel Dekker; 1988.

106. Committee on Nutrition. Aluminum toxicity in infants and children. *Pediatrics.* 1986;78:1150–1154.

107. Chadwick D, Whelan J, eds. *Aluminum in Biology and Medicine.* Chichester, England: Wiley and Sons Ltd; 1992.

108. Perl D. Aluminum and Alzheimer's disease, methodologic approaches. In: Sigel H, ed. *Metal Ions in Biological Systems.* New York, NY: Marcel Dekker; 1988.

109. Kruck R, McLachlan D. Mechanisms of aluminum neurotoxicity: relevance to human disease. In: Sigel H, ed. *Metal Ions in Biological Systems.* New York, NY: Marcel Dekker; 1988.

110. McDermott J, Smith I, Iqbal K, et al. Brain aluminum in aging and Alzheimer disease. *Neurology.* 1979;29:809–814.

111. Markesbery W, Ehmann W, Hosain T, et al. Instrumental neutron activation analysis of brain aluminum in Alzheimer's disease and aging. *Ann Neurol.* 1981;10:511–516.

112. Epstein M. Effects of aging on the kidney. *Fed Proc.* 1979;38:168–171.

113. Ganrot P. Metabolism and possible health effects of aluminum. *Environ Health Perspect.* 1986; 65:363–441.

114. Nielsen F. Other trace elements. In: Ziegler K, Filer L Jr, eds. *Present Knowledge in Nutrition.* 7th ed. Washington, DC: ILSI Press; 1996.

115. Kramer S, Johnson I, Ribeiro A, et al. The structure of the molybdenum cofactor. *J Biol Chem.* 1987;262:16357–16363.

116. Mills C, Davies G. Molybdenum. In: Mertz W, ed. *Trace Elements in Human and Animal Nutrition.* 5th ed. San Diego, Calif: Academic Press; 1987.

117. Rajagopalan K. Molybdenum: an essential trace element in human nutrition. *Annu Rev Nutr.* 1988;8:401–427.

118. Abumrad N, Schneider A, Steel D, et al. Amino acid intolerance during prolonged total parenteral nutrition reversed by molybdate therapy. *Am J Clin Nutr.* 1981;34:2551–2559.

119. Tsongas T, Meglen R, Walravens P, et al. Molybdenum in the diet: an estimate of average daily intake in the United States. *Am J Clin Nutr.* 1980;33:1103–1107.

120. Pennington J, Jones J. Molybdenum, nickel, cobalt, vanadium, and strontium in total diets. *J Am Diet Assoc.* 1987;87:1644–1650.

121. Keen C, Zeidenberg-Cherr S. Manganese. In: Ziegler E, Filer L Jr, eds. *Present Knowledge in Nutrition.* 7th ed. Washington, DC: ILSI Press; 1996.

122. Doisy E. Micronutrient controls on biosynthesis of clotting proteins and cholesterol. In: Hemphill D, ed. *Trace Substances in Environmental Health.* Vol. 6. Columbia, Mo: University of Missouri Press; 1972.

123. Friedman B, Freeland-Graves J, Bales C. Manganese balance and clinical observations in young men fed a manganese-deficient diet. *J Nutr.* 1987;117:133–143.

124. Strause L, Saltman P, Smith K, et al. Spinal bone loss in postmenopausal women supplemented with calcium and trace minerals. *J Nutr.* 1994;124:1060–1064.

125. Leach R Jr. Biochemical role of manganese. In: Hoeckstra W, Suttie J, Ganther J, et al, eds. *Trace Element Metabolism in Animals—2.* Baltimore, Md: University Park Press; 1974.

126. Hurley L, Keen C. Manganese. In: Mertz W, ed. *Trace Elements in Human and Animal Nutrition.* 5th ed. San Diego, Calif: Academic Press; 1987.

127. Gibson R, MacDonald A, Martinez O. Dietary chromium and manganese intakes of a selected sample of Canadian elderly women. *Hum Nutr Appl Nutr.* 1985;39A:43–52.

128. Freeland-Graves J, Behmardi F, Bales C, et al. Metabolic balance in young men consuming diets containing five levels of dietary manganese. *J Nutr.* 1988;118:764–773.

129. Hallfrisch J, Powel A, Carafelli C, et al. Mineral balances of men and women consuming high fiber diets with complex or simple carbohydrates. *J Nutr.* 1987;117:48–55.

130. Freeland-Graves J, Bales C, Behmardi F. Manganese requirements in humans. In: Kies C, ed. *Nutritional Bioavailability of Manganese.* Washington, DC: American Chemical Society; 1987.

131. Schwartz R, Apgar B, Wien E. Apparent absorption and retention of Ca, Cu, Mg, Man, and Zn

from a diet containing bran. *Am J Clin Nutr*. 1986;43:444–455.

132. Bales C, Freeland-Graves J, Lin P-H, et al. Plasma uptake of manganese: response to dose and dietary factors. In: Kies C, ed. *Nutritional Bioavailability of Manganese*. Washington, DC: American Chemical Society; 1987.

133. Lin P-H, Freeland-Graves J. Effects of simultaneous ingestion of calcium and manganese in humans. In: Bales C, ed. *Mineral Homeostasis in the Elderly*. New York, NY: Alan R Liss Inc; 1989.

134. Dougherty V, Freeland-Graves J, Behmardi F, et al. Interactions of iron (Fe) and manganese in

males fed varying levels of dietary manganese. *Fed Proc*. 1987;46:914.

135. Nieboer E, Tom R, Sanford W. Nickel metabolism in man and animals. In: Sigel H, ed. *Metal Ions in Biological Systems*. New York, NY: Marcel Dekker; 1988.

136. Nielsen F. Nickel. In: Mertz W, ed. *Trace Elements in Human and Animal Nutrition*. 5th ed. San Diego, Calif: Academic Press; 1987.

137. Stanbury J. Iodine deficiency and the iodine deficiency disorders. In: Ziegler E, Filer L Jr, eds. *Present Knowledge in Nutrition*. 7th ed. Washington, DC: ILSI Press; 1996.

# CHAPTER 6

# Oral Health in the Elderly

*Wendy E. Martin*

As the first segment of the gastrointestinal system, the oral cavity provides the point of entry for nutrients. The condition of the oral cavity, therefore, can facilitate or undermine nutritional status. If dietary habits are unfavorably influenced by poor oral health, then nutritional status may be compromised. However, nutritional status can also contribute to or exacerbate oral disease. General well-being is related to health and disease states of the oral cavity as well as the rest of the body. An awareness of this interrelationship is essential when the clinician is working with the older patient, since the incidence of major dental problems and the frequency of chronic illness and pharmacotherapy increase dramatically in older people.

## REVIEW OF ANATOMY AND FUNCTIONS OF THE ORAL CAVITY

### Anatomy of the Oral Cavity

The major parts of the oral cavity (Figure 6–1) are lips; vestibules; teeth; maxilla and mandible (upper and lower jaws, respectively); alveolar bone (termed *residual bone* if there are no teeth); gingivae (gums); hard and soft palates (roof of the mouth); tongue and mucous membranes (floor of the mouth);

temporomandibular joint (TMJ); buccal mucosa (lining of the cheeks); salivary glands; and muscles of mastication and facial expression (orofacial musculature). Throughout the mouth, there are blood vessels, lymphatics, and nerves to ensure rapid communication between the oral cavity and other major organ systems.

At the lips, the skin of the face is continuous with the mucous membranes of the oral cavity. The bulk of the lips is formed by skeletal muscles and a variety of sensory receptors that judge the taste and temperature of foods. Their reddish color is due to an abundance of blood vessels near their surface.

The vestibule is the cleft that separates the lips and cheeks from the teeth and gingivae. When the mouth is closed, the vestibule communicates with the rest of the mouth through the space between the last molar teeth and the rami of the mandible.

Thirty-two teeth normally are present in the adult mouth: two incisors, one canine, two premolars, and three molars in each half of the upper and lower jaws. The teeth in the upper jaw are termed *maxillary*, and the teeth in the lower jaw are termed *mandibular*. The mandible is the movable member of the two jaws, whereas the maxilla is stationary. The components of an individual tooth provide a framework within which to appreciate

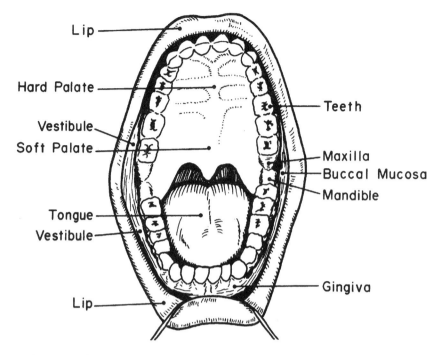

**Figure 6–1** Major parts of the oral cavity.

changes that occur with age (Figure 6–2). Teeth are highly calcified structures composed of four parts: (1) enamel, the hard, brittle substance covering the outer surface of the crown of the tooth; (2) dentin, a bonelike substance forming the main body of the tooth, surrounding the pulp cavity, and covered by enamel on the crown and cementum on the root; (3) cementum, a bonelike substance that covers the tooth root; and (4) pulp chamber and canal(s), the soft central parts of the tooth that contain the blood vessels, nerves, and lymphatics. Each tooth in the mouth is surrounded and supported by alveolar bone. The visible portion of the tooth is termed the *crown*. The portion submerged below the gum line is the *root*. The region where these portions meet is called the *neck* of the tooth. The gingiva surrounds the necks of the teeth and covers the alveolar bone. It is composed of dense, fibrous tissue covered by

a smooth vascular mucosa. The tooth roots are joined to the alveolar bone by periodontal ligaments.

The hard palate forms the roof of the mouth in the chewing area, and the soft palate lies just posterior to it. The floor of the mouth is formed by the tongue, which nearly fills the oral cavity when the mouth is closed, and mucous membranes. The tongue is a mobile mass of mostly skeletal muscle covered by a mucous membrane with numerous papillae on the surface.

The TMJ, located just anterior to the earlobe, is the only joint needed for chewing. A hingelike movement occurs bilaterally in the TMJ during mouth opening and closing. During chewing, the mandible also exhibits protrusive and lateral movements.

The buccal mucosa forms the side walls of the oral cavity and contains numerous mucous glands. The secretions from these glands

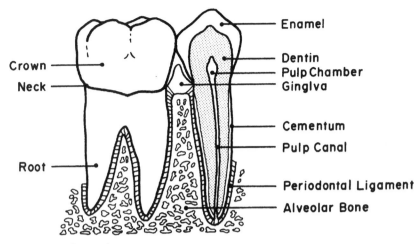

**Figure 6–2** Components of a tooth.

mix with food in the mouth to aid in both chewing and swallowing.

There are three major (bilateral) salivary glands, which secrete saliva into the mouth: parotid, submaxillary, and sublingual. The parotid glands are the largest, and their ducts open into the vestibules opposite the upper second molar teeth. The submaxillary (or submandibular) gland ducts open into the floor of the mouth under the tongue from their location in the angles of the mandible. The sublingual glands, the smallest of the major salivary glands, are embedded in the mucous membranes of the floor of the mouth. Their ducts open under the tongue as well. The major salivary glands contribute about 95% of the total daily volume of saliva; the remaining 5% comes from numerous minor salivary glands in the mucous membranes of the lips, tongue, palates, and cheeks.[1] The primary role of saliva is to protect and maintain oral health.[2,3] In that regard, human saliva contains lubricatory factors (mucins) to keep oral tissues hydrated, pliable, and insulated; contains many antibacterial proteins that regulate colonization of oral bacteria; buffers the acid produced by oral bacteria to maintain tooth integrity; aids in carbohydrate diges-

tion; mediates taste acuity; and is necessary for mastication and preparation of food for swallowing.[4-8]

The orofacial musculature consists of 4 muscles of mastication—the masseter, the lateral pterygoid, the medial pterygoid, and the temporalis muscles—and almost 20 muscles of facial expression. One of these facial muscles, the *buccinator*, acts as an accessory muscle of mastication by eliminating the space of the vestibule between the cheek and the jaws during chewing.

**Functions of the Oral Cavity**

The oral cavity serves in the masticating, tasting, and swallowing of food; as a phonetic box for speech; and as a secondary pathway for breathing. The major and minor salivary glands provide moisture to soften foods as well as supplying carbohydrate-digesting enzymes.

*Mastication (Chewing)*

The teeth are designed for chewing; the anterior teeth provide a strong cutting action, and the posterior teeth provide a grinding action. The names of the teeth demarcate their four basic functions. The *incisors* cut or slice food, the *canines* tear food, the *premolars* shred food, and the *molars* grind food in preparation for swallowing.

Proper chewing is important in the digestion of all foods, especially most fruits and raw vegetables, which contain undigestible cellulose membranes that must be broken down before the food can be used by the body. Also, since digestive enzymes act only on the surfaces of food particles, the rate of digestion is highly dependent on the total surface area of the chewed food that is exposed to intestinal secretions.

The act of chewing has more significance than the mere preparation of food for swallowing. The food is moved around the mouth so that the taste buds are stimulated, and odors are released that stimulate the olfactory receptors. Much of the satisfaction and pleasure of eating depends on these stimuli.

### Digestion in the Mouth

Saliva contains the digestive enzyme ptyalin (amylase), which functions to hydrolyze starches into two disaccharides, maltose and isomaltose. This is the first step in the digestion of carbohydrates. However, since food stays in the mouth for such a limited amount of time, only 3% to 5% of the starches that are eaten are hydrolyzed by the time the food is swallowed.[9] Most naturally occurring starches are digested poorly by ptyalin because they are protected by a thin cellulose cover. Cooking destroys these cellulose membranes and facilitates digestion in the mouth.

In general, swallowing can be divided into three stages: (1) the *voluntary stage*, which initiates the swallowing process; (2) the *pharyngeal stage*, which is involuntary and involves the muscular contractions for the passage of food through the pharynx to the esophagus; and (3) the *esophageal stage*, another involuntary phase that promotes the passage of food from the pharynx to the stomach. The oral cavity is involved with only the first (voluntary) stage of swallowing, which takes about 1 second.[10] When the food is ready to be swallowed, pressure from the tongue upward and backward against the palate forces the bolus of food posteriorly into the pharynx. From here on, the process of swallowing becomes automatic and usually cannot be stopped.

### Speech

Speech is a complex behavior that integrates the processes of respiration, phonation, oral sensation, resonation, and articulation.[10] The mouth is one of the resonators for speech and other vocalizations. The three major organs of articulation are the lips, tongue, and soft palate. Speech, therefore, relies heavily on the anatomic structures of the oral cavity.

## ORAL HEALTH STATUS AND NEEDS IN THE ELDERLY

### Oral Health Status

*Oral health* implies a state that is stable, relatively disease free, and comfortable and that permits adequate functioning for mastication, swallowing, and speech. Poor oral health may be viewed as a state of inadequate functioning resulting from decayed teeth; periodontal disease; ill-fitting dentures or lack of dentures; neglect of oral hygiene; and the presence of pain, inflammation, or infection in the oral cavity. Although few of these conditions pose mortality risks, they may lead to physical dysfunction, pain, and psychologic anguish in the older patient.

A major criterion of successful aging is how well the individual maintains oral health, the ability to chew, the ability to talk, and personal satisfaction with appearance.[11] Unfortunately, the mouth often becomes one of the first areas of the body to be neglected by people who have chronic diseases and infirmities in old age.

There have been only three national surveys indicating the oral status of the elderly, and the older aged were excluded in two of the studies: the National Health Examination Survey of 1960–1962 excluded participants older than 79 years,[12] and the National Health and Nutrition Examination Survey (HANES I) of 1971–1974 included no subjects older than 74 years.[13]

In 1978, the National Institutes of Health (NIH) introduced an oral physiology and aging component to the Baltimore Longitudinal Study of Aging.[14] In Iowa, a longitudinal survey was initiated in 1981 to determine the prevalence and incidence of oral conditions in noninstitutionalized rural elderly Iowans. In 1987, the National Institute of Dental Research (NIDR) published national and regional data on the prevalence of oral conditions in 15,000 working adults and 5600 elderly people who attended multipurpose senior centers.[15] Useful data were obtained from this survey of adult oral health, even though the older participants were not entirely representative of the nation's elderly population. The findings disclosed that

Americans are keeping their teeth longer, are going to the dentist more often for preventive checkups, are reducing the number of cavities in their mouths, and have practically eliminated edentulousness in middle age. Serious dental problems, however, still exist among the elderly (Table 6–1).

## Oral Health Needs

In general, studies reveal that many unmet treatment needs are affecting a large portion of the noninstitutionalized elderly population. This is true whether the study has been conducted by direct examination of patients or by survey. Data from HANES I indicated that 60% of elderly subjects had at least one dental treatment need.[13] The survey of rural elderly Iowans also found a high level of treatment needed: 40% required at least one restoration, 16% at least one extraction, and 27% some prosthodontic treatment; more than 60% of the dentate subjects needed some periodontal treatment.[16–18]

Many local studies and one statewide survey have documented the large need for dental care among institutionalized residents.[19–23] The results have ranged from 2.3 dental services needed per person, with 3.2 services re-

**Table 6–1** Comparison of Oral Health Status of Employed Adults and Older Adults

| Oral Status/Treatment Need | % of Employed Adults | % of Older Adults |
|---|---|---|
| Calculus deposits | 83.9 | 88.9 |
| Edentulousness | 4.2 | 41.1 |
| Gingival bleeding (after probing) | 43.6 | 46.9 |
| Gingival recession (1+ mm) | 51.1 | 88.3 |
| Periodontal attachment loss (1+ sites) | 76.7 | 95.1 |
| Retention of all teeth | 36.7 | 2.1 |
| Root caries | 21.1 | 56.9 |
| Visited dentist in past 2 years | 79.6 | 56.4 |
| Perceived need for dental care | 50.4 | 36.0 |

*Source:* Reprinted from National Survey of Adult Dental Health, *Oral Health of United States Adults: National Findings*, 1987, National Institute of Dental Research.

quired for those having remaining natural dentition,[19] to 82.5% of 3247 patients screened in Vermont nursing homes in 1982.[20] In the latter study, examiners found that 37.2% of the residents required immediate attention to eliminate pain, infection, concern of malignancy, or a combination of these symptoms.

## CHANGES IN ORAL AND CIRCUMORAL STRUCTURES WITH AGING

### Overview

Differentiation of normal aging changes from disease processes in old age is of paramount importance. Not knowing the changes that occur with age might lead to excessive or unnecessary treatment. Erroneously evaluating a disease process as normal aging might have equally serious consequences. Unfortunately, lack of research on the aging oral cavity has resulted in a number of stereotypes and generalizations.[24] Standard graphs, tables, and information in many geriatric medical and dental textbooks show inevitable decrements with age. However, these studies included subjects who, although superficially healthy, in fact had some disease or were taking medication that affected oral function.[25] Most of this early information therefore probably reflects oral changes due to disease or its treatment rather than dysfunctions related directly to increased age.

### Hard Tissues

#### Bone

In the developmental years, bone resorption and deposition occur synchronously in the process of growth and remodeling. Alveolar bone, however, has a remodeling rate greater than that of the other bones of the body.[26] With maturity, bone is notably less active, although there is still some degree of continuing resorption and deposition. After age 35 to 40 years, approximately 1% of bone mass is lost per year in both men and women.[26]

As physical activity diminishes in the later years, so too does the demand for new bone formation. Resorption exceeds deposition, resulting in a net loss of bone. By the time old age is reached, atrophy has resulted from slow resorption with very little remodeling. Not only is there a generalized decline in bone volume,[27] but the composition of bone gradually alters also, resulting in reduced resilience and increased brittleness and fragility[28] (Chapter 12).

Alveolar bone is one of the first bones to be affected by loss of mass. The periosteal and periodontal surfaces of alveolar bone become less resistant to harmful local oral trauma, inflammation, or disease.[29] This is a major factor contributing to periodontal disease, loss of teeth, and, in the edentulous patient, inability to obtain adequate support and stability for dentures.[24,30] In both the maxilla and the mandible, the amount, extent, and uniformity of the bone loss differ with varying etiologies and health status.[31,32] It is now recognized that alveolar bone or residual ridge resorption is confounded by such factors as age, sex, race, and health status of the patient when the teeth are extracted; the tooth extraction technique; the diet of the patient; the presence of local factors; and the frequency of denture use.[31]

#### Teeth

It is frequently reported that the teeth themselves undergo changes with age (Table 6–2). Teeth differ from most other parts of the body in that the reparative or regenerative capacity of their constituent tissues is extremely limited. Also, the blood vessels and nerves become less active with age; as a result, the vi-

**Table 6–2** Anatomic Changes in the Teeth with Age

*Enamel*
   Regeneration/repair—incapable
   Permeability—decreased
*Dentin*
   Permeability—decreased
   Sensitivity—decreased
   Calcification—increased
   Pain conduction—decreased
   Repair—capable with vital tooth pulp
*Pulp chamber and canal(s)*
   Cellularity—decreased
   Innervation—decreased
   Tooth drainage—decreased
   Vascularity—decreased
   Volume—decreased (due to deposition of reparative dentin)
*Apical foramen*
   Size—decreased (may cause decreased pulp vascularity and innervation)
*Cementum*
   Deposition—continuous (major cause of decreased apical foramen size)
   Repair—capable with vital tooth pulp
   Resorption—increased susceptibility
*Entire tooth*
   Brittleness—increased (predisposing tooth to cracks, fractures, shearing)
   Darkening—increased
   Pain sensitivity—decreased
   Thermal sensitivity—decreased
   Translucency—decreased

tality of the average human tooth pulp lasts approximately 70 years.[28]

*Attrition.* The remaining natural teeth are likely to exhibit some flattening of the chewing surfaces induced by repeated contact with opposing teeth during masticatory movements. To compensate for the natural wear of these surfaces, human teeth erupt with their supporting structures throughout adult life.[33–35]

The patterns of tooth wear vary with each patient and are cumulative, since the enamel is incapable of repair or regeneration. The wear can range from minimal faceting to extreme loss of tooth substance, sometimes extending to the gingiva. However, there is no agreement on the point at which physiologic attrition becomes pathologic or contributes to pathologic conditions.[36] In areas of excessive wear, reparative (or secondary) dentin is deposited on the walls of the pulp chamber and canals for protection. This, as well as reduced innervation, helps to explain the reduced tooth pain sensitivity and higher pain threshold in elderly people.

### Temporomandibular Joint

The TMJ is a complex, diarthrodial joint capable of both swinging (hingelike) and sliding motions on many axes. It undergoes functional remodeling throughout life, usually in response to changes in articulation of the teeth or alterations in the space between the maxilla and mandible. The functional changes in the TMJ are by no means confined to elderly individuals.

Signs of TMJ change include joint clicking, limitation of jaw opening, and deviation of the mandible during function, with the major symptom being pain. Researchers with the Baltimore Longitudinal Study of Aging assessed all of these for arteriosclerosis or obliteration of the capillaries.[37] More research into the aging TMJ is needed since these age-related changes may explain some of the masticatory problems in this age group.

## Soft Tissues

### Mucous Membranes

The stereotypic effect of aging on the oral mucosa is that atrophic changes occur. Clinically, these changes involve the surface epithelium's becoming thinner, drier, less elastic, less vascular, less firmly attached to the underlying connective tissue and bone, and more susceptible to injury from mild stresses.[28,38–40] Other changes occur as well with reduction in connective tissue and subcutaneous fat and increased linkage of collagen molecules. Some symptoms have been associated with these alterations, including xerostomia (mouth dryness) and sensations of pain or burning on the tongue, palate, or oral mucosa.[24] These changes, however, must be interpreted with caution. In critical reviews of the literature, Baum[24] and Hill[41] suggested that no conclusions could be drawn about whether atrophy of the oral mucosa is associated with aging. Other researchers have concluded that specific alterations of the oral tissues may instead be induced by a host of environmental factors, such as tobacco smoking or chronic systemic disease.[42]

### Periodontium

*Gingiva.* The gum tissue of the elderly individual gradually recedes from the tooth, with subsequent exposure of more of the tooth surface and root. The degree that gingival recession progresses is related to age, tooth movement, inflammatory changes due to disease, oral care habits, and heredity.

*Periodontal Ligament.* The periodontal ligament is not one ligament but a series of short, dense ligaments connecting the cementum of the tooth root to alveolar bone. Since the ligament is made up of connective tissues, aging affects it in the same way as it does other connective tissues in the body.[43] The result is a progressive loss of soft tissue attachment, leading to exposure of the root and loosening of the teeth within their bony sockets.

### Tongue

The status of the tongue in aging, independent of diseased states and taste acuity, has not been studied in detail. Tongue vascularity changes very little compared with that of other organs because there is little tendency in this tissue for atherosclerosis or obliteration of the capillaries.[42] There is much controversy about whether aging is associated with atrophy of the papillae, increased formation of fissures, and decreasing sensitivity to gustatory stimuli in the tongue.[23,42,44–48]

## Circumoral Tissues

### Oral Musculature

Changes in aging oral musculature are consistent with those in aging muscle tissue in the body as a whole.[49] In general, there are reductions in muscle tone,[10] muscle performance,[50] number and activity of muscle cells, and number and size of the muscle fibers. Replacement of the muscle mass by fat or fibrous connective tissue results in generalized atrophy of the musculature attached to the bones in the oral cavity.[51]

*Mastication.* The muscles of mastication atrophy with age; this decreases the biting force and slows chewing performance.[52–54] The atrophy is probably due in part to disuse, since less muscular effort is required for chewing as a result of failing dentition or a progressively softer diet or both. In either case, the generalized loss of muscle mass decreases the biting force and can make chewing difficult.

*Deglutition.* Aging does not significantly affect the transit of the prepared food bolus through the mouth and pharynx.[55] However, the impact of decreased muscle mass and tone can make swallowing difficult and can alter the ability to form and prepare a bolus in the oral stage of swallowing.[10] Several studies[52–54,56] have demonstrated that as people age they take longer and expend more effort to prepare a food bolus before swallowing.

## Other Changes

### Salivary Glands

In early reports, decreased salivary flow was generally considered to be concomitant with increased age.[24,57,58] Recent evidence indicates that the diminished salivary flow often noted in studies of elderly subjects is due to pathologic conditions or pharmacologic effects of medications, rather than aging.[2,5–7,59,60] Since diminished salivary flow does not occur in healthy, nonmedicated individuals,[61] these findings emphasize that the elderly person may be susceptible to situations and therapies that result in a reduction of saliva availability.

### Sense of Taste

The sense of taste is a function of the taste buds in the mouth. Its importance in nutrition lies in the fact that it allows a person to select food in accord with personal desires and needs of the tissues for specific nutritive substances.

*Taste Buds.* The taste buds are found predominantly on three of the four different types of the tongue papillae (circumvallate, fungiform, and foliate), although they are also located in the epithelium of the palate, tonsillar pillars, and other points around the nasopharynx.[62,63] In early anatomic studies, marked decreases in the numbers and atrophy of the taste buds with aging were reported.[64,65] However, more recent investigations indicate there is no significant loss of taste buds in old age.[66,67]

*Taste Sensitivity.* Elderly people often complain of altered taste sensations (dysgeusia), decreased ability to perceive taste (hypogeusia), or complete loss of taste (ageusia). Few studies, however, have been able to determine the reasons for these decrements in taste sensitivity.[63,68] One explanation is decreased salivary flow, since taste buds react only to dissolved compounds.

Although there is some agreement that taste sensitivity begins to decline after age 55 years, differences in research methods have produced different results.[69] Some studies have indicated that older adults need higher concentrations of the four primary sensations of taste (salty, sour, sweet, bitter) for identification than do children and younger adults.[62,70,71] Others have found that the taste buds detecting saltiness and sweetness are the first to deteriorate and that sensitivity to sour and bitter tastes declines later.[62,65,70–74] The use of psychophysical procedures found only minimal changes in taste sensitivity,[44–46,48] even though a steady decline in taste sensitivity with increasing age is still being found.[46,47]

### Sense of Smell

Smell is the least researched and understood sense. This is due in part to the location of the olfactory sensory receptors in specialized epithelial tissue of the nasal cavity and in part to the fact that the sense of smell is a subjective phenomenon that is not easily measured. In fact, much of what we call taste is actually smell, which largely determines the flavor and palatability of foods and beverages.[75]

Evidence of a decline in olfactory sensitivity with age is still very limited, and the cause of any decrement remains speculative.[76,77] Some investigators have found reduced smell sensitivity, with the greatest problems in recognition and identification of odors among persons older than 80 years.[78] Others have reported age-related losses with significant individual differences.[79-81] It has also been suggested that poor health and smoking may cause an even greater decline in smell sensitivity than does age alone.[81,82]

## CHANGES IN ORAL AND CIRCUMORAL STRUCTURES WITH DISEASE

### Overview

There are three major characteristics of dental diseases: universality, irreversibility, and cumulativeness (Table 6–3). Although these diseases are rarely debilitating or life threatening, there are indications that they have a significant impact on social, economic, and psychologic areas of life, including the quality of life.[83,84] Older adults, however, tend to place minimal importance on their oral health and accept functionally inadequate dentition as an unavoidable consequence of the aging process.

Many of the oral diseases that afflict the elderly are diseases of all age groups. Therefore, preventive dentistry remains an important aspect of their oral health care and should involve all three levels of prevention: (1) preventing initiation of disease, (2) preventing the progression and recurrence of disease, and (3) preventing the loss of function and loss of life.[85]

The prevention of dental disease requires that all individuals see a dentist at least yearly, whether they have natural teeth, no teeth, complete dentures, or teeth and dentures. First, this allows primary prevention procedures to be evaluated and reinforced regularly. Detrimental habits, environmental factors, and nutritional status all affect the likelihood that oral pathology will occur. As an example, poor oral hygiene significantly contributes to the diseases caused or aggravated by bacterial plaque infection,[86] and it is well known that the level of oral hygiene deteriorates with age.[87] Second, regular dental care can lead to early diagnosis and treatment of the pathologic conditions described below.

### Hard Tissues

#### *Bone*

*Resorption.* Bone resorption is associated with the loss of mineral content, increase in porosity, and generalized atrophy. Clinical observation of alveolar bone resorption has so far failed to provide a clear understanding of the mechanisms responsible. There is a portion of the population that shows bone loss without the other findings usually associated with active periodontal disease. This loss is also seen in the absence of dentition.[88]

Resorption of alveolar bone occurs in two dimensions: The mandible resorbs primarily in a vertical direction, resulting in loss of bone height. The maxilla resorbs primarily in a horizontal direction away from the covering lips and cheeks. This means that the chin will appear to protrude because the maxilla has receded horizontally. This leads to the characteristic "toothless look": a shortening of the

**Table 6–3** The Major Characteristics of Dental Diseases[51]

1. *Universality*—Diseases of the oral cavity are the most prevalent of all diseases; dental caries and periodontal disease usually affect most people throughout life.

2. *Irreversibility*—The damage derived from the common oral diseases, such as dental decay or bone loss, is irreversible, although treatment can usually intercept its spread.

3. *Cumulativeness*—The structural losses induced in the teeth and their supporting alveolar bone by oral diseases are cumulative.

---

distance between the chin and nose and a pulling inward of the lips.

Resorption is greater in the mandible than in the maxilla, and, when severe, constitutes a major problem in the wearing of dentures. The residual bony ridge may become thin and knifelike and unable to withstand the downward compressive forces of a conventional denture.

*Osteopenia and Osteoporosis. Osteopenia* refers to metabolic bone diseases that are characterized by X-ray findings of a subnormal amount of mineralized bone mass (Chapter 12). The most common osteopenia is osteoporosis, generally defined as a decrease in the quantity of bone, with an increased incidence of fractures from minimal trauma.[89] Osteoporosis is observable within the oral cavity as dental osteopenia.

One of the first signs of osteoporosis is alveolar bone loss, followed by loss in the vertebrae and long bones.[90,91] Indeed, there is a significant correlation between skeletal osteopenia and density of alveolar bone and residual ridges.[92] Radiographically, it appears as diminished bone mass in the mandibular angular cortex, decreased trabeculae, and a diminished alveolar crest.[93,94] Subsequently, it leads to an inadequate amount of bone mass in the mandible, loss or mobility of teeth, edentulousness, and inability to wear dentures.[32] The loss of teeth and the use of ill-fitting dentures also cause extensive alveolar bone or residual ridge atrophy.[95,96]

Although calcium deficiencies and calcium-phosphorus imbalances are contributing factors in the pathogenesis of osteoporosis,[97] prevention and management include not only increased calcium intake but estrogen therapy, bone-building or antiresorptive agents, dietary vitamin D, and exercise.[91,98–101] Although fluoride therapy is used extensively in preventive dentistry, its widespread use in the prevention of osteoporosis is still being investigated.[102,103]

### Teeth

*Dental Caries (Tooth Decay): Coronal and Root Surfaces.* Dental caries has been considered a disease of young people that stabilizes in the mid-20s and remains dormant until periodontal disease or gingival recession exposes the roots of the teeth and caries of the root surfaces occurs.[85,104,105] However, more recent research indicates that a significant increase in caries, including recurrent decay around restorations, cervical caries at the gingival margin, and root caries, is associated with aging.[15,106,107] Most of the recurrent caries are in the proximal regions of the teeth.[108] Root caries occurs following exposure of the tooth root.[107,109–112]

The diagnosis of dental caries is based on X-ray examination and clinical observation, since there is no absolute correlation between the presence or extent of dental decay and symptoms. It is generally recognized that four things are necessary to produce a carious lesion: cariogenic bacteria, a substrate of dietary carbohydrates, a susceptible host (tooth), and time. However, factors that contribute to high caries risk include poor oral hygiene, gingival recession, reduced salivary flow (which increases plaque accumulation), bacterial virulence, and diet.[108,113]

Conditions that predispose to xerostomia (dry mouth), such as medications, Sjögren's syndrome, and head and neck irradiation, can promote rampant dental caries in all age groups.[114] In fact, the incidence of root surface caries in elderly people is significantly correlated with a low rate of salivary secretion.[115,116]

Historically, the most effective strategy for preventing dental caries has been increasing tooth resistance to pathogenic plaque through the use of fluorides by systemic introduction (water, diet) and topical application (professional or self-applied).[117,118] Even fluoridation of other vehicles, such as salt, milk, and sugar, has been considered in areas where no reticulated water supplies exist.[102] In patients with xerostomia, the development of caries has been avoided largely by daily topical application of either 0.5% sodium fluoride or 0.5% stannous fluoride solutions.[119,120]

Unfortunately, there are few clinical data supporting the use of topical fluoride for prevention of dental caries in geriatric patients with adequate salivary flow.[121–124] Newbrun,[125] however, believes that the elderly population would benefit from the use of fluoride dentifrices, mouth rinses, and gels applied by brush, finger applicator, or plastic tray. The method to be used is dictated by the anticipated susceptibility to decay and the ability of the patient to manage the regimen.

Since both coronal and root caries are plaque-related diseases, measures that limit or inhibit plaque formation should be effective in prevention. Mechanical oral hygiene techniques and chemical antimicrobial agents such as chlorhexidine[126,127] reduce bacterial flora and substrate. Even dietary modification decreases the amount of substrate, acid production, and decalcification of teeth if individuals eliminate or reduce the intake of foods that are soft, sticky, retentive, or high in sugar and if they chew firm foods.[13]

*Abrasion and Erosion.* An aging population with longer retention of teeth is at increased risk for both abrasion (wear of tooth structure by nonmasticatory mechanical forces) and erosion (wear of tooth structure by chemical dissolution). The incidence of both of these conditions increases with age, simply because any damage to the teeth is cumulative. In patients with xerostomia, the diminution in the mucin level of the oral cavity provides less lubrication and protection, posing an even greater risk for abrasion and erosion.

A major etiologic factor of abrasion is overzealous and improper toothbrushing with a hard-bristle brush or an abrasive dentifrice.[128,129] The damage appears as transverse scoring of the tooth surface and tends to be asymmetric in its severity, depending on whether the patient is right-handed or left-handed.[28] Prevention is largely a matter of proper toothbrushing and the use of a soft-bristle brush and toothpaste with minimal abrasivity. Other forms of abrasion result from holding objects with the teeth, chewing tobacco, and using dental floss and toothpicks improperly.

Erosion is a chemical process that occurs when the concentration of acid in the mouth is too high for the saliva to neutralize. The most common causes are chronic ingestion of fruits, fruit juices, and carbonated beverages[130–132]; sucking candies containing phosphorus or citric acid; and gastroesophageal reflux.[133] Erosion can also result from working in an industry that uses or produces acidic materials.[134,135] To prevent dietary erosion, the use of straws with fruit juices and carbonated beverages and the substitution of sugar-free candies or gums are indicated.

The lesions of abrasion and erosion look different: The former are characteristically narrow in relation to depth, and areas of erosion are usually saucer shaped.[28,136] Generally, these lesions do not require restorative treatment unless they are extensive or symptomatic.[136]

*Hypersensitive Dentin and Cementum.* Exposure of dentin or cementum from abrasion, erosion, acute or chronic trauma, or various restorative treatment procedures can lead to hypersensitive dentin and cementum. The teeth are exquisitely sensitive with exposure to any chemical, thermal, tactile, or osmotic stimulus. Although there is great individual variation in pain sensation, hypersensitivities to sour, sweet, cold, hot, and mechanical irritations are most common.[137]

Since hypersensitivity may deter a person from establishing or maintaining adequate oral hygiene procedures, decreasing sensitivity is the first step in treatment. One method is "sealing" the exposed tooth surfaces by applying agents or dentifrices such as fluoride gels and rinses.[138–141] In some cases, dental restoration and even endodontic therapy may be necessary to arrest the progress of the lesion, restore the function and shape of the tooth, and relieve pain.[142]

*Tooth Loss and Edentulousness.* Tooth loss is an irreversible, cumulative process that is no longer considered a natural consequence of aging. Instead, it is known to be the ultimate sequela of the two most common dental diseases, dental caries and periodontal disease. Nevertheless, tooth loss increases in frequency with age. By age 65 years, approximately 40% of Americans have lost all their teeth; another 20% have lost more than half their teeth.

In all age groups, the total loss of teeth is historically related to increased sugar consumption, combined with ignorance of prevention and insufficient dental manpower resources at the time.[34] Tooth loss in adults older than 35 years has been consistently attributed to periodontal diseases.[143–145] However, recent studies of tooth loss in adult populations indicate that caries is most often the cause for tooth extractions.[146–149]

The rate of edentulousness, or total lack of teeth, is declining in the elderly population of the United States. In 1957, 67.3% of persons older than 65 years were edentulous, whereas only 45.5% were so in 1971.[150] This was largely due to the introduction of preventive and restorative dental procedures. Today, less than 40% of elderly people are edentulous, and this number is rapidly decreasing.

In the recent national survey of employed and older adults, in the group aged 55 to 64 years, less than 15% were edentulous.[15] However, the prevalence of lost teeth was still extensive enough to compromise the employed adults' dentition and to impair function in most of the older adults.[15,151] This means that the fewer missing teeth predicted to occur in the future will lead not only to an increase in tooth-related diseases, but also to the continuing need for regular dental care.[152]

### Temporomandibular Joint

Dysfunctions of the TMJ have their primary base in the joint mechanism, even though the actual dysfunction may involve the ligaments, the muscles, or the bone itself. One half of the edentulous and one third of the dentulous older population have signs and symptoms of TMJ disorders,[153] including soreness of the jaw; dull, aching facial pain; severe pain in the joint area; tenderness or pain of the masticatory and facial muscles; dizziness; headaches; impaired hearing or earache; eye pain; chronic fatigue; and popping, clicking, or cracking noises near the ear while opening and closing the mouth.[154–157] These manifestations are dynamic, characterized by periods of quiescence and exacerbation, and have a wide range of expression among patients.[158] However, elderly individuals appear to have more symptoms than do younger persons.[159]

The causes of TMJ dysfunction may be external or internal or both. External causes include degenerative joint disease; alveolar bone resorption; and injuries to the head, neck, or mandible. Internally, attrition, malocclusion, and bruxism, in either natural or artificial teeth, can cause the facial muscles and TMJ to quit working together correctly.[160,161]

Diagnostic and treatment decisions are based on symptom reports and clinical examination findings. Management therapies advocated for TMJ dysfunction include applying moist heat to the face; using prescribed muscle relaxants or other medications; massaging the muscles; eating soft and nonchewy foods; undergoing counseling; training in biofeedback or relaxation procedures; correcting the "bite" of the teeth; and, in severe cases, undergoing surgery.

## Soft Tissues

### Mucous Membranes/Epithelium

The oral mucosa is composed of both keratinized and nonkeratinized epithelium. In addition, the mouth has a dark, moist environment that is replete with microorganisms. The oral mucosa also may be subjected to several environmental influences, such as smoking; chewing of the lips and cheeks; eating a variety of foods; and sources of trauma, allergy, and carcinogenesis.[162]

*Aphthous Ulcer (Canker Sore, Aphthous Stomatitis, Ulcerative Stomatitis).* Aphthous ulcers appear as shallow white macules or papules with flat, fairly even borders surrounded by an intense erythematous halo. Each ulcer often is covered with a pseudomembrane. One or more ulcers may be present. They tend to recur and are usually very painful during their acute phase. The pain may interfere with eating, swallowing, and moving the tongue. Aphthous ulcers occur more frequently in women than in men.

Aphthae are found on oral mucosal surfaces that are not bound to underlying bone, especially the buccal and labial mucosa, dorsum of the tongue, floor of the mouth, soft palate, gingivae, lips, and oropharynx. The diagnosis depends mainly on exclusion of similar but more readily identifiable diseases, a history of recurrence, and inspection of the ulcer.

The etiology is still unclear, as it has never been adequately demonstrated that this lesion is due to a virus or any other specific chemical, physical, psychologic, or hormonal cause.[163] Nuts, coffee, chocolate, and citrus fruits often cause flare-ups, but abstinence will not prevent recurrence. Trauma, nutritional deficiencies, stresses of various types, food components, and allergies have been shown to be contributory to the disease.[163–166]

Healing, which usually occurs in 1 to 3 weeks without scarring, may be accelerated slightly by treatment. A new film-forming medication, hydroxypropyl cellulose (Zilactin), brings impressive pain relief and is able to protect the areas of ulceration from irritants, thus allowing patients to eat and drink more normally.[167] Bland antibiotic or anesthetic mouth rinses, topical steroid-antibiotic therapy, and surface protectants can also reduce pain. Sedatives, analgesics, and vitamins may help indirectly. Good oral hygiene and the minimization of mucosal trauma are helpful. Systemic antibiotics are contraindicated.

*Ulcerative stomatitis* is a general term for multiple ulcerations on an inflamed oral mucosa. It may be secondary to blood dyscrasias, erythema multiforme, bullous lichen planus, acute herpes simplex infection, pemphigoid, pemphigus, and drug reactions. If the lesions cannot be classified, they are referred to as *aphthae*.

*Candidiasis (Moniliasis, Thrush).* Candidiasis is the most common opportunistic infection of the mouth, caused by overgrowth of a species of the fungus *Candida*. The species most frequently implicated in oral infections is *C. albicans*. The yeast phase of the fungus is a component of the normal oral flora of most people.[168] It exists in a symbiotic relationship with many of the other oral microorganisms. Because it has such low virulence in the yeast phase, some change must take place in the local environment to produce conditions favorable for its overgrowth and tissue invasion. The change commonly occurs when there is a reduction in host resistance caused by bacterial and viral infection, systemic disease, or medications.

Oral candidiasis generally presents in one of three distinct clinical forms: acute pseudomembranous candidiasis (thrush), acute atrophic candidiasis (antibiotic sore mouth), or chronic atrophic candidiasis (denture sore mouth). Rare forms include chronic hyperplastic candidiasis and chronic mucocutaneous candidiasis.

The lesions of acute pseudomembranous candidiasis consist of either multifocal or diffuse, white, superficial curdlike plaques occurring anywhere in the oral cavity. The infection is called pseudomembranous because the plaques can be scraped off easily, leaving an erythematous or bleeding base. Most other white mucosal lesions cannot be rubbed off.

Acute atrophic candidiasis often follows prolonged antibiotic or steroid therapy and results, clinically, in a painful erythematous mucosa, particularly involving the tongue. The problem usually resolves with cessation of the medications, but antifungal therapy will hasten recovery.

Chronic atrophic candidiasis presents as a slightly granular or irregularly eroded erythematous mucosa under dentures.

Any of these types of candidiasis can be accompanied by angular cheilitis. The diagnosis is based on the varied clinical picture of the surface white patches or erythematous changes and may be confirmed by laboratory culture. Treatment includes elimination of the causative or predisposing factor, if practical, and administration of antifungal agents.[169–173]

*Leukoplakia (Benign Keratosis, White Patch).* The term *leukoplakia* is used to describe a thickened, white plaque that will not rub or strip off and is not identifiable clinically or pathologically as any other disease. The lesions may be found on all oral mucous membrane surfaces, varying from a small circumscribed area to an extensive lesion involving a large area of mucosa. They are usually asymptomatic and are discovered on routine dental examination or by patients who feel the thickened plaques in their mouths. Leukoplakia occurs more often in men, and the highest incidence is in the fifth to seventh age decade.[174]

The most common cause of leukoplakia is epithelial hyperplasia, hyperkeratosis, hyperorthokeratosis, dyskeratosis, or acanthosis. These terms refer specifically to reactive conditions of the oral mucosal epithelium, usually in response to an irritant or chronic irritation. The specific etiology is often unknown, but there are risk factors: tobacco, alcohol, deficiency of vitamin A or B complexes, and chronic irritating conditions or habits.[175,176]

Treatment consists of removing all irritants. Failure of a keratotic lesion to regress within 2 weeks after elimination of the apparent cause should arouse suspicion, and the lesion should be biopsied or surgically excised. About 5% of patients with leukoplakia eventually develop squamous cell carcinoma in the area of the white lesion.

*Mucositis (Stomatitis). Mucositis* and *stomatitis* are clinical terms describing inflammation, breakdown, and ulceration of the oral mucosal tissues. The disease can vary in its clinical presentation from focal or patchy erythema or ulceration to complete sloughing of the oral mucosa. Secondary hemorrhage is relatively common.

There is a wide variety of causative factors, including chronic mouth breathing, medications, systemic diseases, radiotherapy of the head and neck, and nutritional deficiencies. Patients complain of intense pain, burning, and dysphagia, which lead to an inability to eat or even drink.

Treatment relies heavily on palliation of symptoms, which can be provided by local anesthetic and antacid preparations used singly or in combination. Relief is short-lived, however, since the effect of these agents lasts less than 20 minutes. Benzydamine hydrochloride, a local anesthetic and anti-inflammatory drug, is effective for 1 to 2 hours. The use of any toothpastes or mouthwashes accentuates the problem because of their irritating and desiccating properties.

Radiation-induced mucositis initially appears as reddened and swollen mucosa, but the tissue becomes denuded and ulcerated as therapy continues. The patient experiences pain, burning, and discomfort that is greatly intensified by contact with coarse or highly seasoned foods. Involvement of the pharyngeal mucosa produces difficulties in swallowing and speaking. When therapy ends, spontaneous remission occurs in most patients within several weeks. In the meantime, the use of liquid topical anesthetics in the mouth before mealtimes frequently facilitates eating without discomfort.

*Oral Cancer.* Oral cancer is clearly a disease of older people: Over 98% of cases occur in persons older than 40 years[177,178]; the average age at the time of diagnosis is about 60 years.[179] The male-to-female ratio is approximately 2:1. It was estimated that in 1997 more than 31,000 new cases of cancer of the lips, tongue, floor of the mouth, palate, gingiva, buccal mucosa, and oropharynx would be diagnosed in the United States.[180] These oral cancers account for about 3.1% of all malignancies.

The most common type of oral cancer is squamous cell carcinoma, accounting for more than 90% of all oral malignancies.[181,182] The remaining 10% are predominantly malignant tumors of minor salivary gland tissue and (rarely) lymphomas, sarcomas, and melanomas.[178]

Clinically, an early cancer may appear as a small white patch (leukoplakia); a red velvety patch (erythroplakia); an aphthouslike, crusting, or traumatic ulcer; an erythematous plaque; a slightly raised lesion with central ulceration and a raised border; a verruciform growth; or a small swelling.[183–185] The most common signs and symptoms of oral cancer are listed in Table 6–4.

Frequently, it is impossible to differentiate between squamous cell carcinomas and the benign non-neoplastic lesions seen in aphthous ulceration, herpes simplex infection, or traumatic ulceration. However, the non-neoplastic lesions are usually painful, and most early oral cancers are painless, becoming symptomatic only after they are large enough to impinge on the sensory nerves.[186]

**Table 6–4** Oral Cancer Warning Signals

- Swelling
- Lumps, growths, exophytic masses
- White, scaly patches
- Red patches
- Oral ulcers (bleed easily, nonhealing)
- Atypical facial pain
- Persistent numbness or pain
- Persistent bleeding
- Difficulty in chewing
- Restricted jaw movement
- Trismus
- Restricted tongue movement
- Difficulty in swallowing
- Sore throat that does not heal
- Hoarseness
- Change in denture fit
- Loose teeth

The cause of oral cancer is not known. A genetic factor is not apparent, but there is a definite increased risk with the use of tobacco and alcohol.[178,179,184,185,187–191] Independently, each agent is believed to be associated with an increased incidence of the disease, and the two together may in fact act synergistically.[192] Oral leukoplakia (benign keratosis) is an important precancerous lesion, turning into oral cancer in about 3% to 5% of cases.[193,194] Malignant transformations arising from the oral mucosa are mostly observed between ages 40 and 69 years. Although the peak prevalence is between ages 50 and 59 years, decline is gradual thereafter.[195] Other risk factors for oral cancer include exposure to sunlight, chronic trauma, diet, poor dentition, and history of syphilis infection.[179,182,196,197]

Oral cancer is a devastating disease with significant morbidity and mortality. Curative treatment consists of surgery, radiation, and chemotherapy, alone or in combination. Unfortunately, despite advances in these therapeutic approaches, only about 50% of patients with oral cancer survive the disease.[198] Of course, survival rates vary substantially depending on the site, ranging from 32% for cancer of the oropharynx to 91% for lip cancer, and on how early in the disease treatment is instituted. The poor overall prognosis for oral cancer is due to the fact that the disease is often detected at advanced stages, after the visual detection of tissue changes or the development of symptoms.

Until the process of carcinogenesis is completely understood and true prevention is possible, early detection and treatment remain the best weapons against malignant disease. However, because there are no reliable methods for early diagnosis of squamous cell carcinoma, biopsy is the only definitive means of diagnosis. A biopsy should be done on any oral lesion that has not responded to therapy or resolved in a 2-week period.

Many of the predisposing factors for oral cancer are potentially avoidable. Preventive education should include delineation of the hazards of tobacco and alcohol and the need for regular dental care to reduce irritation and mechanical injury and for early detection.

*Traumatic Ulcers.* Acute trauma (mechanical, thermal, or chemical) is probably the most common cause of oral ulceration[199] and is a frequent problem in the geriatric patient. Ulcers can occur on any mucous membrane surface and are variable in size and shape. The ulcers are raised and have yellow-gray centers surrounded by an erythematous halo. Secondary infections with bacteria or *C. albicans* can occur.

The diagnosis is made primarily by history, since most patients can identify the cause of the trauma. The patient typically complains of an isolated intraoral "sore" with pain or tenderness in the area of the lesion. Symptoms rarely exceed 3 or 4 days, and the lesion heals within 10 to 14 days.[200]

Chronic irritation from decayed or broken teeth and inadequate dentures may lead to chronic ulcers that persist indefinitely. Cheek and tongue biting produce a thin, rough, keratotic film in the area traumatized. Fragments of epithelium are often seen in these cases, as a result of the continuous chewing on the same area.

Treatment is instituted by avoiding the cause of the trauma and contact with any irritants. Dental care is usually necessary to relieve sources of irritation. Surgical repair of any extensive laceration may be necessary.

*Denture-Related Oral Pathology.* Dental prosthetic appliances are intended to restore the health and well-being of patients, but they are responsible for many of the most commonly occurring oral lesions among the elderly. Removable appliances (complete or partial dentures) are implicated with greater frequency than are fixed appliances (bridges) because they may become distorted or broken with use and are frequently abused by the patient.[161] Older patients often do not or cannot comply with instructions for proper removal, placement, maintenance, and cleanliness of their appliances.

Because dentures fit next to teeth and soft tissue, they must be kept clean to maintain oral health. Plaque, food debris, and calculi collect on dentures just as they do on natural teeth. If left uncleaned, the dentures can be a source of irritation, inflammation, infection, or halitosis.

Partial dentures contribute to increased plaque formation around abutment teeth, which increases gingival inflammation over time.[201–203] Since these appliances can also increase tooth mobility and accelerate bone loss,[204] the reduction of plaque becomes even more important.

Frequently, patients perform their own repairs, relines, or adjustments, which can harm the dentures or oral mucosa. Additionally, all denture wearers should be advised that some servicing or readjustment of dentures is necessary occasionally because of normal changes in the supporting tissues and bone.

Common pathologic changes associated with denture wearing include the problems described below.

*Candidiasis.* Denture-related candidiasis is by far the most common type of oral candidal infection.[205] The characteristic appearance is that of a slightly granular or irregularly eroded erythematous mucosa that corresponds exactly to the area covered by the upper denture. In some cases, the denture fits poorly and serves as a nutrient reservoir to foster fungal growth.[206] In patients with well-fitting dentures, the stability and peripheral seal of the upper denture allow the fungus to flourish in the absence of normal salivary flow. The condition seldom causes any discomfort.

These fungi are capable of growing on denture surfaces, from which they can infect and reinfect the soft tissues. Management therefore requires that both the denture and the mucosal surfaces be treated. Dentures should be kept scrupulously clean and soaked frequently in antifungal agents, germicides, or chlorhexidine.[206,207] The infected tissue is treated with topical antifungal agents.[169–171,173]

*Denture Stomatitis (Denture Sore Mouth, Stomatitis Prosthetica).* The true etiology of denture stomatitis, a generalized inflammation associated with denture wearing, is unknown. It has been ascribed to contact hypersensitivity to dental materials, bacterial and candidal infections, tissue reaction to ill-fitting or unclean dentures, residual denture cleanser, medication use, and systemic diseases.[177,205,208,209] It is known to worsen in patients who do not remove their dentures at night or are negligent in denture hygiene.[210,211]

The disease is characterized by a very discrete erythematous reaction that closely follows the outline of the denture. Resolution of the inflammation may be obtained by thoroughly cleaning the denture if it fits well or by constructing a new one if it is ill-fitting. If candidal organisms are a contributing factor to the stomatitis, the denture may be covered with an antifungal ointment before insertion or soaked in an antifungal solution at night.

*Traumatic Ulcers (Denture Sore Spots).* An unstable or unretentive denture will cause tissue irritation or ulceration because of excess movement. Overextended denture flanges, bone spicules under the dentures, and foods—especially seeds—trapped between the denture and mucosa can also cause ulcerative lesions. The ulcers are small, painful, irregularly shaped lesions usually covered by a necrotic membrane and surrounded by an inflammatory halo. Treatment consists of correcting the underlying cause. Most lesions usually heal promptly.

### Periodontium

*Periodontal Disease.* The most common disease of the periodontium is periodontal disease, a term generally used to describe specific chronic disorders that affect the gingiva, supporting connective tissue, and alveolar bone.[212] It is a chronic, progressive, and destructive condition, and its incidence and severity typically increase with age.[213–215] There is considerable question, however, about whether the increase in severity with age represents age-dependent pathology or the cumulative effects of a lifetime of intermittent destruction.[1]

Periodontal disease commonly develops in two stages, gingivitis and periodontitis. As with dental caries, the major etiologic factor is plaque, which accumulates more rapidly and heavily in elderly people.[216] If the plaque is not removed daily, it will calcify into calculus (tartar). Accumulation of plaque, food, bacteria, and calculi on the tooth surfaces between the tooth and gingiva produces a low-grade inflammation of the gingiva (gingivitis). This is clinically characterized by gingival redness, enlargement, tenderness, and bleeding. Although gingivitis develops more rapidly and with greater severity in older adults,[216] it is reversible with adequate plaque control.

If the inflammatory process is allowed to progress, there is formation of pus (pyorrhea) with or without discomfort or other symptoms. Without drainage, the accumulation of pus leads to acute swelling (periodontal abscess) and pain. When the inflammation extends to the underlying alveolar bone and connective tissue (periodontitis), it loosens the teeth and causes them to be extruded. However, once the teeth are lost, the inflammatory symptoms subside.

The diagnosis depends on a combination of findings, including localized pain, loose teeth, the presence of periodontal pockets, erythema, and swelling or suppuration. A severe case results in a foul odor, inflamed and ulcerated gums, fibrotic tissue, and bleeding. Roentgenograms may reveal the destruction of alveolar bone. Margins of overextended fillings often play a role as local irritating factors. Occlusal trauma, particularly from grinding and teeth-clenching habits, and systemic factors may contribute to periodontal disease, but they do not initiate the disease.[217,218]

The prevention of periodontal disease depends largely on plaque control through meticulous oral hygiene.[219,220] Although there are indications that periodontal breakdown progresses slowly in elderly persons,[215] progression of the disease can be retarded by oral hygiene[215,221,222] and use of antimicrobial agents.[126,127,152] Local drainage and oxygenating mouth rinses (3% hydrogen peroxide in an equal volume of water) will usually reverse any acute symptoms and allow for routine follow-up procedures. In some cases, surgery to reduce excess gum tissue helps prevent the formation of periodontal pockets that predispose to periodontal infections. In advanced disease, extraction of teeth may be necessary.

*Necrotizing Ulcerative Gingivitis (Vincent's Infection, Trench Mouth)*. Necrotizing ulcerative gingivitis is an acute, recurring, noncommunicable inflammatory disease of the gingiva resulting from local irritation and organisms in the normal oral flora that invade the gingival tissue when its resistance is lowered. The disease is characterized by redness, swelling, ulceration, bleeding, and pain. The yellowish-gray pseudomembrane that usually covers the ulcerated surface can be removed easily, leaving a raw, bleeding base. In severe cases, there is a fetid odor and foul taste in the mouth. Recurrent attacks can lead to bone loss. Treatment includes eliminating local irritants by careful and thorough oral hygiene procedures. Local anesthetics, as well as antibiotic therapy, may serve as adjuncts to treatment. Caustics are contraindicated.

### Tongue

*Fissured Tongue.* The prevalence of fissured tongue, characterized by cracks on the dorsolateral surfaces of the tongue, increases progressively in each decade of adult life. Fissured tongue is found in varying degrees in approximately 5% of the population. It occurs in 60% of persons after age 40 years.

The fissures are deep, tend to collect food debris and microorganisms, and cause the tongue to be inflamed often. However, the tongue is usually pain free or only mildly tender, even if the fissures become secondarily infected from retained debris and microbes.

Fissuring of the tongue sometimes is asso-ciated with deficiency of vitamin $B_{12}$ complex, or it may be genetic. Another cause is correlation with long-standing glossitis.

Treatment consists of brushing the tongue or rubbing it vigorously with a moistened washcloth to provide relief. The scarring is irreversible.

*Glossitis.* Inflammation of the tongue, usually manifested by considerable atrophy of the filiform papillae, creates a red, smooth appearance. It may be secondary to a variety of diseases, such as anemia, nutritional deficiency, drug reactions, systemic infection, and physical or chemical irritations. The diagnosis is usually based on the history and laboratory studies, including cultures as indicated.

Treatment is based on identifying and correcting the primary cause, if possible, and palliating the tongue symptoms as required. When the cause cannot be determined and there are no symptoms, therapy is not indicated.

*Glossodynia, Glossopyrosis (Burning Tongue, Chronic Lingual Papillitis)*. Glossodynia, or painful, burning, itching, stinging tongue, is a distressing symptom that predominantly affects older women.[223] It can accompany atrophy of the tongue papillae and is a prominent feature of the "burning mouth" syndrome. Involvement of the entire tongue or isolated areas, occurring with or without glossitis, may be the presenting symptoms of hypochromic or pernicious anemia, nutritional disturbances, emotional upset, hormonal imbalance, allergies, psychosomatic syndromes (grief, loneliness, despair), or other systemic disorders.[224] Smoking, xerostomia, medication use, and candidiasis may also be causative.

In most cases, a primary cause cannot be identified. Cultures are of no value, since the offending organisms usually are also present in the normal oral flora. Dental prostheses, caries, and periodontal disease are usually of no causative significance. Although certain foods may cause flare-ups, they are not the primary causes. Dentifrice ingredients are rare causes of burning and pain of the tongue.

Treatment is mainly empiric, since causative factors usually are not identified. Important approaches include ruling out systemic conditions associated with these symptoms, changing the individual's drug regimen, and reassuring the patient that there is no evidence of infection or neoplasia. Ointments and mouth rinses are of no value.

*Hairy Tongue.* Hairy tongue is characterized by elongated, thick, densely matted, and stained filaments on the dorsum of the tongue that resemble hair. The filaments are hypertrophied or hyperplastic filiform papillae that can be stained yellow, brown, or black.

Normally, the developing papillary tissue cells slide off the tongue during mechanical stimulation. When desquamation is diminished, the papillae become elongated and provide a nidus for materia alba to accumulate, for stains to collect, and for bacteria and fungi to lodge and produce minor infections.[176] Common causes of staining are coffee, tobacco, medications, foods, and chromogenic microorganisms.

Hairy tongue is not a serious condition and is easily eliminated by improving tongue hygiene and promoting desquamation. If candidal organisms are present, the use of antifungal agents is indicated.

*Macroglossia.* Macroglossia (large tongue) may be congenital or acquired. It is significant in the elderly population because individuals who have been edentulous for many years may develop this condition. The marked use of the tongue to aid in mastication of food results in muscular hypertrophy, a common type of acquired macroglossia. If the patient is able to wear dentures, the tongue muscle may regress, with reduction in the size of the tongue.

## Circumoral Tissues

### *Lips*

*Angular Cheilitis (Cheilosis, Pseudocheilosis, or Perlèche).* Angular cheilitis is a nonspecific inflammation at the oral commissure area bilaterally. It proceeds to a cracking of the angles of the mouth, with well-defined fissures present. The drooling of saliva often aggravates the condition.

The etiology of angular cheilosis is often complex. The combination of bone resorption, muscle atrophy, and tooth loss decreases the distance between the nose and chin, which causes the skin to wrinkle and fold around the mouth. The wrinkling can also accompany a change of bite with old, ill-fitting, or even new dentures. The wrinkled folds collect saliva, *C. albicans*, bacteria, and other contaminants that can cause the infection. Contributing factors include vitamin B complex deficiency, iron deficiency, or both.[57]

Treatment is directed toward unfolding the skin by the fitting of proper dentures; culturing and treating all infections; initiating measures of local hygiene; and, if necessary, giving iron and vitamin supplements.

*Squamous Cell Carcinomas.* A high risk of lip cancer is associated with the use of tobacco, particularly pipe tobacco, and exposure to ultraviolet radiation. Almost 95% of these cancers develop in the lower lip, where trauma and heat from the pipestem and exposure to the sun are greatest.[225] Atrophy of the lip, thinning of the lip border, and loss of elasticity are early clinical features. Carcinoma of the lip may appear as a crack in the lip surface, a crusting ulcer, or a tumorous growth. The prognosis is very good unless the lesion is extensive, since metastases develop later and less frequently than from intraoral sites.[178]

### Oral Musculature

*Dysphagia.* Dysphagia (difficulty in swallowing) may render a patient vulnerable to aspiration of saliva or oral intake. Indicators that a swallowing problem is likely to be present include dysarthria, poor control of oral secretions, inability to swallow spontaneously, drooling or gurgling aspirations or regurgitation through the nose, and frequent reflexive coughing.[226,227]

The causes of dysphagia may be neurologic, neuromuscular, or structural. In one study,[53] a significant increase in swallowing dysfunction was seen among older persons taking prescription medications. Conditions that alter the ability to form and prepare a bolus in the oral stage of swallowing can also cause dysphagia.[10]

*Dyskinesia.* Oral dyskinesia is a movement disorder characterized by severe, dystonic, involuntary movement of the facial, oral, and cervical musculature.[228,229] The involuntary abnormal contractions, mainly of the tongue, lips, and mandible, occur frequently with age in patients who exhibit disturbances of the cerebral stroma or stromal changes of the extrapyramidal motor system.[230,231] Because the movements disappear when the mouth is opened wide, during sleep, or when the patient's attention is distracted, oral dyskinesia tends to be regarded as a disease of the central nervous system.[228,232]

Some studies have reported a close correlation between oral dyskinesia and poor oral conditions.[228,232] One study describing the clinical appearance of this disease in the aged[228] found that its occurrence was associated with missing teeth and use of uncomfortable dentures. It has also been demonstrated that the symptoms of oral dyskinesia respond favorably to dental treatment, such as extractions, new dentures, and adjustment of old dentures.[229,232]

Drug-induced oral dyskinesia, or tardive dyskinesia, is a permanent side effect of long-term neuroleptic (antipsychotic) drug therapy that does not resolve on withdrawal of the drug. The most common movements are tongue protrusion, licking and smacking of the lips, puffing of the cheeks, sucking and chewing, and facial grimacing.[233,234]

*Trismus.* Trismus is a condition in which tonic spasms of the masticatory muscles limit opening of the mouth. It may develop during or after radiation therapy if these muscles are included in the treatment field. Management is directed toward exercises and various prosthetic appliances to increase the opening capacity of the muscles.

## Other Changes

### Salivary Glands

*Sialolithiasis.* Sialoliths, or salivary stones, may form in any of the major or minor salivary glands or their excretory ducts. The most common manifestation of ductal stones, which do not generally cause complete obstruction, is enlargement of the gland and subsequent pain during eating. Both the glandular swelling and pain subside between meals as the entrapped saliva is gradually excreted.

*Tumors.* Benign and malignant tumors of the salivary glands are more common in older patients, and both the major and minor salivary glands are involved.[235] Overall, neoplasms arising from the minor salivary glands are relatively uncommon compared with those arising from the major salivary glands.[179,236,237] However, most tumors of the minor salivary glands are malignant.[237,238]

Both elderly men and elderly women appear to have an increased risk of salivary gland malignancies; however, little information about the causative factors exists. Radiotherapy is an infrequent etiologic factor.[239] Trauma, infection, stone formation, and the use of alcohol or tobacco are not associated with these tumors.[240]

The survival rates for patients with malignant salivary gland tumors are generally higher than they are for persons with most other oral cancers. Usually, diagnosis and treatment are rendered early, and metastasis occurs late in the course of the disease. Long-term follow-up is essential, however, because there is a high rate of recurrence.

*Xerostomia (Dry Mouth, Decreased Salivary Flow).* Xerostomia, although not a disease concomitant with aging, is a symptom that is often evident in older patients. The main cause is use of xerogenic medications; other causes include vitamin deficiencies, dehydration, mouth breathing, stress, and a variety of systemic diseases and their therapies.

Without the antibacterial, cleansing, lubricating, remineralizing, and buffering actions of saliva, the individual with xerostomia is at increased risk of developing coronal and root surface caries; abrasion and erosion of tooth surfaces; periodontal disease; atrophic glossitis; traumatic injuries to the mucous membranes; mucosal lesions; infections of the pharynx and salivary glands; and dysfunctions of speech, chewing, swallowing, and taste.[30,241–244] In addition to the damage to teeth and supporting structures, problems with prostheses are also magnified when the mouth is dry. Saliva provides a thin, fluid film between the denture base and underlying soft tissues necessary for the retention and stability of dentures during function.[58,245] Additionally, saliva prevents the hard acrylic or metal surfaces from abrading the oral mucosa. Consequently, frequent denture problems and sores arise, and the patient complains of generalized intraoral soreness during mastication.

Patients may express one or all of the signs and symptoms associated with xerostomia in varying degrees of severity. Some of these include mouth dryness; a fissured tongue; glossodynia or glossopyrosis; candidiasis; rampant caries; oral soreness; sticking of food or lips to the teeth; cracking of lips; difficulty in speaking, chewing, and swallowing; a generalized burning sensation; and ageusia, dysgeusia, or hypogeusia.[58,245] The mucosa becomes dry, rough, and sticky; bleeds easily; and is subject to ulceration or infection.

Prevention and management of xerostomia depends on its etiology (Table 6–5). With drug-induced xerostomia, the responsible drug may be able to be eliminated, reduced in dosage or frequency of administration, or replaced by a substitute drug. Management of xerostomia that is irreversible, such as radiation-induced xerostomia, is essentially palliative and accommodative. Small, frequent mouthfuls of water are palatable and inexpensive and moisten the mouth fairly well. To facilitate chewing and swallowing, most patients with xerostomia moisten and thin foods with sauces, gravies, milk, and other fluids.

Artificial saliva preparations provide relief by coating and lubricating the mucosa. Saliva substitutes containing fluoride and fluoride gels are helpful for patients with xerostomia who are at high risk for dental caries. For the lips and dentures, a constant coating of petroleum jelly and frequent oral application of artificial salivas should alleviate some of the problems. However, lemon glycerine swabs should be avoided because of their cariogenic and drying effects. Also, commercial mouthwashes should be avoided because they have a high alcohol content and dry the oral mucosa. Similarly, ingestion of alcoholic beverages should be minimized.[246]

**Table 6–5** Prevention and Management of Xerostomia

Determine etiology
Alter medication regimen
    Eliminate medication
    Reduce dosage or frequency of administration
    Replace with medication for another with less severe oral side effects
Alleviate complaints
    Increase fluid intake (water or low-sugar beverages); avoid caffeinated drinks
    Avoid dry, bulky, spicy, salty, or highly acidic foods
    Avoid tobacco and alcohol intake
    Humidify air
    Use saliva stimulants (local and systemic agents)
      Local agents
        Sugarless hard candy or lozenges
        Sugarless gum
      Systemic agents
        Pilocarpine drops
        Oral pilocarpine (2.5–5.0 mg three times daily before meals)
      Use artificial saliva preparations (containing fluoride)
        Glycerine
        Methylcellulose
      Coat lips and dentures with petroleum jelly
Increase resistance to dental disease
    Have frequent dental examinations
    Use fluorides frequently
    Modify diet
    Control plaque

---

### Sense of Taste

Taste acuity may be affected by oral pathologic conditions, dental diseases, olfactory deficits, medications, malnutrition, smoking, radiation therapy, neurologic deficits, and other systemic disorders.[5] Cues that may indicate alterations in taste sensitivity include decreased or increased appetite, excessive use of seasoning, and excessive use of sugar.

### SYSTEMIC DISEASES AND MEDICATIONS AFFECTING ORAL HEALTH

The elderly population suffers from many concurrent acute and chronic diseases, some of which may have oral manifestations or adversely affect oral health. Since 86% of all elderly persons suffer from at least one chronic disease, oral health problems secondary to these diseases may be important.[247] Systemic diseases that affect the oral and circumoral structures are listed in Table 6–6.

Many of the most commonly experienced chronic disease conditions found in the elderly are symptomatically controlled with the proper use of medications. The increased use of medications with advancing age, therefore, is not surprising. Geriatric patients take more drugs because they have more chronic illnesses than do younger patients. Not only does the problem of multiple drug use among

**Table 6–6** Oral Manifestations of Systemic Diseases

| Disease/Condition | Oral Manifestations |
|---|---|
| Achlorhydria | Tongue—glossitis |
| Adrenal insufficiency | Oral infections—increased risk<br>Oral mucosa—pigmentation<br>Taste—loss or distortion<br>Wound-healing response—poor |
| Agranulocytosis | Gingiva—spontaneous bleeding<br>Hemorrhagic tendency—petechiae<br>Periodontal disease—high incidence<br>Ulcerations—painful, persistent, necrotic |
| Alcoholism | Breath odor of alcohol<br>Dental caries—high incidence<br>Facial neuralgia, edema<br>Hemorrhagic tendency—ecchymoses, petechiae<br>Lips—angular cheilosis<br>Oral cancer—increased risk<br>Oral hygiene—poor<br>Oral infections—increased risk<br>Oral mucosa—jaundiced, ulcerated<br>Parotid salivary glands—chronic swelling<br>Periodontal disease—chronic (with frequent acute exacerbations)<br>Taste—decreased sensitivity<br>Teeth—attrition, erosion, loss<br>Tongue—glossitis, ulcerated<br>Wound-healing response—delayed<br>Xerostomia |
| Alzheimer's disease | Dysphagia<br>Oral hygiene—poor, neglected<br>Taste sensitivity—decreased<br>Xerostomia |
| Amyotrophic lateral sclerosis | Dysarthria<br>Tongue fasciculations—atrophic |
| Anemia | Burning/sore mouth—mucositis/stomatitis<br>Filiform papillae—atrophic<br>Oral mucosa—pale, atrophic, thin, tender<br>Tongue—glossitis, glossodynia<br>Xerostomia |

*continues*

**Table 6–6** continued

| Disease/Condition | Oral Manifestations |
| --- | --- |
| Anxiety disorders | Burning/sore mouth<br>Dysphagia<br>Xerostomia |
| Arthritis | TMJ involvement—limited jaw movement |
| Biliary tract obstruction | Bleeding—excessive, spontaneous<br>Hemorrhagic tendency—petechiae, hematomas |
| Bipolar disorders | Depressive phase—oral hygiene neglected<br>Facial pain syndromes due to mood swings<br>Manic phase—self-inflicted mucosal abrasion |
| Bleeding disorders | Intraoral bleeding—ecchymoses, hematomas, petechiae<br>Oral mucosa—jaundiced |
| Cerebrovascular accident | Chewing difficulty/inability<br>Dysarthria<br>Dysphagia<br>Facial drooping—affects denture fit<br>Gag reflex—decreased<br>Oral motor apraxia<br>Oral sensation—decreased unilaterally |
| Chorea | Dysarthria<br>Oral dyskinesia |
| Congenital heart disease | Cyanosis<br>Intraoral hemorrhages, infections<br>Leukopenia, polycythemia, thrombocytopenia |
| Congestive heart failure | Intraoral bleeding—ecchymoses, petechiae<br>Lips—cyanosis, thinning of vermilion border<br>Oral infections |
| Coronary arteriosclerotic heart disease | Oral or facial pain—referred |
| Crohn's disease | Aphthous ulcers—high frequency<br>Burning/sore mouth<br>Dental caries—high frequency<br>Oral hygiene—poor |

*continues*

**Table 6–6** continued

| Disease/Condition | Oral Manifestations |
| --- | --- |
| Cyclic neutropenia | Mucositis/stomatitis<br>Oral infections—increased risk<br>Periodontal disease—high incidence<br>Ulcerations—aphthous type |
| Dementia | Bruxism<br>Burning/sore mouth<br>Dysphagia<br>Facial pain—atypical<br>Oral injuries—increased susceptibility<br>Periodontal disease—accelerated<br>Poor oral hygiene—chronic |
| Depression | Burning/sore mouth<br>Dental caries—rapid progression<br>Facial pain syndromes—numerous<br>Oral hygiene—poor<br>Periodontal disease—accelerated<br>Tongue—glossodynia<br>Xerostomia |
| Diabetes mellitus | Breath odor of ketone<br>Burning/sore mouth—mucositis/stomatitis<br>Candidiasis<br>Dental caries—rampant<br>Gingiva—inflammation<br>Lips—angular cheilitis<br>Mucomycosis<br>Oral infections—increased susceptibility<br>Oral paresthesias<br>Periodontal disease—accentuated, abscesses<br>Taste sensitivity—decreased<br>Teeth—sensitivity<br>Tongue—glossodynia<br>Ulcerations<br>Wound-healing response—delayed<br>Xerostomia |
| Epilepsy | Gingiva—drug-induced hyperplasia<br>Ulcerations—traumatic |
| Gonorrhea | Gingivitis |

*continues*

**Table 6–6** continued

| Disease/Condition | Oral Manifestations |
|---|---|
| Gonorrhea (continued) | Oral abscesses/mucosal lesions/ulcerations<br>Oral mucosa—erythematous<br>Parotitis<br>Pharyngitis/tonsillitis<br>Stomatitis—generalized |
| Hepatitis | Intraoral bleeding<br>Oral mucosa—pigmentation<br>Taste—loss or distortion |
| Herpes zoster | Bone—osteoradionecrosis<br>Neuralgia—trigeminal<br>Oral mucosa—lesions, ulcerations, pain<br>Teeth—devitalization, exfoliation |
| Hypertension | Neuritis |
| Hyperthyroidism | Dental caries—extensive<br>Periodontal disease—progressive<br>Tongue—tumors (midline of posterior dorsum) |
| Hypoparathyroidism | Candidiasis |
| Hypothyroidism | Candidiasis<br>Taste—loss or distortion<br>Teeth—malocclusion<br>Tongue—macroglossia<br>Xerostomia |
| Immunosuppression | Increased susceptibility to candidiasis; dental caries; infections, local and systemic; intraoral bleeding; periodontal disease; recurrent aphthous ulcers; tumor development |
| Leukemia | Bone—lesions<br>Burning/sore mouth—mucositis/stomatitis<br>Candidiasis<br>Gingiva—hyperplasia, spontaneous bleeding<br>Hemorrhagic tendency—ecchymoses, hematomas, petechiae<br>Herpetic stomatitis<br>Infections—increased risk |

*continues*

**Table 6–6** continued

| Disease/Condition | Oral Manifestations |
|---|---|
| Leukemia (continued) | Lymphadenopathy<br>Oral mucosa—pallor, lesions<br>Oral paresthesias<br>Ulcerations—painful, persistent, necrotic |
| Leukopenia | Oral infections—increased risk |
| Liver disease | Bleeding—excessive, spontaneous<br>Hemorrhagic tendency—ecchymoses, hematomas, petechiae |
| Lupus erythematosus | Burning/sore mouth<br>Candidiasis<br>Mandible—immobility<br>Oral lesions—bullae, erosions<br>Oral mucosa—sloughing<br>TMJ deviation, pain with movement or palpation, joint sounds, locking or dislocation<br>Tongue—fissuring, atrophic papillae<br>Ulcerations<br>Xerostomia |
| Lymphomas | Burning/sore mouth<br>Candidiasis<br>Cervical lymphadenopathy<br>Extranodal oral tumors<br>Hemorrhagic tendency—ecchymoses, petechiae<br>Infections—increased risk |
| Malabsorption syndrome | Bleeding—excessive, spontaneous<br>Candidiasis<br>Hemorrhagic tendency—ecchymoses, hematomas, petechiae |
| Malignant hypertension | Facial paralysis |
| Multiple myeloma | Amyloid deposits in soft tissue<br>Bone—lesions, pain<br>Soft tissues—tumors<br>Teeth—unexplained mobility |

*continues*

**Table 6–6** continued

| Disease/Condition | Oral Manifestations |
| --- | --- |
| Multiple sclerosis | Dysarthria<br>TMJ—pain with movement or palpation, joint sounds<br>Trigeminal neuralgia<br>Xerostomia, drug-induced |
| Muscular dystrophy | Mouth breathing<br>Muscles—weakness, decreased biting force<br>Tongue—hypertrophy |
| Myasthenia gravis | Chewing difficulty<br>Dysphagia<br>Gingiva—poor health<br>Mouth breathing<br>Muscles—weakness, inability to close mouth<br>Tongue—flaccid |
| Narcolepsy | Candidiasis<br>Xerostomia |
| Nephritis | Burning/sore mouth<br>Xerostomia |
| Neurofibromatosis | Oral neurofibromatous lesions<br>Oral paresthesias<br>Soft tissues—pigmentation<br>Tongue—macroglossia, enlarged lingual papillae |
| Organ transplants | Intraoral bleeding—increased susceptibility<br>Oral infections—increased susceptibility<br>Tumor development—increased susceptibility |
| Osteoarthritis | Bone—resorption<br>TMJ—unilateral involvement, dysfunction |
| Paget's disease | Bone—progressive enlargement |
| Parkinson's disease | Chewing difficulty<br>Drooling of saliva due to swallowing difficulty (not excessive production)<br>Dysarthria |

*continues*

**Table 6–6** continued

| Disease/Condition | Oral Manifestations |
| --- | --- |
| Parkinson's disease (continued) | Dysphagia<br>Facial paresthesias, tremors<br>Lips—angular cheilitis, tremors<br>Oral hygiene—poor<br>Oral mucositis—stomatitis<br>Tardive dyskinesia, drug-induced<br>Teeth—involuntary bruxism<br>Tongue—tremors<br>Xerostomia, drug-induced |
| Pemphigus vulgaris | Burning/sore mouth<br>Candidiasis<br>Halitosis<br>Hypersalivation<br>Oral lesions, erosions—bleed easily, painful<br>Ulcerations—raw, red, eroded |
| Pneumonia | Aspiration—increased susceptibility with dysphagia, poor dentition, poor oral hygiene |
| Polycythemia | Oral mucosa—cyanosis |
| Posttraumatic stress disorder | Bruxism<br>Dental caries—increased incidence<br>Oral hygiene—poor<br>Periodontal disease—increased incidence<br>Tongue—glossodynia |
| Progressive bulbar palsy | Chewing difficulty<br>Dysarthria<br>Jaw muscles—spasticity |
| Radiation therapy to head/neck | Candidiasis<br>Mucositis<br>Muscles—dysfunction, trismus<br>Oral infections—increased susceptibility<br>Osteoradionecrosis<br>Pulp—pain, necrosis<br>Taste—lost or distorted<br>Teeth—hypersensitivity, radiation caries<br>Xerostomia |
| Renal disease/dialysis/transplants | Breath odor of urea<br>Calculus—increased formation |

*continues*

**Table 6–6** continued

| Disease/Condition | Oral Manifestations |
|---|---|
| Renal disease/dialysis/transplants (continued) | Candidiasis<br>Dental caries—low incidence<br>Gingiva—pale, undefined, bleeds spontaneously<br>Oral infections—frequent retrograde infectious parotitis<br>Oral mucosa—pallor, uremic stomatitis<br>Renal osteomalacia/osteodystrophy<br>Salivary flow—decreased<br>Taste—metallic<br>Teeth—mobility<br>Tongue—macroglossia, glossodynia<br>Ulcerations—ulcerative stomatitis<br>Wound-healing response—poor |
| Rheumatoid arthritis | Bone—resorption<br>Muscles—atrophic<br>TMJ—dysfunction<br>Xerostomia |
| Sjögren's syndrome | Burning/sore mouth—mucositis/stomatitis<br>Candidiasis<br>Dental caries—increased susceptibility<br>Lips—angular cheilosis, lesions<br>Oral mucosa—lesions<br>Parotid gland—enlargement<br>Periodontal disease—accelerated<br>Saliva—composition changes: increased sodium, potassium, manganese; decreased calcium<br>Taste—loss, distortion<br>Tongue—glossitis, glossodynia<br>Xerostomia |
| Smokeless tobacco use | Gingiva—recession<br>Halitosis<br>Oral cancer—increased risk<br>Oral mucosa—leukoplakia<br>Periodontal disease—accentuated<br>Smell sensitivity—decreased<br>Taste sensitivity—decreased<br>Teeth—abrasion, attrition, erosion, loss |

*continues*

**Table 6–6** continued

| Disease/Condition | Oral Manifestations |
|---|---|
| Syphilis | Oral lesions—chancre, mucous patch, gumma<br>Tongue—interstitial glossitis |
| Temporal arteritis | Orofacial pain |
| Thrombocytopenia | Hemorrhagic tendency—ecchymoses, hematomas, petechiae |
| Tobacco smoking | Calculus—increased<br>Gingivitis—increased<br>Hairy tongue<br>Halitosis<br>Smell sensitivity—decreased<br>Taste—loss or distortion<br>Teeth—abrasion<br>Wound-healing response—delayed |
| Tuberculosis | Lymph node involvement (scrofula)<br>Ulcerations, especially on tongue |
| Urticaria (angioneurotic anemia) | Swelling—soft tissues |
| von Willebrand's disease | Hemorrhagic tendency—ecchymoses, hematomas, petechiae<br>Intraoral bleeding—spontaneous |

elderly people have serious implications due to pharmacokinetic and pharmacodynamic considerations with aging, but also there are iatrogenic oral manifestations of many drugs (Table 6–7).

In addition to the oral signs and symptoms from elderly people's use of properly prescribed and over-the-counter medications, there are oral manifestations of recreational drug abuse, including advanced generalized periodontal disease, bruxism, numerous abscessed or missing teeth, poor oral hygiene, rampant caries, tooth attrition (secondary to bruxism), and xerostomia.[248–251]

## IMPACT OF NUTRITIONAL STATUS ON ORAL HEALTH

Nutritional status has an important role in oral health. A sophisticated system of nutrient interaction is essential to the formation of healthy teeth and the maintenance of oral and circumoral tissues throughout life.[252–254] The systemic effects of nutrients on oral health, growth and development, cell integrity and renewal, proper function of the tissues and saliva, tissue repair, and resistance and susceptibility to oral diseases (Table 6–8) have been studied by very few researchers and need

**Table 6–7**  Drug-Induced Oral Manifestations

Candidiasis
  Antibiotics
  Antineoplastics
  Corticosteroids
  Diuretics
  Immunosuppressives
  Steroid inhalers

Contact hypersensitivity
  Iodine
  Menthol
  Topical analgesics
  Topical antibiotics

Erythema multiforme
  Anticonvulsants
  Antimalarials
  Barbiturates
  Busulfan
  Chlorpropamide
  Clindamycin
  Codeine
  Isoniazid
  Meprobamate
  Minoxidil
  Penicillins
  Phenolphthalein
  Phenylbutazone
  Propylthiouracil
  Salicylates
  Sulfonamides
  Tetracyclines

Fixed drug eruptions
  Barbiturates
  Chlordiazepoxide
  Sulfonamides
  Tetracyclines

Gingival hyperplasia
  Cyclosporine
  Nifedipine
  Phenytoin sodium

Glossodynia
  Diuretics

Hairy tongue
  Antibiotics
  Corticosteroids
  Sodium perborate
  Sodium peroxide

Hypersalivation/sialorrhea
  Antianxiety agents
  Anticholinesterases
  Apomorphine
  Iodides
  Lithium
  Mercurial salts
  Nitrazepam

Infections
  Antineoplastics
  Corticosteroids (high dose)
  Immunosuppressives

Intraoral bleeding/petechiae/purpura
  Antiarrhythmics
  Antibiotics (broad spectrum)
  Anticoagulants
  Aspirin
  Warfarin sodium

Lichenoid mucosal reactions
  Allopurinol
  Antihypertensives
  ß-blockers
  Chloroquine
  Chlorothiazide
  Chlorpropamide
  Dapsone
  Diuretics
  Gold salts
  Mercury compounds
  Nonsteroidal anti-inflammatory agents
  Penicillamine
  Phenothiazines
  Quinidine
  Streptomycin
  Sulfamethoxazole

*continues*

**Table 6–7** continued

Lichenoid mucosal reactions (continued)
  Tetracyclines
  Tolbutamide
  Doxorubicin hydrochloride
  Gold salts
  Mercurial diuretics
  Minocycline
  Phenolphthalein
  Phenothiazines
  Phenytoin
  Silver compounds

Lupus erythematosus (oral mucosa) reactions
  Gold salts
  Griseofulvin
  Hydralazine hydrochloride
  Isoniazid
  Methyldopa
  Penicillin
  Phenytoin
  Primidone
  Procainamide
  Streptomycin
  Sulfonamides
  Tetracyclines
  Thiouracil

Mucositis/stomatitis
  Antineoplastics
  Lithium
  Mercurial diuretics

Oral dyskinesias
  Buspirone

Orofacial neuropathies (numbness, tingling, burning of the face or mouth)
  Acetazolamide
  Antineoplastics
  ß-blockers
  Chlorpropamide
  Ergotamine
  Hydralazine hydrochloride
  Hypoglycemics (oral)
  Isoniazid

Methysergide
Nalidixic acid
Nitrofurantoin
Phenytoin
Streptomycin
Tolbutamide
Tricyclic antidepressants

Pigmentation (soft tissue)
  Antimalarials
  Busulfan
  Chlorhexidine

Salivary gland enlargement
  Antipsychotics
  Insulin
  Iodides
  Isoproterenol
  Methyldopa
  Phenylbutazone
  Potassium chloride
  Thiocyanate
  Thiouracil
  Warfarin sodium

Salivary gland pain and/or swelling
  Antihypertensives
  Antithyroid agents
  Cytotoxic agents
  Ganglion-blocking agents
  Insulin
  Iodine
  Isoproterenol
  Oxyphenbutazone
  Phenothiazines
  Phenylbutazone
  Potassium chlorate
  Sulfonamides
  Warfarin sodium

Spontaneous oral bleeding
  Anticoagulants
  Antineoplastics

*continues*

**Table 6–7** continued

Tardive dyskinesias
  Butyrophenone antipsychotics
  Levodopa
  Phenothiazines
  Thioxanthene

Taste dysfunction
  Amphetamines
  Benzodiazepines
  Carbimazole
  Chlorhexidine
  Chlorpromazine
  Clofibrate
  Ethionamide
  Gold salts
  Griseofulvin
  Levodopa
  Lincomycin
  Lithium carbonate
  Methocarbamol
  Metronidazole
  D-Penicillamine
  Penicillin
  Phenformin hydrochloride
  Phenindione
  Propranolol
  Quinidine
  Tranquilizers
  Vitamins (excessive use)

Tooth decay (rampant)
  Tricyclic antidepressants

Tooth discoloration
  Chlorhexidine
  Gentian violet
  Stannous fluoride
  Tetracyclines

Ulcerations
  Antiarrhythmics
  Antineoplastics
  Aspirin
  Gold salts
  Indomethacin
  Meprobamate

Xerostomia
  Amphetamines
  Analgesics
  Anorexiants
  Antiallergics
  Antianxiety agents
  Antiarrhythmics
  Anticholinergics
  Anticonvulsants
  Antidepressants
  Antidiarrheals
  Antihistamines
  Antihypertensives
  Anti-inflammatory agents
  Antinauseants
  Antineoplastics
  Antiparkinsonism agents
  Antipsychotics
  Antispasmodics
  Atropine
  Barbiturates
  Benzodiazepines
  Bronchodilators
  Central nervous system stimulants
  Congestive heart failure medications
  Decongestants
  Diuretics
  Ganglion-blocking agents
  Hypnotics
  Lithium
  Monoamine oxidase inhibitors
  Muscle relaxants
  Narcotics
  Nonsteroidal anti-inflammatory agents
  Phenylbutazone
  Scopolamine
  Sympathomimetics
Barbiturates (continued)
  Tranquilizers

*continues*

**Table 6–7** continued

Ulcerations (continued)
  Mercurial diuretics
  Methotrexate
  Methyldopa
  Naproxen
  D-Penicillamine
  Phenylbutazone
  Potassium chloride
  Propranolol
  Spironolactone
  Thiazide diuretics
  Tolbutamide

more attention and understanding. The local effects of food on plaque formation and the resultant oral disease processes, including coronal and root caries, gingivitis, and periodontitis, have been relatively well described.

**Plaque Formation**

Plaque consists mainly of bacteria and a matrix produced by them that is composed primarily of carbohydrate, protein, salts, and water. From a dietary standpoint, carbohydrates have an important role in initiating plaque formation. Once plaque is present, carbohydrates from food and beverages can diffuse into it and be fermented by the plaque bacteria. The acid produced can dissolve tooth structure, thus leading to carious lesions. Although acids present in food and beverages may also diffuse into the plaque, the result is usually erosion of the tooth surface and not dental caries.

If fermentable carbohydrates are not part of the diet, the acid-producing activity of the plaque will be low. Plaque is still demonstrable in subjects eating a diet devoid of fermentable carbohydrates, but the plaque is thin and structureless.[255] In contrast, subjects eating a sucrose-rich diet have voluminous, turgid plaque formation.

The texture of the diet may also influence dental plaque. Diets containing soft foods increase plaque formation more than those composed of firmer foods. In a study of women on a low-calorie diet, the rate of plaque formation increased.[256]

Plaque initially forms along the tooth-gum margin and gradually spreads across the tooth surface as the bacterial matrix grows. Since dietary carbohydrates contribute to this supragingival plaque formation, they have been implicated as an etiologic agent in the resulting gingival inflammation.[100,257,258]

**Dental Caries**

Although dental caries is generally accepted as primarily a microbial disease, diet plays a crucial secondary role. The dietary component contributing most to the initiation and progression of the caries process is fermentable carbohydrates.[259] Biochemical, microbiologic, and animal and human clinical and epidemiologic studies support a causal relationship. Even root surface caries in human populations is enhanced by the ingestion of dietary sugars.[113,260]

Normally, before eating, the pH of tooth surface plaque exposed to saliva is close to neutrality (pH 6.5–7.0).[261] The ingestion of

**Table 6–8** Systemic Effects of Nutrients on Oral Health

| Nutrient | Systemic Effect |
|---|---|
| Barium | Tooth decay resistance |
| Boron | Tooth decay resistance |
| Calcium | Bone formation/maintenance<br>Muscle tone maintenance<br>Nerve impulse transmission<br>Tooth formation/maintenance |
| Calcium-phosphorus balance | Bone maintenance<br>Periodontal maintenance |
| Copper | Bone formation/maintenance<br>Collagen synthesis<br>Periodontal maintenance<br>Wound healing |
| Fluorine | Tooth decay resistance |
| Folic acid | Epithelial integrity<br>Wound healing |
| Gold | Tooth decay resistance (mild) |
| Iron | Epithelial integrity<br>Periodontal maintenance |
| Lead | Tooth decay promotion |
| Lithium | Tooth decay resistance |
| Magnesium | Bone formation/maintenance<br>Tooth decay promotion<br>Tooth formation<br>Wound healing |
| Manganese | Cell membrane formation<br>Tooth decay resistance |
| Molybdenum | Tooth decay resistance (mild) |
| Nickel | Wound healing |

*continues*

**Table 6–8** continued

| Nutrient | Systemic Effect |
|---|---|
| Phosphorus | Bone formation/metabolism<br>Tooth decay resistance<br>Tooth formation/metabolism |
| Protein | Epithelial integrity<br>Taste bud renewal<br>Tooth formation<br>Wound healing |
| Selenium | Tooth decay promotion |
| Silicon | Bone formation |
| Strontium | Tooth decay resistance |
| Sulfur | Bone maintenance |
| Vanadium | Bone maintenance<br>Tooth decay resistance |
| Vitamin A | Epithelial integrity<br>Tooth formation<br>Wound healing |
| Vitamin $B_1$ | Wound healing |
| Vitamin $B_2$ | Wound healing |
| Vitamin $B_6$ | Wound healing |
| Vitamin C | Epithelial integrity<br>Periodontal maintenance<br>Tooth formation<br>Wound healing |
| Vitamin D | Bone formation/maintenance<br>Tooth formation |
| Zinc | Epithelial integrity/metabolism<br>Periodontal maintenance<br>Taste bud renewal<br>Wound healing |

foods containing fermentable carbohydrates leads to acid production by the cariogenic plaque bacteria on tooth surfaces. The acids cause a rapid drop in pH that can result in demineralization of the tooth substance. If the plaque pH falls below the critical point of about 5.5 and remains there for an appreciable time, the food causing the decrease is likely to support caries initiation and progression.[262,263]

The greatest concentration of acid, or lowest pH, occurs in 5 to 15 minutes,[261] but teeth are attacked by acids for 20 minutes or more. Saliva has a buffering effect that helps to control acid production to some degree, and it contains proteins that act as antibacterial agents. However, in elderly persons, who may have reductions in salivary flow and therefore reduced buffering and antibacterial capacity, each acid attack is significantly prolonged.

### Dietary Control

There is compelling evidence that dietary control of dental caries requires modification in the form, quantity, frequency, and timing of consumption of carbohydrates.[264,265] Sucrose traditionally has been regarded as the form of carbohydrate most detrimental to teeth.[266,267] However, recent research indicates that many of the common simple sugars (glucose, dextrose, fructose, maltose, and lactose) can contribute to the rapid formation of acid by dental plaque.[268,269] Some studies even suggest that complex carbohydrates, such as starches, have the potential to promote caries under certain conditions.[270,271]

Reducing the quantity of fermentable carbohydrates ingested deprives the potentially pathogenic plaque of necessary substrates for growth. It also limits the numbers of cariogenic microorganisms found in the dental plaque.[272,273]

Frequency of consumption is important, since each encounter of bacteria with fermentable carbohydrates can result in acid production, tooth surface demineralization, and the formation of carious lesions.[274,275] There is a strong association between root caries lesions in adults and the frequency of fermentable carbohydrate intake.[113,276] Restricting between-meal snacks containing cariogenic carbohydrates is advised, since frequent sugar consumption, especially between meals, is associated with increased dental caries activity.

The best time to ingest fermentable carbohydrates is with meals. Eating these foods at mealtime will produce less caries than eating the same foods eaten between meals. One reason for this may be that saliva, the production of which is increased during meals, helps neutralize acid production and clears food from the mouth. This is not true for between-meal snacks. Recently, however, it has been established that increasing salivary flow rates after meals, as with sugarless gum chewing, helps reduce plaque acids that can cause caries.[277]

### Cariogenicity

*Cariogenicity* refers to the potential that a specific food or diet has for dental caries formation. The local acidogenic activity of the food, not its nutrient content, largely determines its cariogenic potential.[278] Clinical trials to evaluate the cariogenicity of foodstuffs are expensive processes.[263] Studies must last 2 or 3 years, since dental caries develop slowly and are not clinically discernible for many months.

A key determinant of cariogenicity is oral clearance time.[279] When sugar is consumed in foods that adhere to or between tooth surfaces, caries activity has been shown to increase.[280] However, if the fermentable carbohydrate source is eaten with a beverage or in liquid form, the time needed for oral clearance is reduced, resulting in a lower net cariogenic potential. Thus, solid or retentive sugar-containing foods are more cariogenic than sugar-containing foods that are liquid or nonretentive.[278] Likewise, fermentable carbohydrates eaten at meals are less cariogenic than the same ones eaten between meals.[265]

Another indication of cariogenicity is the change in plaque pH associated with food consumption.[273] This measure has been used by a number of investigators to monitor the cariogenicity of particular foods and has been found to relate to oral clearance time. In one study, foods that adhered to the teeth depressed the plaque pH for longer periods than did foods that were removed from the teeth more quickly.[281,282]

The cariogenic potential of preparations of liquid medications is of particular concern for the geriatric patient. These medications frequently include high levels of sucrose, glucose, or fructose as sweeteners. Studies of patients taking sweetened liquid medications demonstrate a significant increase in dental caries, especially with long-term therapy.[283] Sweetened liquid iron supplements, cough syrups, antibiotics, and anticonvulsants have been shown to decrease plaque pH after ingestion.[284,285]

### Artificial Sweeteners

Research has been focused on identifying and developing substances that serve as taste-competitive, noncariogenic sugar substitutes. Aspartame and saccharin are the two agents currently available. Cyclamate was banned by the Food and Drug Administration in 1970 because of concerns over its safety. That ban currently is being reconsidered.

Aspartame is noncariogenic, but it is not noncaloric.[286] However, its sweetness is of sufficient intensity (180 times sweeter than sucrose) that only small amounts are required, resulting in a very significant reduction in calories.

Saccharin is 300 times sweeter than sucrose but is not metabolized by the body and is therefore noncaloric and non-nutritive.[287] Although it has been periodically labeled potentially carcinogenic, studies to date support its safety for human consumption.

### Sugar Alcohols

Technically, the sugar alcohols are not sugars, but they are closely related both chemically and biochemically. Since their degrees of sweetness, compared with those of sugars, are similar, they are used as sugar substitutes.

Sorbitol, mannitol, and xylitol have been used in sugarless chewing gums and candies. Sorbitol- and xylitol-sweetened products appear to be noncariogenic in clinical trials.[263,288–290] Apparently, xylitol is not metabolized by plaque microorganisms at all, and sorbitol is not metabolized rapidly enough to support an active carious process.

In one study, chewing sorbitol gum after consuming potentially cariogenic snacks helped in counteracting the adverse plaque pH measurements.[291] The investigator postulated that the gum not only stimulated salivary flow, which is known to have a high buffering capacity, but allowed the saliva to penetrate between the tooth surfaces to neutralize acid production by plaque microorganisms.

## Periodontal Disease

Nutrition has never been implicated as a primary etiologic agent in gingivitis or periodontitis. However, it does play a secondary role by influencing or altering the resistance of the periodontium to the noxious agents and irritants that have a primary etiologic role.[291] The importance of both diet and nutrition in maintaining effective host defense mechanisms to withstand periodontal microbial challenge is well established.[292,293]

Nutrient deficiencies can affect the rate and degree of periodontal disease rather than its initiation. Research suggests that the disease progresses faster and is more severe in patients whose diets do not supply the necessary nutrients.[294,295] However, there is insufficient evidence at this time to justify nutritional therapy as part of periodontal treatment.[254]

## Other Oral Conditions

The role, if any, of diet and nutrition in edentulous ridge resorption, mucosal lesions, glossodynia, and taste perception is poorly defined,[254] although research is evolving in the area of diet as a risk factor for oral cancer.[197] Positive associations have been found with increasing consumption of meats, liver, sodium, and retinol.[296,297] Intakes of vitamins A, C, and E, as well as consumption of raw fruits and vegetables, are associated with a reduced risk of oral cancer.[197,297–302]

A major reason for poor adaptation to dentures by elderly persons is reduced tissue tolerance resulting from an inadequate diet.[303,304] Thin and friable epithelium covering the edentulous area may not tolerate the forces imposed on it by the hard, unyielding base of the denture.

The composition of saliva is critically dependent on flow rate from the glands, and numerous studies have demonstrated that both the physical consistency and the nutritional quality of the diet influence the structure of the glands, as well as the flow rate of saliva.[305,306]

## Nutrient Intake and Malnutrition

Inadequate amounts of nutrients can result in fragile, friable oral tissues, with a loss of adaptability and tolerance to irritants and a loss of repair potential.[307] For many nutrient deficiencies, the oral cavity serves as an early warning system.

Because of the rapid tissue turnover and easy visibility of the oral mucosa, it is possible to identify signs of inadequate intake or improper absorption before other organ systems are affected.[308] Although not all nutrient deficiencies have oral manifestations, the most common ones are listed in Table 6–9. Oral signs indicative or suggestive of malnutrition are listed in Table 6–10.

## IMPACT OF ORAL HEALTH ON NUTRITIONAL STATUS

There is general agreement that poor oral health is a risk factor contributing to malnutrition, weight loss, poor general health, and loss of strength.[309,310] Although the impact of oral health status alone on dietary intake and nutritional status of the elderly is virtually unknown, any alteration in the anatomic structures or physiologic functions of the oral cavity may play an important role in deterring the elderly from attaining or maintaining a proper diet and nutritional state.

Dietary intake, with respect to food selection, chewing, and swallowing, is integral to the health of the geriatric patient. Many factors influence food selection, including social customs, taste preferences, amount of preparation, and cost.[56,311,312] Chewing is influenced by the status of the oral cavity and the efficiency of the masticatory apparatus. Swallowing depends on adequate lubrication and moisture provided by the salivary glands, as well as sufficient functioning of the oral musculature to form and prepare a food bolus. Clearly, any factor that interferes with food selection, chewing, or swallowing can restrict food intake and thus affect nutritional status.

**Table 6–9** Nutritional Deficiencies and Related Oral Manifestations

| Nutrient Deficiency | Oral Manifestations |
| --- | --- |
| Vitamin A | Candidiasis<br>Gingiva—hypertrophy, inflammation<br>Oral mucosa—keratosis, leukoplakia<br>Periodontal disease<br>Taste—decreased acuity<br>Xerostomia |
| Vitamin B complex | Lips—angular cheilosis<br>Oral mucosa—leukoplakia<br>Periodontal disease<br>Tongue—papillary hypertrophy, magenta color, fissuring, glossitis |
| Vitamin $B_2$ (riboflavin) | Filiform papillae—atrophic<br>Fungiform papillae—enlarged<br>Lips—shiny, red, angular cheilosis<br>Tongue—magenta color, soreness |
| Vitamin $B_3$ (niacin) (*pellagra*) | Lips—angular cheilosis<br>Mucositis/stomatitis<br>Oral mucosa—intense irritation/inflammation, red, painful, denuded, ulcerated<br>Tongue—glossitis, glossodynia<br>Tongue (dorsum)—smooth, dry<br>Tongue (tip/borders)—red, swollen, beefy<br>Ulcerative gingivitis |
| Vitamin $B_6$ (pyridoxine hydrocholoride) | Burning/sore mouth<br>Lips—angular cheilosis<br>Tongue—glossitis, glossodynia |
| Vitamin $B_{12}$ (cyanocobalamin) (*pernicious anemia*) | Bone loss<br>Burning/sore mouth—mucositis/stomatitis<br>Gingiva—hemorrhagic<br>Halitosis<br>Hemorrhagic tendency—petechiae<br>Lips—angular cheilosis<br>Oral mucosa—epithelial dysplasia<br>Oral paresthesias—burning, numbness, tingling<br>Periodontal fibers—detachment<br>Taste—loss or distortion |

*continues*

**Table 6–9** continued

| Nutrient Deficiency | Oral Manifestations |
| --- | --- |
| Vitamin B$_{12}$ (cyanocobalamin) (*pernicious anemia*) (continued) | Tongue—beefy red, glossy, smooth; glossitis, glossodynia, loss of papillae<br>Ulcerations—aphthous type<br>Wound-healing response—delayed<br>Xerostomia |
| Vitamin C (*scurvy*) or megavitamin C withdrawal | Blood vessels—fragility<br>Bone—abnormal osteoid formation, fragility, loss<br>Burning/sore mouth<br>Candidiasis<br>Gingiva—friability, raggedness, swelling, redness, hemorrhagic tendency<br>Hemorrhagic tendency—petechiae, subperiosteal<br>Oral infections—decreased resistance<br>Periodontal disease—increased susceptibility<br>Teeth—marked mobility, spontaneous exfoliation<br>Wound-healing response—delayed |
| Vitamin D | Periodontal disease |
| Vitamin K | Candidiasis<br>Gingiva—bleeding |
| Calcium | Bone—excessive resorption, loss of mineral, fragility, osteoporosis<br>Hemorrhagic tendency<br>Periodontal disease<br>Teeth—mobility, early loss, edentulism |
| Copper | Bone—decreased trabeculae, decreased vascularity, fragility |
| Folic acid | Burning/sore mouth—mucositis/stomatitis<br>Candidiasis<br>Filiform/fungiform papillae—atrophic, loss<br>Gingiva—inflammation<br>Lip—angular cheilosis<br>Tongue—glossitis |

*continues*

**Table 6–9** continued

| Nutrient Deficiency | Oral Manifestations |
| --- | --- |
| Folic acid (continued) | Tongue (dorsum)—slick, bald, pale, or fiery<br>Tongue (tip/borders)—red, swollen<br>Ulcerations—aphthous type |
| Iron | Bleeding complications—increased risk<br>Burning/sore mouth<br>Candidiasis<br>Dental caries—increased susceptibility<br>Dysphagia<br>Filiform papillae—atrophic<br>Lips—angular cheilosis, pallor<br>Oral infections—increased risk<br>Oral mucosa—pallor<br>Oral paresthesias<br>Tongue—atrophic, pale; glossitis, glossopyrosis<br>Ulcerations—aphthous type<br>Xerostomia |
| Magnesium | Bone—fragility<br>Gingiva—hypertrophy |
| Phosphorus | Dental decay—increased susceptibility<br>Periodontal disease |
| Protein | Bone—decreased repair<br>Epithelium—fragility, burning sensation<br>Lips—angular cheilosis<br>Oral infections—decreased resistance<br>Periodontal disease—increased susceptibility<br>Wound-healing response—delayed |
| Protein-calorie | Bone loss<br>Candidiasis<br>Necrotizing ulcerative gingivitis<br>Periodontal disease |
| Water | Burning/sore mouth<br>Epithelium—dehydration, fragility<br>Muscle strength—diminished<br>Tongue—glossopyrosis<br>Xerostomia |

*continues*

**Table 6–9** continued

| Nutrient Deficiency | Oral Manifestations |
| --- | --- |
| Zinc | Candidiasis |
| | Dental caries—increased susceptibility |
| | Epithelial thickening |
| | Oral mucosa—atrophic |
| | Periodontal disease—increased suscepti-bility |
| | Smell acuity—decreased |
| | Taste acuity—loss or distortion |
| | Wound-healing response—delayed |
| | Xerostomia |

## Dentition Status

Dentition status, inasmuch as it contributes to masticatory efficiency, may exert potent effects on dietary intake. Research suggests that the number of occluding teeth, especially in the posterior segments of the mouth, is correlated with masticatory efficiency.[52,56,313–318] Masticatory efficiency is dependent not only on the number and condition of teeth present but also on the length of time spent in chewing a bolus of food and the force exerted when biting.[319]

Impaired masticatory efficiency and biting force have been associated with many oral conditions.[10,54,318] These include atrophy of orofacial musculature; oral dyskinesia; trismus; bone loss; tooth attrition, brittleness, mobility, pain, or loss; advanced carious lesions; TMJ dysfunction or dislocation; mucosal atrophy; generalized periodontal disease; gingival enlargement; and ill-fitting dentures.

One commonly held belief is that optimal masticatory efficiency allows an individual to select a wider variety of foods, which leads to a more nutritionally balanced diet.[320,321] It is also suggested that the loss of mechanical chewing efficiency leads to a preference for soft, easy-to-chew foods,

which may increase the risk of nutritional deficiencies.[56,100,311,322-327] These foods tend to be high in carbohydrates, cholesterol, and calories but low in fiber, protein, iron, calcium, and essential vitamins. Such a diet routinely contains salt and saturated fats in unhealthy amounts for persons with heart disease and usually lacks vitamin K, which leads to calcium loss in bone.[328]

Edentulousness can affect masticatory function and dietary choice, but its influence on nutritional status is controversial. Some researchers have found that tooth loss is a strong predictor of inadequate nutrition, resulting from problems with biting, chewing, or swallowing foods.[329] Other investigators have found little evidence to indicate that adequate dentition is necessary for geriatric patients to maintain a satisfactory nutritional state.[330,331]

Even the incidence of malnutrition, weight loss, and gastrointestinal disturbances in the older adult appears to be unrelated to impaired masticatory function.[319,320,332-335] In these studies, the percentage of individuals with significantly reduced or inefficient masticatory ability was similar to the percentage of persons with and without overt signs of malnutrition or undernutrition. In addition, various changes in blood chemistry usually

**Table 6–10** Oral Signs Suggestive of Malnutrition

| Oral Area | Normal Appearance | Signs Associated with Malnutrition |
|---|---|---|
| Teeth | Bright; no caries; no pain | Dental caries; may be missing or erupting abnormally |
| Gums | Healthy; red; not swollen; no bleeding | Receding; spongy; bleed easily |
| Tongue | Deep red; not swollen or smooth | Scarlet or magenta color; smooth; raw; swelling; sores; atrophic, hyperemic, or hypertrophic papillae |
| Lips | Smooth; not swollen or chapped | Redness; swelling of mouth and lips |
| Face | Uniform color; smooth; pink; healthy appearance; not swollen | Lumpiness or flakiness of skin around mouth |
| Salivary | Face not swollen in gland areas | Parotid enlargement (swollen glands, cheeks) |

*Source:* Adapted with permission from G. Christakis, *Nutritional Assessment in Health Programs,* 7th printing, p. 19, © 1984, American Public Health Association.

associated with malnutrition have not been routinely found in individuals with significantly reduced masticatory ability.[336]

It would appear that replacing missing teeth with partial or complete dentures would improve chewing and limit the risk of nutritional problems. Indeed, the change from poor natural dentition or edentulousness to complete dentures is generally accompanied by improved chewing efficiency and nutritional status,[333,337,338] but there are conflicting observations in the literature.[314,331]

Properly fitted dentures may allow one to choose from a wider selection of food textures. However, denture wearing has been reported to interfere with the ability to eat satisfactorily, talk clearly, and laugh freely.[339,340] Elderly denture wearers also require more time to chew before swallowing than do those with natural teeth.[54]

It is well known that the denture wearer does not have the chewing efficiency enjoyed by the individual with natural teeth. Several studies have shown that significant differences in chewing ability occur among persons with intact natural dentition, individuals with partial prosthetic replacements, and individuals with complete dentures.[314–316,323,341–345] Dental studies have established that the chewing efficiency of an average complete denture wearer is only 15% to 25% of that of an individual with natural teeth.[312,322,341,342,346,347]

Even so, a chewing efficiency as low as 23%, a level attainable with just the 12 maxillary and mandibular anterior teeth, was sufficient to digest the 28 experimental foods in one study of masticatory efficiency and food assimilation.[348] Since the masticatory efficiency attained by the average denture wearer is in this range, most people with dentures should be able to chew food adequately for proper digestion.

The condition of dentures has a direct bearing on an individual's ability to chew. Well-fitting dentures in a healthy mouth can result in better chewing, swallowing, and digestion.[330,333,349] Problems with denture fit, bone shrinkage, and the gum tissues supporting the denture compromise masticatory function and may negatively alter dietary intake.[54] In fact, many denture wearers avoid foods that tend to slip under dentures or are too difficult to manipulate and chew.[350]

Other studies[321,346,351–354] have reported significant variation in the masticatory performance of people who wear dentures. Some individuals are barely able to comminute a test food, whereas others with similar prostheses have a relatively high degree of masticatory proficiency. Furthermore, approximately five times more effort is required for the average person wearing complete dentures to pulverize a test food to the same degree that a person with natural dentition can. This agrees with previous reports that impaired chewing ability is not usually improved by chewing food longer or by increasing the rate of chewing, but rather by ingesting foods that are softer and easier to chew[323] or by swallowing larger particles.[314,317] Therefore, denture wearers may be more prone to accidental choking from improper mastication.[355–357]

Data from dietary surveys before and after the insertion of new dentures are inconclusive about associated changes in essential nutrient intake.[333,338,358–365] Before the insertion of new dentures, several essential nutrients were consumed in quantities significantly lower than the recommended daily allowance. After new dentures were placed, shifts in nutrient intake occurred, although the changes were not necessarily beneficial. Subjective evaluations, however, indicated im-

proved chewing efficiency, which aided food digestion, particularly of fibrous foods.

### Self-Perceived Chewing Ability

Experimental subjects' evaluations of their own chewing ability have been examined as possible predictors of masticatory efficiency, but most reported results are conflicting.[56,315,316,342,344,345,364,366–369] There appears to be wide individual variation in the subjective assessment of chewing problems that is not always related to dentition status. For those with poor masticatory efficiency, the lack of a perceived problem is probably due in part to the selection of foods that are easy to chew or to preparation of food in such a way as to facilitate chewing. In fact, perceived ease of chewing is related to subjective estimates of food preference.[315,316,343,344,350,370] In general, denture wearers give lower preference ratings to hard-to-chew foods than do persons with intact or even compromised natural dentition.

### Dietary Control of Chewing Difficulties

For those with chewing problems due to dentures or tooth loss, the key is to modify food selection habits and methods of preparing foods for easier chewing. Specific ways to overcome chewing difficulties are listed in Table 6–11.

## Oral Cancer

Neoplasms in the oral cavity can interfere with chewing and swallowing because of both pain and infiltration of tissues. Antineoplastic drugs and radiation therapy can alter the character and volume of saliva. In addition, the balance of the oral flora is disrupted, allowing overgrowth of opportunistic organisms such as *Candida* species.

Many patients who undergo radiation therapy for oral cancer become nutritional ca-

**Table 6–11** Dietary Control of Chewing Difficulties

- Drink fluids with meals to aid in chewing and swallowing.
- Chop, grind, or mechanically blend foods that are hard to chew.
- Add sources of dietary fiber (stems of vegetables, whole grains, skins of fruits and vegetables, and seeds or berries) that can be cooked, shredded, mashed, ground, or softened with liquids without affecting the fiber content.
- Shred or chop raw vegetables and use them in salads.
- Mash or strain cooked vegetables.
- Buy prechopped vegetables and meat.
- Prepare meats and vegetables in soups, stews, and casseroles.
- Trim meats to remove fat and tough fibers.
- Substitute softer, protein-rich foods such as fish, eggs, peanut butter, cheese, baked beans, ground meats, or yogurt for regular meat.

- Use melted cheese as a sauce on vegetables or toast, to increase protein intake.
- Add extra nonfat dry milk powder to cream soups, cooked cereals, puddings, custards, creamed vegetables, casseroles, and milk beverages to increase protein and calorie content.
- Use cooked whole-grain cereals such as oatmeal or mixed grains.
- Add bran to hot cereals, baked breads, meatloaf, and casseroles.
- Use fruit juices in place of fruits. Most fruits can be pureed in a blender and the pulp added to juices.
- Avoid sticky foods that adhere to teeth and dentures.
- Use menus from cookbooks written for people with chewing problems.
- Most important, eat a variety of foods from the major food groups each day.

---

sualties. Profound loss of appetite is an early and sustained reaction to radiation-induced soreness, xerostomia, taste loss, dysphagia, and nausea and vomiting.[371] Eating becomes a pleasureless and painful chore, and food selection is restricted to items that do not aggravate the oral discomfort, often at the expense of adequate nutrition. When prolonged and severe enough, lack of nutrients can precipitate a nutritional deficiency stomatitis.

**Oral Pain**

Oral pain can reduce food intake in both texture and amount. In fact, many patients experiencing dental or facial pain avoid certain foods.[372] As an example, mucositic tissues are sensitive to temperature and pressure, so a semisoft diet that is low in sucrose and citric acid is advised.[373]

Masticatory ability, biting force, and tongue movements are impaired in painful oral conditions, thus influencing the ability to chew many foods. Oral pain can also interfere with swallowing. Conditions that can cause oral pain are listed in Table 6–12.

**Saliva**

Saliva is essential for taste perception, mastication, and swallowing of foods. It provides the environment for optimal functioning of taste buds and contributes to ingestion and digestion by forming a mucin-coated food bolus and adequate fluid volume to allow for ready passage along the chewing and swallowing surfaces. The bolus is then digested in the gastrointestinal tract.

When salivary flow is deficient, it causes various stresses on the hard and soft tissues of

**Table 6–12** Oral Conditions That Can Be Painful

- Angular cheilosis
- Aphthous ulceration
- Benign mucous membrane pemphigoid
- Burning mouth syndrome
- Candidiasis
- Contact stomatitis
- Dental caries
- Denture stomatitis
- Erythema multiforme
- Glossodynia
- Glossopharyngeal neuralgia
- Herpes labialis
- Herpetic stomatitis
- Hypersensitive teeth
- Lichen planus
- Mucositis
- Necrotizing ulcerative gingivitis
- Oral cancer (advanced)
- Periodontal disease
- Pulpal infection
- TMJ dysfunction
- Traumatic ulceration
- Trigeminal neuralgia

the mouth, leading to increased oral disease and dysfunction of chewing, swallowing, and taste.[54] The greater concentration of electrolytes in a diminished amount of saliva can result in a salty or metallic taste in the mouth. In addition, decreased ptyalin levels in the reduced salivary flow may affect digestion of chewed particles.

Most patients with xerostomia have difficulty eating solid and dry foods,[57,58] which can contribute to changes in nutritional intake patterns.[374–377] Oral pain associated with sialadenitis or sialolithiasis can also impair oral intake. In response, elderly individuals reduce the intake of various foods or switch to foods more easily chewed.

To facilitate chewing and swallowing in severe xerostomia, food must be lubricated with artificial saliva or prepared in liquid or semiliquid form. Saliva substitutes have been shown to improve both chewing and swallowing.[378,379] Many patients moisten foods with sauces, gravies, milk, and other fluids.

**Taste and Smell Sensitivity**

For the most part, taste and smell determine the flavor of foods and beverages.[379] Reduced acuity of either of these senses may significantly lessen the ability to enjoy food and thus decrease appetite. Declines in gustation and olfaction, whether with age, chronic disease, or drug use, decrease the flavor and palatability of foods and beverages. Because of this, the senses of both taste and smell are important in food selection and nutrient intake.[375,378,380]

Decreased taste sensitivity is compounded by dental disease or poor oral hygiene.[5,381,382] The causes can be physical, such as debris covering the taste buds, or chemical, such as taste fatigue from constant stimulation by decaying matter in the mouth.[63] Also, chronic dental or periodontal infections can result in the continuous discharge of purulent matter into the mouth, creating a constantly unpleasant taste. Routine oral hygiene has been shown to improve sensitivity to salty and sweet tastes and may improve the elderly patient's appetite.[79]

Saliva has modulating effects on taste sensitivity. A salty taste is detected only when the concentration is above salivary levels of sodium chloride. Saliva diminishes the effect of a sour taste as a result of buffering by salivary bicarbonate. Decreased salivation also alters the taste of many foods.[381,382]

Diminished taste also may result from altered taste perception.[307] It has long been suspected that denture wearers have a lowered ability to taste,[307,343,383] and edentulous individuals experience a reduction in taste sensitivity after the insertion of complete dentures.[384] Perhaps the taste buds in the hard palate are more insensitive to taste, especially sour and bitter, when covered with dentures.[44,307,385]

Giddon and colleagues[386] compared the ability of denture wearers and persons with natural dentition to differentiate the sweetness of a solid food. It was found that the denture wearers took more than twice as long to render a judgment as did subjects with natural dentition. The denture wearers were unable to distinguish among cookies containing various levels of sucrose.

## CONCLUSION

The cumulative effects of aging, disease, and trauma contribute to the wide variety of oral health problems prevalent in the older adult. Although many of these problems can be neither prevented nor cured by diet alone, to ignore nutritional considerations in the oral disease process would be a serious error. Many of the oral problems mentioned previously are associated with dietary deficiencies, excesses, or practices that are detrimental to the oral and circumoral structures. It is imperative that dietary intake provide adequate nutrients to support oral health and function.

There is also a strong association between oral health status and food selection, chewing efficiency, and ability to swallow. Clearly, oral health problems that interfere with any aspects of these factors can restrict food intake and ultimately affect nutritional status.

## REFERENCES

1. Somerman MJ, Hoffeld JT, Baum BJ. Basic biology and physiology of oral tissues: overview and age-associated changes. In: Tryon AF, ed. *Oral Health and Aging*. Littleton, Mass: PSG Publishing Co Inc; 1986.

2. Baum BJ. Salivary gland function during aging. *Gerodontics*. 1986;2:61–64.

3. Mandel ID. The role of saliva in maintaining oral homeostasis. *J Am Dent Assoc*. 1989;119:298–304.

4. Mandel ID, Wotman S. The salivary secretion in health and disease. *Oral Sci Rev*. 1976;8:25–47.

5. Baum BJ. Normal and abnormal oral status in aging. *Annu Rev Gerontol Geriatr*. 1984;4:87–105.

6. Baum BJ, Bodner L, Fox PC, et al. Therapy-induced dysfunctions of salivary glands. *Spec Care Dent*. 1985;5:274–277.

7. Fox PC, Heft MW, Herrera M, et al. Secretion of antimicrobial proteins from the parotid glands of different aged healthy persons. *J Gerontol*. 1987;42:466–469.

8. Spielman AI. Interaction of saliva and taste. *J Dent Res*. 1990;69:838–843.

9. Guyton AC. Secretory functions of the alimentary tract. In: Guyton AC, ed. *Textbook of Medical Physiology*. 5th ed. Philadelphia, Pa: WB Saunders Co; 1976.

10. Sonies BC, Stone M, Shawker T. Speech and swallowing in the elderly. *Gerodontology*. 1984;3:115–123.

11. Kiyak HA. Psychosocial factors in dental needs of the elderly. *Spec Care Dent*. 1981;1:22–30.

12. Johnson ES, Kelly JE, Van Kirk LE. *Selected Dental Findings in Adults, by Age, Race and Sex: United States: 1960–1962*. Washington, DC: US Public Health Service; 1965. US Dept of Health, Education, and Welfare PHS publication No. 1000, Series 11.

13. *Basic Data on Dental Examination Findings for Persons 1–74 years, US 1971–1974*. Washington, DC: National Center for Health Statistics; 1979.

Vital and Health Statistics series 11, data from National Health and Nutrition Examination Survey (HANES), No. 214.

14. Baum BJ. Characteristics of participants in the oral physiology component of the Baltimore Longitudinal Study of Aging. *Community Dent Oral Epidemiol.* 1981;9:128–134.

15. *Oral Health of United States Adults: National Findings.* Bethesda, Md: National Institute of Dental Research; 1987. National Institutes of Health publication 87-2868.

16. Hand JS, Hunt RJ. The need for restorations and extractions in a non-institutionalized elderly population. *Gerodontics.* 1986;2:72–76.

17. Hunt RJ, Srisilapanan P, Beck JD. Denture-related problems and prosthodontic treatment needs in the elderly. *Gerodontics.* 1985;1:226–230.

18. Hunt RJ. Periodontal treatment needs in an elderly population in Iowa. *Gerodontics.* 1986;2:24–27.

19. Bagramian R, Heller P. Dental health assessment of a population of nursing home residents. *J Gerontol.* 1977;32:168–174.

20. Council on Dental Health and Health Planning, Bureau of Economic and Behavioral Research. Oral health status of Vermont nursing home residents. *J Am Dent Assoc.* 1982;104:68–69.

21. Empey G, Kiyak HA, Milgrom P. Oral health in nursing homes. *Spec Care Dent.* 1983;3:65–67.

22. Yamagata PA, Brattebo SC, Steifel DJ. Use of a dental service in a nursing home. *Spec Care Dent.* 1985;5:64–67.

23. Gordon SR. Survey of dental need among veterans with severe cognitive impairment. *Gerodontics.* 1988;4:158–159.

24. Baum BJ. Research on aging and oral health: an assessment of current status and future needs. *Spec Care Dent.* 1981;1:156–165.

25. Williams TF. Patterns of health and disease in the elderly. *Gerodontics.* 1985;1:284–287.

26. Ramazzotto LJ, Curro FA, Gates PE, et al. Calcium nutrition and the aging process: a review. *Gerodontology.* 1986;5:159–168.

27. Somerman MJ. Mineralized tissues in aging. *Gerodontology.* 1984;3:93–99.

28. Cohen B. Ageing in teeth and associated tissues. In: Cohen B, Thomson H, eds. *Dental Care for the Elderly.* London, England: Year Book Medical Publishers Inc; 1986.

29. Heeneman H, Brown DH. Senescent changes in and about the oral cavity and pharynx. *J Otolaryngol.* 1986;15:214–216.

30. Langer A. Oral changes in the geriatric patient. *Compend Contin Educ Dent.* 1981;2:258–264.

31. Ettinger RL. *Oral Changes Associated with Aging, Module 2.* Iowa City, Iowa: University of Iowa College of Dentistry; 1982. Geriatric Curriculum Series.

32. Shapiro S, Bomberg TJ, Benson BW, et al. Postmenopausal osteoporosis: dental patients at risk. *Gerodontics.* 1985;1:220–225.

33. Fishman LS. Dental and skeletal relationships to attritional occlusion. *Angle Orthod.* 1976;46:51–63.

34. Ainamo A, Ainamo J. The dentition is intended to last a lifetime. *Int Dent J.* 1984;34:87–92.

35. Begg PR. Stone age man's dentition. *Am J Orthod.* 1984;4:298–312.

36. Hand JS, Beck JD, Turner KA. The prevalence of occlusal attrition and considerations of treatment in a noninstitutionalized elderly population. *Spec Care Dent.* 1987;7:202–206.

37. Heft MW. Prevalence of TMJ signs and symptoms in the elderly. *Gerodontology.* 1984;3:125–130.

38. Klein DR. Oral soft tissue changes in geriatric patients. *Bull NY Acad Med.* 1980;56:721–727.

39. Kahane JC. Anatomic and physiologic changes in the aging peripheral speech mechanism. In: Beasley DS, Davis GA, eds. *Aging: Communication Processes and Disorders.* New York, NY: Grune & Stratton; 1981.

40. Koopman CF, Coulthard SW. The oral cavity and aging: symposium on geriatric otolaryngology. *Otolaryngol Clin North Am.* 1982;15:293–312.

41. Hill MW. The influence of aging on skin and oral mucosa. *Gerodontology.* 1984;3:35–45.

42. Breustedt A. Age-induced changes in the oral mucosa and their therapeutic consequences. *Int Dent J.* 1983;33:272–280.

43. Mackenzie IC, Holm-Pedersen P, Karring T. Age changes in the oral mucous membranes and periodontium. In: Holm-Pedersen H, Loe H, eds. *Geriatric Dentistry: A Textbook of Oral Gerontology.* St. Louis, Mo: CV Mosby Co; 1986.

44. Hermel J, Schonwetter S, Samueloff S. Taste sensation identification and age in man. *J Oral Med.* 1970;25:39–42.

45. Hyde RJ, Feller RP, Sharon IM. Tongue brushing, dentifrice, and age effects on taste and smell. *J Dent Res*. 1981;60:1730–1734.

46. Weiffenbach JM, Cowart BJ, Baum BJ. Taste intensity perception in aging. *J Gerontol*. 1986;41:460–468.

47. Satoh Y, Seluk LW. Taste threshold, anatomical form of fungiform papillae and aging in humans. *J Nihon Univ Sch Dent*. 1988;30:22–29.

48. Bartoshuk LM. Clinical psychophysics of taste. *Gerodontics*. 1988;4:249-255.

49. Newton JP, Abel RL, Robertson EM, et al. Changes in human masseter and medial pterygoid muscles with age: a study by computed tomography. *Gerodontics*. 1987;3:151–154.

50. Newton JP, Yemm R, Abel RW, et al. Changes in human jaw muscles with age and dental state. *Gerodontology*. 1993;10:16–22.

51. Vergo TJ Jr, Papas A. Physiological aspects of geriatric dentistry. *J Dent*. 1984;4:10–14.

52. Feldman FS, Kapur K, Alman JE, et al. Aging and mastication: changes in performance and in the swallowing threshold with natural dentition. *J Am Geriatr Soc*. 1980;28:97–103.

53. Baum BJ, Bodner L. Aging and oral motor function: evidence for altered performance among older persons. *J Dent Res*. 1983;62:2–6.

54. Idowu AT, Graser GN, Handelman SL. The effect of age and dentition status on masticatory function in older adults. *Spec Care Dent*. 1986;6:80–83.

55. Elliott JL. Swallowing disorders in the elderly: a guide to diagnosis and treatment. *Geriatrics*. 1988;43:95–113.

56. Chauncey HH, Kapur KK, Feller RP, et al. Altered masticatory function and perceptual estimates of chewing experience. *Spec Care Dent*. 1981;1:250–255.

57. Langer A. Oral signs of aging and their clinical significance. *Geriatrics*. 1976;31:63–69.

58. Massler M. Xerostomia in the elderly. *NY J Dent*. 1986;56:260–261.

59. Tylenda JA, Ship JA, Fox PC, et al. Evaluation of submandibular salivary flow rate in different age groups. *J Dent Res*. 1988;67:1225–1228.

60. Navazesh M, Brightman VJ, Pogoda JM. Relationship of medical status, medications, and salivary flow rates in adults of different ages. *Oral Surg Oral Med Oral Pathol*. 1996;81:172–176.

61. Baum BJ. Evaluation of stimulated parotid saliva flow rate in different age groups. *J Dent Res*. 1981;60:1292–1296.

62. Zegeer LJ. The effects of sensory changes in older persons. *J Neurosci Nurs*. 1986;18:325–332.

63. Whitehead MC. Neuroanatomy of the gustatory system. *Gerodontics*. 1988;4:239–243.

64. Cooper RM, Bilash MA, Zubek JP. The effect of age on taste sensitivity. *J Gerontol*. 1959;14:56–58.

65. Erickson RI. The elderly patient: a new challenge for dentists. *J Calif Dent Assoc*. 1982;10:49–50.

66. Bradley RM. Effects of aging on the anatomy and neurophysiology of taste. *Gerodontics*. 1988;4:244–248.

67. Kullaa-Mikkonen A, Kaponen A, Seilonen A. Quantitative study of human fungiform papillae and taste buds: variation with aging and in different morphological forms of the tongue. *Gerodontics*. 1987;3:131–135.

68. Weisfuse D, Catalanotto FA, Kamen S. Gender differences in suprathreshold scaling ability in an older population. *Spec Care Dent*. 1986;6:25–28.

69. Kiyak HA. Psychological changes associated with aging: implications for the dental practitioner. In: Tryon AF, ed. *Oral Health and Aging*. Littleton, Mass: PSG Publishing Co Inc; 1986.

70. Richter CP, Campbell KH. Sucrose taste thresholds of rats and humans. *Am J Physiol*. 1940;128:291–297.

71. Byrd E, Gertman S. Taste sensitivity in aging persons. *Geriatrics*. 1959;14:381–384.

72. Grzegorczyk PB, Jones SW, Mistretta CM. Age-related differences in salt taste acuity. *J Gerontol*. 1979;34:834–840.

73. Massler M. Geriatric nutrition: the role of taste and smell in appetite. *J Prosthet Dent*. 1980;43:247–250.

74. Baker KA, Didcock EA, Kemm FR, et al. Effect of age, sex and illness on salt taste detection thresholds. *Age Ageing*. 1983;12:159–165.

75. Doty RL. A review of olfactory dysfunctions in man. *Am J Otolaryngol*. 1979;1:57–79.

76. Mistretta CM. Aging effects on anatomy and neurophysiology of taste and smell. *Gerodontology*. 1984;3:131–136.

77. Weiffenbach JM. Taste and smell perception in aging. *Gerodontology*. 1984;3:137–146.

78. Venstrom D, Amoore JE. Olfactory threshold in relation to age, sex or smoking. *J Food Sci.* 1968;33:264–265.

79. Kimbrell GM, Furchgott E. Effect of aging on olfactory threshold. *J Gerontol.* 1963;18:364–365.

80. Schiffman S, Pasternak M. Decreased discrimination of food odors in the elderly. *J Gerontol.* 1979;34:73–79.

81. Doty RL, Shaman P, Applebaum SL, et al. Smell identification ability: changes with age. *Science.* 1984;226:1441–1443.

82. Chalke HD, Dewhurst JR, Ward CW. Loss of sense of smell in old people. *Public Health.* 1958;72:223–230.

83. Ettinger RL. Oral disease and its effect on the quality of life. *Gerodontics.* 1987;3:103–106.

84. Nikias M. Oral disease and quality of life. *Am J Public Health.* 1985;75:11–12.

85. Mandel ID. Preventive dentistry for the elderly. *Spec Care Dent.* 1983;3:157–163.

86. Nystrom GP, Adams RA. Oral hygiene and the elderly. In: Tryon AF, ed. *Oral Health and Aging.* Littleton, Mass: PSG Publishing Co Inc; 1986.

87. Kandelman D, Bordeur JM, Simard P, et al. Dental needs of the elderly: a comparison between some European and North American surveys. *Community Dent Health.* 1986;3:19–39.

88. Goldberg AF, Gergans GA, Mattson DE, et al. Radiographic alveolar process/mandibular height ratio as a predictor of osteoporosis. *Gerondontics.* 1988;4:229–231.

89. Richards M. Osteoporosis. *Geriatr Nurs (New York).* 1982;3:98–102.

90. Krook L, Whalen JP, Lesser GV, et al. Human periodontal disease and osteoporosis. *Cornell Vet.* 1972;62:371–391.

91. Lutwak L. Continuing need for dietary calcium throughout life. *Geriatrics.* 1974;29:171–178.

92. Kribbs PJ, Smith DE, Chestnutt CH III. Oral findings in osteoporosis, part II: relationship between residual ridge and alveolar bone resorption and generalized skeletal osteopenia. *J Prosthet Dent.* 1983;50:719–724.

93. Bras J, van Ouij CP, Abraham-lnpijn L, et al. Radiographic interpretation of the mandibular angular cortex: a diagnostic tool in metabolic bone loss. *Oral Surg Oral Med Oral Pathol.* 1982; 53:541–545.

94. Scileppi KP. Bone and joint disease in the elderly. *Med Clin North Am.* 1983;67:517–530.

95. Tallgren A. The continuing reduction of the residual alveolar ridges in complete denture wearers: a mixed-longitudinal study covering 25 years. *J Prosthet Dent.* 1972;27:120–132.

96. Kribbs PJ, Chesnutt CH. Osteoporosis and dental osteopenia in the elderly. *Gerodontology.* 1984; 3:101–106.

97. Wical EE, Swoope CC. Studies of residual ridge resorption, part II: the relationship of dietary calcium and phosphorus to residual ridge resorption. *J Prosthet Dent.* 1974;32:13–22.

98. Recker RR, Saville PD, Heaney RP. Effect of estrogens and calcium carbonate on bone loss in postmenopausal women. *Ann Intern Med.* 1977; 87:649–655.

99. Heaney RP, Gallagher JC, Johnston CC, et al. Calcium nutrition and bone health in the elderly. *Am J Clin Nutr.* 1982;36(suppl 5):986–1013.

100. Jakush J. Diet, nutrition, and oral health: a rational approach for the dental practice. *J Am Dent Assoc.* 1984;109:20–32.

101. Goodman CE. Osteoporosis: protective measures of nutrition and exercise. *Geriatrics.* 1985;40:59–70.

102. Schamschula RG, Barmes DE. Fluoride and health: dental caries, osteoporosis, and cardiovascular disease. *Annu Rev Nutr.* 1981;1:427–435.

103. Riggs BL, O'Fallon WM, Lane A, et al. Clinical trial of fluoride therapy in postmenopausal osteoporotic women: extended observations and additional analysis. *J Bone Miner Res.* 1994;9:265–275.

104. Banting DW. Epidemiology of root caries. *Gerodontology.* 1986;5:5–11.

105. Katz RV. Assessing root caries in populations: the evolution of the Root Caries Index. *J Public Health Dent.* 1980;40:7–16.

106. Axelsson P, Lindhe J. Effect of controlled oral hygiene procedures on caries and periodontal disease in adults: results after six years. *J Clin Periodontol.* 1981;8:239–248.

107. Beck JD, Hunt RJ, Hand JS, et al. Prevalence of root and coronal caries in a noninstitutionalized older population. *J Am Dent Assoc.* 1985; 111:964–967.

108. Goldberg J, Tanzer J, Munster E, et al. Cross-sectional clinical evaluation of recurrent enamel car-

ies, restoration of marginal integrity, and oral hygiene status. *J Am Dent Assoc*. 1981;102:635–641.

109. Billings RJ, Brown LR, Kaster AG. Contemporary treatment strategies for root surface dental caries. *Gerodontics*. 1985;1:20–27.

110. Seichter U. Root surface caries: a critical literature review. *J Am Dent Assoc*. 1987;115:305–310.

111. Yanover L. Root surface caries: epidemiology, etiology, and control. *J Can Dent Assoc*. 1987;53:842–859.

112. Wallace MC, Retief DH, Bradley EL. Prevalence of root caries in a population of older adults. *Gerodontics*. 1988;4:84–89.

113. Hix JO, O'Leary TJ. The relationship between cemental caries, oral hygiene status, and fermentable carbohydrate intake. *J Periodontol*. 1976; 47:398–404.

114. Slome BA. Rampant caries: a side effect of tricyclic antidepressant therapy. *Gen Dent*. 1984; 32:494–496.

115. Ravald N, Hamp SE. Prediction of root surface caries in patients treated for advanced periodontal disease. *J Clin Periodontol*. 1981;8:400–414.

116. Kitamura M, Kiyak HA, Mulligan K. Predictors of root caries in the elderly. *Community Dent Oral Epidemiol*. 1986;14:34–38.

117. Arnold FA Jr. Fluorine in drinking water: its effect on dental caries. *J Am Dent Assoc*. 1948; 136:28–36.

118. Ripa LW. Professionally (operator) applied topical fluoride therapy: a critique. *Clin Prevent Dent*. 1982;4:3–10.

119. Dreizen S, Brown LR, Handler S, et al. Radiation-induced xerostomia in cancer patients. *Cancer*. 1976;38:273–278.

120. Rothwell BR, Richard EL. Diabetes mellitus: medical and dental considerations. *Spec Care Dent*. 1984;4:58–65.

121. Swango PA. The use of topical fluorides to prevent dental caries in adults: a review of the literature. *J Am Dent Assoc*. 1983;107:447–450.

122. Burt BA, Ismail AI, Eklund SA. Root caries in an optimally fluoridated and a high fluoride community. *J Dent Res*. 1986;65:1154–1158.

123. Ripa LW, Leske GS, Forte F, et al. Effect of a 0.05% neutral NaF mouth rinse on coronal and root caries of adults. *Gerodontology*. 1987;6:131–136.

124. Sinkford JC. Oral health problems in the elderly: research recommendations. *Gerodontics*. 1988; 4:209–211.

125. Newbrun E. Prevention of root caries. *Gerodontology*. 1986;5:33–41.

126. Bain MJ. Chlorhexidine in dentistry: a review. *NZ Dent J*. 1980;76:49–54.

127. Tonelli PM, Hume WR, Kenney EB. Chlorhexidine: a review of the literature. *Periodont Abstr*. 1983;31:5–10.

128. Saxton CA, Cowell CR. Clinical investigation of the effects of dentifrices on dentin wear at the cementoenamel junction. *J Am Dent Assoc*. 1981;102:38–43.

129. Hand JS, Hunt RJ, Reinhardt JW. The prevalence and treatment implications of cervical abrasion in the elderly. *Gerodontics*. 1986;2:167–170.

130. Reussner GH, Coccodrilli G Jr, Thiessen R Jr. Effects of phosphates in acid-containing beverages on tooth erosion. *J Dent Res*. 1975;54:365–370.

131. Mueninghoff LA, Johnson MH. Erosion: a case caused by unusual diet. *J Am Dent Assoc*. 1982;104:51–52.

132. Linkosalo E, Markkanen H. Dental erosions in relation to lactovegetarian diet. *Scand J Dent Res*. 1985;93:436–441.

133. White DK, Hayes RC, Benjamin RN. Loss of tooth structure associated with chronic regurgitation and vomiting. *J Am Dent Assoc*. 1978; 97:833–835.

134. Malcolm D, Paul E. Erosion of the teeth due to sulphuric acid in the battery industry. *Br J Ind Med*. 1961;26:249–266.

135. ten Bruggen Cate HJ. Dental erosion in industry. *Br J Ind Med*. 1968;25:249–266.

136. Levy SM. The epidemiology and prevention of dental caries in adults. *Compend Contin Educ Dent*. 1988;(suppl 11):S390–S398.

137. Hong F, Nu Zhong-ying XX. Clinical classification and therapeutic design of dental cervical abrasion. *Gerodontics*. 1988;4:101–103.

138. Hodosh M. A superior desensitizer: potassium nitrate. *J Am Dent Assoc*. 1974;88:831–832.

139. Collins JF, Gingold J, Stanley H, et al. Reducing dentinal hypersensitivity with strontium chloride and potassium nitrate. *Gen Dent*. 1984;32:40–43.

140. Council on Dental Therapeutics. Acceptance of promise with fluoride and Sensodyne-F toothpastes for sensitive teeth. *J Am Dent Assoc.* 1986;113:673–675.

141. Berman LH. Dentinal sensation and hypersensitivity: a review of mechanisms and treatment alternatives. *J Periodontol.* 1985;56:216–222.

142. Dayton RE, deMarco TJ, Swedlow D. Treatment of hypersensitive root surfaces with dental adhesive materials. *J Periodontol.* 1974;45:873–878.

143. Brekhus PJ. Dental disease and its relation to the loss of human teeth. *J Am Dent Assoc.* 1929; 16:2237–2247.

144. Allen EF. Statistical study of the primary cause of extractions. *J Dent Res.* 1944;23:453–458.

145. Pelton WJ, Pennell EH, Druzina A. Tooth morbidity experience in adults. *J Am Dent Assoc.* 1954;49:439–445.

146. Bailit HL, Braun R, Maryniuk GA, et al. Is periodontal disease the primary cause of tooth extraction? *J Am Dent Assoc.* 1987;114:40–45.

147. Niessen LC, Weyant RJ. Causes of tooth loss in a veteran population. *J Public Health Dent.* 1989;49:19–23.

148. Johnson TE. Factors contributing to dentists' extraction decisions in older adults. *Spec Care Dent.* 1993;13:195–199.

149. Stephens RG, Kogon SL, Jarvis AM. A study of reasons for tooth extraction in a Canadian population sample. *J Can Dent Assoc.* 1991;57:501–504.

150. National Center for Health Statistics. *Edentulous Persons, US 1971.* Baltimore, Md: Health Resources Administration; 1974. US Dept of Health, Education, and Welfare publication series 10, No. 29.

151. Brown LJ, Meskin LH. Sociodemographic differences in tooth loss patterns in United States employed adults and seniors, 1985–1986. *Gerodontics.* 1988;4:345–362.

152. Yanover L, Elanling D, Grainger R, et al. Effect of a daily 0.2% chlorhexidine rinse on the oral health of an institutionalized elderly population. *J Can Dent Assoc.* 1988;54:595–598.

153. Budtz-Jorgensen E, Luan WM, Holm-Pedersen P, et al. Mandibular dysfunction related to dental, occlusal and prosthetic conditions in a selected elderly population. *Gerodontics.* 1985;1:28–33.

154. Franks AST. Masticatory muscle hyperactivity and temporomandibular joint dysfunction. *J Prosthet Dent.* 1965;15:1122–1131.

155. Hansson T, Nilner M. A study of the occurrence of symptoms of diseases of the TMJ, masticatory musculature and related structures. *J Oral Rehabil.* 1975;2:313–324.

156. Greene CS, Marbach JJ. Epidemiologic studies of mandibular dysfunction: a critical review. *J Prosthet Dent.* 1982;48:184–190.

157. Rugh JD, Solberg WK. Oral health status in the United States: temporomandibular joint disorders. *J Dent Educ.* 1985;49:398–406.

158. Jeanmonod A. The diagnosis and treatment of temporomandibular dysfunctions in older partially or totally edentulous patients. *Int Dent J.* 1982;32:339–344.

159. Helkimo M. Epidemiologic surveys of dysfunction of the masticatory system. *Oral Sci Rev.* 1976;7:54–69.

160. Granados JI. The influence of the loss of teeth and attrition on the articular eminence. *J Prosthet Dent.* 1979;42:78–85.

161. Richards LC, Brown T. Dental attrition and degenerative arthritis of the temporomandibular joint. *J Oral Rehabil.* 1981;8:293–307.

162. Nesbit SP, Gobetti JP. Multiple recurrence of oral erythema multiforme after secondary herpes simplex: report of case and review of literature. *J Am Dent Assoc.* 1986;112:348–352.

163. Antoon JW, Miller RL. Aphthous ulcers: a review of the literature on etiology, pathogenesis, diagnosis, and treatment. *J Am Dent Assoc.* 1980; 101:803–808.

164. Wray D, Ferguson MM, Mason DK, et al. Recurrent aphthae: treatment with vitamin $B_{12}$, folic acid, and iron. *Br Med J.* 1975;2:490–493.

165. Nally FF, Blake GC. Recurrent aphthae: treatment with vitamin $B_{12}$, folic acid, and iron. *Br Med J.* 1975;3:308.

166. Hay KD, Reade PC. The use of an elimination diet in the treatment of recurrent aphthous ulceration of the oral cavity. *Oral Surg Oral Med Oral Pathol.* 1984;57:504–507.

167. Rodu B, Russell CM, Ray KL. Treatment of oral ulcers with hydroxypropyl cellulose film (Zilactin® D). *Compend Contin Educ Dent.* 1988;9:420–422.

168. Mackowiak PA. The normal microbial flora. *N Engl J Med.* 1982;307:83–93.

169. Borelli D, Fuentes J, Leiderman E, et al. Ketoconazole, an oral antifungal: laboratory and clinical assessment of imidazole drugs. *Postgrad Med J.* 1979;55:657–661.

170. Yap BS, Bodey GP. Oropharyngeal candidiasis treated with troche form of clotrimazole. *Arch Intern Med.* 1979;139:656–657.

171. Dreizen S. Oral candidiasis. *Am J Med.* 1984; 77(4D):28–33.

172. Gallagher FJ, Taybos GM, Terezhalmy GT. Clinical diagnosis and treatment of oral candidiasis. *J Indiana Dent Assoc.* 1985;64:26–28.

173. Johnson JD, George DI Jr. Treatment of chronic atrophic oral candidiasis with ketonazole (Nizoral): a case report. *J Oral Med.* 1986; 41:138–144.

174. Waldron CA, Shafer WG. Leukoplakia revisited: a clinicopathologic study of 3256 oral leukoplakias. *Cancer.* 1975;36:1386–1392.

175. Gupta PC. Epidemiologic study of the association between alcohol habits and oral leukoplakia. *Community Dent Oral Epidemiol.* 1984;12:47–50.

176. Christen AG, McDonald JL Jr, Klein IA. A primer of relevant facts for smokers. *Dent Teamwork.* 1989;2:25–26.

177. Alexander WN. Oral lesions in the elderly. In: Tryon AE, ed. *Oral Health and Aging.* Littleton, Mass: PSG Publishing Co Inc; 1986.

178. Binnie WH, Wright JM. Oral mucosal disease in the elderly. In: Cohen B, Thomson H, eds. *Dental Care for the Elderly.* London, England: Year Book Medical Publishers Inc; 1986.

179. Silverman S Jr, ed. *Oral Cancer.* 2nd ed. New York, NY: American Cancer Society; 1985.

180. Parker SL, Tong T, Bolden S, et al. Cancer statistics, 1997. *CA.* 1997;47:5–27.

181. Hill MW, Rowe DJ. Influence of aging on oral cancer. *Dent Hyg.* 1982;56:26–30.

182. Little JW, Falace DA. Oral cancer. In: Little JW, Falace DA, eds. *Dental Management of the Medically Compromised Patient.* 3rd ed. St Louis, Mo: CV Mosby Co; 1988.

183. Shedd DP. Clinical characteristics of early oral cancer. *JAMA.* 1971;215:955–956.

184. Rothman K, Keller A. The effect of joint exposure of alcohol and tobacco on risk of cancer of the mouth and pharynx. *J Chronic Dis.* 1972; 25:711–716.

185. Mashberg A. Erythroplasia: the earliest sign of asymptomatic oral cancer. *J Am Dent Assoc.* 1978;96:615–620.

186. Wynder L, et al. Tobacco and alcohol consumption in relation to the development of multiple primary cancers. *Cancer.* 1977;40:1872–1878.

187. Moore C. Smoking and mouth-throat cancer. *Am J Surg.* 1964;108:565–569.

188. Silverberg S Jr, Griffith M. Smoking characteristics of patients with oral carcinoma and the risk for second oral primary carcinoma. *J Am Dent Assoc.* 1972;85:637–640.

189. Mashberg A, Garfinkel L, Harris S. Alcohol as a primary risk factor in oral squamous carcinoma. *CA.* 1981;31:146–155.

190. Elwood JM, Pearson JC, Skippen DH, et al. Alcohol, smoking, social and occupational factors in the aetiology of cancer of the oral cavity, pharynx and larynx. *Int J Cancer.* 1984;34:603–612.

191. Brugere J, Guenel P, Leclerc A, et al. Differential effects of tobacco and alcohol in cancer of the larynx, pharynx, and mouth. *Cancer.* 1986;57:391–395.

192. Rothman KJ. The proportion of cancer attributable to alcohol consumption. *Prev Med.* 1980;9:174–179.

193. Einhorn J, Wersall J. Incidence of oral carcinoma in patients with leukoplakia of the oral mucosa. *Cancer.* 1967;20:2189–2193.

194. Squier CA. Smokeless tobacco and oral cancer: a cause for concern? *CA.* 1984;34:242–247.

195. Shi HB, Xu GQ, Shen ZY. A retrospective study of oral mucosal diseases in three age groups. *Gerondontics.* 1988;4:235–237.

196. Lindqvist C, Teppo L. Epidemiological evaluation of sunlight as a risk factor of lip cancer. *Br J Cancer.* 1978;37:983–989.

197. Hebert JR, London J, Miller DR. Consumption of meat and fruit in relation to oral and esophageal cancer: a cross-national study. *Nutr Cancer.* 1993;19:169–179.

198. Silverman S Jr, Gorsky M. Epidemiologic and demographic update in oral cancer: California and national data—1973 to 1985. *J Am Dent Assoc.* 1990;120:495–499.

199. Peterson DE. Oral mucosal ulcerative lesions. *Pharmacol Dent.* 1986;2:1–4.

200. Greer RO. A problem-oriented approach to evaluating common mucosal lesions in the geriatric patient: a survey of 593 lesions in patients over 60 years of age. *Gerodontics*. 1985;1:68–74.

201. Ghamrawy EE. Quantitative changes in dental plaque formation related to removable partial dentures. *J Oral Rehabil*. 1976;3:115–120.

202. Brill N, Tryde G, Stoltze K, et al. Ecologic changes in the oral cavity caused by removable partial dentures. *J Prosthet Dent*. 1977;38:138–148.

203. Chandler JA, Brudvik JS. Clinical evaluation of patients eight to nine years after placement of removable partial dentures. *J Prosthet Dent*. 1984;51:736–743.

204. Rissin L, House JE, Conway C, et al. Effect of age and removable partial dentures on gingivitis and periodontal disease. *J Prosthet Dent*. 1979;42:217–223.

205. Budtz-Jorgensen E. Clinical aspects of *Candida* infection in denture wearers. *J Am Dent Assoc*. 1978;96:474–479.

206. Lambert JP, Kolstad R. Effect of a benzoic acid–detergent germicide on denture-borne *Candida albicans*. *J Prosthet Dent*. 1986;55:699–700.

207. Budtz-Jorgensen E, Loe H. Chlorhexidine as a denture disinfectant in the treatment of denture stomatitis. *Scand J Dent Res*. 1972;80:457–464.

208. Nater JP, Groenman NH, Wakkers-Garritsen BG, et al. Etiologic factors in denture sore mouth syndrome. *J Prosthet Dent*. 1978;40:367–373.

209. Koopmans ASF, Kippuw N, de Graaff J. Bacterial involvement in denture-induced stomatitis. *J Dent Res*. 1988;67:1246–1250.

210. Bastian RJ. Denture sore mouth, aetiological aspects and treatment. *Aust Dent J*. 1976;21:375–382.

211. Arendorf TM, Walker DM. Oral candidal populations in health and disease. *Br Dent J*. 1979;147:267–272.

212. Williams RC. Periodontal disease. *N Engl J Med*. 1990;322:373–382.

213. Anderson DL. Periodontal disease and aging. *Gerodontology*. 1982;1:19–23.

214. Douglass CW, Gillings D, Sollecito W, et al. National trends in the prevalence and severity of the periodontal diseases. *J Am Dent Assoc*. 1983;107:403–412.

215. Page RC. Periodontal diseases in the elderly: a critical evaluation of current information. *Gerodontology*. 1984;3:63–70.

216. Holm-Pedersen P, Agerbaek N, Theilade E. Experimental gingivitis in young and elderly individuals. *J Clin Periodontol*. 1975;2:14–24.

217. Glickman I, Smulow JB. The combined effects of inflammation and trauma from occlusion in periodontitis. *Int Dent J*. 1969;19:393–407.

218. Ramfjord SP, Ash MM. Significance of occlusion in the etiology and treatment of early, moderate, and advanced periodontitis. *J Periodontol*. 1981;52:511–516.

219. Axelsson P, Lindhe J. Effect of controlled oral hygiene procedures on caries and periodontal disease in adults. *J Clin Periodontol*. 1978;5:133–151.

220. Axelsson P, Lindhe J. The significance of maintenance care in the treatment of periodontal disease. *J Clin Periodontol*. 1981;8:281–294.

221. Lindhe J, Haffajee AD, Socransky SS. Progression of periodontal disease in adult subjects in the absence of periodontal therapy. *J Clin Periodontol*. 1983;10:433–442.

222. Lindhe J, Nyman S. The effect of plaque control and surgical pocket elimination on the establishment and maintenance of periodontal health: a longitudinal study of periodontal therapy in cases of advanced periodontitis. *J Clin Periodontol*. 1975;2:67–79.

223. Schmitt RJ, Sheridan PJ, Rogers RS III. Pernicious anemia with associated glossodynia. *J Am Dent Assoc*. 1988;117:838–840.

224. Powell FC. Glossodynia and other disorders of the tongue. *Dermatol Clin*. 1987;5:687–693.

225. Hill JH, Deitch RL. Early detection of cancers of the head and neck. *VA Pract*. 1986;2:57–72.

226. Venus CA. Interacting with patients who have communication disorders. *Tex Dent J*. 1990;107:11–16.

227. Zimmerman JE, Oder LA. Swallowing dysfunction in acutely ill patients. *Phys Ther*. 1981;61:1755–17.

228. Watanabe I, Sato M, Yamane H, et al. Oral dyskinesia of the aged, I: clinical aspects. *Gerodontics*. 1985;1:39–43.

229. Watanabe I, Yamane G, Yamane H, et al. Oral dyskinesia of the aged, II: electromyographic appearances and dental treatment. *Gerodontics*. 1988;4:310–314.

230. Pakkenberg H, Fog R. Spontaneous oral dyskinesia. *Arch Neurol*. 1974;31:352–353.

231. Altrocchi PH, Forno LS. Spontaneous oralfacial dyskinesia: neuropathology of a case. *Neurology.* 1983;33:802–805.

232. Sutcher HD, Underwood RB, Beatty RA, et al. Orofacial dyskinesia: a dental dimension. *JAMA.* 1971;216:1459–1463.

233. Kamen S. Tardive dyskinesia: a significant syndrome for geriatric dentistry. *Oral Surg Oral Med Oral Pathol.* 1975;39:52–57.

234. Nishioka GJ, Montgomery MT. Masticatory muscle hyperactivity in temporomandibular disorders: is it an extrapyramidally expressed disorder? *J Am Dent Assoc.* 1988;116:514–520.

235. Eneroth CM. Salivary gland tumors in the parotid gland, submandibular gland, and the palate region. *Cancer.* 1971;27:1415–1418.

236. Richardson GS, Dickason WL, Gaisford JC, et al. Tumors of salivary glands: an analysis of 752 cases. *Plast Reconstr Surg.* 1975;55:131–138.

237. Eveson JW, Cawson RA. Salivary gland tumours: a review of 2410 cases with particular reference to histological types, site, age and sex distribution. *J Pathol.* 1985;146:51–58.

238. Eveson IW, Cawson RA. Tumours of the minor (oropharyngeal) salivary glands: a demographic study of 336 cases. *J Oral Pathol.* 1985;14:500–509.

239. Sener SF, Scanlon EF. Irradiation induced salivary gland neoplasia. *Ann Surg.* 1980;191:304–306.

240. McKenna RJ. Tumors of the major and minor salivary glands. *CA.* 1984;34:24–39.

241. Ettinger RL. Xerostomia: a complication of aging. *Aust Dent J.* 1981;26:365–371.

242. Dove J, Sheridan P. Advances in dental research: pilocarpine used to stimulate normal saliva production. *J Am Dent Assoc.* 1985;111:310.

243. Atkinson JC, Fox PC. Clinical pathology conference: xerostomia. *Gerodontics.* 1986;2:193–197.

244. Niessen LC, Jones JA. Professional dental care for patients with dementia. *Gerodontology.* 1987;6:67–71.

245. Lloyd PM. Xerostomia: not a phenomenon of aging. *Wis Med J.* 1983;82:21–22.

246. Jolly DE, Paulson RB, Paulson GW, et al. Parkinson's disease: a review and recommendations for dental management. *Spec Care Dent.* 1989;9:74–78.

247. Kelly JF, Winosgrad CH. A functional approach to stroke management in elderly patients. *J Am Geriatr Soc.* 1985;33:48–60.

248. Rosenbaum CH. Did you treat a drug addict today? *Int Dent J.* 1981;31:307–312.

249. Verlander JM, Johns ME. The clinical use of cocaine. *Otolaryngol Clin North Am.* 1981;14:521–531.

250. Carter EF. Dental implications of narcotic addiction. *Aust Dent J.* 1978;23:308–310.

251. Friedlander AH, Mills MJ. The dental management of the drug-dependent patient. *Oral Surg Oral Med Oral Pathol.* 1985;60:489–492.

252. McBean LD, Speckmann EW. A review: the importance of nutrition in oral health. *J Am Dent Assoc.* 1974;89:109–114.

253. DePaola DP, Kuftinec MN. Nutrition in growth and development of oral tissues. *Dent Clin North Am.* 1976;20:441–459.

254. Alfano MC. Diet and nutrition in the etiology and prevention of oral disease. *J Dent Res.* 1980; 59:2194–2202.

255. Carlsson J, Egelberg J. Effect of diet on early plaque formation in man. *Odontol Rev.* 1965; 16:112–125.

256. Johansson I, Ericson T, Steen L. Studies of the effect of diet on saliva secretion and caries development: the effect of fasting on saliva composition of female subjects. *J Nutr.* 1984;114:2010–2020.

257. Brown AT. The role of dietary carbohydrates in plaque formation and oral disease. *Nutr Rev.* 1975;33:353–361.

258. Theilade E, Theilade T. Role of plaque in the etiology of periodontal disease and caries. *Oral Sci Rev.* 1976;9:23–63.

259. Gibbons RJ, van Houte J. Dental caries. *Annu Rev Med.* 1975;26:121–136.

260. Marthaler TM, Froesch ER. Hereditary fructose intolerance: dental status of eight patients. *Br Dent J.* 1967;123:597.

261. Englander HR. Anticaries and antiplaque agents. In: Neidel EA, Kroeger DC, Yagiela JA, eds. *Pharmacology and Therapeutics for Dentistry.* St Louis, Mo: CV Mosby Co; 1980.

262. Binns NM. Caries and carbohydrates: a problem for dentists and nutritionists. *Dent Health.* 1981;20:5–10.

263. Snacks and caries. *Nutr Rev.* 1987;45:169–172.

264. Scheinen A, Makinen KK. The Turku sugar studies I–XXI. *Acta Odontol Scand.* 1971;32:383–412.

265. Katz S. A diet counseling program. *J Am Dent Assoc.* 1981;102:840–845.

266. Falender LG, Leban SG, Williams FA. Postoperative nutritional support in oral and maxillofacial surgery. *J Oral Maxillofac Surg.* 1987; 45:324–330.

267. Sheiham A. Sucrose and dental caries. *Nutr Health.* 1987;5:25–29.

268. Makinen KK. The role of sucrose and other sugars in the development of dental caries: a review. *Int Dent J.* 1972;22:363–386.

269. Schachtele CF, Jensen ME. Comparison of methods for monitoring changes in the pH of human dental plaque. *J Dent Res.* 1982;61:1117–1125.

270. Mormann JE, Muhlemann HR. Oral starch degradation and its influence on acid production in human dental plaque. *Caries Res.* 1981;15:166–175.

271. Jensen ME, Schachtele CF. The acidogenic potential of reference foods and snacks at interproximal sites in the human dentition. *J Dent Res.* 1983;62:889–892.

272. de Stoppelaar JD, van Houte J, Backer-Dirks O. The effect of carbohydrate restriction on the presence of *Streptococcus mutans, Streptococcus sanguis* and iodophilic polysaccharide-producing bacteria in human dental plaque. *Caries Res.* 1970;4:114–123.

273. Firestone A, Imfeld T, Schmid R, et al. Cariogenicity of foods. *J Am Dent Assoc.* 1980; 101:443.

274. Mandel ID. Effectiveness of biomedical and biosocial research on improving oral health. *J Public Health Dent.* 1978;38:312.

275. Shaw JH. Dietary considerations in oral health. *Fam Community Health.* 1980;3:51–60.

276. Papas A, Palmer C, McGandy R, et al. Dietary and nutritional factors in relation to dental caries in elderly subjects. *Gerodontics.* 1987;3:30–37.

277. Council on Dental Therapeutics. Consensus: oral health effects of products that increase salivary flow rate. *J Am Dent Assoc.* 1988;116:757–759.

278. Hefferren JJ, Harper DS, Osborn JC. Foods, consumption factors and dental caries. *Gerodontics.* 1987;3:26–29.

279. Bibby BG, Mundorff SA, Zero DT, et al. Oral food clearance and the pH of plaque and saliva. *J Am Dent Assoc.* 1986;112:333–337.

280. Lundquist C. Oral sugar clearance: its influence on dental caries activity. *Odontol Rev.* 1952; 3(suppl 1):121–123.

281. Jenkins GN, Kleinberg I. Studies on the pH of plaque in interproximal areas after eating sweets and starch foods. *J Dent Res.* 1956;35:964. Abstract 24.

282. Ludwig TG, Bibby BG. Acid production from different carbohydrate foods in plaque and saliva. *J Dent Res.* 1957;36:56–60.

283. Roberts IF, Roberts GJ. Relation of medicines sweetened with sucrose and dental disease. *Br Med J.* 1979;2:14–16.

284. Lokken P, Birkeland JM, Sannes E. pH changes in dental plaque caused by sweetened, iron-containing liquid medicine. *Scand J Dent Res.* 1975;83:279–283.

285. Feigal RJ, Jensen ME. The cariogenic potential of liquid medications: a concern for the handicapped patient. *Spec Care Dent.* 1982;2:20–24.

286. Matsukobo T, Myake S, Takaesu Y. Evaluation of aspartame as a non-cariogenic sweetener. *Clin Nutr.* 1984;65:193–196.

287. Alfin-Slater RB, Pi-Sunyer FX. Sugar and sugar substitutes: comparisons and indications. *Postgrad Med.* 1987;82:46–56.

288. Glass RL. A two-year clinical trial of sorbitol chewing gum. *Caries Res.* 1983;17:365–368.

289. Birkhed D, Edwardsson S, Kalfas S, et al. Cariogenicity of sorbitol. *Swed Dent J.* 1984; 8:147–154.

290. Jensen ME. Responses of interproximal plaque pH to snack foods and effect of chewing sorbitol-containing gum. *J Am Dent Assoc.* 1986;113: 262–266.

291. Spolsky VW, Wolinsky L. The relationship between nutrition and diet and dental caries periodontal disease. *J Calif Dent Assoc.* 1984; 12:12–18.

292. Alfano MC. Controversies, perspectives and clinical implications of nutrition in periodontal disease. *Dent Clin North Am.* 1976;20:519–548.

293. Slavkin HC. The aging process and nutrition: conception to senescence. *Spec Care Dent.* 1981; 1:31–36.

294. Suomi JD. Prevention and control of periodontal disease. *J Am Dent Assoc.* 1971;83:1271–1287.

295. Charbeneau TD, Hurt WC. Gingival findings in spontaneous scurvy: a case report. *J Periodontol.* 1983;54:694–697.

296. Marshall JR, Graham J, Haughey BP, et al. Smoking, alcohol, dentition and diet in the epidemiol-

ogy of oral cancer. *Eur J Cancer B Oral Oncol.* 1992;28B:9–15.

297. Day GL, Shore RE, Blot WJ, et al. Dietary factors and secondary primary cancers: a follow-up of oral and pharyngeal cancer patients. *Nutr Cancer.* 1994;21:223–232.

298. Marshall J, Graham S, Mettlin C, et al. Diet in the epidemiology of oral cancer. *Nutr Cancer.* 1982;3:145–149.

299. Winn DM, Ziegler RG, Pickle LW, et al. Diet in the etiology of oral and pharyngeal cancer among women from the southern United States. *Cancer Res.* 1984;44:1216–1222.

300. McLaughlin JK, Gridley G, Block G, et al. Dietary factors in oral and pharyngeal cancer. *J Natl Cancer Inst.* 1988;80:1237–1243.

301. Gridley G, McLaughlin JK, Block G, et al. Diet and oral and pharyngeal cancer among blacks. *Nutr Cancer.* 1990;14:219–225.

302. Barone J, Taioli E, Hebert JR, et al. Vitamin supplement use and risk for oral and esophageal cancer. *Nutr Cancer.* 1992;18:31–41.

303. Dreizen S. Nutrition and aging. *Spec Care Dent.* 1982;2:263–267.

304. Massler M. Influence of diet on denture-bearing tissues. *Dent Clin North Am.* 1984;28:211–221.

305. Buchner A, Screebny LM. Enlargement of salivary glands: review of the literature. *Oral Surg Oral Med Oral Pathol.* 1972;34:209–222.

306. Enwonwu CO. Biochemical and morphologic changes in rat mandibular gland in experimental protein-calorie malnutrition. *Exp Mol Pathol.* 1972;16:244–269.

307. Cutter CR. Nutrition in the advanced years. *J Tex Dent Hyg Assoc.* 1979;17:5–7.

308. Nakamoto T, Mallek HM. Significance of protein-energy malnutrition in dentistry: some suggestions for the profession. *J Am Dent Assoc.* 1980;100:339–342.

309. Sullivan DH, Martin W, Flaxman N, et al. Oral health problems and involuntary weight loss in a population of frail elderly. *J Am Geriatr Soc.* 1993;41:725–731.

310. Jette AM, Feldman HA, Douglass C. Oral disease and physical disability in community-dwelling older persons. *J Am Geriatr Soc.* 1993;41:1102–1108.

311. Nizel AE. Role of nutrition in the oral health of the aging patient. *Dent Clin North Am.* 1976; 20:569–584.

312. Epstein S. Importance of psychosocial and behavioral factors in food ingestion in the elderly and their ramifications on oral health. *Gerodontics.* 1987;3:23–25.

313. Yurkstas AA. The effect of missing teeth on masticatory performance and efficiency. *J Prosthet Dent.* 1954;4:120–123.

314. Helkimo E, Carlsson GE, Helhmo M. Chewing efficiency and state of dentition: a methodological study. *Acta Odontol Scand.* 1978;36:33–41.

315. Wayler AH, Kapur KK, Feldman RS, et al. Effects of age and dentition status on measures of food acceptability. *J Gerontol.* 1982;37:294–299.

316. Wayler AH, Chauncey HH. Impact of complete dentures and impaired natural dentition on masticatory performance and food choice in healthy aging men. *J Prosthet Dent.* 1983;49:427–433.

317. Oosterhaven SP, Westert GP, Schaub RMH, et al. Social and psychologic implications of missing teeth for chewing ability. *Community Dent Oral Epidemiol.* 1988;16:79–82.

318. Jenike MA. Tardive dyskinesia: special risk in the elderly. *J Am Geriatr Soc.* 1983;31:71–73.

319. Mumma RD Jr, Quinton K. Effect of masticatory efficiency on the occurrence of gastric distress. *J Dent Res.* 1970;49:69–74.

320. Berry WTC. Mastication, food, and nutrition. *Dent Pract Dent Rec.* 1972;22:249–253.

321. Hartsook EI. Food selection, dietary adequacy, and related dental problems of patients with dental prostheses. *J Prosthet Dent.* 1974;32:32–40.

322. Yurkstas AA, Emerson WH. Dietary selections of persons with natural and artificial teeth. *J Prosthet Dent.* 1964;14:695–697.

323. Chauncey HH, House JE. Dental problems in the elderly. *Hosp Pract.* 1977;12:81–86.

324. Osterberg T, Steen B. Relationship between dental state and dietary intake in 70-year-old males and females in Göteborg, Sweden: a population study. *J Oral Rehabil.* 1982;9:509–521.

325. Chen MK, Lowenstein F. Masticatory handicap, socioeconomic status, and chronic conditions among adults. *J Am Dent Assoc.* 1984;109:916–918.

326. Sastry RS. Nutrition study, III: nutritional status of edentulous patients subsequent to complete denture treatment. *J Indiana Dent Assoc.* 1984; 56:145–147.

327. Brodeur JM, Laurin D, Valleer RE, et al. Nutrient intake and gastrointestinal disorders related to masticatory performance in the edentulous elderly. *J Prosthet Dent.* 1993;70:468–473.

328. Ramsey WO. Nutritional problems of the aged. *J Prosthet Dent.* 1983;49:16–19.

329. Joshipura KJ, Willett WC, Douglass CW. The impact of edentulousness on food and nutrient intake. *J Am Dent Assoc.* 1996;127:459–467.

330. Neill DJ, Phillips HI. The masticatory performance and dietary intake of elderly edentulous patients. *Dent Pract.* 1972;22:384–389.

331. Baxter JC. The nutritional intake of geriatric patients with varied dentitions. *J Prosthet Dent.* 1984;51:164–168.

332. Rodriquez-Olleros A. Gastritis in the toothless. *Rev Gastroenterol.* 1947;14:180–186.

333. Neill DJ, Philips HIB. The masticatory performance, dental state and dietary intakes of a group of elderly army pensioners. *Br Dent J.* 1970; 128:581–585.

334. Hunt RJ, Beck JD, Lemke JH, et al. Edentulism and oral health problems among elderly rural Iowans: the Iowa 65+ rural health study. *Am J Public Health.* 1985;75:1177–1181.

335. Horn VJ, Hodge WC, Treuer JP. Dental condition and weight loss in institutionalized demented patients. *Spec Care Dent.* 1994;14:108–111.

336. Kapur KK. Optimum dentition in the elderly. In: Chauncey HH, Epstein S, Rose CL, et al, eds. *Clinical Geriatric Dentistry: Biomedical and Psychosocial Aspects.* Chicago, Ill: American Dental Association; 1985.

337. Anderson EL. Eating patterns before and after dentures. *J Am Diet Assoc.* 1971;58:421–426.

338. Baxter CJ. Nutrition and the geriatric edentulous patient. *Spec Care Dent.* 1981;1:259–261.

339. Straus R, Sandifur JC, Hall DS, et al. Behavioral factors and denture status. *J Prosthet Dent.* 1977; 37:264–273.

340. Smith JM. Oral and dental discomfort: a necessary feature of old age? *Age Ageing.* 1979; 8:25–31.

341. Yurkstas AA, Emerson WH. Decreased masticatory function in denture patients. *J Prosthet Dent.* 1964;14:931–934.

342. Heath MR. The effect of maximum biting force and bone loss upon masticatory function and dietary selection of the elderly. *Int Dent J.* 1982; 32:345–356.

343. Chauncey HH, Muench ME, Kapur KK, et al. The effect of the loss of teeth on diet and nutrition. *Int Dent J.* 1984;34:98–104.

344. Wayler AH, Muench ME, Kapur KK, et al. Masticatory performance and food acceptability in persons with removable partial dentures, full dentures and intact natural dentition. *J Gerontol.* 1984;39:284–289.

345. Carlsson GE. Masticatory efficiency: the effect of age, the loss of teeth and prosthetic rehabilitation. *Int Dent J.* 1984;34:93–97.

346. Kapur KK, Soman SD. Masticatory performance and efficiency in denture wearers. *J Prosthet Dent.* 1964;14:687–694.

347. Haraldson T, Karlsson U, Carlsson GE. Bite force and oral function in complete denture wearers. *J Oral Rehabil.* 1979;6:41–48.

348. Farrell JH. The effect of mastication on the digestion of food. *Br Dent J.* 1956;100:149–155.

349. Idowu AT, Handelman SL, Graser GN. Effect of denture stability, retention, and tooth form on masticatory function in the elderly. *Gerodontics.* 1987;3:161–164.

350. Ettinger RL. Diet, nutrition, and masticatory ability in a group of elderly edentulous patients. *Aust Dent J.* 1973;18:12–19.

351. Farrell JH. Biological aspects of prosthetic dentistry: masticatory effects in patients with and without dentures. *Int Dent J.* 1964;14:226–237.

352. Ann L. Biting forces in edentulous patients. *Malays Dent J.* 1966;6:18–31.

353. Slagter AP, Olthoff LW, Bosman F, et al. Masticatory ability, denture quality, and oral conditions in edentulous subjects. *J Prosthet Dent.* 1992; 68:299–307.

354. Slagter AP, Bosman F, Va der Bitt A. Comminution of two artificial test foods by dentate and edentulous subjects. *J Oral Rehabil.* 1993; 20:159–176.

355. Bunker PG. The role of dentistry in problems of foreign bodies in the air and food passages. *J Am Dent Assoc.* 1962;64:782–787.

356. Wengraf C. Pharyngo-esophageal foreign bodies in denture wearers. *Dent Pract.* 1969;19:281–282.

357. Anderson DL. Death from improper mastication. *Int Dent J.* 1977;27:349–354.

358. Baxter CI. The nutritional intake of complete denture patients: a computerized study. *J Indiana Dent Soc.* 1980;59:14–17.

359. Renaud M, Mercier P, Vinet A. Does the rehabilitation of the masticatory function influence the nutritive value of the diet? *St Mary's Hosp Med Bull*. 1982;24:186.

360. Gunne HS, Wall AK. The effect of new complete dentures on mastication and dietary intake. *Acta Odontol Scand*. 1985;43:257–268.

361. Gunne HS. The effect of removable partial dentures on mastication and dietary intake. *Acta Odontol Scand*. 1985;43:269–278.

362. Rosenstein DI, Chiodo G, Ho IW, et al. Effect of proper dentures on nutritional status. *Gen Dent*. 1988;36:127–129.

363. Elmstahl S, Birkhed D, Christiansson U, et al. Intake of energy and nutrients before and after dental treatment in geriatric long-stay patients. *Gerodontics*. 1988;4:6–12.

364. Vinton P, Manly RS. Masticatory efficiency during the period of adjustment to dentures. *J Prosthet Dent*. 1955;5:477–480.

365. Sebring NG, Guckes AD, Li SH, et al. Nutritional adequacy of reported intake of edentulous subjects treated with new conventional or implant-supported mandibular implants. *J Prosthet Dent*. 1995;74:358–363.

366. Agerberg G, Carlsson GE. Chewing ability in relation to dental and general health: analyses of data obtained from a questionnaire. *Acta Odontol Scand*. 1981;39:147–153.

367. Lappalainen R, Nyyssonen V. Self-assessed chewing ability of Finnish adults with removable dentures. *Gerodontics*. 1987;3:238–241.

368. Ekelund R. Dental state and subjective chewing ability of institutionalized elderly people. *Community Dent Oral Epidemiol*. 1989;17:24–27.

369. Greksa LP, Parraga IM, Clark CA. The dietary adequacy of edentulous older adults. *J Prosthet Dent*. 1995;72:142–145.

370. Gordon SR, Kelley SL, Sybyl IR, et al. Relationship in very elderly veterans of nutritional status, self-perceived chewing ability, dental status, and social isolation. *J Am Geriatr Soc*. 1985;33:334–339.

371. Chencharick JD, Mossman KL. Nutritional consequences of the radiotherapy of head and neck cancer. *Cancer*. 1983;51:811–815.

372. Locker D, Grushka M. The impact of dental and facial pain. *J Dent Res*. 1987;66:1414–1417.

373. Fattore LD, Baer R, Olsen R. The role of the general dentist in the treatment and management of oral complications of chemotherapy. *Gen Dent*. 1987;35:374–377.

374. Cohen T, Gitman L. Oral complaints and taste perception in the aged. *J Gerontol*. 1959;14:294–298.

375. Schiffman SS, Moss J, Erickson RP. Thresholds of food odors in the elderly. *Exp Aging Res*. 1976;2:389–398.

376. Rhodus NL, Brown J. The association of xerostomia and inadequate intake in older adults. *J Am Diet Assoc*. 1990;90:1688–1692.

377. Ernst SL. Dietary intake, food preferences, stimulated salivary flow rate, and masticatory ability in older adults with complete dentitions. *Spec Care Dent*. 1993;13:102–106.

378. Vissink A, Schaub RMH, van Rijn LJ, et al. The efficacy of mucin-containing artificial saliva in alleviating symptoms of xerostomia. *Gerodontology*. 1987;6:95–101.

379. Moeller TP. Sensory changes in the elderly. *Dent Clin North Am*. 1989;33:23–31.

380. Griep MI, Verleye G, Franck AH, et al. Variation in nutrient intake with dental status, age and odour perception. *Eur J Clin Nutr*. 1996;50:816–825.

381. Corso JF. The sensory effects of aging on man. *Scientia*. 1968;103:362–393.

382. Corso JF. Sensory processes and age effects in normal adults. *J Gerontol*. 1971;26:90–105.

383. Henkin RI, Christiansen RL. Taste thresholds in patients with dentures. *J Am Dent Assoc*. 1967;75:118–120.

384. Chauncey HH, Wayler AH. The modifying influence of age on taste perception. *Spec Care Dent*. 1981;1:68–74.

385. Henkin RI, Christiansen RL. Taste localization on the tongue, palate, and pharynx of normal man. *J Appl Physiol*. 1967;22:316–320.

386. Giddon DB, Dreisbach ME, Pfaffman C, et al. Relative abilities of natural and artificial dentition patients for judging the sweetness of solid foods. *J Prosthet Dent*. 1954;4:263–268.

# CHAPTER 7

# Smell, Taste, and Somatosensation in the Elderly

*Valerie B. Duffy*

Smell, taste, and somatosensation (touch, pain, and temperature sensations), contribute to the sustenance of nutritional health and food enjoyment by receiving and processing information from the food world. The quality of this sensory information can influence whether we choose a food or beverage. The aroma of food may stimulate our appetite even if we are not hungry. Once the food is in the mouth, the taste, smell, and somatosensory sensations blend into a composite food flavor. Foods and beverages that are appealing and diverse in flavor may stimulate us to eat more. Conversely, we may have less desire to eat if the quality of the sensory experience is less appealing or void of diversity. Thus, our desire to eat, what we eat, and, ultimately, our nutritional status may be influenced by the smell, taste, and somatosensation. Understanding the physiological and psychological processes of these senses and how these processes may change with aging is important to understanding maintenance of nutritional health and the food enjoyment in older adults.

This chapter aims to review the physiology of these sensory systems and the psychology of our perceptual response. These processes are reviewed within the context of normal function and of changes associated with aging and disease. The chapter ends with a discussion of the association between nutrition and smell, taste, and somatosensation in older adults.

## SMELL VERSUS TASTE VERSUS SOMATOSENSATION IN THE PROCESSING OF FOOD FLAVOR

The chemosenses are so named because they respond to chemicals such as those that make up foods and beverages. The sense of smell allows detection, recognition, and exact identification of odors both from the environment and from the oral cavity (see Figure 7–1). For example, we use the sense of smell to detect the off-odors of souring milk, to recognize that cookies are flavored with vanilla or rum extract, or to distinguish a Bordeaux from a Pinot Noir (and, with a very fine tuned sense of smell, to identify even the region and year of the wine's production!). True taste is the perception of salt, sweet, sour, and bitter (although some claim *umami*, the meaty fla-

I was supported in the preparation of this manuscript by grants from the National Institutes of Health (DC00283, Linda M. Bartoshuk, Principal Investigator) and the United States Department of Agriculture (NRICGP/USDA 9603745, Valerie B. Duffy, Principal Investigator).

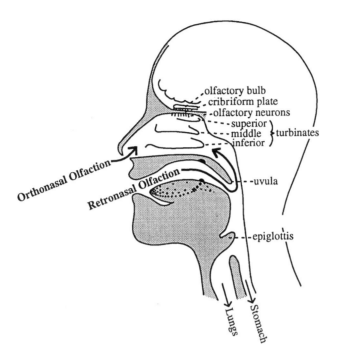

**Figure 7–1** The two pathways for olfactory perception. Odors are perceived through the nostrils (ie, orthonasal olfaction) and through the oral cavity (ie, retronasal olfaction). Both pathways carry the odor to the olfactory neurons, where the chemical signal (ie, odor) is transduced into a nerve signal. *Source:* VB Duffy and LM Bartoshuk, Sensory Factors in Feeding, in ED Capaldi, *Why We Eat What We Eat: The Psychology of Eating*, Figure 1, pp. 147, © 1996, American Psychological Association.

vor of glutamate, is the fifth basic taste quality). The somatosensory system is responsible for processing the feel, texture, temperature, and pungent or irritating chemicals of food.

Although functionally similar, each chemosense has a separate neurochemical system to carry sensory information from the receptors to the brain. Chemosensory stimuli must reach and be adsorbed to a specific receptor cell. These receptor cells have long extensions (cilia or microvilli) that provide enough surface area for adsorption. The high level of specificity of the receptor cells makes it possible for the chemosensory system to detect and differentiate the slightest variation in chemical stimuli. Chemicals that differ only in chiral form can generate radically different

perceptions. For example, *d*- and *l*-isomers of carvone produce the olfactory sensations of caraway and spearmint.[1] While the human olfactory system has the potential to distinguish an unlimited number of chemicals, in reality the odorants that people differentiate number only in the hundreds.[2] The same chemical specificity is also true for taste; a number of compounds may produce a sweet taste, but the quality of each sweet taste may vary slightly. The receptor cells also transduce the chemical stimuli into electrical signals, transforming chemical signals into nerve signals. Throughout life, receptor cells undergo birth, maturation, and death. The majority of taste receptors live 10 days[3] and are continually replaced. Olfactory receptor cells take between 30 and 120 days to regenerate.[4]

## THE PHYSIOLOGY OF THE CHEMOSENSES

### Sense of Smell

Olfactory stimuli reach the olfactory system through two pathways: from the environment through the nostrils (orthonasal route) and from the mouth through the nasopharynx (retronasal route) (see Figure 7–1). Both routes transport odorants to the olfactory epithelium, which is located on the dorsal aspect of the nasal cavity in the septum and in part of the superior turbinate of the sinuses.[5] The eating experience perfectly exemplifies the dual nature of olfactory perception. We may perceive food odors passively through normal breathing. Sniffing increases the intensity of odors by causing turbulent airflow through the nasal cavity and an increase in the concentration of odor molecules that reach the olfactory receptors.[6] We can appreciate the full bouquet of a wine by holding the glass close to the nose and sniffing (orthonasal olfaction). In the mouth, foods and beverages present a complex mixture of smell, taste, and somatosensory sensations. Foods and beverages that are cold or have flavoring embedded may provide little olfactory stimulation until actually placed in the mouth. Chewing and mouth movements warm and release olfactory volatiles and, with the addition of swallowing, create sufficient oral pressure to pump these olfactory volatiles up through the oropharynx and nasopharynx to the olfactory epithelium (retronasal olfaction).[7] Thus, like the sniffing action, the tongue, cheek, and throat movement must work in harmony to release and transport olfactory volatiles to ensure adequate retronasal olfactory perception.

The olfactory epithelium has olfactory receptor cells, supporting cells, and basal cells (see Figure 7–2). The olfactory receptors are actually the olfactory neurons, which transmit the duration of exposure to, the identity, and the concentration of thousands of different odors to the central nervous system. The supporting cells secrete mucus, and basal cells serve to generate new olfactory receptors. The size of the human olfactory epithelium is approximately 10 cm$^2$, 1/100 of the size of that of the dog, an animal that possesses a much keener sense of smell. Nonetheless, a 2-cm$^2$ area of human olfactory tissue is estimated to contain 6 million ciliated olfactory cells.[8] Individuals with congenital anosmia (ie, without a sense of smell) have greatly reduced or absent olfactory epithelium.[9]

Odorants must travel through a fluid phase to reach the olfactory receptors (Figure 7–2). The odorants are dissolved in the olfactory mucus, which may serve to concentrate and amplify the chemical message.[10] The odorants pass through this mucus layer either by diffusion[11] or by facilitated diffusion with a transport protein.[12] The cilia of the olfactory receptors are distributed through the epithelium. The odorant binding to the receptor proteins initiates the transduction cascade (ie, the conversion of the chemical signal to an electrical signal). The mechanism of transduction involves the cAMP (cyclic adenosine 3′,5′-monophosphate) second-messenger system (see Hildebrand and Shepherd[13] for a review). The odorant binding with receptor proteins activates a G-protein to stimulate the adenylate cyclase enzyme cascade and the production of cAMP. The cAMP mediates depolarization of the olfactory receptor cell. The action potential is carried by the nonmyelinated axon of the receptor cell (ie, olfactory nerve) through the cribriform plate to the olfactory bulb. The receptor cells synapse on the dendrites of the mitral or tufted cells in the glomeruli of the olfactory bulb (see Greer[14] for a review). The axons of the mitral

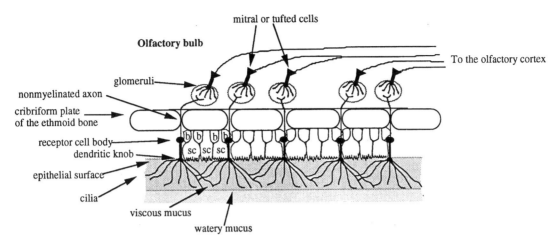

**Figure 7–2** Peripheral olfactory pathways. The olfactory mucosa has the olfactory receptor cells (receptor cell body, dendritic knob, and cilia noted), the supporting cells (sc), and basal cells (b). The nonmyelinated axons of the olfactory receptor cells project centrally through the cribriform plate of the ethmoid bone and terminate in the glomeruli of the olfactory bulb. The olfactory bulb neurons (mitral or tufted cells) project centrally to the olfactory tract. *Source:* Data from S. Schiffman, Taste and Smell Losses in Normal Aging and Disease, *Journal of the American Medical Association*, Vol. 278, pp. 1357–1362, © 1997; C. Greer, Structural Organization of the Olfactory System, in T. Getchel, et al., eds., *Smell and Taste in Health and Disease*, pp. 65–81, © 1991, Raven Press; S. Kinnamon and R. Margolskee, Mechanisms of Taste Transduction, *Current Options in Neurobiology*, Vol. 6, pp. 506–513, © 1996.

and tufted cells transmit the sensory message to the olfactory cortex and to other broader cortical regions and limbic brain structures, including the hippocampus (memory) and the hypothalamus (feeding center).

**Sense of Taste**

True tastants (salt, sugar, sour, bitter) stimulate taste receptors located in special end organs (taste buds) on the tongue, soft palate, pharynx, larynx, and epiglottis. (Data exist to support that qualities like umami, the savory taste of glutamate, are true tastants.[15,16]) Taste buds on the tongue are found within gustatory papillae: the fungiform papillae on the anterior tongue, the foliate papillae on the posterior lateral sides of the tongue, and the circumvallate papillae, which extend in an inverted "V". across the root of the tongue (see Figure 7–3). Humans show large variation in both number of fungiform papillae and number of taste buds on these papillae (see Miller and Bartoshuk[17] for a review). This variation appears to relate to sensory abilities. Genetic supertasters, who rate 6-*n*-propylthiouracil as extremely bitter, have the highest density of fungiform papillae and taste buds upon them.[18] Compared with nontasters, supertasters give the highest ratings to a number of bitter (eg, calcium chloride, potassium chloride) and sweet (eg, sucrose, fructose) compounds[19] and a number of somatosensory sensations (see below).

Taste buds contain between 50 and 150 cells that form an ovoid structure. These cells are divided into basal cells (from which new taste cells originate) and three types of elongated bipolar cells (dark, intermediate, and light), which have microvilli that extend

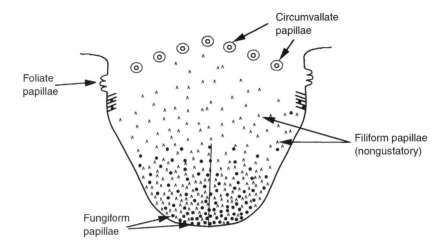

**Figure 7–3** The human tongue, showing the gustatory papillae (fungiform, foliate, and circumvallate papillae) and the nongustatory filiform papillae.

through a taste pore into the oral environment. The microvilli appear to contain the taste receptors. To reach microvilli, tastants become dissolved in saliva and a mucus layer. The saliva and mucus layer may contain proteins that aid in the transport of the tastants to the microvilli. A single taste cell can respond to more than one taste quality. Thus, gustatory papillae, which contain several taste cells, respond to more than one quality. (Humans can perceive salt, sweet, sour, and bitter on all parts of the oral cavity that contain taste receptors. As pointed out by Bartoshuk,[20] the idea of a "tongue map"—the ability to perceive certain taste qualities on a specialized area of the tongue—is an "enduring scientific myth" that continues to show up in children's books and even some professional references. By painting taste solutions on the areas of cranial nerve innervation, one can easily disprove the tongue map.) However, the mechanism of taste transduction is specific for the type of gustatory stimuli.[21] The gustatory stimuli interact with the taste receptor, which results in depolarization of the receptor and transmission of the electrical signal. Taste transduction involves sodium and potassium ion channels and two second-messenger systems (eg, adenylate cyclase and phosphatidylinositol systems).

Branches of three cranial nerves innervate the taste buds on each side of the tongue and transmit the electrical signal to the medulla (as reviewed by Pritchard[22]):

- The chorda tympani nerve (branch of cranial nerve VII) innervates taste buds in the fungiform papillae and in the anterior foliate papillae.
- The lingual branch of the glossopharyngeal nerve innervates the taste buds in the posterior foliate papillae and in the circumvallate papillae.
- The superficial petrosal branch of cranial nerve VII innervates taste buds on the soft palate.
- The superior branch of the vagus nerve (cranial nerve X) innervates taste buds in the epiglottis.

These cranial nerves project to the nucleus of the solitary tract (NST). This region receives information from the somatosensory and the olfactory systems. From the NST, the axons travel to the ventrobasal thalamus and then to the gustatory cortex.

## Somatosensation

Cranial nerve V, the trigeminal nerve, transmits the largest amount of somatosensory sensations from the face. Branches of this cranial nerve innervate the mucous membranes of the nasal cavity, the oral cavity, and the eye (see Silver and Finger[23] for a comprehensive review of the anatomy of the trigeminal system). Foods and beverages stimulate three of the four classes of sensory fibers and receptors in the trigeminal nerve: (1) tactile sensations such as particle size, texture, and creaminess stimulate mechanoreceptors; (2) temperature of foods and beverages stimulates thermoreceptors; and (3) irritants and pungent foods stimulate nociceptors. Somatosensory sensations are integrated with but separate from smell and taste sensations. Odor compounds, if concentrated enough, cause intranasal stimulation of both the olfactory and trigeminal nerves.[24] Concentrated or noxious odors also irritate the eyes and can affect change in the respiratory and circulatory systems (this warns the organism that a harmful substance is present). Individuals with olfactory dysfunction may still be able to distinguish the presence of concentrated odors through intranasal stimulation of the trigeminal nerve. The taste and somatosensory systems are also integrated. Strong tastants (eg, concentrated citric acid or sodium chloride) can also stimulate the nociceptors and produce irritation on the tongue. In fact, up to 75% of the innervation of the fungiform papillae on the anterior tongue is from the lingual branch of the trigeminal nerve.[25] On the posterior tongue, the glossopharyngeal nerve carries sensory fibers for pain, touch, and temperature. Licking, as described by Green,[26] integrates the chemosensory systems and can provide a highly enjoyable experience. For example, while a person is licking maple walnut ice cream, the trigeminal nerve senses coolness, creaminess, and texture of the ice cream and added nuts, and the chorda tympani nerve senses the sweetness. As the ice cream is moved to the back of the tongue, the melting and mouth movements release and pump the maple and walnut flavor volatiles to cranial nerve I for olfactory perception.

Individuals show genetic variation in ability to perceive oral somatosensory sensations. Supertasters of 6-*n*-propylthiouracil, as compared with nontasters, give higher intensity to a variety of oral irritants, including chili peppers (ie, capsaicin), black pepper (ie, piperine), ginger (ie, zingerone), carbonation, and alcohol.[27] Supertasters also give highest tactile sensations to high-fat milk products,[28] salad dressings,[29] and viscous agents such as guar gum.[30] The genetic variation in ability to perceive oral somatosensory sensations has an anatomical basis. Supertasters have the highest density of fungiform papillae,[18] and since taste and trigeminal fibers innervate fungiform papillae, they also may have the most trigeminal innervation to the anterior tongue. Genetic supertasters may also have the highest propensity to experience oral pain in response to conditions and therapies that impair oral health (eg, chemotherapy, radiation therapy).

## CHEMOSENSORY PSYCHOPHYSICS

Psychophysics, a branch of psychology, involves the study of how perception relates to physical stimulation. This includes how smell, taste, and somatosensory sensations vary with the quality, concentration, and duration of exposure to odorants, tastants, and a range of touch, temperature, and pain stimuli.

Psychophysical investigation can characterize both the relationship between the physical world and the perceptual world and the changes in that relationship as the result of aging. Examples of two psychophysical procedures include the determination of the concentration required for detection or recognition of a chemical (threshold) and how perceived intensity varies with changing concentration (suprathreshold). In olfaction, odor identification tasks (ie, the ability to identify correctly a number of odorants) are a standard psychophysical procedure. Psychophysical evaluation can also include measuring the liking or disliking of chemosensory stimuli.

Valid psychophysical techniques are necessary to understand fully the effect of age-related physiological changes on chemosensory perception. Below is a description of the common psychophysical techniques.

### Threshold

Threshold is sensitivity to a particular chemosensory stimulus and represents the lowest concentration needed to elicit a sensation (detection threshold) or to recognize a sensation (recognition threshold). Individuals' thresholds are very simple to compare, whether within a cohort of elderly individuals or across age cohorts. A high threshold (or low sensitivity) indicates that an individual requires a high concentration to first perceive a chemosensory stimulus.

For olfactory thresholds, the procedure must ensure delivery of a consistent concentration (ie, parts per billion) of odorant through devices such as porous paper dipped in odorant, sniff or squeeze bottles containing the odorant diluted in water or oil, or an olfactometer (as reviewed by Doty[31]). One technique for assessing threshold is the two-alternative forced-choice version of the ascending method of limits (see Stevens and Dadarwala[32]). In olfactory threshold testing, for example, the subject is presented with two squeeze bottles, one with odorant at the weakest concentration and the other with only the diluent (the order of presentation is random). The subject is asked to squeeze and sniff one bottle at a time and to judge which bottle contains the stronger odorant (forced choice). If correct, he or she is tested again with the same concentration. If the individual judges incorrectly, a stronger concentration is presented (ascending method of limits). The threshold is the concentration at which the subject makes four or five consecutive correct choices.

The staircase procedure, a variant of the method of limits, is another threshold method used frequently in clinical and experimental procedures. In this procedure, the subject responds to stimuli that are above and below the threshold level. For taste thresholds, for example, the subject is presented with two solutions, one, the stimulus (nondetectable level), the other, diluent (usually water). If the subject judges correctly, the tester decreases the concentration and makes the task more difficult. This is a reversal or a change in the concentration tested. If the subject judges incorrectly, the tester increases the concentration and makes the task easier. This also is a reversal. The threshold value is calculated as the mean concentration of all reversals (generally six). (For more information about these procedures, see McBurney and Collings[33] or Doty.[31])

When one is interpreting threshold elevations in aging, it is important to note that the process relies on both sensory and nonsensory data. A falsely elevated threshold could result from conservative judgments and the unwillingness of subjects to identify a stimulus as present until they are absolutely sure.[34] As well, thresholds can show large variability, which makes repeat testing highly recommended to ensure the validity of the measurement.[32]

**Suprathreshold**

By measuring suprathreshold perception, one attempts to describe an individual's full sensory world. The clinician or experimenter can measure how perceived intensity varies with concentration of an odorant, a tastant, or an irritant (using concentrations that range from barely detectable levels to strong, very strong, and even strongest imaginable sensation). This is referred to as *direct scaling,* or measuring the relationship between perceived intensity and concentration. The primary concern with this measurement is the valid comparison of intensity judgments across individuals. That is, how does one subject's judgment of "strong" compare with another's? Are the two sensations equal? How can you be sure if you cannot share the same sensory experiences? Identification tasks are another measure of suprathreshold perception, used most frequently in the measurement of olfactory perception.

### Scaling: Measuring Perceived Intensity

The general techniques for measuring perceived intensity are (1) category scales, (2) magnitude estimation, (3) line scales with and without labels, and (4) magnitude matching (the gold standard method). The literature on taste and smell in aging includes a variety of these scaling methods (see Bartoshuk and Duffy[35] for a review of the scaling techniques in literature on aging). Understanding the use and limitations of each type of scaling method will support the appropriate interpretation of studies on chemosensory perception and aging. The following briefly describes each scaling technique. Correct use of scaling techniques has application beyond measuring sensory perception, including measuring hedonic feelings toward foods and even feelings of satisfaction with patient care services and detecting changes in behavior and quality of life over time or in response to an intervention.

*Category Scales.* One familiar scale is the Natick 9-point category scale (1 = *very weak*, 5 = *medium*, 9 = *very strong*).[36] The subjects assign a number between 1 and 9 to indicate the intensity of the stimulus. This type of scale is quickly administered and easy to understand. However, when a person gives one stimulus a rating of 3 and another a rating of 6, the only conclusion permissable is that the second stimulus was stronger than the first. Thus, category scales only order the intensity of stimulus.[37] This method of scaling does not reflect how much stronger one stimulus is than another (ie, does not measure relative intensity). Category scales also do not measure absolute intensity, for the clinician or experimenter can never assume that "moderate" means the same thing to all individuals. These scales therefore may not allow valid comparison of perceived intensity across individuals or groups.

*Magnitude Estimation.* Magnitude estimation requires a subject to assign a number to represent the intensity of a stimulus, according to the following instructions:

> Please tell me how strong or weak a series of tastes and sounds are to you by providing a number to represent the intensity. The larger the number, the stronger the taste or sound. Conversely, the smaller the number, the

weaker the taste or sound. You can use any numbers that you desire. However, I will ask you to judge the tastes and sounds relative to the first one you perceive. That is, if the second stimulus is three times stronger than the first, provide a number that is three times larger than the first number. If the second stimulus is a third as strong, then give a number that is a third as large.

With this scale, a rating of 8 reflects an intensity twice that of a rating of 4 (the intensities are relative). Magnitude estimation prevents a ceiling effect or the inability of the subject to express the true increase in the perceived intensity of increasing concentrations. For example, in line with the above instructions, the subject might feel that he or she would use a 1-to-10 scale to judge the intensity of salt solutions. Upon tasting the solutions, the subject gives a 4 to the first solution and an 8 to the second solution. The subject feels that the third solution is twice as strong as the second solution. Magnitude estimation allows subjects the freedom to give a rating of 16 even though they might have originally thought they would use a 1-to-10 scale. Some line scales may not afford this freedom and thus are subject to ceiling effects (ie, ceiling effects limit the individual from expressing the true intensity of the stimuli).

Magnitude estimation assumes that individuals can use numbers appropriately. The practice task of judging the distance between two points can quickly train the subject to assign numbers that represent magnitude with ratio properties. The following is a practice setting (the order of presentation can be varied): "Please assign a number to represent the distance between my two fingers [eg, 5 inches in space], between my two hands [eg, shoulder width apart], again between my two

hands [eg, full arm span], between my two fingers [eg, 1 inch apart], and again between my two fingers [eg, 1/2 inch apart]."

Magnitude estimation does not allow comparison of perceived intensity across subjects unless the meaning and use of the number scale is standardized. One subject may have used a 1-to-50 number scale, another a 1-to-15 scale. The clinician or experimenter cannot assume that one subject's rating of 15 equals another subject's rating of 50 because the numbers have meaning only to the subject. The problem may be addressed by asking the subject the meaning of his or her scale *after* the session is completed.[38] For this technique, subjects are asked, "If you did or had experienced something as 'very strong,' what number would you have provided?" The subject then generates numbers for all the desired adjectives of intensity. The only limitation is the assumption that the adjectives mean the same thing to all of the subjects. Another way to standardize the number scale or magnitude estimate data is through the use of magnitude matching (see below).

*Line Scales.* Line scales, either labeled with adjectives or not, equate the length of the line with the intensity of the stimuli. Figure 7–4 shows three different labeled lines that vary in type and placement of adjectives: a standard visual analogue scale, the Marks scale,[39] and the Green scale.[40] The tape-pull method is a variant of the line length, but without adjective labels. In this procedure,[41] the subjects pull a retractable metal tape (up to 3 m), with the length of the tape reflecting the intensity of stimuli.

These scales provide a visual frame of reference and are easy for naive subjects to use. The visual analogue scale can have the same inherent problems of a category scale. The Marks[39] and Green[40] scales were designed to limit ceiling effects (described above)

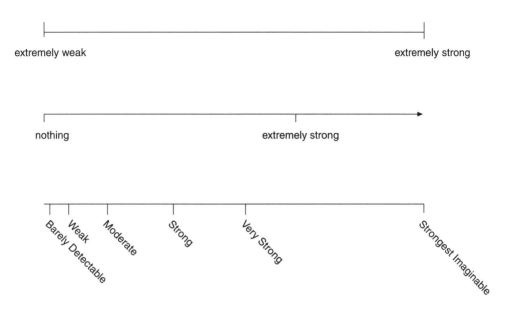

**Figure 7–4** Three labeled lines for scaling the perceived intensity of chemosensory stimuli. The top scale is the standard visual analogue scale. The middle scale was constructed by Marks.[39] The bottom scale, the label magnitude scale, was constructed by Green and colleagues.[40] *Source:* Adapted with permission from L. Marks, Sensory and Cognitive Factors in Judgments of Loudness, *Journal of Experimental Psychology,* Vol. 5, pp. 426–443, © 1972, American Psychological Association, and B. Green et al., A Semantically-Labeled Scale of Oral Sensation with Apparent Ratio Properties, *Chemical Senses,* Vol. 18, pp. 683–702, © 1993, Oxford University Press.

through the positioning of "extremely" in the Marks line or "strongest imaginable" in the Green scale. The Green scale also includes instructions to subjects in the use of the scale that include the statement that the meaning of "strongest imaginable" might be a sensation so strong as to cause pain (eg, the pain of burning your mouth on hot pizza).

Line scales can provide a measure of *absolute intensity* only if it is assumed that individuals treat the meaning of adjectives similarly (if the line is labeled) and use the same line length to represent the same gradations of intensity. Magnitude matching eliminates the need to make these assumptions.

*Magnitude Matching.* This procedure matches the intensity judgments from one sensory continuum to another, or across qualities within a sensory continuum (also called *cross-modality matching*). One sensory stimulus serves as the standard, and the assumption is that all individuals experience the standard equally. Marks and Stevens[42,43] developed this procedure to use with magnitude estimate data. For example, in measuring perceived odor intensity in young and older adults, the standard could be the intensity of sodium chloride (with the assumption that intensity of NaCl shows less risk of loss with aging and thus is perceived equally in both age groups). In the session, subjects judge the intensity of a concentration series of odors and NaCl solutions, usually presented in a random order. The experimenter instructs the subject to provide magnitude estimate data *and* to use the same number scale to judge the intensity of odors and tastes. For comparison within and between cohorts, the odor intensities are standardized with the NaCl intensities.

The primary limitation of magnitude matching is the identification of an appropriate standard. If the perceived intensity of the standard shows an association with age, finding a difference between young and elderly subjects in the perceived intensity of the sensation of interest is nearly impossible. The results of intensity measured with labeled lines may be improved by normalizing the line data with a standard.[44] That is, the example above could be repeated using the Green scale and NaCl intensity to examine perceived odor intensity in young and older adults.

*Misuse of Standards in Psychophysical Testing.* Some experimental designs have included the use of standards that inappropriately force subjects to assign similar ratings for very different perceptual experiences. A complete explanation of this error can be found in the literature.[35] While a number of aging studies have used these inappropriate standards, following are the details of one study.[45] In this experiment, investigators were interested in determining the perceived saltiness of tomato juices that varied in NaCl and citric acid concentration. Before sampling the tomato juices, the subjects (young and elderly) were given standards for the "least salty" as "tomato juice with no added salt" and "most salty" as "tomato juice with 1.5% NaCl." The subjects were told to make their intensity judgment on a 10-cm line relative to these two standards. This is a very different procedure than magnitude matching. In this procedure, subjects are forced to comply with these set standards. What if the standards were not perceived equally by all sub-

jects? What if the 1.5% NaCl in the tomato juice was not the saltiest stimulus? Citric acid can add to the perceived intensity of saltiness, and the highest concentration of citric acid in tomato juice might have created the perception of the most intense saltiness for some subjects. This paradigm could accommodate neither these possibilities nor the difference between young and elderly cohorts.

### Identification Tasks

Identification tasks are frequently used in the clinical assessment of olfactory functioning. Subjects perceive and identify odorants, usually being prompted with a list of odors (tested odors and those that are distracters). Odor identification requires cognition, memory, and familiarity with the odorants. Correct odor identification requires sufficient sensory information to detect and recognize the odor as familiar, retrieve the odor name from long-term memory, and form the odor-word relationship.[46] Individuals with sensory impairment have difficulty linking an odor to a verbal description,[2] the "tip of the nose" phenomenon.[47]

Experimental designs should control for the potential of cognitive difficulties exaggerating the degree of age-related olfactory impairment.[48] Odor identification procedures can be constructed to measure primarily sensory functioning. Screening subjects for cognitive functioning can provide information as to whether an identification task is appropriate for the individual. The odors in the test should be familiar to the age cohort. Previous research shows that the elderly perform better on odor identification tasks that include odors from their childhood.[46] The task should minimize difficulties with retrieving odor names by providing a list of odors to choose from. Allowing individuals to select the correct odor name from a list and retesting missed items after correct feedback can decrease the cognitive challenges of odor identification tasks.[49]

## Summary of the Psychophysical Techniques To Measure Chemosensory Functioning in Aging

Thresholds provide a measure of sensitivity but may or may not reflect the ability to perceive stimuli at concentrations relevant to eating. Suprathreshold tasks measure perception of real-world stimuli. For perceived intensity measures, the scaling method must (1) allow subjects to express the range of their sensations (which will eliminate the ceiling effect), (2) only use standards not related to the measure of interest, and (3) provide a valid way to compare perceived intensity across subjects (eg, magnitude matching). In the performance of identification tasks (primarily for olfaction), the method must attempt to separate sensory influences from cognitive influences. Psychophysical tasks that utilize foods and beverages may have the most application in the exploration of the relationship between chemosensory functioning and nutritional outcomes.

## CHEMOSENSORY CHANGES AND AGING

Clinicians can assess normal sensory functioning (ie, normosmic, normogeusic) and reveal a range of disorders in olfaction, taste, and somatosensation (see Snow et al[50] for a complete characterization of chemosensory disorders). In olfaction, individuals can suffer from diminished (hyposmia) or absent (anosmia) ability to perceive one, a few, or all tested odorants. Specific anosmia may be a genetic variation and not a disorder. For example, up to 30% of the population have a specific anosmia to the musky compounds galoxide and androstenone.[51] Individuals can

also show altered olfactory perception, or dysosmia. Dysosmia can be the distortion of odor quality (parosmia—eg, smelling burnt paper instead of baby powder) or a phantom olfactory sensation with no apparent olfactory stimulus (olfactory hallucinations, phantosmia).

In taste, individuals can also show diminished (hypogeusia) or absent (ageusia) taste perception. Total ageusia is very rare[52]: The ability to taste with the whole mouth is maintained despite major damage to the nerves that subserve taste. As with olfaction, individuals can suffer from altered taste perception (dysgeusia). Chronic dysgeusia or a persistent salt, sweet, sour, or bitter sensation can result from a stimulus in the mouth (eg, the taste of an oral infection) or something that leaks into the mouth from the bloodstream (eg, a bitter taste from medications). The dysgeusia can also be a phantom sensation generated by spontaneous activity in the nervous system in the absence of stimulation (analogous to phantom limb sensations).

Somatosensory perceptions can also be altered. Loss of sensitivity can occur to touch sensations (numbness) and to chemical irritants (desensitization). Chemical desensitization can occur through the application and removal of capsaicin (the burn of chili pepper).[53] This desensitization property can provide an effective means of analgesia for peripheral sources of oral pain.[54] Individuals can also perceive pain or hypersensitivity to somatosensory stimuli.

The following is a review of the findings from studies on chemosensory perception in aging. This review is cautious in presenting some of the findings, as some reflect the limitations of the psychophysical procedures outlined above. With this consideration, the data support that age-related olfactory dysfunction is more common than taste dysfunction. Somatosensory sensations also appear stable across age, although there are some age-related declines in touch sensation in the mouth. It is important to mention that complaints of "taste loss," if sensory, are olfactory problems. Individuals usually are unable both to separate and to distinguish taste from smell when a chemosensory stimulus is placed in the mouth. They are also unable to distinguish the contributions of taste and smell to the overall intensity of a chemical stimulant.[55,56] Individuals usually attribute the flavor of food as "taste" to resolve the ambiguity of the mutual olfactory-taste stimuli.[56] Clinicians must carefully question older adults to understand their complaint, and if it is sensory, they must assess whether the complaint involves taste or smell (see below).

## The Sense of Smell and Aging

Most studies support the thesis that olfaction shows age-related declines. It is hypothesized that aging alone produces a gradual loss of olfactory function that is often unrecognized (see discussion below). A more precipitous loss of olfactory perception could indicate an overriding environmental insult (eg, nasal/sinus disease). Older adults can show a range of functioning from total loss (anosmia) to diminished ability (hyposmia) to a sense of smell equal to that of younger adults (normosmia). It is difficult to separate olfactory losses of aging from those caused by disease and environmental insults. Analysis of data from the Baltimore Longitudinal Study of Aging by Ship and Weiffenbach[57] shows age-related declines in olfactory perception in a group of successfully aging men and women. However, Barber,[58] from analysis of the National Geographic Smell Survey, showed less olfactory impairment in a sample of elderly subjects who did not report a history of exposure to environmental insults.

The anatomical structure of olfaction makes it more vulnerable to loss than taste. Cowart and colleagues[59] present the following information. Olfactory information is carried by only cranial nerve I; taste is transmitted by branches of three different cranial nerves (VII, IX, X). The olfactory nerve must travel through the ethmoid bone and can be severed with a specifically located head trauma (see description below under "Head Trauma"). As well, the olfactory receptors are embedded in a relatively small region of the superior sinus region, whereas taste has receptors (taste buds) on the tongue, on the palate, and in the throat. Because the olfactory neurons also serve as olfactory receptors, they are directly exposed to environmental insults such as toxins and infectious agents. While olfactory neurons can regenerate, they must do so by reinnervating the olfactory bulb. In taste, the neurons are protected, as there are specialized taste receptors and epithelial cells.

Two large cross-sectional studies of free-living individuals provide data on age-related changes in olfactory perception across the life span. One study included over 1,900 individuals from ages 5 to 99 years[60] and measured olfactory perception with the University of Pennsylvania Smell Identification Test (UPSIT).[61] The UPSIT has 40 odors and a multiple-choice format. Subjects scratch and sniff the odor and try to identify the odor from three distracters. From the data, Doty and colleagues[60] concluded the following: peak olfactory performance occurred between the third and fourth decades; women had higher olfactory performance than men; and up to 50% of individuals older than 65 years had major olfactory impairment. The other large cross-sectional study was the National Geographic Smell Survey.[62] In this survey, 1.2 million people responded to a 6-odor, scratch-and-sniff type of test. The ability to detect and correctly identify each odor showed age-related declines. Average perceived intensity also declined from younger to older cohorts. This survey also showed that women had higher olfactory performance than men did in each age cohort.

The findings from these two large-scale studies and a review by Cain and Stevens[63] highlight a number of important issues related to olfactory functioning and aging:

1. Does the olfactory loss in aging influence the entire range of perceptual experience from an elevation of thresholds (ie, lower sensitivity) to reduced perception of more concentrated stimuli?

2. Is the age-related loss equal for all olfactory stimuli, or are some qualities more vulnerable to losses with aging?

3. Important to geriatric nutrition, does aging influence the perception of odors and olfactory flavors equally? That is, are there factors that impair the ability to perceive the full flavor of food even if the older adult has a normal sense of smell?

The next section presents data to address each of these issues related to olfactory perception in aging.

### Threshold versus Suprathreshold Perception

The elderly, on average, require from 2-fold to 100-fold higher concentration to recognize the presence of an odorant (recognition threshold).[32,62,63] Using magnitude matching, Stevens and colleagues[64] were the first to report reduced odor intensities in the elderly subjects. The testing was first conducted using an auditory standard and was repeated later with the intensity of sodium chloride as a standard.[65] This latter study also showed greater age-related impairment to olfaction than to taste (see further discussion below). In comparing perceived intensities of six odors that varied in quality, Stevens and Cain[66] found that age-related olfactory losses were apparent for both weak and strong odor-

ants. Thus, a substantial elevation in threshold would reflect a reduced ability to perceive more concentrated olfactory stimuli.

### Age-Related Olfactory Losses Appear Quality Specific

Other sensory systems show quality-specific changes associated with aging, including hearing and taste (see discussion below about taste). Complete information about quality-specific olfactory loss with aging may never be fully available. One difficulty is that there are an infinite number of odors to test. It also is difficult to pick an odor that represents the qualities of a group of odors because odors do not appear to conform to a particular categorization scheme.[63] Nonetheless, the data from the National Geographic Smell Survey suggest that age-related losses are not uniform across odors.[62] For example, sweet and fruity odors may be most vulnerable to the physiological changes that accompany aging, while musky and spicy odors are relatively stable.[67] The ability to detect mercaptans (eg, sulfur compounds added to natural gas as warning agents) appears vulnerable to olfactory loss with age[62]; losses were also observed in some middle-aged individuals. Thus, it appears that aging may not influence the ability to perceive all odor compounds equally. Which odors are most vulnerable to changes with aging remains uncertain and may depend on the individual's odor repertoire and whether the olfactory losses are due to aging or a combination of aging with additional environmental insults.

### Retronasal versus Orthonasal Olfaction and Aging

The olfactory epithelium should respond similarly to an odor whether it is delivered through the nostrils or through the mouth. However, consider the anticipation that accompanies a brewing cup of coffee. The aroma permeates the kitchen, and when brewing is finished, the coffee is poured into a cup. The olfactory flavor of the coffee may not be quite the same as the odor. Rozin[68] describes the qualitative differences between olfactory stimuli perceived from the nose and from the mouth. The olfactory flavor components of the coffee mix with the coffee bitterness, the hot temperature, and the feel of the coffee in the mouth. All of these factors modulate perception of the coffee odorants in the mouth differently than those perceived through the nostrils. Retronasal perception is also dependent on mouth and swallowing movements to release and transport olfactory volatiles. Smelling through the nostrils is a more passive process that occurs with normal respiration; smelling through the mouth is a much more active process. Factors that impede mouth and swallowing movements could decrease the perception of olfactory flavors in foods and beverages.

The perception of olfactory food flavor shows age-related declines. Cain et al[69] reported that middle-aged and older individuals were equally unable to discriminate the presence of an olfactory seasoning in a food item. In their study, subjects (young, middle-aged, and older individuals) had to distinguish, in a forced-choice procedure, a soup (cold carrot soup) that contained the spice marjoram from a soup that did not have this seasoning. The elderly also show diminished ability to identify food flavors. Both Schiffman[70] and Murphy[71] showed that the elderly, more than the young, tend to rely solely on olfaction in the identification of blended food items. Stevens and Cain[72] found lower perceived intensity ratings of an orally sampled odorant (ethyl butyrate) in elderly than in young subjects. To control the retronasal stimulation, the subjects perceived the stimulus with and without the nose pinched. The younger subjects, with the nose open, consistently gave stronger ratings to the overall intensity of ethyl butyrate solutions. The elderly subjects

did not notice a difference between the overall intensity with the nose pinched or open. The hypothesis that perceived intensity of retronasal stimuli shows age-related declines is also supported by Dabrila and Duffy.[73] In their study, women rated the intensity of chocolate and orange flavoring delivered both orthonasally in plastic squeeze bottles with a pop-up spout and retronasally in a sucrose-sweetened gelatin. The middle-aged women, on average, exhibited lower orthonasal and retronasal olfactory perception than the young women. These studies all suggest that an age-related decline in olfactory perception decreases the ability to perceive the full flavor of food and that these losses may occur in middle age.

Defects to the olfactory system could impair olfactory perception, regardless of whether the odors were delivered through the nostrils or through the oral cavity. However, clinical conditions might show dissociation between retronasal and orthonasal olfaction. The ability to perceive the full olfactory flavor of food requires sufficient mastication to release olfactory volatiles from foods and mouth and swallowing movements to create enough intraoral pressure to pump the volatiles from the mouth retronasally to the olfactory epithelium.[7] Burdach and Doty[7] hypothesize that the elderly are able neither to release food volatiles effectively nor to generate enough active turbulent airflow to transport these released volatiles to the olfactory cleft. Conditions that impair chewing, mouth, and swallowing movements could diminish retronasal perception, even with an intact olfactory system. The elderly can show impairment in chewing, even with natural dentition.[74] Duffy and colleagues[75] found diminished olfactory flavor sensitivity in older women who wore complete maxillary dentures or dentures that at least covered the palate of the mouth. The denture effect on olfactory flavor sensitivity was independent of the ability to perceive odors through the nostrils. That is, some of the older women had a normal sense of smell but an elevated olfactory flavor sensitivity. The limitation of this study was that the functional ability of the dentures was not directly measured. Factors such as the stability, retention, and occlusion of dentures could be important to perceiving the full olfactory flavor of foods. Many other oral conditions and swallowing disorders could have the potential to diminish retronasal olfactory perception. A number of studies report diminished food enjoyment with oral health problems, such as oral pain and periodontal disease.[76–79] Some of the diminished food enjoyment could stem from impaired olfactory flavor perception.

Interestingly, some subjects with laryngectomies also exhibit a diminished ability to perceive odors through the nostrils, while the ability to perceive olfactory flavors remains intact.[80] The laryngectomy interrupts the normal path of air traveling from the nose or mouth to the lungs and allows the individual to breathe through a stoma in the throat. The patients complained that they could not smell odors but did not notice a diminished flavor of food. Orthonasal olfaction was impaired because the air carrying odors does not pass through the nostrils during breathing. Olfactory flavor perception was intact because eating could have allowed the olfactory volatiles to reach the olfactory epithelium retronasally.

## The Sense of Taste and Aging

Total ageusia is rarely seen. Data from the University of Pennsylvania Smell and Taste Center serve as compelling evidence in support of this statement. Of the 750 individuals presenting to this center with "taste loss," less than 4% had measurable taste impairment, while 71% had measurable olfactory dysfunction.[52] There is debate, however, about the extent of taste impairment with aging. Researchers appear to agree that aging is associated with elevated taste thresholds, although some qualities show more elevations than others do. However, unlike olfactory perception, taste threshold may not reflect the ability to perceive concentrated tastes, such as those one would experience during eating.[35] Some of the studies that hypothesize taste impairment in the elderly incorporate elements that retain the psychophysical problems mentioned above. Aging can be associated with loss of taste perception on individual areas of cranial nerve innervation. However, this does not usually result in noticeable changes in the ability to taste and is more relevant to the understanding of interactions between the cranial nerves that subserve taste.

This section discusses (1) age-related elevations in taste thresholds, (2) suprathreshold taste perception and aging, and (3) cranial nerve interactions that maintain whole-mouth taste perception.

### Elevated Taste Threshold in Aging

Taste losses associated with aging are most commonly found at the threshold level (see Murphy[81] for a review). Some qualities show greater threshold elevations than others[82]: Salt thresholds show age-related elevations, while sucrose thresholds appear stable across age cohorts. Within bitter compounds, the degree of age-related threshold elevation also varies.[83] The elderly can show elevated thresholds for tastes in taste mixtures (eg, NaCl threshold in citric acid).[84]

There is no conclusive evidence to support that taste anatomical changes necessarily occur with aging. It is difficult to see change in the number of taste receptors (ie, taste buds) with aging.[85] Some of this uncertainty is due to the large variation in density of taste buds normally seen in humans (particularly the density of fungiform papillae taste buds).[18,85]

Even within animal models, there is no support for changes in peripheral taste system with aging (see Mistretta[86,87] for reviews).

### Suprathreshold Taste Perception and Aging

In taste, threshold level may not indicate the ability to perceive concentrated tastes or suprathreshold perception (see Bartoshuk and Duffy[35] for a review). That is, an older adult may show an elevated threshold for NaCl but rate concentrated NaCl for saltiness exactly as would a younger adult. Attention to suprathreshold taste function may provide the most information about the taste world of older adults. The scientific literature reflects that the primary method used to assess suprathreshold function in aging is perceived intensity (identification tasks are less interesting because there are a limited number of taste qualities). Many of the studies examining taste and aging have methodological issues that make interpreting the findings difficult (see Bartoshuk and Duffy[35] for a review).

A number of studies, with magnitude matching as the psychophysical method, have reported that older adults rate concentrated tastants as intensely as do younger adults. The validity of this gold standard psychophysical method hinges on the ability to find a standard that does not show loss with aging. Using a valid standard allows comparison of taste intensity between young and elderly subjects. A number of studies have been conducted using an auditory standard.[65,88,89] The auditory standard was low frequency and relatively high intensity (aging is associated with largest losses to the perception of high-frequency, low-intensity sounds). With these studies, the primary finding was that the perceived intensity judgments of young and elderly subjects overlapped. In some of the studies, the elderly subjects gave higher ratings than did young

subjects to the lowest concentrations of tastant. Bartoshuk and colleagues[88] explain that some elderly may have an underlying dysgeusia that adds to the intensity of tastants. Alternatively, the elderly may report perceiving a sensation even if one is not present (ie, false-positive responding).[90]

Throughout all of the intensity studies with aging (see Bartoshuk and Duffy[35]), there is little support for perceived intensity changes in taste associated with aging. However, the studies are primarily cross-sectional in design, which always leaves room for debate as to which are the most appropriate methods for comparing taste intensity judgments across age cohorts. One study provides longitudinal data to examine changes with aging; preliminary analyses of these data do not support that taste changes with aging.[91]

There is uncertainty as to how variation in taste, such as with genetics and sex hormonal status, interacts with the aging process. Do genetic supertasters show a differential rate of taste loss with aging because they have more taste receptors? Taste, as well as olfaction and oral somatosensations, appears to be under the control of sex hormone variation. Young women are statistically more likely than young men to be supertasters.[18] Data also show that there are taste changes across pregnancy[92] and that oral sensations vary with menstruation.[93] Taste may decline with decreases in sex hormone levels in the menopausal process. Lucchina[94] found fewer genetic supertasters in a sample of elderly women than in young women. If considered as a whole, these data may suggest that taste is upregulated in women of childbearing age. The sex hormones may also modulate olfactory[95,96] and somatosensory[93] sensations. These sensory changes may support a healthy pregnancy by modulating response to the food world (eg, upregulation of bitter taste helps the mother avoid ingesting bitter poisons). During the perimenopausal period, the diminishing levels of sex hormones may alter chemosensory sensations. The role of sex hormones in altering oral sensations has been hypothesized.[97]

### Taste Losses to Areas of Cranial Nerve Innervation

Cranial nerves VII, IX, and X work together to respond to tastes in the foods and beverages that are sampled with the whole mouth, as during eating. Individuals can show loss of taste functioning on individual areas of cranial nerve innervation. This taste loss is revealed by unilaterally applying or painting taste solutions on each of the oral loci innervated by the cranial nerves that subserve taste.[98] These losses are associated with pathologies that can cause unilateral or bilateral damage to these cranial nerves (see "Pathologies of the Middle Ear," below). Study of the separate cranial nerves that innervate taste has increased understanding of how these nerves interact to maintain normal taste functioning and how damage can disrupt the normal interaction between these nerves.

Whole-mouth taste perception is maintained, even with extensive damage to the taste system. A dramatic example of the resilience of the taste system is explained by Bartoshuk[20] from an anecdote in *The Physiology of Taste*, written by Brillat-Savarin in the early 1800s. In this case, a prisoner had the anterior portion of his tongue cut off as punishment. This removed the chorda tympani (cranial nerve VII) innervation of taste. However, the prisoner did not complain of taste problems and instead reported intense or painful sensations from very sour or bitter substances. Thus, the innervation from cranial nerves IX and X compensated for the loss of cranial nerve VII to maintain whole-mouth taste perception. This has been shown clinically in patients who had their chorda tympani nerve severed in surgery to remove acoustic neuromas.[98] These individuals had loss of taste on the anterior tongue (cranial nerve VII) but heightened taste sensations on the posterior tongue (cranial nerve IX).

Heightened sensations from the posterior tongue may result from the overcompensation of cranial nerve IX for damage done to cranial nerve VII. This phenomenon might be the basis of a dysgeusia that exists in the absence of apparent taste stimulation.[99] This overcompensation has been shown clinically not only in patients who have undergone chorda tympani nerve cuts but also experimentally in subjects who have had their chorda tympani nerve temporarily anesthetized. The elderly can show discrete losses of taste to areas of cranial nerve innervation.[100] It is uncertain whether these losses occur with aging or because of conditions that damage individual cranial nerves. Because of the redundancy in nerve innervation, the discrete losses of taste go unnoticed. If the damage to one cranial nerve is substantial, the elderly can have a dysgeusia that can add to the intensity of taste stimuli. This was described by Bartoshuk[100]: Elderly subjects perceived weak taste solutions as more intense than did young subjects.

## Somatosensation and Aging

Older adults show lower touch sensitivity than younger adults on various body loci, including the tongue.[101] However, this may not influence perceived intensity of oral tactile stimuli. Weiffenbach et al[102] reported that age was not associated with a difference in perceived intensity of thickened liquids (thickened with methylcellulose). Perception of temperature in the mouth also does not appear to show age-related changes.[102,103]

There appears to be change with aging in the perception of chemical irritation. Perception of irritation through the nasal cavity shows age-related declines. In comparison with younger adults, older individuals report less pungency in carbon dioxide inhaled through the nostrils.[64] However, response to oral irritation may show age-related increases, especially in women. Bartoshuk and colleagues[104] found that older women ($\geq$53 years) reported the highest burn from oral capsaicin. The rated capsaicin burn was especially high in those older women who were genetic supertasters (measured by perceived bitterness of 6-$n$-propylthiouracil-impregnated paper). With menopause, there may be some loss of bitterness perception, especially to the anterior tongue. The loss of taste on the anterior tongue (cranial nerve VII) could make the response to the irritation (cranial nerve V) on the anterior tongue even more pronounced. This may have clinical relevance. Age associates with a dramatic increase in the incidence of neuropathic pain conditions, including postherpetic neuralgia and trigeminal neuralgia.[105] As well, burning mouth syndrome, a syndrome characterized by excruciating oral pain, afflicts primarily postmenopausal women. It may be that taste and pain interactions play a role in the etiology of burning mouth syndrome.[104]

## CAUSES OF CHEMOSENSORY DYSFUNCTION

Interest in the causes of chemosensory dysfunction was stimulated in the 1970s, when the National Advisory Neurological and Communicative Disorders and Stroke Council estimated that 2 million adults suffered from taste or smell disorders.[106] This figure may not reflect the level of dysfunction seen in the elderly. Some individuals are so distraught about the disorder that they seek out one of the few clinical research centers specializing in chemosensory evaluation. The following section reviews the causes of chemosensory disturbances, including changes specifically associated with aging.

The most common causes of chemosensory dysfunction in patients without major systemic diseases are upper respiratory tract infections, head trauma, and chronic nasal/sinus disease.[52,107] These diseases can diminish olfactory perception through one or a combination of these factors: (1) reduced ability to transport odorants to the olfactory receptors, (2) damage to the sensory receptors that receive and transduce the olfactory message, and (3) damage to the peripheral or central neurophysiological systems. More common in the aged are the degenerative diseases of the central nervous system (Alzheimer's disease and Parkinson's disease) that have olfactory dysfunction as a comorbidity. Less common causes of olfactory dysfunction are congenital disorders, toxic exposures, and medications. Individuals with chronic systemic disease can also show chemosensory disorders.

Taste disorders can also result from conditions that disrupt the transport of stimuli to the receptors and those that disrupt the neural pathways necessary for taste perception.[50] Taste loss can occur to specific areas of cranial nerve innervation, but these usually go unnoticed. Individuals are most troubled by dysgeusia (persistent salty, sweet, sour, or bitter sensation), especially if chronic.[52] If the patient cannot describe the sensation as salty, sweet, sour, or bitter, then it is a dysosmia or parosmia. Most troubling is the fact that these disorders may not be evaluated correctly and may be instead treated as psychiatric problems.

The primary causes of chemosensory disorders are discussed below. For a more extensive description, see Doty et al.[108]

## Upper Respiratory Tract Infections

Upper respiratory tract infections (URIs) can diminish olfactory perception through nasal obstruction and damage to the olfactory receptors by the virus. The effect of the common cold on olfactory abilities has been shown through direct experimental investigation.[109] After inoculation with a common cold virus, volunteers showed elevated butanol odor thresholds. The level of threshold elevation was predicted by the degree of nasal obstruction. The URI virus primarily affects the peripheral olfactory processes. Through electron-microscopic observations,[9] individuals with post-URI olfactory dysfunction had reduced numbers of olfactory receptor cells with cilia. Patients may take several years to show improved olfactory function after a URI, although over 50% can show some improvements.[110] Patients with URI-related olfactory loss (and head trauma; see below) may exhibit parosmia (the distortion of an odor when an odor is present).[111] This could represent damage to the olfactory receptor cells.[112] Prevention of URIs (or the flu) may be the best way to avoid this risk of olfactory dysfunction.

The viruses that cause URI can also damage areas of the taste system while leaving whole-mouth taste perception intact.[113]

## Pathologies of the Middle Ear

A number of pathologies can damage the chorda tympani nerve as it passes through the middle ear (eg, otitis media). Some surgeries may also involve damage to the chorda tympani nerve (eg, acoustic neuroma surgery). Patients with pathological or surgical damage of the chorda tympani nerve can show unilateral or bilateral taste impairment to the anterior tongue for one or all taste qualities, depending on the extent of the nerve damage.[98,114] However, patients rarely report a change in taste perception,[17] even when the chorda tympani nerve is cut.[115] Whole-mouth taste perception is maintained because the remaining taste nerves appear to compensate for the loss of taste in one area of the mouth. In fact, surgical or experimental manipulation of the chorda tympani nerve can result in increased taste sensations from the area of cranial nerve IX (this may be the basis of dysgeusia that results from nerve stimulation and not from a substance present in the mouth).

## Head Trauma

Head trauma can cause more severe chemosensory losses than either URIs or nasal sinus disease.[52] Approximately 5% of all individuals with head injuries suffer from posttraumatic anosmia (as reviewed by Costanzo and Becker[116]). More severe head trauma results in a higher frequency of anosmia, especially in those injuries involving frontal and occipital blows.[117] Head injury–related olfactory loss can be caused by peripheral damage to the olfactory nerves and the nose and central damage to the olfactory centers in the brain.[118] The most common cause of olfactory loss is thought to be the severing of the olfactory nerves where they pass through the cribriform plate of the ethmoid bone (see Figure 7–1) as the result of the coup-contrecoup forces (impact that causes the brain to bump the opposite side of the skull).[118] Patients with head trauma–related olfactory dysfunction can show disorganization of cells in the olfactory epithelium and few olfactory cilia that reach the epithelial surface[9]; damage to the olfactory bulb and tracts; and damage to the inferior frontal lobes.[119] Only a few patients (up to 35%)

show slight improvements in olfactory perception over time.[110,120]

Head trauma can also cause taste loss, but the incidence is very low (0.4% to 0.5%).[118] More common is the loss of taste to areas of taste perception.[121] Head trauma may damage the chorda tympani nerve more frequently than the glossopharyngeal nerve because the former is more vulnerable to injury where it passes through the temporal bone.[118] Because of the compensating interactions between the taste nerves, patients do not usually complain of taste loss with head trauma unless the loss is extensive.

**Chronic Nasal and Sinus Disease**

These conditions are associated with swollen tissues, polyps, tumors, and deformities, all of which can obstruct the odorant from traveling through the nasal passages to the olfactory epithelium. According to the National Health Interview Survey of 1994, 15% of older adults report chronic sinusitis.[122] Age also associates with increased nasal resistance (decreased nasal airflow), physical changes in the nasopharynx, and changes to the relationship between nasal and pulmonary airflow.[123] Some clinical research centers find chronic nasal/sinus disease to be the most common form of olfactory dysfunction.[124] Allergic rhinitis can elevate olfactory thresholds by modifying the amount and chemical composition of the mucus secretion,[125] through the allergic response,[126] and through the level of inflammation in the sinus tissues.[127] Up to 23% of individuals who suffer from allergic rhinitis suffer from elevated olfactory thresholds,[127] and according to the National Health Interview Survey of 1994, 8% of older adults report allergic rhinitis without asthma.[122]

Nasal/sinus disease may be the only treatable form of olfactory dysfunction. Diagnosis of this condition must be done by a trained ear, nose, and throat physician and usually includes the patient history, physical examination, and computed tomagraphy (CT) scans.[107] If patients notice fluctuations in their sense of smell with exacerbation of nasal/sinus conditions, they may benefit from aggressive therapy to prevent the olfactory disturbances associated with more chronic conditions.[107] Medical management of nasal/sinus disease includes controlling both the causes of the inflammation (eg, allergens causing allergic rhinitis, nasal infections) and the level of the inflammation (eg, topical corticosteroids).[124] These therapies may cause improvement to olfactory functioning. Some nasal/sinus diseases require surgical interventions (eg, severe sinusitis and nasal polyposis). Just over half of the individuals with progressive sinusitis had olfactory improvements with endoscopic sinus surgery.[128]

**Menopause**

Diminished estrogen may have an influence on chemosensory functioning and the normal balance of oral sensation. Hormone replacement has been hypothesized to aid in the preservation of olfactory functioning with aging.[52] (See the above discussion on taste and somatosensory sensations in postmenopausal women.)

**Dementia**

Olfactory dysfunction is reported in both Alzheimer's disease and Parkinson's disease. From a meta-analysis of 43 studies in this area, Mesholam and colleagues[129] concluded that these neurodegenerative disorders are associated with olfactory dysfunction. Both showed a similar pattern of olfactory dysfunction: impaired odor identification and elevated recognition and detection thresholds.

## Systemic Diseases

A number of diseases have been associated with chemosensory disorders. However, this association is often drawn from patient reports and is without valid measures of chemosensory functioning. The level of chemosensory impairment associated with these chronic diseases may relate to the severity of the disease, how the disease complications impair the chemosensory processes, and the side effects of the medications. As well, these chronic diseases impair nutritional health, which can also affect chemosensory functioning. The following is a review of some of the systemic diseases and the associated chemosensory alterations.

### Liver Disease

Individuals with liver disease can show elevated detection and recognition thresholds for both odorants[130] and tastes.[130,131] Recovery from the illness or correcting the nutrient deficiency (eg, vitamin A[130]) may improve chemosensory functioning (see Deems et al[132] for a review).

### Kidney Disease

With kidney disease, individuals on either hemodialysis or peritoneal dialysis had significantly higher olfactory thresholds than those of matched controls, and the level of olfactory impairment correlated with the severity of disease.[133] The individuals who had renal transplantation did not show these threshold elevations. Although patients on dialysis present with a high frequency of complaints about food "taste" and enjoyment, the response may be hedonic as opposed to sensory.[132]

### Cancer

Patients with cancer frequently report changes in the taste of food and changes in appetite. However, the cancer itself does not appear to cause a reduction in taste or olfactory perception unless it directly interrupts receptor sites or neural transmission (see Duffy et al[134] for a review). Cancer therapies may influence chemosensory perception. More research is needed on the influence of cancer (and its therapies) on olfactory perception. Ophir et al[135] did report olfactory impairment extending beyond 6 months after radiation therapy. Chemotherapy, through eliciting nausea and vomiting, can cause conditioned food aversions (see below under "Medications"). Because of the psychophysical errors in the study procedures, taste changes with chemotherapy are difficult to determine. As well, olfactory changes with chemotherapy have not really been investigated. Radiation therapy, especially if localized to the head and neck region, can result in "blindness of the mouth,"[136] although the loss is not seen in all individuals; some may actually show intensified taste sensations (see Duffy et al[134] for a review).

### Diabetes Mellitus

The effects of the neuropathic and vascular complications of this chronic disease appear to influence the level of chemosensory dysfunction. For example, individuals with diabetes mellitus complicated by macrovascular disease show higher risk of olfactory impairment, as measured with an odor identification task.[137] In type II diabetes, hedonic response to sweet beverages may be a function of dietary intake rather than a change in the ability to taste sweetness.[138]

## Other Diseases/Conditions

Some disease states can decrease olfactory perception by changing the quantity and quality of the mucus secretion and thus physically or chemically modifying olfactory perception (see Getchell and Mellert[139] for a review). For example, patients with cystic fibrosis exhibit olfactory dysfunction. This disease changes the chemical makeup and viscosity of mucus secretions. These changes could impede the odorant from reaching the olfactory receptors. Individuals with Sjögren's syndrome can complain of taste and olfactory problems.[140,141] This condition impairs salivary gland and mucus production. This could impair the oral manipulation of food that releases flavor volatiles and thus decrease the level of odorant from reaching the olfactory receptors. However, no measured smell disturbance was reported by use of an olfactometer.[142] With taste, Sjögren's syndrome can elevate taste thresholds but leave the ability to perceive real-world taste concentrations (ie, suprathreshold concentration) unimpaired.[140]

## Exposures

Exposures to pollutants may cause the replacement of olfactory neurons with respiratory neurons in the olfactory cleft and may result in decreased olfactory perception.[143] Elevated olfactory thresholds have been observed in past and present cigarette smokers[144] and in people exposed to airborne chemicals (see, eg, Schwartz et al[145]).

## Medications

The elderly are at risk for drug-nutrient interactions because they often take multiple medications to control chronic diseases. It is important to determine whether medications influence food intake in older adults through the alteration of chemosensory perception. Medications that alter taste and olfactory perception have been reviewed.[146] Below is a description and summary of some of the effects of medication on chemosensory perception.

Medications can have a direct effect on chemosensory functioning. They can impair the transport of stimulus to the receptor and change the peripheral structures and sensory transduction mechanisms. For example, medications with the side effect of xerostomia and/or drying of the nasal mucous membranes could impair the tastant or odorant from reaching the receptors. This could result in diminished olfactory or taste perception, although this has not been shown clinically (see above discussion on Sjögren's syndrome) and may not affect suprathreshold taste or olfactory function (see Catalanotto and Sweeney[147] for a review). Xerostomia can increase the risk of oral infections and periodontal disease and can produce altered taste (ie, dysgeusia) and olfactory sensations (ie, parosmia).[147] Medications can enter the mouth through the saliva (see, eg, Steele et al[148]) and gingival fluid.[149] This could produce a dysgeusia (the quality of which may be bitter to match the usual taste of medications), an olfactory sensation,[150] and even tactile sensations (eg, metallic). Medications that are not introduced to or through the mouth but rather in the blood may also stimulate both taste (venous taste phenomenon)[151] or olfactory sensations.[150]

Medications can influence our preference for foods through conditioned aversions. Conditioned food aversions can occur with medications that induce nausea and vomiting[152]: The individual associates the discomfort of the nausea and vomiting with the food eaten directly before the illness, even if the cause of the illness was not the food. These aversions are reported frequently in the literature as one mechanism for the loss of appetite and the change in preference for foods as the result of cancer and its therapies.

The clinician should take caution in interpreting the reports of chemosensory changes with medications. Patient reports may represent a combination of sensory and non-sensory issues, as well as confusions between taste, olfaction, and somatosensory changes. Thorough investigations on the effect of medications on chemosensory mechanisms are yet to be completed. This would include studies with valid psychophysical measurements to characterize the threshold and suprathreshold influences of medications on chemosensory functioning. Each patient should receive an individual assessment of chemosensory-related complaints. Careful interviewing of the patient will help the clinician determine if the change is sensory or nonsensory (see below). Working with the health care team and changing medications can alleviate some of the chemosensory complaints and lower the risk of drug-nutrition interactions.

**Oral Health**

Oral health is necessary for adequate oral sensations. Ship[153] provides a review of some of the oral conditions that can alter oral chemosensations. These include infections, oral lesions, xerostomia, poorly fitting dental prostheses, and oral problems associated with systemic disease. These conditions can cause parosmia (smelling the infection in the mouth), dysgeusia (tasting the byproducts of the oral infection), and diminished retronasal olfactory sensations.

**IMPACT OF NUTRITIONAL STATUS ON CHEMOSENSORY FUNCTION IN AGING**

Nutritional deficiencies or toxicities could influence any of the neurological or biochemical processes in chemosensation. However, as reviewed by Friedman and Mattes,[154] chemosensory disturbances are not consis-tently seen with minimal malnutrition and instead are associated with marked nutritional deficiencies or toxicities.

However, a special note on zinc is required. Zinc deficiency has been associated with taste loss; zinc supplementation may improve taste perception in individuals with zinc deficiency related to chronic diseases[155,156] and in persons with head and neck cancer treated with irradiation.[157] It may be that the disease,[158] other nutrient deficiencies (eg, magnesium,[131] and/or protein status[159]) may be more important than zinc nutrition to maintain taste functioning. However, most of the studies on taste and nutritional status are conducted with threshold measures that may not indicate ability to perceive tastes usual to foods and beverages. Thus, the documented taste disorders may have little association with food behaviors, as shown by Madden and colleagues.[131]

Individuals can show chemosensory disorders without dietary inadequacies or obvious nutritional risk.[160,161] Thus, does the zinc deficiency cause chemosensory disturbances in aging? Zinc supplementation for otherwise healthy individuals with chemosensory disorders appears to be of no benefit. Most individuals who have reported taking zinc for chemosensory disorders report no improvement in their condition[162] and show no difference in chemosensory function than those not taking zinc.[52] The ineffectiveness of zinc supplementation for chemosensory functioning was also demonstrated in two double-blinded studies.[163,164] As well, lower zinc status was not associated with taste acuity in elderly subjects.[165] However, elderly individuals with biochemically measured zinc deficiency may show improved taste acuity with zinc supplementation.[166] In summary, the benefit of zinc supplementation to improve food flavor perception in the elderly is still not substantiated. Olfactory perception shows the greatest age-related dysfunction, yet the benefit of zinc supplementation to olfactory functioning is questionable. It is also not clear whether aged individuals would notice improved gustatory sensitivity in response to the zinc supplementation *and* whether this improvement would have a positive impact on their dietary behaviors.

## IMPACT OF CHEMOSENSORY FUNCTION ON NUTRITIONAL STATUS IN AGING

The sensory qualities of food play an important role in influencing what we choose to eat. Olfactory information may be critical in shaping what we like to eat, as it allows the exact identification of foods and beverages. Orthonasal olfaction may play a role in stimulating appetite through the perception of odors in the environment. Once food is in the mouth, the sense of taste, retronasal olfaction, and somatosensory sensations combine to provide the composite sensation of flavor. Our preference for foods and beverages smelled through the nostrils may be very different than our preference for foods and beverages experienced as the composite sensation of flavor.[68] For example, the Jamaican fruit "sticking toe" has a very unpleasant aroma but, when placed in the mouth, produces a wonderful sensation.

Very little of food preference is innate. Human beings are born liking sweet and disliking bitter (see Mennell and Beauchamp[167] for a review). The rest of what we like and dislike in food is learned. (See *Why We Eat What We Eat*[168] for a review of the research on physiological, developmental, biological, and cultural factors that shape our eating habits.) Humans use chemosensory experience from the food world to learn an individual array of food likes and dislikes. We couple the

flavor of food with a positive learning experience (see Capaldi[169] for a review). We may like the olfactory flavor of a food because it is paired with sweetness, a quality we are predisposed to like. Basic to life is learning to like foods and beverages that provide a source of calories. We can very rapidly learn to like a particular flavor that is associated with calories from starch and from fat. Negative learning also occurs and produces food dislikes. We couple the specific olfactory flavor of a food with the negative experience of nausea and vomiting (see Schafe and Bernstein[170] for a review). These learned food aversions can be very powerful and can last for years. It is important to note that sociocultural factors can modulate the biological factors that drive food likes and dislikes and thus what is actually consumed.[171]

It is important to ask whether the chemosensory profile of the food and beverage world changes enough with aging to alter food preferences and the patterns of food selection that have developed over a lifetime. This discussion focuses on the impact of olfactory dysfunction on nutritional outcomes in older adults, as olfaction seems most vulnerable to age-related loss. Theoretically, olfactory dysfunction could modify the sensory profile of foods and beverages. This modification might alter food preference, the desire to eat (appetite), and satiety responses to food and beverage sensations (see "Appetite and Satiety in Olfactory Dysfunction" below). A change in food preference, appetite, and satiety response could influence food selection. Ultimately, olfactory dysfunction could change nutritional status parameters, such as body weight. This hypothesized association between olfactory dysfunction and nutritional outcomes is shown in Figure 7–5 (based on a model presented by Shepherd[172]). This conceptual model also includes the interaction between measured and self-rated ol-

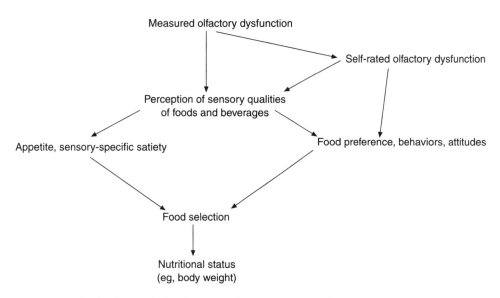

**Figure 7–5** Hypothesized association between chemosensory dysfunction and nutritional outcomes.

factory dysfunction in association with nutritional outcomes.

Much of the initial research on olfactory dysfunction and nutritional outcomes was conducted with individuals who sought help from one of the few National Institutes of Health–funded clinical research centers that specialized in chemosensory disorders. These individuals are troubled enough by their disorders to seek out one of a few of these centers, even if there is little hope for a cure. Most report a change in their eating habits because of the disorder, although the specific response varies with the disorder and with the individual. Applying the nutrition findings from this group of health-seeking individuals to the elderly is not appropriate, as the elderly may experience overall changes in functional ability with age and may neither notice nor seek medical treatment for olfactory disturbances. Older adults may notice neither a loss of olfactory perception nor a change in the sensory quality of foods. They also may merely maintain food habits that were established over their lifetime. However, older

adults could consciously or unconsciously modify well-established food preferences and behaviors in response to the olfactory impairment. The modification could fit two general patterns: "indiscriminate eating" and "compensation eating."[173] These patterns serve only as a description of the potential nutritional response to olfactory dysfunction.

1. *Indiscriminate eating*—Older adults with olfactory dysfunction eat less for pleasure. They experience fewer olfactory cues to stimulate an appetite. The flavor of food is diminished, and everything has a "blah" flavor. This decreases enjoyment of eating and may decrease the drive for flavor diversity (ie, decreased sensory-specific satiety[174]). Nutritional risk can result if the diet becomes monotonous, decreasing the ability to meet nutritional requirements and, in the extreme, causing weight loss.

2. *Compensation eating*—Older adults with olfactory dysfunction use sensory and nonsensory strategies to compensate for

the loss of olfactory food flavor. This may include relying on the taste (eg, sweet and salty foods) and somatosensory components of food for enjoyment. Nutritional risk could occur with excessive intake of sweet and salty foods that also often provide an excess intake of fat, which could cause an energy imbalance and the risk of obesity. In the nonsensory domain, individuals may select food more for its ability to maintain health and manage chronic disease than for sensory qualities.

This section addresses the following questions related to this conceptual model and general nutrition patterns:

- Do the elderly notice changes in olfactory functioning with aging, and how does this influence nutritional outcomes?
- Does the olfactory dysfunction interfere with perception of the sensory qualities of foods and beverages?
- Do olfactory disorders influence food preference and food intake in elderly individuals?
- Does olfactory dysfunction increase nutritional risk in elderly individuals?

**Self-Rated Olfactory Changes with Aging**

One's perception of health can provide clinicians with a useful proxy for measured health status. Perception of health and feelings of change with age may provide an understanding of the processes through which an individual evaluates and acts on symptoms. Study of these perceptions will ultimately enhance the understanding of how olfactory losses affect nutritional health and eating enjoyment. Questions about the taste and smell problems are asked on the Minimum Data Set for long-term care facilities. Obtaining rated change can also provide a

historical complement to a single measure of functioning.

Although ratings of olfactory perception show age-associated declines, many of the elderly do not notice even major olfactory impairments. Data from the National Geographic Survey (1.2 million responses, 20% older than 60 years) show a decline in mean rated smell perception with increasing age.[62] Males rated smell perception lower at each age from teens to the ninth decade, whereas with females, mean rating increased to a peak rating in the fourth decade and then declined at a slope equal to that of males. Most elderly do not notice diminished olfactory sensitivity.[175] The only exception is individuals who have been diagnosed with sinusitis. These individuals may expect to have olfactory impairment.[175] Nearly all individuals with sinusitis and diminished olfactory sensitivity report the impairment. Ship and Weiffenbach[57] examined the sensitivity and specificity of self-rated olfactory functioning. They found that impaired individuals were less likely to report a dysfunction and that normosmic individuals were not likely to complain of an olfactory dysfunction.

The self-rating of sensory function requires individuals to evaluate their own sense of well-being, rate a perceptual experience, and compare current function to that of an earlier age. Because this entails private and subjective responses, the quality of the result ultimately relies on individuals' being able to accurately rate their impressions.[34] Discordance between rated and measured perception could stem from an unwillingness to disclose the sensory loss or the rate and magnitude of the loss. The individuals' attention to their sensory function or to their own health could also affect the discrepancy between rated and measured sensory function. Some elderly subjects may not want to admit a loss of smell perception or may assume that their smell function is good considering their age. Individuals may notice a sudden loss (as with an insult such as head trauma) more than the gradual loss of smell associated with aging. However, if the amount of loss exceeded a certain theoretical point, a person might notice it even if the decline occurred gradually. Finally, some people may not assign value to their sense of smell or may not exhibit overall health-seeking tendencies. Therefore, they may just assume that their sense of smell is adequate without really giving it any thought.

Asking individuals to rate their perception of physical difficulty may help understand the impact of the difficulty on health outcomes. For example, Wayler and colleagues[176] reported that the perception of difficulty in chewing a food with any type of prosthesis was a larger determinant of food acceptance than actual mastication abilities. Mattes et al[177] also reported that an individual's perception of a disorder potentiates the negative effects on nutrition. In a group of individuals who sought treatment for a chemosensory disorder, they found a greater nutritional risk (eg, weight changes) in individuals who reported that the disorder changed their interest in eating or who felt that eating exacerbated the intensity of the chemosensory disorder.

## Perception of the Sensory Attributes of Food Flavor with Olfactory Dysfunction

Foods and beverages present a complex mixture of chemosensory stimuli. "Normal" taste, smell, and somatosensory sensations blend into a composite perceptual experience. With a change in ability to perceive some or all of the olfactory components, the taste and somatosensory components may become more apparent. The strong, bitter taste of a food may be more apparent with a less-ened olfactory component. For example, dark chocolate may have a subtle blending of rich chocolate olfactory flavor, plus the correct balance of the bitter chocolate with sweetness. Removing the chocolate flavor may only exaggerate the bitterness of the chocolate, even in the presence of sweetness.

Most individuals who seek treatment for olfactory dysfunction report that food is less flavorful and less enjoyable.[161,178] The reports of olfactory flavor changes with aging vary. Stevens[179] reported the responses of younger and older participants ($N = 276$) to the following "yes/no" questions: (1) Do you have a problem tasting? (2) Do you have a problem smelling? (3) Have you noticed changes in tastes of foods? (4) Do you enjoy food? The food complaints appear low considering the large olfactory loss displayed with aging: Only 17% of the elderly subjects answered "yes" to one or more of questions 1 through 3 and/or "no" to question 4; only 5.8% of the total complained of weakened food enjoyment all or some of the time. In contrast, nearly the entire younger group stated that eating was a great pleasure. The elderly individuals who did report "yes" to the above questions attributed the problem to a lifelong lack of interest in food, restricted diets, the expense of foods, and denture problems. Todhunter[180] reports more complaints of changes in food flavor with aging. Of 529 older adults, over 50% believed that food had "less taste" than when they were younger.

## Food Preference, Food Intake, and Olfactory Dysfunction

Most odors that we experience are complex mixtures of odor molecules. A change in the ability to perceive one or some of the odor molecules could change the hedonic response to the odorant. For example, the elderly may rate characteristically unpleasant odors (eg, mercaptans or the smell of sulfur) as less pleasant[62] because they are unable to perceive some of the odor compounds in the mercaptans.

Most individuals who seek treatment for olfactory dysfunction report using food and non–food-related strategies to maintain food appreciation.[161] The most commonly mentioned strategies involved the use of primary taste qualities, spices, and trigeminal stimulants,[161] especially increased use of salt and/or sugar.[177] The taste or somatosensory properties of food may carry more importance in determining food preference and intake in individuals with olfactory impairment. Duffy and colleagues[181] reported that elderly women with poorer olfactory functioning reported less preference for and intake of foods with strong sour (eg, citrus fruits) and bitter (eg, *Brassica* vegetables) tastes. With olfactory dysfunction, the sour or bitter taste may become more apparent and make the food less appealing. Texture is also an important component of food acceptance and is rated as the most important component of food identification and food enjoyment in individuals with congenital anosmia.[182]

An older person with olfactory dysfunction may compensate for this loss by preferring foods with a pleasant primary taste, those with a stronger olfactory component, or even those with a pungent sensation. Some of these preference patterns have been shown experimentally. In taste, elderly subjects report higher concentrations of salt and sweet as more preferable than do younger subjects.[183] However, in a recent study, Drewnowski and colleagues[184] found no difference in salt preference between young and elderly subjects. The lack of agreement on salt preference between the two studies may relate to a number of factors, including different psychophysical procedures. Unfortunately, neither study employed magnitude matching; instead, both used scales that have many psychophysical limitations. In olfaction, de Graaf and colleagues[185] showed that elderly subjects, in comparison with young subjects, reported lower perceived intensities of many olfactory flavorings in common food products and subsequently showed higher preferences for the higher concentrations of these flavorings in these foods. It is unclear from this study and the study by Drewnowski et al[184] if the elderly with the poorer sense of smell preferred the highest concentration of taste and olfactory flavorings. The elderly may compensate for the olfactory loss by preferring and consuming more sweets. In a sample of free-living elderly women, intake of sweet and high-fat foods showed a significant association with olfactory ability.[181] Those with a poorer sense of smell showed the most frequent intake of these foods. Interestingly, elderly persons with probable Alzheimer's disease also show higher preference for sweets than do elderly persons without this dementia.[186] The authors suggest a neurochemical basis for this pattern of food preference. However, olfactory dysfunction, an early marker for Alzheimer's disease, may also contribute to this sweet preference. The combination of sweet and fat is pleasurable for many but may be especially so in those with olfactory impairment.

Changes in oral sensations from foods and beverages associated with aging may cause older adults to be less discriminating in their food choices. Experimentally, Pelchat and LaChaussee[187] have shown that older adults with measured olfactory dysfunction are less finicky and more willing to try novel food items. As a risk, these older adults may be less able to use olfactory cues to tell that foods are spoiled. Those with olfactory dysfunction may also be less willing to cook for themselves or to eat a variety of foods.[181] This finding may emphasize the importance of senior meal opportunities that aim to provide older adults with at least one nourishing meal each day. Chemosensory changes with aging may be advantageous to some older adults. These changes may make it easier for the older adult to base food selection on the nutritional value of foods instead of only the sensory qualities. For example, Warwick and Schiffman[188] show that the elderly may be less aware of changes in level of fat in milk products. In their study, the elderly and young rated liking for sweet/fat and salt/fat mixtures that varied in the level of fat. The level of fat did not influence preference for these mixtures in the elderly; the younger subjects showed differing preference with variation in level of fat in these mixtures. These findings suggest that decreasing the level of fat in diets of older adults does not have to disrupt food enjoyment.

**Appetite and Satiety in Olfactory Dysfunction**

In animals, olfactory dysfunction can disrupt dietary behaviors[189] and cause loss of appetite and weight.[190] Clinically, the relationship between appetite and olfactory dysfunction is not consistent. Up to 48% of individuals seen for a chemosensory disturbance report a decreased appetite with the onset of the disorder.[178] In this same sample, food aversions were highest in those with multiple chemosensory disorders and altered taste or olfactory sensations, such as dysgeusia and parosmia.[178] Some researchers claim that chemosensory losses play a major role in the anorexia often observed in the elderly.[191] However, in a sample of free-living elderly women, even those with poorest olfactory function did not report less enjoyment of food or a poor appetite.[181]

Food flavor could influence both the kinds of foods selected and the total food intake,

possibly through "sensory-specific satiety."[174] According to this theory, as a person eats a food, the pleasantness of its flavor decreases, while the pleasantness of other foods not consumed decreases much less or remains constant. Sensory-specific satiety has an effect on the quantity of food eaten at a meal[192] and may promote diversity of dietary intake. Therefore, olfactory dysfunction and a large change in flavor perception could modify the physiologic response to food, decrease the drive for flavor diversity, and increase the likelihood of consuming a monotonous diet.[193]

The association between olfactory perception and sensory-specific satiety in young and older subjects was tested by Rolls and McDermott.[194] In this study, subjects from four age cohorts (adolescent, young adult, middle-aged, and elderly) participated in sensory-specific satiety measures and in a standard measure of orthonasal olfaction (UPSIT).[61] For the sensory-specific satiety measures, subjects sampled and rated the pleasantness of the taste, odor, appearance, and texture of a number of foods (including the first serving of low-fat strawberry yogurt). They then consumed a second serving of low-fat strawberry yogurt and provided pleasantness ratings of eaten (yogurt) and uneaten foods (other sampled foods). Elderly subjects did not show sensory-specific satiety; they rated as much pleasantness and desire to eat the second serving of the strawberry yogurt as they did the first serving. Interestingly, there was no significant relationship between measured orthonasal olfaction and the sensory-specific response in the elderly (even though elderly subjects had lower olfactory functioning than was tested in the other age cohorts). However, the lack of association might relate to a combination of orthonasal and retronasal difficulties. Some of the middle-aged and elderly subjects wore dentures, and these subjects did not appear to report as great a change in the "taste" of yogurt from first to second exposures. The presence of dentures could diminish retronasal olfaction (even more than that observed for orthonasal olfaction) and blunt the sensory-specific satiety response in the elderly subjects.

### Nutrient Intake and Body Weight in Olfactory Dysfunction

Most individuals who seek evaluation for a chemosensory disorder report that they change their eating habits in response to the chemosensory disorder.[161,177,178] The majority of these individuals report consuming an adequate total nutrient intake (intakes >66% of the RDA, derived from dietary analysis of 3-day food records).[161] Free-living elderly women with lower olfactory perception had higher intakes of nutrients that can increase the risk of cardiac disease (higher intake of saturated fatty acid calories, lower polyunsaturated to saturated fatty acid intake, higher total fat).[181] Ferris and Duffy[161] found a strong relationship between a reported increased food intake, obesity (greater than 120% of the Metropolitan Relative Weight), and smell dysfunction, especially in elderly women. Individuals with olfactory dysfunction and increased food intake often reported "not feeling satisfied with eating. . . . I eat more because I hope that the next bite will taste better." The association between olfactory dysfunction and weight gain was also uncovered by Mattes and Cowart.[178] Males may show a different association between weight and olfactory dysfunction. Ferris and Duffy[161] reported that of the underweight males, the majority were anosmic. A higher risk of weight loss was also observed in individuals who suffer from multiple chemosensory dis-

orders.[178] As well, patients with burning mouth syndrome may show risk for being underweight.[52]

### ASSESSING CHEMOSENSORY COMPLAINTS IN OLDER ADULTS

An older person may complain that food just does not "taste" good anymore. He or she may also report not enjoying eating. The following section summarizes questions and psychophysical tools that dietetics practitioners can use to assess the chemosensory complaint and determine whether a chemosensory disorder contributes to the lack of enjoyment from eating. If a chemosensory dysfunction is suspected, additional physical examinations, including otolaryngological, neurological, and dental evaluations, can assess the probable cause of the disorder.

### Determining If the Complaint Is Sensory or Nonsensory

Individuals may complain about the "taste" of foods for a number of reasons other than problems with chemosensory perception. Pleasure from eating and appetite can act separately from the sensory input of foods and beverages. Simple questions may help the clinician start to distinguish a sensory from a nonsensory problem.

1. *Questions about the Complaint*
   - "What does the food 'taste' like to you? Can you taste salt, sweet, sour (eg, lemon or vinegar), and bitter (eg, strong coffee or even a medication)?" Answers to these questions help determine if the complaint is sensory and help rule out a taste problem.
   - "How long have you had the problem? Was the change gradual or sudden?" Answers to these questions help deter-

mine if the complaint is a chronic or an acute problem.

- "Do you associate the complaint with any specific problem?" Answers to this and the two preceding questions may help determine if the condition is associated with one of the pathologies that cause chemosensory disorders. The question could then be expanded to request a history of specific chemosensory-related conditions.
- "Does the problem change? Is the problem better on some days than on others?" Individuals with olfactory dysfunction associated with nasal/sinus disease may report fluctuations in the ability to smell. Individuals may benefit from a complete evaluation by an otolaryngologist to rule out nasal/sinus disease, which is the only treatable cause of olfactory disorders.
- "Do odors smell as they should? For example, does peanut butter smell like peanut butter? Do you think you could tell what you were eating if your eyes were closed?" These questions address the sense of smell—not only diminished orthonasal olfaction but also odor distortions and retronasal perception.
- "Do you have a persistent taste in your mouth, such as a persistent salty, sweet, sour, or bitter taste?" This question should help determine if the individual has a dysgeusia. The individual may not be able to describe the quality as salty, sweet, sour, or bitter and may instead describe the quality as something vague (eg, "yuk" or "foul"). This may be an olfactory sensation related to the smell of an infection.
- "Are you suffering from oral pain, burning, prickling, or numbness on your tongue or in your mouth?" These

questions are designed to reveal a somatosensory disturbance associated with the "taste complaint." Individuals who respond positively to this question may benefit from further dental or medical evaluation.

2. *Nutritional Consequences of the "Taste Complaint"*

- "Have you changed your eating habits in response to the change in the way food 'tastes'? Are you avoiding any foods because of the problem? Have you changed the types of foods you eat since the problem started? Are you adding anything to your foods to make the 'taste' of the food any better?" A chemosensory disorder may have a negative impact on nutritional health if the individual complains of a chemosensory problem and/or complains that the problem has influenced his or her eating habits.[178]
- "Are you taking any vitamin, mineral, or herbal supplements because of your disorder?" Individuals who present to clinical research centers with chemosensory disorders have reported frequent use of supplements.[161] Because these conditions are usually untreatable, individuals may turn to alternative therapies.
- "How is your appetite? Has your appetite changed since the problem started?"
- "Do you enjoy eating? Has your enjoyment of eating or activities related to food and eating changed since the problem started?"
- "Has your weight changed in response to the problem?"

The client may need to answer additional questions about the disorder and the nutritional outcomes before the clinician can determine if the problem is sensory or nonsensory. These may include specific questions about feelings of health and happiness. Individuals may feel depressed because the chemosensory disorder has disrupted their eating and food behaviors. With olfactory dysfunction, older persons may not feel as confident cooking or may stop entertaining friends and family because of decreased enjoyment in cooking. If the chemosensory dysfunction is disruptive enough to their feelings of well-being, they may need to seek assistance in coping with the disorder.[195]

### Screening for Taste and Olfactory Functioning

The sense of taste is the easiest to test with stimuli readily available (table salt, sugar, sour [lemon or vinegar], and bitter [instant coffee crystals]). The clinician should ask the individual to identify the taste of the four stimuli. A number of odor identification tasks are available to use in a clinical setting. The odor identification task from the Connecticut Chemosensory Clinical Research Center Test[49] can provide a low-cost olfactory screen. The odors are baby powder, chocolate, cinnamon, coffee, mothballs, peanut butter, Ivory soap, and a trigeminal probe (Vicks VapoSteam). The clinician should place the odor in a covered jar and conceal the stimulus to reduce nonolfactory cues. The subjects are asked to identify the odors from a list of odors and distracters (see either Cain[196] or Cain et al[49] for a listing). Correct feedback is provided, and misidentified items are presented a second time. If subjects miss four out of the seven nontrigeminal odors (even after correct feedback is given and missed items are presented a second time), they have probable hyposmia and should have more in-depth olfactory evaluation by an otolaryngologist.

UPSIT[61] is a commercially available test of olfactory functioning (Sensonics, Inc,

Haddonfield, NJ). This test includes 40 "scratch-and-sniff" odorants and a multiple-choice format. Normative data on a large number of subjects according to age and sex allow the determination of the level of olfactory functioning (ie, anosmia, hyposmia) and what the level is relative to age and sex.

Olfactory tests that include measuring the perception of retronasal olfaction might more fully capture the sensory experience of eating. Clinicians can use jellybeans as a way to test retronasal olfaction (gourmet jellybeans may provide the best stimulus, as the olfactory flavors are distinctive). The first task is to distinguish taste from olfactory flavor. The clients should be asked to sample the jellybean with their noses plugged (visual cues as to the flavor of the jellybean should be avoided). Then the client is asked to unplug the nose and is asked if the jellybean "tastes" any different. With the nose plugged, one should be able to sense only the taste and somatosensory cues from foods and beverages. However, opening the nostrils allows retronasal transport of the olfactory flavors to the olfactory epithelium. If the client does not notice a difference with the nose plugged versus unplugged, he or she has retronasal olfactory impairment. The jellybeans can also be used in an identification task. The clinician should select the jellybean flavors that might be most familiar to his or her clients and set up a selection list that includes the correct labels and distracters. The clinician must be sure to give feedback and retest missed items to increase the chance of testing only olfactory perception. Misidentification of more than 50% of the jellybeans probably would constitute olfactory impairment in older adults.

### Assessing the Complaint of Dysgeusia

Dysgeusias are very disturbing disorders to the individual and are difficult to diagnose.

As well, they often do not have a treatment. In practice, clinicians can use a combination of questions and topical anesthesia as tools for diagnosing the origins of dysgeusia, as described by Miller and Bartoshuk.[17] First, the clinician should determine that the patient has a persistent taste. If the topical anesthetic abolishes the taste, then the dysgeusia may result from something present in the mouth (eg, tasting an oral infection) or from a taste seeping into the mouth from the blood (as with a medication). Addressing the cause may alleviate the dysgeusia. If the taste is not changed or intensified by the topical anesthetic, it may be the result of nerve stimulation. The clinician must take care in administering and assessing the results of the topical anesthetic.[17] If the effect of the anesthetic is not total, an inappropriate conclusion can be drawn. To avoid this, the clinician should test the thoroughness of the anesthesia by applying a taste stimulus. Care should be taken as well to avoid any adverse reactions, such as aspiration, from the topical anesthetic. An individual who has intensification of a dysgeusia from a topical anesthetic should have further medical and dental evaluation.

## NUTRITIONAL INTERVENTIONS FOR CHEMOSENSORY DISORDERS IN THE ELDERLY

From the nutritional and chemosensory assessment, clinicians can create an individualized nutritional care plan to help clients maintain their nutritional health and enjoyment of eating despite the olfactory impairment.[197] Individuals can utilize a number of strategies to compensate for loss. Since the ability to taste is stable with aging, the primary taste qualities of foods and beverages can be important predictors of food enjoyment. Sweet or salty foods, especially those that are also high in fat, may be particularly enjoyable to individuals with olfactory dysfunction. Dietetics

practitioners can help older adults incorporate these foods into a healthy diet that is balanced with enjoyable exercise. Acceptance of fruits and vegetables can also be enhanced in the older adult with olfactory dysfunction by masking the bitterness with either salt[198] or sucrose.[199] Thus, the addition of salt may increase the acceptance of green vegetables that have a strong bitter taste component. As well, the addition of table sugar could increase acceptance of fruits with a bitter taste (eg, grapefruit). Somatosensory sensations can also provide another dimension to a meal. Variation in the texture and temperature of foods and even the addition of an irritant (eg, black pepper, chili pepper, ginger) may help maintain interest in eating with diminished or absent olfactory food flavor. The color and presentation of food, or "eating with the eyes," may help stimulate appetite and food enjoyment, especially for those with olfactory dysfunction.

The strategies to compensate for the olfactory dysfunction may be critical to maintain nutritional health and food enjoyment in long-term care residents. The resident may be on a restricted diet, which could limit the use of sweet and salty foods to compensate for olfactory changes. Chewing and swallowing difficulties also limit the ability to use texture as a way to vary the sensory qualities of foods. Pureed food also may not have the vibrant colors of fresh foods. Long-term care residents, especially those with olfactory impairments, may benefit from liberalizing the diet restrictions in order to stimulate appetite and to maintain food enjoyment and the quality of life.[200] Many initiatives in long-term care facilities continue to combat the effects of olfactory dysfunction on nutritional risk of the older adult. These include increasing the visual appeal of texture-modified foods (including pureed foods) and using garnishes to enhance food presentation. Fortifying the olfactory flavor component of food may also improve intake and the nutritional status of long-term care residents with chemosensory disorders.[201] Eating with others in a pleasant atmosphere may divert attention from the sensory aspects of eating to the social aspects of the meal.

## SUMMARY

Nutrition plays a vital role in the health and overall well-being of older adults. Smell, taste, and somatosensation contribute to food enjoyment and nutritional health by allowing individuals to receive taste, smell, and somatosensory sensations from the food world. However, through the process of aging and the continual exposure to environmental insults, the elderly are at risk for loss of olfactory perception. Poorly fitting dentures may further increase the risk of olfactory dysfunction by reducing retronasal processing of olfactory food flavor. Taste and somatosensory systems can show disturbances, such as dysgeusias (ie, persistent tastes with or without oral stimula-

tion) and oral pain syndromes, that can impair the quality of life and the ability to obtain oral nourishment.

Older adults who complain of chemosensory disturbances or complain that eating is not enjoyable deserve a thorough assessment. There are a limited number of treatments for chemosensory disturbances if the sensory system is damaged. Chemosensory disorders can improve if the underlying cause is treatable, such as through the modification of medications or alleviation of the underlying condition (eg, periodontal disease). Treatable or not, chemosensory disorders can influence nutritional health. Dietetics practitioners should assess the nutritional impact of measured or perceived chemosensory disorders on the quality of the eating experience and nutritional health in older adults. The nutritional response to the olfactory loss is not uniform. Dietetics practitioners should develop individualized nutritional care plans for older adults with reported or suspected chemosensory disturbances.

## REFERENCES

1. Pickenhagan W. Enantioselectivity in odor perception. In: Teranishi R, Buttery R, Shahidi F, eds. *Flavor Chemistry: Trends and Development*. Washington, DC: American Chemical Society; 1989: 151–157.

2. Engen T. Remembering odors and their names. *Am Scientist*. 1987;75:497–503.

3. Beidler L, Smith J. Effects of radiation therapy and drugs on cell turnover and taste. In: Getchell T, Doty R, Bartoshuk L, Snow JB Jr, eds. *Smell and Taste in Health and Disease*. New York, NY: Raven Press; 1991:753–763.

4. Costanzo R, Graziadei P. Development and plasticity of the olfactory system. In: Finger T, Silver W, eds. *Neurobiology of Taste and Smell*. New York, NY: John Wiley & Sons; 1987:233–250.

5. Moran D, Rowley J, Jafek B. Electron microscopy of human olfactory epithelium reveals a new cell type: the microvillar cell. *Brain Res*. 1982;253: 39–46.

6. Laing D. Optimum perception of odor intensity by humans. *Physiol Behav*. 1985;34:569–574.

7. Burdach K, Doty R. The effects of mouth movements, swallowing and spitting on retronasal odor perception. *Physiol Behav*. 1987;41:353–356.

8. Moran D, Rowley J, Jafek B. The fine structure of olfactory mucosa in man. *J Neurocytol*. 1982; 11:721–746.

9. Moran D, Jafek B, Eller P, Rowley JD. Ultrastructural histopathology of human olfactory dysfunction. *Microsc Res Tech*. 1992;23:103–110.

10. Lancet D. Vertebrate olfactory reception. *Annu Rev Neurosci*. 1986;9:329–356.

11. Getchell T, Getchell M. Regulatory factors in the vertebrate olfactory mucosa. *Chem Senses*. 1990;15:223–231.

12. Pevsner J, Snyder S. Odorant-binding protein: odorant transport function in the vertebrate nasal epithelium. *Chem Senses*. 1990;15:217–222.

13. Hildebrand J, Shepherd G. Mechanisms of olfactory discrimination: converging evidence for common principles across phyla. *Annu Rev Neurosci.* 1997;20:595–631.

14. Greer C. Structural organization of the olfactory system. In: Getchell T, Doty R, Bartoshuk L, Snow JB Jr, eds. *Smell and Taste in Health and Disease.* New York, NY: Raven Press; 1991:65–81.

15. Hellekant G, Danilova V, Ninomiya Y. Primate sense of taste: behavioral and single chorda tympani and glossopharyngeal nerve fiber recordings in the rhesus monkey, *Macaca mulatta. J Neurophysiol.* 1997;77:978–993.

16. Hellekant G, Ninomiya Y, Danilova V. Taste in chimpanzees II: single chorda tympani fibers. *Physiol Behav.* 1997;61:829–841.

17. Miller IJ, Bartoshuk L. Taste perception, taste bud distribution, and spatial relationships. In: Getchell T, Doty R, Bartoshuk L, Snow JB Jr, eds. *Smell and Taste in Health and Disease.* New York, NY: Raven Press; 1991:205–233.

18. Bartoshuk L, Duffy V, Miller I. PTC/PROP tasting: anatomy, psychophysics, and sex effects. *Physiol Behav.* 1994;56:1165–1171.

19. Bartoshuk L, Fast K, Karrer T, Marino S, Price R, Reed D. PROP supertasters and the perception of sweetness and bitterness. *Chem Senses.* 1992; 17:594. Abstract.

20. Bartoshuk L. The biological basis of food perception. *Food Qual Preference.* 1993;4:21–32.

21. Kinnamon S, Margolskee R. Mechanisms of taste transduction. *Curr Opin Neurobiol.* 1996;6:506–513.

22. Pritchard T. The primate gustatory system. In: Getchell T, Doty R, Bartoshuk L, Snow JB Jr, eds. *Smell and Taste in Health and Disease.* New York, NY: Raven Press; 1991:109–125.

23. Silver W, Finger T. The trigeminal system. In: Getchell T, Doty R, Bartoshuk L, Snow JB Jr, eds. *Smell and Taste in Health and Disease.* New York, NY: Raven Press; 1991:97–108.

24. Doty R, Brugger W, Jurs P, Orndorff M, Snyder P, Lowry L. Intranasal trigeminal stimulation from odorous volatiles: psychometric responses from anosmic and normal humans. *Physiol Behav.* 1978;20:175–185.

25. Whitehead MC, Kachele DL. Development of fungiform papillae, taste buds, and their innervation in the hamster. *J Comp Neurol.* 1994;340:515–530.

26. Green B. Thermal perception on lingual and labial skin. *Percept Psychophys.* 1984;36:209–220.

27. Karrer T. *The Effects of Capsaicin Desensitization on Chemical, Thermal, and Tactile Perception in the Human Mouth.* New Haven, Conn: Yale University; 1991. Doctoral dissertation.

28. Duffy V, Lucchina L, Snyder D, Bartoshuk L. Supertasters of PROP (6-*n*-propylthiouracil) rate the highest creaminess to high-fat milk products. *Chem Senses.* 1996;21:598. Abstract.

29. Tepper B, Nurse R. Fat perception is related to PROP taster status. *Physiol Behav.* 1997;61: 949–954.

30. Prutkin J. *Genetic Variation in Oral Sensations.* New Haven, Conn: Yale University; 1997. Undergraduate thesis.

31. Doty R. Olfactory system. In: Getchell T, Doty R, Bartoshuk L, Snow JB Jr, eds. *Smell and Taste in Health and Disease.* New York, NY: Raven Press; 1991:175–203.

32. Stevens J, Dadarwala A. Variability of olfactory thresholds. *Chem Senses.* 1993;13:643–653.

33. McBurney DH, Collings VB. *Introduction to Sensation/Perception.* 2nd ed. Englewood Cliffs, NJ: Prentice Hall; 1984.

34. Weiffenbach J. Assessment of chemosensory functioning in aging: subjective and objective procedures. In: Murphy C, Cain W, Hegsted D, eds. *Nutrition and the Chemical Senses in Aging: Recent Advances and Current Research Needs.* New York, NY: Annals of the New York Academy of Sciences; 1989:56–64.

35. Bartoshuk L, Duffy V. Taste and smell. In: Masoro E, ed. *Aging.* New York, NY: Oxford University Press; 1995:363–375.

36. Kamen J, Pilgrim F, Gutman N, Kroll B. Interactions of suprathreshold taste stimuli. *J Exp Psychol.* 1961;62:348–356.

37. Stevens S. The psychophysics of sensory function. In: Rosenblith W, ed. *Sensory Communication.* Cambridge, Mass: MIT Press; 1961:1–33.

38. Moskowitz H. Magnitude estimation: notes on what, how, when, and why to use it. *J Food Qual.* 1977;1:195–228.

39. Marks L. Sensory and cognitive factors in judgments of loudness. *J Exp Psychol.* 1972;5:426–443.

40. Green B, Shaffer G, Gilmore M. A semantically-labeled scale of oral sensation with apparent ratio properties. *Chem Senses.* 1993;18:683–702.

41. Weiffenbach J, Cowart B, Baum B. Taste intensity perception in aging. *J Gerontol.* 1986;41:460–468.

42. Marks L, Stevens J. Measuring sensation in the aged. In: Poon L, ed. *Aging in the 1980's: Psychological Issues.* Washington, DC: American Psychological Association; 1980:592–598.

43. Stevens J, Marks L. Cross-modality matching functions generated by magnitude estimation. *Percept Psychophys.* 1980;27:379–389.

44. Snyder D, Lucchina L, Duffy V, Bartoshuk L. Magnitude matching adds power to the labeled magnitude scale. *Chem Senses.* 1996;21:673. Abstract.

45. Little A, Brinner L. Taste responses to saltiness of experimentally prepared tomato juice samples. *J Am Diet Assoc.* 1984;84:1022–1027.

46. Wood JB, Harkins SW. Effects of age, stimulus selection, and retrieval environment on odor identification. *J Gerontol.* 1987;42:584–588.

47. Lawless H, Engen T. Association to odors: interference, memories, and verbal labeling. *J Exp Psychol.* 1977;3:52–59.

48. Corwin J. Assessing olfaction: cognitive and measurement issues. In: Serby M, Chobor K, eds. *Science of Olfaction.* Berlin, Germany: Springer-Verlag; 1992:335–354.

49. Cain WS, Gent JF, Goodspeed RB, Leonard G. Evaluation of olfactory dysfunction in the Connecticut Chemosensory Clinical Research Center. *Laryngoscope.* 1988;98:83–88.

50. Snow JJ, Doty R, Bartoshuk L, Getchell T. Categorization of chemosensory disorders. In: Getchell T, Doty R, Bartoshuk L, Snow JB Jr, eds. *Smell and Taste in Health and Disease.* New York, NY: Raven Press; 1991:445–447.

51. Amoore J. Specific anosmia and the concept of primary odors. *Chem Senses Flavor.* 1977;2:267–281.

52. Deems D, Doty R, Settle R, et al. Smell and taste disorders: an analysis of 750 from the University of Pennsylvania Smell and Taste Center. *Arch Otolaryngol Head Neck Surg.* 1991;117:519–528.

53. Green B. Capsaicin sensitization and desensitization on the tongue produced by brief exposures to a low concentration. *Neurosci Lett.* 1989;107:173.

54. Berger A, Bartoshuk L, Duffy V, Nadoolman W. Capsaicin for the treatment of oral mucositis pain. In: DeVita V, Hellman S, Rosenberg S, eds. *Principles and Practice of Oncology—Update.* Philadelphia, Pa: JB Lippincott Co; 1995:243–248.

55. Mozell M, Smith B, Smith P, Sullivan L, Swender P. Nasal chemoreception in flavor identification. *Arch Otolaryngol.* 1969;90:367–373.

56. Murphy C, Cain WS, Bartoshuk LM. Mutual action of taste and olfaction. *Sens Processes.* 1977;1:204–211.

57. Ship J, Weiffenbach J. Age, gender, medical treatment and medication effects on smell identification. *J Gerontol.* 1993;48:M26–M32.

58. Barber C. Olfactory acuity as a function of age and gender: a comparison of African and American samples. *Int J Aging Hum Dev.* 1997;44:317–334.

59. Cowart B, Young I, Feldman R, Lowry L. Clinical disorders of smell and taste. *Occup Med.* 1997; 12:465–483.

60. Doty RL, Shaman P, Applebaum SL, Giberson R, Siksorski L, Rosenberg L. Smell identification ability: changes with age. *Science.* 1984;226:1441–1442.

61. Doty R, Shaman P, Dann M. Development of the University of Pennsylvania Smell Identification Test: a standardized microencapsulated test of olfactory function. *Physiol Behav.* 1984;34:489–502.

62. Wysocki CJ, Gilbert AN. The National Geographic Smell Survey: effects of age are heterogenous. In: Murphy C, Cain W, Hegsted D, eds. *Nutrition and the Chemical Senses in Aging: Recent Advances and Current Research Needs.* New York, NY: Annals of the New York Academy of Sciences; 1989:12–28.

63. Cain WS, Stevens JC. Uniformity of olfactory loss in aging. In: Murphy C, Cain W, Hegsted D, eds. *Nutrition and the Chemical Senses in Aging: Recent Advances and Current Research Needs.* New York, NY: Annals of the New York Academy of Sciences; 1989:29–38.

64. Stevens J, Plantinga A, Cain W. Reduction of odor and nasal pungency associated with aging. *Neurobiol Aging.* 1982;3:125–132.

65. Stevens JC, Bartoshuk LM, Cain WS. Chemical senses and aging: taste versus smell. *Chem Senses.* 1984;9:167–178.

66. Stevens JC, Cain WS. Age-related deficiency in the perceived strength of six odorants. *Chem Senses.* 1985;10:515–529.

67. Russel M, Cummings B, Profitt B, Wysocki C, Gilbert A, Cotman C. Life span changes in the verbal categorization of odors. *J Gerontol B Psychol Sci Soc Sci.* 1993;48:P49–P53.

68. Rozin P. "Taste-smell confusions" and the duality of the olfactory sense. *Percept Psychophys*. 1982; 31:397–401.

69. Cain W, Reid F, Stevens J. Missing ingredients: aging and the discrimination of flavor. *J Nutr Elder*. 1990;9:3–15.

70. Schiffman SS. Food recognition by the elderly. *J Gerontol*. 1977;32:586–592.

71. Murphy C. Cognitive and chemosensory influences on age-related changes in the ability to identify blender foods. *J Gerontol*. 1985;41:47–52.

72. Stevens J, Cain W. Smelling via mouth: effect of aging. *Percept Psychophys*. 1986;40:142–146.

73. Dabrila G, Duffy V. Middle-aged females exhibit lower orthonasal and retronasal olfactory perception than young females. *Chem Senses*. 1996; 21:591–592. Abstract.

74. Feldman R, Kapus K, Alman J, Chauncey H. Aging and mastication: changes in performance and in the swallowing threshold with natural dentition. *J Am Geriatr Soc*. 1980;28:97–103.

75. Duffy V, Cain W, Ferris A. Measurement of sensitivity to olfactory flavor: application in a study of aging and dentures. Submitted.

76. Ship J. Gustatory and olfactory considerations: examination and treatment in general practice. *J Am Dent Assoc*. 1993;124(6):55–62.

77. Lipton J, Ship J, Larach-Robinson D. Estimated prevalence and distribution of reported orofacial pain in the United States. *J Am Dent Assoc*. 1993;124(10):115–121.

78. Ship J, Grushka M, Lipton J, Mott A, Sessle B, Dionne R. Burning mouth syndrome: an update. *J Am Dent Assoc*. 1995;126(7):842–853.

79. Griep M, Verlye G, Franck A, Collys K, Mets T, Massart D. Variation in nutrient intake with dental status, age and odour perception. *Eur J Clin Nutr*. 1996;50:816–825.

80. Ritter F. Fate of olfaction after laryngectomy. *Arch Otolaryngol*. 1964;79:169–171.

81. Murphy C. Taste and smell in the elderly. In: Meiselman HL, Rivlin RS, eds. *Clinical Measurement of Taste and Smell*. Lexington, Mass: Collamore Press; 1986:343–367.

82. Weiffenbach JM, Baum BJ, Burghauser R. Taste thresholds: quality specific variation with aging. *J Gerontol*. 1982;37:372–377.

83. Cowart B, Yokomukai Y, Beauchamp G. Bitter taste in aging: compound-specific decline in sensitivity. *Physiol Behav*. 1994;56:1237–1241.

84. Stevens J, Cain W. Changes in taste and flavor in aging. *Crit Rev Food Sci Nutr*. 1993;33:27–37.

85. Miller IJ. Human taste bud density across adult age groups. *J Gerontol*. 1988;43:B26–B30.

86. Mistretta C. Anatomy and neurophysiology of the taste system in aged animals. In: Murphy C, Cain W, Hegsted D, eds. *Nutrition and the Chemical Senses in Aging: Recent Advances and Current Research Needs*. New York, NY: Annals of the New York Academy of Sciences; 1989:277–290.

87. Mistretta C. Developmental neurobiology of the taste system. In: Getchell T, Doty R, Bartoshuk L, Snow JB Jr, eds. *Smell and Taste in Health and Disease*. New York, NY: Raven Press; 1991:35–64.

88. Bartoshuk LM, Rifkin B, Marks LE, Bars P. Taste and aging. *J Gerontol*. 1986;41:51–57.

89. Lucchina L, Bartoshuk L, Duffy V, Ferris A, Marks L. Preliminary examination of suprathreshold olfactory and taste perception: free-living elderly females exhibit greater olfactory than taste impairment. *Chem Senses*. 1994;19:508. Abstract.

90. Stevens J, Cain W, Demarque A, Ruthruff A. On the discrimination of missing ingredients: aging and salt. *Appetite*. 1991;16:129–140.

91. Weiffenbach J. Taste intensity perception in human aging: preliminary longitudinal results confirm earlier cross-sectional findings. Presented at the annual meeting of the Association for Chemoreception Sciences; April 1991; Sarasota, Fla.

92. Duffy V, Bartoshuk L, Striegel-Moore R, Rodin J. Taste changes across pregnancy. In: Murphy C, ed. *Olfaction and Taste XII*. New York, NY: Annals of the New York Academy of Sciences, 1998:805–809.

93. Bartoshuk L, Duffy V, Fast K, et al. Variability in taste, oral pain, and taste anatomy: evidence for menstrual control over oral perception. *Appetite*. Abstract.

94. Lucchina L. *6-n-Propylthiouracil Status: Genetic Determinants of Diet-Related Behaviors and Nutritional Status in Older Females*. Storrs, Conn: University of Connecticut; 1995. Doctoral dissertation.

95. Doty R, Snyder P, Huggins G, Lowry L. Endocrine, cardiovascular, and psychological correlates of olfactory sensitivity changes during the human menstrual cycle. *J Comp Physiol Psychol*. 1981;95:45–60.

96. Gilbert A, Wysocki C. Quantitative assessment of olfactory experience during pregnancy. *Psychosom Med.* 1991;53:693–700.

97. Zachariasen R. Oral manifestations of menopause. *Compendium.* 1993;14:1584.

98. Kveton J, Bartoshuk L. The effect of unilateral chorda tympani damage on taste. *Laryngoscope.* 1994;104:25–29.

99. Bartoshuk L, Beauchamp G. Chemical senses. *Annu Rev Psychol.* 1994;45:419–449.

100. Bartoshuk L. Taste: robust across the age span? In: Murphy C, Cain W, Hegsted D, eds. *Nutrition and the Chemical Senses in Aging: Recent Advances and Current Research Needs.* New York, NY: Annals of the New York Academy of Sciences; 1989:65–75.

101. Stevens J, Choo K. Spatial acuity of the body surface over the life span. *Somatosens Mot Res.* 1996;13:153–166.

102. Weiffenbach J, Tylenda C, Baum B. Oral sensory changes in aging. *J Gerontol.* 1990;45:M121–M125.

103. Calhoun K, Gibson B, Hartley L, Minton J, Hokanson J. Age-related changes in oral sensation. *Laryngoscope.* 1992;102:109–116.

104. Bartoshuk L, Caseria D, Catalanotto F, et al. Do taste-trigeminal interactions play a role in oral pain? *Chem Senses.* 1996;21:578. Abstract.

105. Heft M. Orofacial pain. *Clin Geriatr Med.* 1992;8:557–568.

106. US Dept of Health, Education, and Welfare, National Institute of Neurological and Communicative Disorders and Stroke, eds. *Report of the Panel on Communicative Disorders to the National Advisory Neurological and Communicative Disorders and Stroke Council.* Bethesda, Md: National Institutes of Health; 1979.

107. Leopold D. Olfactory function and disorders. In: Baily B, ed. *Head and Neck Surgery: Otolarnygology.* Philadelphia, Pa: JB Lippincott Co; 1993:250–261.

108. Doty R, Bartoshuk L, Snow J. Causes of olfactory and gustatory disorders. In: Getchell T, Doty R, Bartoshuk L, Snow JB Jr, eds. *Smell and Taste in Health and Disease.* New York, NY: Raven Press; 1991:449–462.

109. Akerlund A, Bende M, Murphy C. Olfactory threshold and nasal mucosal changes in experimentally induced common cold. *Acta Otolaryngol (Stockh).* 1995;115:88–92.

110. Duncan H, Seiden A. Long-term follow-up of olfactory loss secondary to head trauma and upper respiratory tract infection. *Arch Otolaryngol Head Neck Surg.* 1995;121:1183–1187.

111. Scott A. Clinical characteristics of taste and smell disorders. *Ear Nose Throat J.* 1989;68:297–315.

112. Kimura Y, Miwa T, Sakashita H, Donjyo T, Ishimaru T, Furukawa M. Clinical observations on parosmia [article in Japanese]. *Nippon Jibiinkoka Gakkai Kaiho.* 1992;95:51–57.

113. Bartoshuk L, Catalanotto F, Scott A, Solomon G. Spatial taste losses associated with head trauma, upper respiratory tract infection and nasal symptoms. *Chem Senses.* 1989;14:684. Abstract.

114. Bartoshuk L, Duffy V, Reed D, Williams A. Supertasting, earaches and head injury: genetics and pathology alter our taste worlds. *Neurosci Biobehav Rev.* 1996;20:79–87.

115. Bull T. Taste and the chorda tympani. *J Laryngol Otol.* 1965;79:479–493.

116. Costanzo R, Becker D. Smell and taste disorders in head injury and neurosurgery patients. In: Meiselman H, Rivlin R, eds. *Clinical Measurements of Taste and Smell.* New York, NY: Macmillan Publishing Co; 1986:565–578.

117. Sumner D. Post-traumatic anosmia. *Brain.* 1964;87:107–120.

118. Costanzo R, Zasler N. Head trauma. In: Getchell T, Doty R, Bartoshuk L, Snow JB Jr, eds. *Smell and Taste in Health and Disease.* New York, NY: Raven Press; 1991:711–730.

119. Yousem D, Geckle R, Bilker W, McKeown D, Doty R. Posttraumatic olfactory dysfunction: MR and clinical evaluation. *AJNR Am J Neuroradiol.* 1996;17:1171–1179.

120. Doty R, Yousem D, Pham L, Kreshak A, Geckle R, Lee W. Olfactory dysfunction in patients with head trauma. *Arch Neurol.* 1997;54:1131–1140.

121. Solomon G. *Patterns of Taste Loss in Clinic Patients with Histories of Head Trauma, Nasal Symptoms, or Upper Respiratory Infections.* New Haven, Conn: Yale University School of Medicine; 1991. Thesis.

122. Adams P, Marano M. Current estimates from the National Health Interview Survey, 1994. National Center for Health Statistics. *Vital Health Stat.* 1995;10:81–82.

123. Edelstein D. Aging of the normal nose in adults. *Laryngoscope.* 1996;106:1–25.

124. Mott A. Topical corticosteroid therapy for nasal polyposis. In: Getchell T, Doty R, Bartoshuk L, Snow JB Jr, eds. *Smell and Taste in Health and Disease.* New York, NY: Raven Press; 1991:553–572.

125. Hinriksdottir I, Murphy C, Bende M. Olfactory threshold after nasal allergen challenge. *J Otorhinolaryngol Relat Spec.* 1997;59:36–38.

126. Apter A, Mott A, Frank M, Clive J. Allergic rhinitis and olfactory loss. *Ann Allergy Asthma Immunol.* 1995;75:311–316.

127. Cowart B, Flynn-Rodden K, McGeady S, Lowry L. Hyposmia in allergic rhinitis. *J Allergy Clin Immunol.* 1993;91:747–751.

128. Downey L, Jacobs J, Lebowitz R. Anosmia and chronic sinus disease. *Otolaryngol Head Neck Surg.* 1996;115:24–48.

129. Mesholam R, Moberg P, Mahr R, Doty R. Olfaction in neurodegenerative disease: a meta-analysis of olfactory functioning in Alzheimer's and Parkinson's diseases. *Arch Neurol.* 1998;55:84–90.

130. Garrett-Laster M, Russell R, Jacques P. Impairment of taste and olfaction in patients with cirrhosis: the role of vitamin A. *Hum Nutr Clin Nutr.* 1984;38C:203–214.

131. Madden A, Bradbury W, Morgan M. Taste perception in cirrhosis: its relationship to circulating micronutrients and food preferences. *Hepatology.* 1997;26:40–48.

132. Deems R, Friedman M, Friedman L, Maddrey WC. Clinical manifestations of olfactory and gustatory disorders associated with hepatic and renal disease. In: Getchell T, Doty R, Bartoshuk L, Snow JB Jr, eds. *Smell and Taste in Health and Disease.* New York, NY: Raven Press; 1991:805–816.

133. Griep M, Van der Niepen P, Sennesael J, Mets T, Massart D, Verbeelen D. Odour perception in chronic renal disease. *Nephrol Dial Transplant.* 1997;12:2093–2098.

134. Duffy V, Lucchina L, Fast K, Bartoshuk L. Taste and cancer. In: Berger A, Levy M, Portnoy R, Weissman D, eds. *Principles and Practice of Supportive Oncology.* Philadelphia, Pa: JB Lippincott Co; 1998:141–151.

135. Ophir D, Guterman A, Gross-Isseroff R. Changes in smell acuity induced by radiation exposure of the olfactory mucosa. *Arch Otolaryngol Head Neck Surg.* 1988;114:853–855.

136. MacCarthy-Leventhal E. Post radiation mouth blindness. *Lancet.* 1959;19:1138–1139.

137. Weinstock R, Wright H, Smith D. Olfactory dysfunction in diabetes mellitus. *Physiol Behav.* 1993;53:17–21.

138. Tepper B, Hartfiel L, Schneider S. Sweet taste and diet in type II diabetes. *Physiol Behav.* 1996;60:13–18.

139. Getchell M, Mellert T. Olfactory mucus secretion. In: Getchell T, Doty R, Bartoshuk L, Snow JB Jr, eds. *Smell and Taste in Health and Disease.* New York, NY: Raven Press; 1991:83–95.

140. Weiffenbach J, Schwartz L, Atkinson J, Fox P. Taste performance in Sjögren's syndrome. *Physiol Behav.* 1995;57:89–96.

141. Henkin R, Talal N, Larson A, Mattern C. Abnormalities of taste and smell in Sjögren's syndrome. *Ann Intern Med.* 1972;76:375–383.

142. Rasmussen N, Brofeldt S, Manthorpe R. Smell and nasal findings in patients with primary Sjögren's syndrome. *Scand J Rheumatol Suppl.* 1986;61:142–145.

143. Leopold D, Bartoshuk L, Doty R, Jafek B, Smith D, Snow JJ. Aging of the upper airway and the senses of taste and smell. *Otolaryngol Head Neck Surg.* 1989;100:287–289.

144. Frye R, Schwartz B, Doty R. Chronic dose-related influence of cigarette smoking on olfactory function. *JAMA.* 1990;263:1233–1236.

145. Schwartz B, Doty R, Monroe C, Frye R, Barker S. Olfactory function in chemical workers exposed to acrylate and methacrylate vapors. *Am J Public Health.* 1989;79:613–618.

146. Schiffman S. Taste and smell losses in normal aging and disease. *JAMA.* 1997;278:1357–1362.

147. Catalanotto F, Sweeney E. Oral conditions affecting chemosensory function. In: Getchell T, Doty R, Bartoshuk L, Snow JB Jr, eds. *Smell and Taste in Health and Disease.* New York, NY: Raven Press; 1991:643–651.

148. Steele W, Stuart J, Whiting B. Serum, tear, and salivary concentrations of methotrexate in man. *Br J Clin Pharmacol.* 1979;7:207–211.

149. Alfano M. The origin of gingival fluid. *J Theor Biol.* 1974;47:127–136.

150. Maruniak J, Silver W, Moulton D. Olfactory receptors' response to blood-borne odorants. *Brain Res.* 1983;265:312–316.

151. Matsuyama H, Tomita H. Clinical applications and mechanisms of intravenous taste tests. *Auris Nasus Larynx.* 1986;13:S43–S50.

152. Garb J, Stunkard A. Taste aversions in man. *Am J Psychiatry.* 1974;131:1204–1207.

153. Ship J. Gustatory and olfactory considerations: examination and treatment in general practice. *J Am Dent Assoc.* 1993;124:55–62.

154. Friedman M, Mattes R. Chemical senses and nutrition. In: Getchell T, Doty R, Bartoshuk L, Snow JB Jr, eds. *Smell and Taste in Health and Disease.* New York, NY: Raven Press; 1991:391–404.

155. Weisman K, Christensen E, Dreyer V. Zinc supplementation in alcoholic cirrhosis: a double-blind clinical trial. *Acta Med Scand.* 1979; 205:361–366.

156. Mahajan S, Prasad A, Lambujon J, Abbasi A, Briggs W. Improvement of uremic hypogeusia by zinc: a double-blinded study. *Am J Clin Nutr.* 1980;33:1517–1521.

157. Ripamonti C, Zecca E, Brunelli C, et al. A randomized, controlled clinical trial to evaluate the effects of zinc sulfate on cancer patients with taste alterations caused by head and neck irradiation. *Cancer.* 1998;82:1938–1945.

158. Sturniolo G, D'Inca R, Parisi G, et al. Taste alterations in liver cirrhosis: are they related to zinc deficiency. *J Trace Elem Electrolytes Health Dis.* 1992;6:15–19.

159. Tabuchi R, Econ M, Ohara I, Agr D. Influence of zinc supplementation to diets at graded levels of protein on taste sensitivity, morphological changes of tongue epithelia and serum zinc concentration in growing rats. *J Am Coll Nutr.* 1996;15:303–308.

160. Ferris AM, Schlitzer JL, Schierberl MJ, et al. Anosmia and nutritional status. *Nutr Res.* 1985;5:149–156.

161. Ferris AM, Duffy VB. The effect of olfactory deficits on nutritional status: does age predict individuals at risk? In: Murphy C, Cain W, Hegsted D, eds. *Nutrition and the Chemical Senses in Aging: Recent Advances and Current Research Needs.* New York, NY: Annals of the New York Academy of Sciences; 1989:113–123.

162. Price S. The role of zinc in taste and smell. In: Meiselman H, Rivlin R, eds. *Clinical Measurement of Taste and Smell.* New York, NY: Macmillan Publishing Co; 1986:443–445.

163. Henkin R, Schechter P, Friedwald W, Demets D, Raff M. A double blind study of the effects of zinc sulfate on taste and smell dysfunction. *Am J Med Sci.* 1976;272:285–299.

164. Greger J, Geissler A. Effects of zinc supplementation on taste acuity of the aged. *Am J Clin Nutr.* 1978;31:633–637.

165. Bales C, Stenman L, Freeland-Graves J, Stone J, Young R. The effect of age on plasma zinc uptake and taste acuity. *Am J Clin Nutr.* 1986;44:664–669.

166. Prasad A, Fitzgerald J, Hess J, Kaplan J, Pelen F, Dardenne M. Zinc deficiency in elderly patients. *Nutrition.* 1993;9:218–224.

167. Mennell J, Beauchamp G. The early development of human flavor preferences. In: Capaldi E, ed. *Why We Eat What We Eat.* Washington, DC: American Psychological Association; 1996:83–112.

168. Capaldi E, ed. *Why We Eat What We Eat.* Washington, DC: American Psychological Association; 1996.

169. Capaldi E. Conditioned food preferences. In: Capaldi E, ed. *Why We Eat What We Eat.* Washington, DC: American Psychological Association; 1996:53–80.

170. Schafe G, Bernstein I. Taste aversion learning. In: Capaldi E, ed. *Why We Eat What We Eat.* Washington, DC: American Psychological Association; 1996:31–51.

171. Rozin P. Sociocultural influences on food selection. In: Capaldi E, ed. *Why We Eat What We Eat.* Washington, DC: American Psychological Association; 1996:233–263.

172. Shepherd R. Sensory influences on salt, sugar and fat intake. *Nutr Res Rev.* 1988;1:125–144.

173. Ship J, Duffy V, Jones J, Langmore S. Geriatric oral health and its impact on eating. *J Am Geriatr Soc.* 1996;44:456–464.

174. Rolls B. Sensory-specific satiety. *Nutr Rev.* 1986;44:93–101.

175. Nordin S, Monsch A, Murphy C. Unawareness of smell loss in normal aging and Alzheimer's disease: discrepancy between self-reported and diagnosed smell sensitivity. *J Gerontol B Psychol Sci Soc Sci.* 1995;50:P187–P192.

176. Wayler AH, Muench ME, Kapur KK, Chauncy HH. Masticatory performance and food acceptability in persons with removable partial dentures,

full dentures, and intact natural dentition. *J Gerontol*. 1984;39:284–289.

177. Mattes R, Cowart B, Schiavo M, et al. Dietary evaluation of patients with smell and/or taste disorders. *Am J Clin Nutr*. 1990;51:233–240.

178. Mattes R, Cowart B. Dietary assessment of patients with chemosensory disorders. *J Am Diet Assoc*. 1994;94:50–56.

179. Stevens J. Food quality reports from non-institutionalized aged. In: Murphy C, Cain W, Hegsted D, eds. *Nutrition and the Chemical Senses in Aging: Recent Advances and Current Research Needs*. New York, NY: Annals of the New York Academy of Sciences; 1989:87–93.

180. Todhunter EN. Life style and nutrient intake in the elderly. In: Winick M, ed. *Nutrition and Aging*. New York, NY: John Wiley & Sons; 1976: 119–127.

181. Duffy V, Backstrand J, Ferris A. Olfactory dysfunction and related nutritional risk in free-living, elderly women. *J Am Diet Assoc*. 1995;95:879–884.

182. Doty R. Food preference ratings of congenitally anosmic humans. In: Kare M, Maller O, eds. *Chemical Senses and Nutrition*. New York, NY: Academic Press; 1977:315–325.

183. Murphy C, Withee J. Age-related differences in the pleasantness of chemosensory stimuli. *Psychol Aging*. 1986;1:312–318.

184. Drewnowski A, Henderson S, Driscoll A, Rolls B. Salt taste perceptions and preferences are unrelated to sodium consumption in healthy older adults. *J Am Diet Assoc*. 1996;96:471–474.

185. de Graaf C, Polet P, van Staveren W. Sensory perception and pleasantness of food flavors in elderly subjects. *J Gerontol B Psychol Sci Soc Sci*. 1994;49:P93–P99.

186. Mungas D, Cooper J, Weiler P, Gietzen D, Franzi C, Bernick C. Dietary preference for sweet foods in patients with dementia. *J Am Geriatr Soc*. 1990;38:999–1007.

187. Pelchat M, LaChaussee J. Food cravings and taste aversions in the elderly. *Appetite*. 1994;23:193.

188. Warwick Z, Schiffman S. Sensory evaluation of fat-sucrose and fat-salt mixtures: relationship to age and weight status. *Physiol Behav*. 1990; 48:633–636.

189. Tews J, Repa J, Nguyen H, Harper A. Protein selection by olfactory bulbectomized rats. *Nutr Rep Int*. 1985;31:797–803.

190. May K. Association between anosmia and anorexia in cats. In: Roper SD, Atema J, eds. *Olfaction and Taste IX*. New York, NY: Annals of the New York Academy of Sciences, 1987; 510:480–482.

191. Schiffman S, Warwick Z. Use of flavor-amplified foods to improve nutritional status in elderly persons. In: Murphy C, Cain W, Hegsted D, eds. *Nutrition and the Chemical Senses in Aging: Recent Advances and Current Research Needs*. New York, NY: Annals of the New York Academy of Sciences; 1989:267–276.

192. Rolls BJ, Rolls ET, Rowe EA, Kingston B, Megson A, Gunary R. Variety in a meal enhances food intake in man. *Physiol Behav*. 1981;26:215–221.

193. Rolls B. Aging and appetite. *Nutr Rev*. 1992; 50:422–426.

194. Rolls B, McDermott T. Effects of age on sensory-specific satiety. *Am J Clin Nutr*. 1991;54:988–996.

195. Tennen H, Affleck G, Mendola R. Coping with smell and taste disorders. In: Getchell T, Doty R, Bartoshuk L, Snow JB Jr, eds. *Smell and Taste in Health and Disease*. New York, NY: Raven Press; 1991:787–802.

196. Cain W. Testing olfaction in a clinical setting. *Ear Nose Throat J*. 1989;68:316–328.

197. Duffy V, Ferris A. Nutritional management of patients with chemosensory disturbances. *Ear Nose Throat J*. 1989;68:395–397.

198. Breslin P, Beauchamp G. Suppression of bitterness by sodium. *Chem Senses*. 1995;20:609–623.

199. Schiffman S, Gatlin L, Sattely-Miller E, et al. The effect of sweeteners on bitter taste in young and elderly subjects. *Brain Res Bull*. 1994;35:189–204.

200. Womack P, Breeding C. Position of the American Dietetic Association: liberalized diets for older adults in long term care. *J Am Diet Assoc*. 1998;98:201.

201. Schiffman S, Warwick Z. Effect of flavor enhancement of foods for the elderly on nutritional status: food intake, biochemical indices, and anthropometric measures. *Physiol Behav*. 1993; 53:395–402.

# CHAPTER 8

# The Aging Gut

*John R. Saltzman*

Form and function change in the aged, but because of the functional reserve of most organ systems, changes may not be evident except during stress associated with disease. Function declines with age in various organ systems, but at different rates, and the potential for organ system interaction is high. Sometimes abnormalities are obvious, but nutritional and gut changes are often occult. Organ failure often leads to impaired nutrition because of poor intake, altered metabolic rate, and altered nutritional requirements. Malnutrition contributes to progression of organ failure, making nutrition an important element of treatment.

## AGING AND THE GASTROINTESTINAL SYSTEM

Little is known about the morphologic and functional changes of the gastrointestinal system with aging. Available information is mostly derived from studies involving institutionalized subjects. Because of technical limitations associated with the clinical evaluation of gastrointestinal function to differentiate wellness and disease, it is difficult to measure smaller changes of function in a general population. Tests designed to diagnose disease may not be sensitive enough for the study of normal aging, whereas others may be too sensitive and have no clinical or nutritional significance. Contrary to several other organ systems, many variables affect optimal function of the gastrointestinal tract. Furthermore, the heterogeneity of the older population in response to aging, disease, and medications makes the evaluations difficult.

Overall, there is little change in gastrointestinal function due to aging in the absence of disease because of the large reserve capacity of this multiorgan system. The functional reserve of the gastrointestinal system is greatest in the midgut, pancreas, and liver. Intestinal segments may adapt, and functional reserves tend to buffer change so that only long-term observations may uncover abnormalities. This is less true for the proximal and distal portions of the gut. Esophageal and gastric disorders usually lead to symptoms associated with eating, whereas colon problems cause difficulties with evacuation. Common gastrointestinal symptoms are often nonspecific and do not indicate the exact nature or severity of disease. Clinical skills are necessary to diagnose these disorders, prognosticate, and prescribe treatment.

This chapter provides a practical view of the impact of aging on normal gastrointestinal function and suggests the implications of common chronic conditions—and altered nutritional requirements—brought about by these changes. The challenge in caring for older adults includes understanding changes in nutritional needs with aging and providing adequate nutrition. This chapter describes some of the complex interrelationships involved in the care and feeding of older people.

## ESOPHAGUS

Swallowing functions of the oropharynx and esophagus involve the transport of food from mouth to stomach, while preventing nasal reflux, tracheal aspiration, and gastroesophageal reflux. Impaired swallowing is common in older individuals, but available evidence indicates that this is due more to the effects of associated diseases than to the intrinsic effects of aging per se. Dysphagia (food sticking with swallowing) and eating dependence can have a profound impact on nutrition. Common disorders result in malnutrition because of oropharyngeal and esophageal dysphagia. Gastroesophageal reflux frequently is symptomatic and also can lead to dysphagia. Symptoms of esophageal dysfunction in older people may be difficult to recognize, as they are often atypical and vague, and may not suggest an esophageal problem.[1] Shaker et al[2] have recognized that in older adults the size of the bolus needs to be bigger and thus that older persons may handle liquids less well than they handle soft foods such as pudding.

### Incidence and Character of Feeding/ Swallowing Disorders

The incidence of eating disability in older nursing home residents may reach 50%.[3] In such patients, findings of dysphagia are often accompanied by a higher incidence of pneumonia caused by gram-negative microorganisms.[4,5] In a study of nursing home patients,

Siebens and colleagues[3] evaluated eating dependence, defined as an impairment of the five components of eating, including behavioral and cognitive ability to recognize food and eat it, normal upper extremity function, oral phase of swallowing, pharyngeal phase of swallowing, and esophageal phase of swallowing. Dependent patients who required physical assistance with eating made up 32% of the nursing home population. Only 25% ate regular diets, and they demonstrated a higher prevalence of abnormal oral-stage swallowing behavior, including spitting, choking, inability to chew, drooling, nasal regurgitation, squirreling food (retaining food in the buccal pouch), delayed swallowing, and overstuffing of the mouth. Signs of abnormal pharyngeal swallowing included coughing during meals or while drinking, choking during meals, and speaking in a wet-sounding voice. A large portion of the dependent eaters could not be tested for gag reflex or voice quality because they would not or could not follow instructions. Mortality rates were higher in the dependent eaters. These findings, and the results of nursing care in these patients, which were not correlated with weight loss during a 3-month period, suggest that simple bedside observations are effective in identifying this basic clinical problem.

Symptoms of dysphagia may occur in diverse older populations in the presence of a cerebrovascular accident (CVA), head and neck surgery, and progressive neurologic disease. Warning signs include a confused mental state that may interfere with the complex sensory and motor functions of eating; dysarthric speech due to weakness or poor control of muscles common to both speech and swallowing; excessive drooling, which can follow neuromuscular impairment of these same mechanisms; coughing and choking on food or sputum; excessive time to consume a meal; unexplained weight loss;

difficulty in chewing; pain with swallowing; or lodgment of food. In spite of these correlates, it is important to recognize the extensive differential diagnoses for pharyngeal and esophageal dysphagias, some of which represent reversible, treatable lesions[6] (Table 8–1).

## Oropharyngeal Physiology

There are three phases to swallowing: oral, pharyngeal, and esophageal. Together, the first two take less than 2 seconds; the third takes 3 to 7 seconds. The first two phases involve oropharyngeal transfer. The oral phase begins with the lips closed and the tip of the tongue contacting the upper mouth structure. The tongue is then elevated while a slight elevation of the larynx occurs, resulting in a progressive stripping of the bolus against the hard palate and the tongue into the pharynx. This first phase of swallowing is under voluntary control.

The pharyngeal phase is the most complex neuromuscular aspect of swallowing. The bolus is projected into the esophagus while the airway is protected. When pharyngeal sensation is intact, the medullary swallowing center controls cranial nerve motor impulses, which close the velopharyngeal valve, elevate the larynx, and relax the upper esophageal sphincter. As the bolus passes the upper esophageal sphincter, the vocal cords close, and the base of the tongue is forced against the posterior pharyngeal wall. At the conclusion of the pharyngeal phase of swallowing, there is forceful contraction of the pharyngeal constrictors, followed by descent of the larynx and contraction of the upper esophageal sphincter.[7]

## Assessment of Oropharyngeal Function

Oropharyngeal function is assessed by history and observation. Careful observation of the patient's eating will make the magnitude of the problems clear. Subsequent clinical studies may include direct inspection of the pharyngeal and esophageal anatomy, an X-ray observation of its function by barium, or a cookie swallow with video scintigraphy. Occasionally, esophageal motility studies are necessary for an accurate clinical diagnosis, which permits a proper prescription for diet and eating behavior.

## Oropharyngeal Dysphagia

The symptoms of oropharyngeal dysphagia include reflux of fluid out through the nose, persistent cough, a wet hoarseness, overt choking, and a persistent sense of the need to clear the throat. Clinical signs include progressive wasting, dehydration, and recurrent bronchitis. Oropharyngeal dysphagia occurs in older subjects because of underlying neurologic disease, muscle weakness, or atrophy. Even older asymptomatic adults have demon-

---

**Table 8–1** Causes of Dysphagia

Oropharyngeal
   Cerebrovascular accident
   Neoplasia
   Zenker's diverticulum
   Cricopharyngeal bar
   Parkinsonism
   Neuromuscular disorders
   Local structural lesions
   Thyroid disorders

Esophageal
   Stricture
   Spasm/motility disturbance
   Neoplasia
   Esophagitis
   Rings and webs
   Medication induced

strated abnormal swallowing due to poor tone of the pharynx, inadequate opening of the cricopharyngeal sphincter, pooling of barium in the adjacent laryngeal folds, and aspiration into the trachea.[1] Typically, liquids are handled less well than soft foods.[8]

The commonly held belief that patients can localize accurately the source of dysphagia is not supported by the medical literature. Patients often point to the neck when dysphagia is caused by distal esophageal disease, so this symptom cannot be used to identify pharyngeal dysphagia. However, if a patient points to the epigastric area, the distal esophagus is usually the location of the stricture. Although coughing and choking can indicate either oral or pharyngeal abnormality, the majority of such patients do not cough. Likewise, although coughing during swallowing usually indicates laryngeal penetration, some patients do not cough even though this occurs.

Dysphagia for solid foods is strongly suggestive of anatomic narrowing. Barium swallow studies may be inadequate because of incomplete distention of all segments. Barium X-rays should be done with the use of a barium pill to detect significant narrowed areas. A lower esophageal ring is the most commonly missed cause of dysphagia for solid foods. Progressive dysphagia to solids eventually results in dysphagia to both solids and liquids due to an anatomic narrowing.

Mixed dysphagia for liquids and solids can occur in patients with pharyngeal dysphagia due to neurologic injury as well as esophageal motility disorders. Since oropharyngeal dysphagic patients have more difficulty with thin liquids and also have greater airway penetration, dysphagia for water can be a differential feature.

Regurgitation of undigested food may be of either pharyngeal or esophageal origin. Late regurgitation can be caused by Zenker's diverticulum or achalasia of the esophagus.

Chest pain and heartburn are not reliable in differentiating pharyngeal and esophageal dysphagia.

Drooling and other evidence of oropharyngeal dysfunction are not necessarily accompanied by clinical evidence of more extensive neuromuscular disease. As many as 50% of neurogenic dysphagic patients have no associated abnormalities on screening physical examination, and in many patients no definite neurologic diagnosis can be established at the initial examination.

Combined functional and anatomic abnormalities are common. As many as one third of patients may have multifactorial dysphagia with coincidental abnormalities in both the pharynx and the esophagus.[9] These observations support an integrated and thorough assessment of dysphagic symptoms to include the pharyngeal and esophageal mechanisms.

### Treatment

Although there is considerable evidence to permit prognostication of behavioral patterns for the extremities and for bulbar and higher cortical functions, after CVA similar correlates for swallowing are limited. In a prospective study, Robbins[10] evaluated patients with isolated left and right CVAs and brainstem CVAs by neurologic examination, computed tomography, video fluoroscopy, selected manometry, and magnetic resonance imaging. All patients demonstrated delayed response of the pharyngeal phase and increased penetration of food. Patients with cortical stroke had increased oral-stage durations for liquid and semisolid foods. Patients with unilateral left and right cortical stroke and those with brainstem CVA had the most difficulty with the oral stage of swallowing and with incoordination of the lips, mandible, and tongue. The right unilateral CVA patients had increased penetration of the vocal folds by food and an increased risk of aspiration, according to video fluoroscopy and history. This aspiration occurred during the delay of the pharyngeal stage of swallowing. Patients with brainstem CVA had relatively normal oral phases, but the most frequent occurrence of aspiration was due to poor airway protection during swallowing and large pharyngeal residuals after swallowing. Manometric studies demonstrated incomplete relaxation of the upper esophageal sphincter as well as delay with respect to pharyngeal contraction.[10]

The different oropharyngeal patterns provide important information for treatment planning, but the general observations, as noted by Siebens and associates,[3] are also important for the selection of appropriate treatment measures. Because patients with left unilateral cortical CVA often demonstrate findings of verbal and oral apraxia, they are not able to swallow on command. This interferes with interpretation of the swallowing study. When these patients were placed in a more natural eating situation, their oral-stage durations were more equivalent to normal, and they used postural changes spontaneously to facilitate swallowing. Only 1 of 20 patients required nonoral feeding techniques because of dysphagia.

Patients with right unilateral CVA did not attempt compensation spontaneously for their difficulty in swallowing, even though aspiration was commonly observed. Defense of the airway was not very forceful, and over one third of these subjects required nonvolitional feeding.

The group with brainstem CVA demonstrated forceful reflux attempts at coughing, but most required nonvolitional feeding techniques. These observations effectively prognosticate the outcome of therapeutic maneuvers and the need for nonvolitional nutritional support (Table 8–2). Robbins[10] describes three therapeutic categories: compensatory, rehabilitive, and medical. These treatment categories are based on the thorough clinical evaluation described above.

Compensatory therapy involves the introduction of external factors or new combinations of behavior to substitute for defects. These include postural adjustment, supraglottic swallow, food placement, and diet modification. Choices are available in a complex range and are best implemented with speech therapy consultation. They are most effective in the left unilateral CVA group.

Dietary modifications in combination with posturing are frequently used in the treatment of the stroke patients. Liquids initially are eliminated from the diet because of the likelihood of aspiration during the delayed pharyngeal stage. Occasionally food requiring chewing may need to be eliminated. Tilting the head forward at a 45° angle can facilitate vallecular maintenance of material until the

**Table 8–2** Swallowing Disorders after CVA

| CVA Type | Signs and Symptoms | Aspiration | Need for Enteral Nutrition |
|---|---|---|---|
| Left CVA | Verbal and oral apraxia, spontaneous compensation with swallowing | Present | 1/20 of patients |
| Right CVA | No spontaneous compensation with swallowing | Common | 1/3 of patients |
| Brainstem | Normal oral phase | Most frequent | Almost all patients |

pharyngeal contraction stage is initiated. The size of the bolus must be limited to 2 mL. Patients who cannot carry out instructions often require nonvolitional feeding techniques.

A unique postural compensation was beneficial to the brainstem group. Most of the pooling of the food appeared at the level of the piriform sinuses unilaterally, so that turning the head toward the impaired side facilitated the flow of material through the upper esophageal sphincter, reduced residual material, and reduced or eliminated aspiration.

Rehabilitation therapy involves the retraining of a disordered movement or behavior by repetitive practice. Patients selected for rehabilitative therapy often receive nonvolitional nutritional support because food is not introduced in the treatment regimen until significant progress has been demonstrated. These treatment programs involve oromotor exercises, vocal fold reduction exercises, and thermal sensitization. Several medical/surgical and prosthetic treatments available for the treatment of dysphagia, including intracordal injection, cricopharyngeal myotomy, and palatal reshaping prosthesis, did not prove successful in the study by Robbins.[10] The work done at the Johns Hopkins Swallowing Center demonstrates the necessity of careful clinical and specialized assessment of neurologic deficits and speech pathology combined with nutritional assessment and therapeutic maneuvers.

## Esophageal Dysphagia

Esophageal dysphagia is due to a disturbed swallowing mechanism in the body of the esophagus or in the region of the lower esophageal sphincter, usually causing a lodgment of food or an awareness of the passage of food through the chest, occasionally with pain. Some patients first present with complete blockage of the esophagus following the ingestion of a piece of meat. Most often, esophageal dysphagia is caused by anatomic rather than functional changes.

Esophageal motility is probably normal in aged people. Many patients with motility abnormalities attributed to presbyesophagus demonstrate features most consistent with diffuse esophageal spasm with disorganized esophageal contraction waves rather than the progressive peristaltic patterns normally observed with swallowing.[11] Many patients have other conditions, such as diabetes mellitus, senile dementia, and peripheral neuropathy, that most likely account for these abnormalities on the basis of abnormal neuromuscular function.[12] In very old patients, there is a marked decline in the magnitude of esophageal contractions, suggesting smooth muscle weakness, but the clinical importance of this observation is unclear. Thus, the overall physiologic function of the esophagus is preserved in older persons with the possible exception of the very old (older than 80 years), in whom presbyesophagus may develop.

Gastroesophageal reflux is a common problem and may be more common in older people because of underlying disease and their frequent use of medications that may contribute to it. Gastroesophageal reflux is more common in the upright position and after meals, but it is probably more serious when it occurs in the recumbent position and during sleep. Factors that contribute to its cause include delayed gastric emptying, incompetence of the lower esophageal sphincter, failure of the esophagus to generate waves of peristalsis to clear refluxed material, and the injurious nature of the gastric contents. It is unclear whether age-associated changes may contribute to the frequency of this disorder, but common diseases of older adults and commonly used medications are known to affect this esophageal dysfunction.[13]

Gastroesophageal reflux may produce no symptoms, even while causing severe injury to the esophagus, but commonly patients experience pyrosis or heartburn. Regurgitation may occur with heartburn or independently, with changes in posture, after meals, or at other times. When injury to the esophagus is severe, patients may experience esophageal dysphagia due to esophagitis, or stricture formation. Painful swallowing may accompany dysphagia in some patients. It is increasingly recognized that gastroesophageal reflux may result in pharyngeal reflux or tracheal aspiration and may cause the laryngeal and pulmonary symptoms of change in voice, chronic cough, asthma, and recurrent pulmonary infections. Inflammation of the esophagus may also cause iron-deficiency anemia resulting from occult blood loss from the inflamed mucosa.

Nutrient requirements probably do not change with gastroesophageal reflux, except in the case of iron-deficiency anemia and the metabolic stress brought on by recurrent pulmonary infections. However, dietary modifications are considered an important element of the treatment protocol, which includes postural measures, drug restriction, antacids, motility agents, histamine 2 ($H_2$) blockers, and proton pump inhibitors. Fat, chocolate, peppermint, and alcohol decrease lower esophageal sphincter pressure; coffee, both caffeinated and decaffeinated, stimulates gastric acid secretion; alcohol and fruit drinks irritate the mucosa, probably because of their osmotic effect; and large meals, probably by their volume, delay gastric emptying. Avoiding meals before retiring, and elevating the head of the bed with blocks may be the two most important measures to take to prevent complications of gastroesophageal reflux disease. A low-fat, high-carbohydrate diet with smaller meals is desirable. Drugs that contribute to delayed gastric emptying or that increase gastroesophageal reflux are nicotine,

anticholinergics, calcium-channel blockers, theophylline, diazepam, and β-adrenergic blocker agonists. Antacids used in the treatment of this condition will increase the dietary load of divalent cations and help to alleviate symptomatic constipation.

The above comments about oropharyngeal dysphagia, esophageal dysphagia, and gastroesophageal reflux disease are especially relevant to the nutritionist participating in the care of older patients in acute care hospitals and long-term care facilities, as well as those treated with tube feedings. For older patients with esophageal dysphagia, one must seek a clinical diagnosis, rather than attributing symptoms to old age.[8] For most of these patients, specific treatment for the underlying condition is central to the goal of adequate nutrition through dietary management or nutritional support techniques.

## STOMACH

Changes in gastric morphology and function occur with age, but these changes do not seem to be separate and distinct from those of acquired disease. Gastric secretion does not decrease solely due to advanced age, as thought in the early 1900s.[14] Older adults who have low acid and pepsin secretion have associated atrophic gastritis.[15]

Chronic atrophic gastritis occurs in 11% to 50% of older persons in various studies, depending on the population, diagnostic tests, and definition of atrophic gastritis.[16,17] Although there are several different classification systems for chronic gastritis, the system by Strickland and Mackay[18] has been most widely used due to its clinical utility and simplicity. Type A gastritis involves the body and fundus of the stomach and is associated with autoimmune findings, including parietal cell antibodies and autoimmune conditions of other organs (Table 8–3). Type A atrophic gastritis may also be associated with an autosomal dominant inheritance pattern and is relatively uncommon in the United States. It is found in less than 5% of persons over the age of 60.[19] Type B gastritis predominantly affects the antrum of the stomach without autoimmune associations and is the most common type seen in older persons.[20,21] Krasinski et al[19] showed that in an urban Boston population the prevalence of atrophic gastritis among 60- to 69-year-old people was 24%, among 70- to 79-year-old people was 32%, and among people aged 80 years and older was 37%.

The etiologic factor most strongly associated with the development of type B chronic atrophic gastritis is *Helicobacter pylori*,[22] an organism strongly associated with peptic ulcer disease. Initial infection with *Helicobacter pylori* causes a mild, superficial gastritis that affects both the antrum and body of the stomach. The superficial gastritis progresses with time to a chronic inflammatory gastritis of the antrum and/or the body of the stomach. Eventually the progression of gastritis may lead to atrophic gastritis with loss of gastric glands, a condition in which regression with a return of normal gastric epithelium is unusual. Vitamin $B_{12}$ deficiency is commonly associated with atrophic gastritis type A[19] due to decreased intrinsic factor and acid production. However, vitamin $B_{12}$ deficiency is much less frequent in type B atrophic gastritis, as intrinsic factor production is relatively well preserved and as there is some gastric acid production except in the most extreme cases of gastric atrophy.

Lack or absence of gastric acid due to atrophic gastritis may lead to adverse clinical consequences. One of the major defenses to limit the growth of bacteria in the upper intestines is gastric acid. When gastric acid production is diminished or lost, the bacterial overgrowth syndrome, with symptoms of abdominal discomfort, nausea, diarrhea, and weight loss with malabsorption, may occur. However, this is relatively unusual unless there are other altered host defenses, for the bacteria that colonize the upper gastrointestinal tract solely due to lack of gastric acid are usually not anaerobic, bile salt–splitting organisms. The lack of gastric acid may also lead to altered nutrient absorption for those nutrients that have a pH-dependent uptake mechanism. This will be further discussed in the section "Small Intestine," subsection "Micronutrient Absorption."

**Table 8–3** Differential Features of Atrophic Gastritis

| Characteristics | Type A | Type B |
|---|---|---|
| Site | Body Fundus | Antrum body (patchy) |
| Etiology | Autoimmune | *Helicobacter pylori* |
| Inheritance | Autosomal | Unknown |
| Antibodies | Parietal cell Intrinsic factor | Unusual |
| Prevalence | Rare | Common |

Although the incidence of peptic ulcer disease is declining for the population at large,[23] evidence suggests that the incidence of gastric ulcer has increased among older adults.[24] The incidence of ulcer perforation is also increasing.[25] Ulcer disease is more often complicated in older patients, possibly because of malnutrition and concurrent illness.[26] Antacids are frequently used by older individuals for dyspeptic symptoms.[27] Chronic or high-dose antacid therapy is associated with multiple side effects, including constipation, obstruction, and osteomalacia with use of aluminum antacids; diarrhea, dehydration, and electrolyte disturbances with use of magnesium antacids; and hypercalcemia, kidney stones, and acid rebound with use of calcium antacids.[28–30]

Nonsteroidal anti-inflammatory drugs (NSAIDs) play a major role in the pathophysiology and complications of gastroduodenal disease in older patients. They are the most commonly prescribed medications for patients older than age 65 years.[31,32] A substantial number of patients experience pain, burning, indigestion, nausea, and vomiting while taking these drugs.[33] A variety of mucosal injuries occur with ingestion of NSAIDs, including mucosal hemorrhages, erosions, and acute or chronic ulcers.[34] NSAIDs have also been associated with increased risk of gastrointestinal bleeding.[35]

Gastric emptying of solids by the antrum and of liquids by the fundus is elegantly controlled by gastroduodenal regulatory mechanisms responsive to the composition of ingested foods, duodenal contents, and multiple external influences.[16] Liquid emptying of the stomach, which is vagally mediated, is slowed, whereas solid emptying, which is antrally determined, seems to be preserved with aging.[35] In older adults, the gastric emptying of mixed meals is somewhat delayed. A study demonstrated in 25 older adults that the gastric emptying time ($T_{1/2}$) of a mixed meal was 136 ± 13 minutes compared to 81 ± 4 minutes in younger controls.[36] However, the changes in gastric emptying may be confounded by the presence of atrophic gastritis, as delayed emptying may be attributable to underlying atrophic gastritis.[37,38] Accelerated early gastric emptying of liquids with normal late phases of gastric emptying has been noted.[39] Gastric emptying of a fatty meal may be delayed.[37] However, it is unlikely that these alterations are clinically significant.

## PANCREAS

### Pancreatic Changes with Age

Intraluminal digestion is dependent on pancreatic secretion of enzymes, proenzymes, and bicarbonate. Biliary secretion of bile salts is essential for micelle formation, and biliary bicarbonate contributes to acid neutralization. The functional reserve is so great that 90% of secretory capacity must be lost before significant maldigestion occurs. The complex control of pancreatic secretion involves the central nervous system and gastric and intestinal mediators. Intestinal trophic substances, recurrent cycles of pancreatic secretion, and nutritional state are determinants of the ability of the pancreas to secrete (Figure 8–1). Extrapancreatic factors, such as acid hypersecretory states, decreased or diverted biliary secretions, altered anatomy of the proximal gastrointestinal tract, impaired release of intestinal mediators, and bacterial overgrowth in the small intestine, can adversely influence intraluminal digestion.

It might be expected that there would be age-related changes in both the morphology and the function of the aged pancreas, but the clinical significance of these changes is unclear. In older persons, malnutrition, hepato-

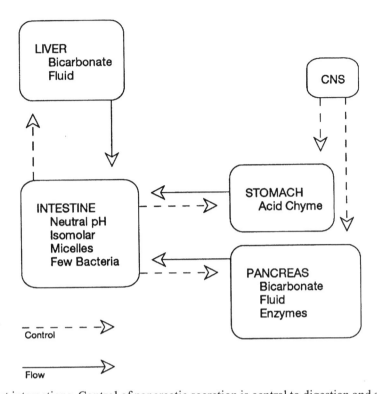

**Figure 8–1** Gut interactions. Control of pancreatic secretion is central to digestion and subject to modulation by the central nervous system (CNS) and intestinal factors.

biliary or gastrointestinal surgery, and other factors affecting digestion and absorption could exacerbate the effects of these changes.

Beyond age 70 years, the pancreas is smaller and weighs less. Pancreatic ducts are dilated, and there is increased parenchymal fibrosis.[40] The diameter of the pancreatic duct increases with advancing age such that after age 50 it expands an average of 8% per decade.[41] However, the tapered appearance and smooth margins of the pancreatic duct are preserved with aging. The development of ductular ectasia in intralobular and interlobular ducts correlates with the development of pancreatic duct dilatation. These age-related changes can be misinterpreted as chronic pancreatitis during endoscopic retrograde cholangiopancreatography (ERCP).[42]

Clinical pancreatic insufficiency, resulting in loss of fat, protein, minerals, and fluid in the feces, occurs when pancreatic secretion is less than 10% of normal. Lesser decreases in pancreatic function are difficult to detect. Although there is controversy about the presence and extent of pancreatic secretory decline with age, most investigators question its clinical significance. In both human and animal studies, there appears to be a linear decline of enzyme output, while volume and bicarbonate concentration increase to a maximum at about the fourth decade of life and then progressively decline.[34,40–44] Perhaps more insightful is the work by Greenberg and Holt,[45] which demonstrated that the pancreatic enzyme concentrations in aging rats did not adapt to dietary changes as well as they did in younger rats. The enzymes lipase and amylase were studied. The findings suggest that age modifies the effect of gastrointestinal hormones on maintenance of pancreatic mass and enzyme content. Although the clinical significance of these observations is unclear, their potential importance cannot be overemphasized because of the magnification of rather small changes in hormone reactivity or responsiveness, potentially reflecting large changes in secretory rate.[45,46]

## Diseases of the Pancreas in the Aged Population

### Acute Pancreatitis

Acute pancreatitis is not uncommon in older people. It is responsible for 5% to 7% of the cases of abdominal pain in older persons.[47] It follows the frequency of gallstone-induced biliary tract disease and occurs most often in women, but drug-induced acute pancreatitis is also frequent.[48] Alcohol is rarely the cause of acute pancreatitis in older adults. Pancreatic cancer is an unusual cause of acute pancreatitis but must be considered in older persons with acute pancreatitis. Age is a negative prognostic factor, as older subjects are more likely to die of shock and sepsis.[49–51] The uncomplicated course of this disease usually involves a period of acute illness characterized by pain, nausea, and vomiting. Older adults may initially present with more subtle symptoms and less marked physical symptoms than younger persons. When the disease is more severe, sepsis, pancreatic abscess, and shock complicate the picture. Less ill patients usually recover in a matter of days with resumption of oral intake, but they may undergo multiple diagnostic and perhaps surgical procedures if retained gallstones are suspected. The management of stress me-

tabolism is the major challenge to the nutritionist. Severely ill patients often face protracted periods of bowel rest. Total parenteral nutrition support is usually provided in patients with moderate or severe pancreatitis (Figure 8–2).

### Chronic Pancreatitis

Chronic pancreatitis is of interest to the nutritionist because episodes of symptoms reduce oral intake, while late stages of the disease result in maldigestion due to pancreatic insufficiency. The most common cause of chronic pancreatitis is alcoholism; however, onset after age 60 years is uncommon. Idiopathic chronic pancreatitis in general is the second most common cause of chronic pancreatitis (20%). In older persons with the new onset of chronic pancreatitis, idiopathic causes predominate. Chronic pancreatitis can principally involve the large ducts, as from tumor or stones, or the small ducts, as is typical of idiopathic chronic pancreatitis. The small duct form may also involve little to no pancreatic calcification, making diagnosis more difficult.[52]

Pancreatic insufficiency in asymptomatic older people may be accounted for by the presence of either painless disease or chronic primary inflammatory pancreatitis. Painless chronic pancreatitis appears to be more frequent in the sixth and seventh decades. These patients frequently have steatorrhea, diabetes, pancreatic calcifications, and weight loss. There is extensive scarring and atrophy of the gland, and response to therapy is unpredictable.[40]

*Nutritional Management.* The management of pancreatic insufficiency due to chronic pancreatitis is based on the replacement of pancreatic enzymes, dietary modification to minimize the consequences of pancreatic insufficiency, and supplementation of

<table>
<tr><td>

ACUTE PANCREATITIS

*Occult*
    No oral intake
    Usual short time



Complicated course
Sepsis
No oral intake
Drainage has high protein
    content
Usually no residual
    pancreatic insufficiency

</td><td>

CHRONIC PANCREATITIS

*Clinical*
    Multiple episodes
    Intake reduced by pain
    Chronic course
    Ethanol as carbohydrate

    Malnutrition as late
      presentation
    Maldigestion
    Steatorrhea

</td></tr>
</table>

**Figure 8–2** Nutrition problems with pancreatitis.

vitamins that may be malabsorbed as a result of this condition. Pancreatic insufficiency most commonly occurs after a long duration of chronic pancreatitis, but it can occur acutely with obstruction of the pancreatic duct by carcinoma and transiently with acute or relapsing acute pancreatitis. It is likely that visceral protein depletion results in pancreatic insufficiency. Steatorrhea is often a more serious problem than creatorrhea because lipase secretion may decrease more rapidly.[53] Carbohydrate malabsorption also occurs, but its quantitative importance has not been established.[54]

Mild steatorrhea may not be associated with any symptoms. Weight loss may be minimal if food intake is adequate. Enzyme replacement is indicated for weight loss, diarrhea, dyspepsia, and fecal fat excretion exceeding 15 g/d. Some patients also experience reduced pain on pancreatic supplementation.[55] Enzyme preparations are usually given with meals, but even in high doses they do not completely resolve the steatorrhea.

Pancreatic extracts may form insoluble complexes with folic acid and interfere with its absorption.[56]

In patients with painful disease, recurrent hospitalizations with reduced or absent oral intake and intake reduced secondary to pain and analgesic use can contribute to the overall picture of malnutrition. Patients who fail to respond may have complicating factors such as primary intestinal disease, bacterial overgrowth, or inactivation of enzyme by gastric acid. Disproportionate acidification of the duodenum because of impaired bicarbonate secretion from the pancreas also occurs. Aluminum hydroxide is effective in reducing steatorrhea during pancreatic enzyme replacement therapy, and $H_2$ blockers have produced variable results.

Fat-soluble vitamin deficiency occurs despite adequate control of steatorrhea.[57] Nondiabetic retinopathy is improved by vitamin A therapy in patients with pancreatic insufficiency, but zinc malabsorption may also play a role.[55] Vitamin $B_{12}$ malabsorption occurs in chronic pancreatic insufficiency and may be due to a deficiency of a pancreatic factor or impaired proteolysis of vitamin $B_{12}$ binders.[58] Clinical evidence of vitamin $B_{12}$ malabsorption is rare. Dietary treatment of chronic pancreatitis is based on the rationale that a high-fat diet exacerbates steatorrhea and abdominal pain and therefore that dietary fat should be restricted to 25% or less of total calories. Malabsorption of protein should be treated with a diet rich in protein. In severe symptomatic chronic pancreatitis, medium-chain triglycerides, which do not require lipolysis but enter the intestinal mucosa directly, can be used as replacement calories. A high-fiber diet is relatively contraindicated in pancreatic insufficiency because fiber may bind as much as 80% to 95% of pancreatic enzymes.[59]

## SMALL INTESTINE

### Morphology

Because passive absorption is dependent on the surface area of the small intestine, studies have been made of the morphologic changes in the intestinal villous and microvillous membranes that might occur with aging. Animal studies have demonstrated a decrease in the number of villi, villous atrophy, and abnormal villous shape with advancing age. However, the validity of these early studies is questionable because of a lack of information on the nutritional state of the animals. In humans there may be minor changes between young adults and older persons, including shorter villi in the older subjects, but this finding has not been consistently demonstrated.[60] Although it is not possible to equate normal appearance with normal function, later studies effectively excluded disease- and nutrition-related variables and did not demonstrate abnormal appearance of the ab-

sorptive surface, suggesting that well-being and nutritional state are predominant factors in determining morphology and function.[61]

The epithelial surface of the intestinal villous membrane is normally regenerated at a rapid rate. Replication occurs in the intestinal crypt; then, as cells migrate toward the apex of the villous, differentiation and maturation occur. No difference in migration rate has been demonstrated, but the activities of several important enzymes are delayed in aged rats. Although results from older studies conflict with those of more recent studies, on the basis of current information it can be concluded that otherwise healthy, well-nourished older individuals have no substantial differences in intestinal morphology; however, they may have functional abnormalities because of altered enzyme activity of epithelial cells due to delayed maturation.[61]

### Integrity

Integrity and permeability of the small intestine may be altered by a variety of diseases, including Crohn's disease and celiac sprue. If the small intestinal mucosa is disrupted, there may be increased antigen access and abnormal nutrient transport. The lactulose-manitol absorption test measures the relative absorptions of lactulose, a large molecule absorbed paracellularly to manitol, a relatively small molecule absorbed transcellularly, and provides an assessment of overall small intestinal permeability. When healthy adults older than 60 years are compared with younger adults, there are no significant changes as measured in the lactulose-manitol absorption test.[62] The $\alpha_1$-antitrypsin clearance measures intestinal integrity by assessing the "leakiness" of the gut and measuring lost $\alpha_1$-antitrypsin in the stool. The $\alpha_1$-antitrypsin clearance is unchanged with advancing age when older adults are compared to younger adults.[63] Thus, small intestinal integrity does not seem to be altered due to the aging process alone.

## Function

### Carbohydrate Absorption

The potential for malabsorption is suggested by the alteration of enzyme activity of epithelial cells. Dietary carbohydrates, which approximate 40% of ingested calories, require digestion from the constituent polysaccharides to monosaccharides before intestinal absorption. The initial phase of digestion occurs in the intestinal lumen by pancreatic amylase, the secretion of which is well preserved in older people. Further hydrolysis of disaccharides and short-chain polysaccharides is accomplished by mucosal cell enzymes. However, overall carbohydrate absorption seems to remain intact with advancing age.

The absorption of glucose is difficult to study in older subjects because glucose metabolism, body size, and body composition are altered. In vitro studies do not suggest an abnormality of glucose absorption in aged mice.[64,65] One method used to evaluate glucose absorption is to measure hydrogen excretion in the breath. Hydrogen, a product of bacterial fermentation of carbohydrate, is absorbed in the colon and excreted in the breath. Postprandial breath hydrogen excretion studies of older patients consuming meals with different amounts of carbohydrate demonstrate excessive excretion of breath hydrogen in one third of people older than 65 years given a 100-g carbohydrate meal. Excessive excretion of hydrogen is also seen in some older subjects given as little as 25 to 50 g of carbohydrate.[66] In young adults, ingestion of a 200-g carbohydrate meal is not associated with elevated breath hydrogen excretions, whereas elevated breath hydrogen excretions

can be detected in over 60% of older adults.[66] The excess hydrogen produced may be from malabsorption of carbohydrate, with subsequent hydrogen production by colonic bacteria or from bacterial metabolism of carbohydrate in the small intestine due to bacterial overgrowth.

Carbohydrate absorption is often evaluated by the D-xylose test. D-xylose, a pentose sugar, is absorbed mainly by diffusion that parallels intestinal absorptive capacity, and it is excreted in urine. Low values may result from incomplete urine collections, impaired renal function, or malabsorption. Earlier studies suggesting impaired D-xylose excretion in older subjects have been dismissed because of the known reduction in urine clearance rate with advanced age. Overall absorption of D-xylose is not affected by age alone except in the very old (those older than 80 years).[67] In the absence of disease, it appears that the aged small intestine has normal carbohydrate absorption within the range of clinically important parameters such as symptoms and evidence of malabsorption. Although dietary carbohydrate has no recommended daily allowance (RDA), several organizations, including the American Heart Association and the U.S. Department of Agriculture, recommend dietary carbohydrate (regardless of age) to make up 55% to 60% of calories, as well as an increased proportion of complex carbohydrates to simple sugars.

### Fat Absorption

The absorption of dietary fats is biochemically more complex than that of other nutrients. Malnutrition associated with steatorrhea and appropriate laboratory studies confirm the diagnosis of malabsorption. A 72-hour fecal fat collection while the patient is on a fixed high–dietary fat intake is the standard measure of fat absorption. The absorption of long-chain triglycerides, fatty acids, monoglycerides, and vitamin D occurs as passive diffusion after intraluminal digestion. The limiting factors are dependent on the concentration of bile salts and the unstirred water layer.[68]

The absorbed triglycerides and vitamin D are transferred from the intestinal cell to the lymphatics as chylomicrons and very–low-density lipoproteins (VLDLs). In aged animals, the absorption of radioactively labeled glycerol and vitamin $D_3$ is decreased, suggesting a defect in the synthesis of chylomicrons and lipoproteins by the enterocyte.[69] This problem may be related to impaired synthesis of essential apoproteins and phospholipids.[70]

In older adults, the capacity for fat absorption is well maintained. Arora et al[67] measured fat absorption in healthy adults aged 20 to 59 years and found fecal fat excretions of 3.3 ± 2.3 g/d compared with 2.5 ± 1.8 g in those aged 60 to 69 years and 2.9 ± 1.9 g in those aged 70 to 91 years. In a Scandinavian population, similar results were found between young and older adults when dietary fat intake was 85 to 90 g/d.[71] Thus, with normal levels of fat consumption, fat digestion and absorption in older adults are equivalent to those in young persons.[72]

At high levels of fat intake (115 to 120 g/d), older adults have less fat absorption than younger adults.[71] In older adults who are institutionalized, there may be even less fat absorption.[73] When fat malabsorption occurs in older adults without an obvious cause, the small intestinal bacterial overgrowth syndrome is often the reason, with bacterial deconjugation of bile acids. Simko and Michael[74] evaluated very high-fat intakes in debilitated older, malnourished hospitalized patients and found that although there was an increase in fecal fat content, these patients were capable of absorbing an average of 329 g of fat per day. Thus, although older persons have a somewhat diminished reserve capacity of the small intestine to absorb dietary fats compared with that of younger adults, it is still significant.

### Protein Absorption

Protein turnover in the intestine is very high, with respect to the total protein content of the intestine, because of the high synthetic activity related to cell renewal and enzyme production. Few studies to date provide information in older adults about quantitative absorptive changes for amino acids and peptides. However, older persons may digest and absorb high-protein diets less well than younger adults, as demonstrated by a small increase in fecal nitrogen content after ingestion of a protein load.[75] Although the 1989 RDA for protein is 0.8 g of protein per kilogram of body weight per day, in older adults this may be adequate only with high energy intakes (≥40 kcal/kg per day).[76] Older adults typically have intakes of about 30 kcal/kg per day, at which more than half of older persons do not obtain nitrogen balance.[77] In Boston, free-living older persons were noted by Munro et al[78] to have an average protein consumption of 1.05 g/kg per day, with no evidence that protein-energy malnutrition correlated with lower intakes. Daily protein intakes of 1 g of protein per kilogram of body weight in the older person will usually provide adequate nutrition.

### Micronutrient Absorption

It is unclear whether deficiency or disease occurs because of vitamin malabsorption in otherwise healthy older people. Research in this area is hampered by the interpretation of blood levels and how they may relate to biochemical effects or tissue stores. Without disease, it is unlikely that malabsorption of vitamins results in significant vitamin depletion.[79] Inadequate dietary intakes are likely responsible for much of the poor vitamin nutriture in older adults.[80] It is now recognized that the RDAs for dietary nutrients established for younger adults cannot be simply extrapolated to older adults.[81] The RDAs are correctly being reevaluated in older adults, not only to provide adequate nutrients such that deficiency states do not occur, but also to prevent chronic disease or treat a marker of chronic disease.

The fat-soluble vitamins may be absorbed more readily by older individuals. This is also true of other lipids.[82–84] In older animals, vitamin A uptake is increased due to a decrease in the thickness of the unstirred water layer. Krasinski et al[85] studied why older adults have higher vitamin A tolerance curves than younger adults. Using plasmapharesis after ingestion of vitamin A–rich meals with subsequent reinfusion of chylomicrons and chylomicron remnants, they showed that older adults had about half the vitamin A clearance rates of young adults. It is reasonable to recommend to older adults to obtain a large proportion of the vitamin A requirement from the precursor carotene, found in fruits and vegetables, as carotenes may have a beneficial effect on cancer prevention.

The absorption of vitamin D in older persons appears to be impaired. Blood levels of 25-hydroxycholecalciferol are lower in older subjects, and malabsorption of labeled cholecalciferol has been reported. The importance of this observation is emphasized by evidence that calcium absorption appears to be lower in older people than it is in younger people and that osteoporosis and osteomalacia frequently occur in older individuals. The mechanism of this malabsorption and the relationship of circulating vitamin D metabolites are unclear, but it appears that there is a reduced adaptation to low dietary intake of calcium. Decreased intakes of vitamin D by older adults are in part responsible for low vitamin D levels, as over three quarters have vitamin D intakes less than two thirds of the 1989 RDA of 5 µg/d. In addition, older adults have decreased renal synthesis of 1,25-dihydroxyvitamin D and decreased skin synthesis of vitamin D.[86] The decrease in skin synthesis of vitamin D is due to reduced sunlight exposure (especially common in institutionalized older adults) and decreased efficiency of skin synthesis.[87,88] In older adults who are institutionalized or homebound, it is reasonable to supplement with 400 IU/d.

Vitamin K levels may be altered with advancing age. Plasma phylloquinone (vitamin $K_1$) concentrations are decreased in older adults compared with younger adults.[89] Small intestinal bacterial overgrowth can result in the synthesis and absorption of menaquinones (vitamin $K_2$).[90] Although menaquinones may contribute to vitamin K nutriture, they typically are not sufficient to replete vitamin K in a deficient patient.

Water-soluble vitamin absorption is probably normal in older adults. Low plasma levels of vitamin C have been correlated with reduced oral intake. No differences of thiamin excretion have been seen in young or older subjects. The absorption for folate in the small intestine is pH dependent, with an optimum pH of about 6.3.[91] In older adults with atrophic gastritis, the pH of the small intestine is higher than in those with normal acid production, pH 7.1 ± 0.1 versus pH 6.6 ± 0.1.[92] This small increase in the pH of the small intestine in older adults with atrophic gastritis results in a significant diminution of folate absorption. The administration of dilute acid along with oral folate improves folate absorption in those with atrophic gastritis. But paradoxically, older adults with atrophic gastritis have higher serum folate values than those with normal gastric acid production.[19] Folate-synthesizing bacteria in the small intestine of older adults with atrophic gastritis are responsible for the additional folate.[93]

Folate deficiency may also increase serum homocysteine levels, as folate is needed to convert homocysteine to methionine. High homocysteine levels are a risk factor for atherosclerotic heart and cerebrovascular disease. In the Framingham Heart Study, plasma folate levels below 11.6 µmol/L, a value well within the normal range, were associated with elevated homocysteine levels.[94] Future guidelines for folate supplementation will need to take into consideration how much dietary folate is required to reduce homocysteine levels to normal.

Serum and plasma vitamin $B_6$ values tend to decrease with advancing age. Vitamin $B_6$ is primarily absorbed in the proximal small intestine, and even with supplementation, up to 40% of older adults may remain vitamin $B_6$ deficient.[95] The average vitamin $B_6$ requirement for older adult males and females is about 2.0 mg/d.[96] Low vitamin $B_6$ levels can also lead to elevated homocysteine values by an altered ability to convert homocysteine to cystathionine.[97]

Age does not seem to be an independent variable for the ileal absorption of vitamin $B_{12}$ (Chapter 3). However, vitamin $B_{12}$ absorption is complex and dependent on multiple factors, including salivary R binders, gastric secretion of acid and intrinsic factor, pancreatic exocrine sufficiency, and intact terminal ileal mucosa. Disruptions of any of these factors may lead to decreased vitamin $B_{12}$ absorption. The classic cause of vitamin $B_{12}$ deficiency is autoimmune type A atrophic gastritis (pernicious anemia). Type B atrophic gastritis also limits the bioavailability of vitamin $B_{12}$ due to diminished protein-bound vitamin $B_{12}$ release from lack of gastric acid.[98]

Tests of protein-bound vitamin $B_{12}$ absorption have shown that older adults with type B atrophic gastritis have decreased absorptions.[99] However, when subjects with type B atrophic gastritis are given free (crystalline) vitamin $B_{12}$, absorption is normalized. Patients treated with potent acid-reducing medications such as the proton-pump inhibitors (ie, omeprazole) also malabsorb protein-bound vitamin $B_{12}$.[100] Ingestion of acidic beverages such as cranberry juice along with protein-bound vitamin $B_{12}$ can normalize vitamin $B_{12}$ absorption. In addition, bacteria that colonize the upper gastrointestinal tract in subjects with type B atrophic gastritis can take up and bind vitamin $B_{12}$, but antibiotic treatment can normalize vitamin $B_{12}$ absorption.[101]

Vitamin $B_{12}$ is also involved in homocysteine metabolism, with low vitamin $B_{12}$ levels causing elevated homocysteine levels. In the Framingham Heart Study, vitamin $B_{12}$ levels below 296 µmol/L were associated with rising homocysteine levels.[102] Although vitamin $B_{12}$ deficiency often results in anemia, the neuropsychiatric manifestations of vitamin $B_{12}$ deficiency may occur even in the absence of anemia.[103]

Low serum concentrations of iron and transferrin in aged individuals do not seem to be related to malabsorption of iron, as no such age-related changes have been demonstrated.[104] Iron deficiency in older subjects is most often accounted for by intestinal blood loss due to malignant or benign disease, although gastric achlorhydria may account for the reduction of the absorption of nonheme iron (Chapter 11)[105].

Calcium absorption appears to decline with advancing age.[106] However, decreased calcium absorption in older adults is primarily due to poor vitamin D nutriture and inactivity. Older adults also have poor calcium intakes in the diet, which are partially due to the high prevalence of lactase deficiency. Certain types of calcium, such as calcium carbonate, are poorly absorbed in older adults with atrophic gastritis.[106–108] However, several studies have not shown any significant change in calcium absorption when calcium is ingested from or with food in subjects with atrophic gastritis.[109,110] Lifetime intake of calcium is a major factor in the development of osteoporosis.

## Motility

Small bowel motility appears to be intact in healthy older people.[111,112] This is not true, however, for the changes seen with medical illness or drug effects. In an intestinal motility study of fasting and fed older subjects, all three phases of the migrating motor complex were present, and there were no differences in the motility index or duration or velocity of phase III contractions. There was a slight decrease in the motility index and the frequency of contractions after feeding, but there were no differences in the mean amplitude of contractions. It is not known whether these latter changes have clinical significance or alter intestinal transit time.[113] Several clinical studies suggest that subclinical pancreatic insufficiency and bacterial overgrowth in the small intestine are a common cause of malabsorption. However, the results are clouded by problems of patient selection and concomitant systemic or gastrointestinal disease. Therefore, when malabsorption is suspected, a specific diagnosis should be pursued, since it is unlikely that major clinical problems of malabsorption are unique to older people.[79,114–116]

## INTESTINAL DISORDERS

### Disaccharidase Deficiency

Deficiency of the disaccharidase lactase is the most common disorder of carbohydrate digestion. Its appearance with aging and maturation can be considered normal in most people, with the exception of some northern Europeans, as there is a steady decline in brush border enzymes after weaning.[117] Adults retain about 10% to 30% of intestinal lactase activity and develop symptoms only when they ingest sufficient lactose to exceed lactase production. Lactase deficiency also occurs in the presence of primary intestinal diseases such as viral gastroenteritis, tropical and nontropical sprue, Crohn's disease, bacterial and parasitic infections of the intestine, and cystic fibrosis.

The symptoms of lactase deficiency are nonspecific. Even so, most adults who have this condition are aware of their intolerance to milk because of abdominal cramping, bloating, distention, flatulence, and possible diarrhea. Symptoms are due to the osmotic effect of unhydrolyzed and unabsorbed lactose shifting fluid into the intestinal tract, resulting in a rapid passage of contents through the intestine into the colon. Colonic bacteria hydrolyze the lactose to lactic acid and short-chain fatty acids, lowering the pH of the stool. Hydrogen produced by this fermentation is absorbed and excreted in the breath, which is a useful test for detecting lactose intolerance. The diagnosis can be confirmed by administering an oral dose of lactose, observing symptoms, and measuring blood glucose levels. When 0.75 to 1.5 g of lactose per kilogram of body weight is administered, the presence of symptoms and a rise in blood glucose concentration of less than 20 mg/dL above the fasting level are considered diagnostic of the disorder. Measurement of breath hydrogen after the ingestion of 50 g of lactose is a more sensitive and specific test. Lactase deficiency in older adults is important because of the potential for chronic deficiency of calcium and protein intake. The appearance of lactose intolerance as a new symptom should prompt consideration of other underlying gastrointestinal disease.[118,119]

Although lactase activity commonly declines with advancing age, the concentrations of intestinal sucrase and maltase are unchanged. In the rat, there appears to be an age-related decline in small intestinal glucose transport activity.[120] In humans, small intestinal sodium-glucose transport has not consistently been demonstrated to be altered with aging.[120,121] There is no known clinical consequence of altered sodium-glucose cotransport with aging.

## Celiac Disease (Gluten-Sensitive Enteropathy)

Celiac disease, also known as gluten-sensitive enteropathy, results from small intestinal mucosal injury caused by dietary exposure to wheat gluten. The classic symptoms of this disease include diarrhea, bloating, and weight loss, which are a result of the profound malabsorption and steatorrhea seen in these patients. Celiac disease is more common in females, found in a female-to-male ratio of approximately 3:1.[122] The occurrence of this disease in older adults is not widely recognized, and its manifestations may be atypical. In contrast to earlier descriptions, recent reports suggest that as many as 25% of patients with celiac disease may be first diagnosed in later years.[123–125] Most patients with this disease do not present with the classic symptoms of diarrhea with steatorrhea, osteomalacia, or anemia, but they may have more subtle findings, including nonspecific gastrointestinal complaints that may be transient or acute. In over half the reported cases, abnormalities of the blood count, including macrocytosis and mild anemia, prompted further investigation. In older patients, an abnormally low serum folate level may also indicate the presence of celiac disease.[126]

Cachexia, depression, fatigue, and anemia in older individuals usually lead to consideration of occult malignancy rather than primary gastrointestinal disease. Although the mimicking of malignancy appears to be a more common feature of celiac disease in older patients, other manifestations are typical but often misdiagnosed (eg, edema attributed to heart disease, osteomalacia attributed to osteoporosis, and wasting due to occult malignancy elsewhere). Older patients may present with small intestinal ulcerations, a syndrome of splenic atrophy, villous atrophy and cavitation of mesenteric lymph nodes, or subacute intestinal pseudo-obstruction.[127–129] Occult gastrointestinal bleeding may occur in about half of patients with celiac disease and may result in iron deficiency.[130] The diagnosis of celiac disease is dependent on a small bowel biopsy that demonstrates the typical features of a flat mucosa due to villous atrophy. The presence of antigluten or antireticulin immunoglobulin A or immunoglobulin G antibodies in the plasma has long been used as a screening test in adults.[131] However, more recently it has been recognized that the IgA antiendomysial antibody test is the most sensitive and specific noninvasive diagnostic test available.[132] The breath hydrogen test differentiates patients with celiac disease from normal subjects but does not identify those who have bacterial overgrowth.[133]

The laboratory features of celiac disease reflect the profound disturbance of absorption in the proximal intestine, resulting in steatorrhea and malabsorption of iron and folic acid but typically preservation of vitamin $B_{12}$ and bile salt absorption. This dysfunction of intestinal digestion and absorption due to enzyme depletion is secondary to the early exfoliation of maturing enterocytes. These abnormal findings return to normal after treatment with a gluten-free diet, although lactase deficiency may persist or be slow to improve.[134]

The treatment of celiac disease in older patients consists of the removal of gluten from the diet. Most patients will respond, but those patients with profound malnutrition and debility are at risk for death due to infection and hemorrhage. In such extreme cases, nutritional support measures may be necessary to facilitate the establishment of adequate oral feeding. Older patients may require additional training to successfully alter their dietary intake. Management of calcium and vitamin D metabolism needs to be attended to and may require oral supplementation. Failure to respond to a gluten-free diet should prompt consideration of underlying complicating diagnoses, such as intestinal lymphoma.

## Bacterial Overgrowth

The small intestinal bacterial overgrowth syndrome is one of the most important clinical conditions that more frequently occurs in older adults. The upper gastrointestinal tract is normally considered sterile, with fewer than $10^3$ organisms per milliliter of intestinal secretions. Occult malabsorption caused by bacterial contamination of the small intestine is more common in older individuals than is generally recognized. Of 24 patients with unrecognized malabsorption in the presence of clinical malnutrition, 17 were found to have bacterial contamination associated with duodenal-jejunal diverticula, postgastrectomy syndrome, or otherwise normal gastrointestinal anatomy.[135] This condition of overgrowth of abnormal microflora in the small intestine is variously called the *blind loop syndrome, stagnate loop syndrome,* or *small intestinal stasis syndrome.* The condition can occur in patients who have abnormal bacterial flora without stasis. The overgrowth

of microflora disturbs intraluminal digestion and mucosal function and results in malabsorption of fat, protein, carbohydrate, electrolytes, and vitamin $B_{12}$. Malnutrition due to steatorrhea and macrocytic anemia due to vitamin $B_{12}$ deficiency frequently develop.

The normal human jejunum is populated by a variable number of transient organisms derived from oral pharyngeal sources. Ileal bacterial populations are somewhat higher and reflect a colonic origin. Protective mechanisms in the proximal gut include acidity of the stomach and the normal cleansing activity of proximal small intestinal motility. Diseases, operations, or medications that reduce gastric acidity are correlated with high levels of bacterial contamination, as are conditions that reduce small intestinal motility, such as scleroderma, diabetes and pseudo-obstruction. Older adults are at increased risk to develop small intestinal bacterial overgrowth due to the high prevalence of atrophic gastritis with hypochlorhydria or achlorhydria. Immunologic secretions (from the intestines, liver, and pancreas), the mucous barrier, and bile acids probably play a lesser role in protecting against or reducing bacterial overgrowth. When bacterial contamination of the proximal intestine occurs, anaerobic organisms form a large proportion of the total and result in multiple disturbances of intraluminal digestion and mucosal absorption. The contaminating bacteria deconjugate bile acids, reducing their concentration, and thus interfere with fat digestion. Malabsorption of the fat-soluble vitamins (vitamins A, D, E, and K) may occur in association with generalized fat malabsorption. Bacterial overgrowth also contributes to denaturation of ingested protein, disturbed function of brush border enzymes, and probable protein loss from injured mucosa. In adults, the D-xylose tolerance test may become abnormal because of bacterial fermentation and impaired mucosal absorption. As a result of malabsorption, the end products of bacterial metabolism contribute to diarrhea and water and electrolyte losses.

Although pathogenic bacteria in the upper gastrointestinal tract cause the bacterial overgrowth syndrome, not all bacteria that can grow in the upper gastrointestinal tract result in adverse clinical conditions. Coliforms and anaerobes are the typical organisms responsible for the bacterial overgrowth syndrome. However, bacterial colonization of the upper gastrointestinal tract that occurs solely from a lack of gastric acid, whether due to atrophic gastritis or medications, may have few adverse clinical manifestations.[136] Thus, "simple" colonization of the upper gastrointestinal tract is clinically silent and is not typically detected. However, most older persons with steatorrhea of unclear etiology will have occult intestinal bacterial overgrowth.[137]

The clinical symptoms of the bacterial overgrowth syndrome include abdominal pain, bloating, diarrhea, and weight loss. Older adults often have nonspecific symptoms such as bloating and nausea with manifestations of weight loss or malnutrition. Thus, a high index of suspicion is required to diagnose the bacterial overgrowth syndrome in older adults who present in a subtle manner.

Clinical investigation of these patients is directed toward defining anatomic defects or disturbed motility that would contribute to stasis and identifying conditions that reduce bacterial defenses. In addition to the usual diagnostic studies for malabsorption (such as stool examination for fecal fat and D-xylose absorption studies), hydrogen breath tests, small bowel biopsy, and collection of intestinal contents for microbiologic analysis may be done.[138] However, the diagnosis may be difficult, as the noninvasive tests are not totally accurate and the invasive tests are rarely performed. The most widely accepted noninvasive tests are the glucose- and lactulose-hydrogen breath tests, with sensitivities of about 80%. The most accurate noninvasive test is the 1-g [14]C D-xylose breath test, with a sensitivity of 95%, but unfortunately it is not available at most centers.[99] However, the "gold standard" test is considered to be intestinal intubation with a sterile tube, with aspiration of intestinal contents and subsequent microbiologic quantitative assays. Typically, this is done at the time of upper endoscopy. It is relatively expensive and has potential side effects. Thus, most clinicians will empirically diagnose the bacterial overgrowth syndrome and initiate a diagnostic trial of antibiotics.

The underlying cause of the small intestinal bacterial overgrowth syndrome should be corrected if possible. As most conditions that cause this syndrome are not easily correctable, antibiotics are the mainstay of treatment. Antibiotics are typically given in 2-week courses that may have to be repeated at varying intervals, or rotating antibiotic courses may be necessary depending on the situation. Nutrition support is also important with appropriate therapy for micronutrient deficiency, fat malabsorption, lactose maldigestion, and fat-soluble vitamin deficiency.

## Inflammatory Bowel Disease

Ulcerative colitis and Crohn's disease represent two diagnostic categories of inflammatory diseases of the bowel of unknown etiology. Ulcerative colitis is a mucosal disease limited to the colon and involves the rectum and contiguous parts of the colon proximally to varying degrees. Crohn's disease more typically affects the ileum and proximal portions of the colon and tends to be more segmental, with skipped areas of normal-appearing bowel. Because of the involvement of the small intestine and the propensity for perforation of the bowel with fistula and abscess formation, Crohn's disease has, for most patients, a greater negative impact on nutritional state than does chronic ulcerative colitis. Both diseases occur more frequently in young patients, with onset during the teenage years and the 20s. Onset after age 60 years probably accounts for less than 10% of patients. Published studies of the epidemiology of inflammatory bowel disease may underestimate the true prevalence by 27% to 38%; examination of asymptomatic patients between the ages of 50 and 75 years during a screening study for colorectal cancer uncovered 8 people with previously undiagnosed inflammatory bowel disease among approximately 18,000 participants.[139] Many patients diagnosed with inflammatory bowel disease after age 60 years are probably suffering from ischemic colitis or infectious colitis instead.[140,141]

Of patients older than 60 years who have inflammatory bowel disease, some have had early onset and survived to advanced age with potential complications of intestinal and extraintestinal involvement, sequelae of surgical treatment, and side effects of earlier or continuing medical treatment. Others have had recent onset of this disease, often in the presence of other acute and chronic diseases common in older people. Analysis of the nutritional needs of these patients relies on an understanding of the clinical spectrum of the disease, the extent and severity of intestinal involvement, the duration of illness, and the side effects of medical and surgical treatment. In older adults, typical presentations of diseases are overall less common, and this disparity can lead to delays in both proper diagnosis and treatment.[142]

There is a suggestion that some features of late-onset ulcerative colitis distinguish it from early-onset disease. Late-onset disease is less extensive, being more frequently limited to the rectum and the left colon rather than involving the entire colon. Diarrhea is more severe and is accompanied by less bleeding. At the onset of the disease, the illness is more protracted, is perhaps less responsive to treatment, and has shorter remissions. Of great importance in older patients is that significant weight loss, anemia, and frequent hospitalizations are more common.[143]

In older adults, many of the symptoms of Crohn's disease, including diarrhea, cramping abdominal pain, fatigue, weight loss, and low-grade fever, might easily be attributed to underlying malignancy. Features that usually alert the clinician to the presence of Crohn's disease include the anorectal manifestations of fistulas and abscesses. Anemia, hypoproteinemia, and malnutrition are caused by the chronic inflammatory process, poor oral intake, increased gastrointestinal losses, and malabsorption. Older patients with Crohn's disease are more likely to have left-sided colonic involvement than are younger cohorts, who more commonly have isolated ileal disease.[144]

The treatment of inflammatory bowel disease in older patients does not differ substantially from that in younger patients. 5-Aminosalicylate medications, corticosteroids, and metronidazole are commonly used drugs. Other immunosuppressants are used for patients with intractable disease. Sulfasalazine has an antifolate effect and may contribute to gastrointestinal side effects that include epigastric discomfort and chronic headache. Corticosteroids can exacerbate diabetes mellitus, cause hypertension, accelerate osteoporosis, and complicate conditions marked by salt and water retention, such as congestive heart failure and renal failure. As in younger patients, older patients with late-onset disease often require surgery.[145]

## Radiation Enteritis

Radiation enteritis results from a dose-related injury to the intestine, most commonly associated with radiation treatment of cancer of the cervix, uterus, prostate, rectum, sigmoid, and bladder. As the population ages and more patients become candidates for radiation therapy, this side effect will become more prevalent. In the acute form, radiation enteritis typically causes diarrhea but is usually self-limited; when severe, it may be sufficient to interrupt treatment.[146] When the disease has continued beyond 3 months, it is considered chronic, and its importance probably is underestimated. Most patients do not seek medical help until serious complications occur.[147]

Radiation therapy typically injures cells that divide rapidly, so crypt cells in the small intestine are particularly vulnerable. The chronic form of the disease is thought to be due to a progressive, irreversible ischemia that results in a fibrinous peritonitis in which loops of intestine are bound together. Fibrosis, submucosal edema of the bowel wall, and perforation occur. Ulceration of the mucosa is common; deeper ulcerations are associated with perforation. Mucosal areas of atrophy are also present, and scarring results in luminal narrowing.

The severity of radiation injury based on findings and symptoms is categorized as mild, consisting of diarrhea controlled by diet and reassurance; marked, noted by diarrhea and rectal pain and relieved by medications; or severe, characterized by fistulization, perforation, and stricture. Patients with diabetic vascular disease and atherosclerosis are at greatest risk of developing severe radiation enteritis.

The latent period between radiation therapy and the onset of symptoms can be years. Initial symptoms include postprandial fullness, nausea, and cramping, which progress to distention and vomiting. In a retrospective review of 3900 patients at risk for chronic radiation enteritis, O'Brien and colleagues[148] documented the typical course of these patients. Patients with early symptoms were hospitalized and treated with nasogastric suction and intravenous fluids; there were clinical findings of incomplete bowel obstruction. Diets were advanced as tolerated, and patients were discharged on a soft diet. Repeated episodes of partial small bowel obstruction followed, and patients continued to deteriorate over time. Once this cycle of recurrent small bowel obstruction occurred, all patients ultimately required surgical treatment. Bowel obstruction was due to narrowed, thickened bowel wall rather than to associated adhesions. Resection and anastomosis of bowel often were not possible, and bypass of affected segments was required.[148]

Multiple factors contribute to the risk of chronic radiation injury to the bowel, including adhesions due to prior surgery, pelvic inflammatory bowel disease, extremely low body weight, diabetes mellitus, cardiovascular disease, preexisting vascular compromise of the bowel, and combined chemotherapy and radiation therapy.[149] Some surgeons advise wide excision of affected bowel rather than bypass.[150,151]

## Acute Radiation Enteritis

The treatment of acute radiation enteritis consists of the symptomatic use of antidiarrheal agents, including opiates and anticholinergic drugs. Cholestyramine, a bile salt–binding agent, is used on the basis of the hypothesis that injured distal small bowel fails to resorb bile salts. Bile salts entering the colon have a profound secretory effect; binding the salts reduces these effects.[152] The use of elemental diet therapy to prevent radiation injury has led to conflicting results. McArdle and associates[153] studied the effect of elemental diets before and during radiation therapy for invasive bladder cancer, using retrospective controls. A peptide-based formula was given orally, by nasoenteric tube, or by needle jejunostomy; symptoms improved, and small bowel function returned promptly with early passage of flatus and feces. Patients treated with nutritional support had no microscopic damage to the ileum. On electron microscopic examination, there was preservation of the normal glycocalyx, preservation of cell microstructure and tight cell junctions, and greater preservation of brush border enzymes. It is not certain what role, if any, other factors, such as pancreatic biliary secretions or mechanical effects of regular diet, have in the pathophysiology of intestinal injury.[153]

### Chronic Radiation Enteritis

Unfortunately, the lesions of chronic radiation enteritis, including mucosal injury, evidence of stricture with bowel stasis, and perforation with fistula formation, are probably not reversible. A variety of treatment programs have been tried, with a mixture of results. These include treatments for bile salt diarrhea and bacterial stasis syndrome and the use of a variety of anti-inflammatory agents. Unfortunately, many pathophysiologic factors are probably operating, so the efficacy of low-fat diets, low-residue diets, gluten-free or lactose-deficient diets, and elemental diets remains to be established. Parenteral nutrition has been used to induce weight gain, to correct hypoproteinemia, and to close fistulas.[154]

As noted above, many of these patients eventually have surgical treatment. Resection and bypass often result in short bowel syndrome. During the management of the patient with radiation enteritis, it is important to recognize that premorbid malnutrition often is present. Radiated tissues heal

poorly, and dehiscence of wounds and infection are common complications. Nutritional rehabilitation must await metabolic recovery from surgery and the initiation of the convalescent phase.

## LIVER

Significant morphologic and functional changes in the liver due to aging are of interest to the clinician because alterations in synthetic, excretory, or metabolic processes can affect the response to disease and the disposition of drugs. However, most hepatic changes are due to systemic disease and the liver diseases commonly seen in older individuals.

Liver weight decreases after age 50 years, parallel to the anthropometric changes of decreased body weight and muscle mass. In advanced age, the liver becomes disproportionately small.[155] On the basis of microscopic observations, these changes appear to be due to diminished numbers of hepatocytes.[156] Other changes in liver morphology are nonspecific and may be due to extrahepatic processes. There is an increase in portal and periportal fibrosis, and liver cells tend to be larger, with larger or multiple nuclei and nucleoli. Enlargement of the liver cells may be due to compensatory hypertrophy. An increased amount of lipofuscin pigment is present in the Kupffer cells,[157,158] and changes in the Golgi apparatus and rough and smooth endoplasmic reticulum may parallel hepatic functional changes seen in older subjects.[159]

### Liver Function and Aging

Decreases in liver blood flow from 0.3% to 1.5% per year occur with age.[160,161] Alterations in serum bilirubin, transaminases, alkaline phosphatase, dye tests of hepatic excretion (sulfobromophthalein sodium), and radioactive labeled excretion tests (Rose Bengal) do not occur in older people with histologically normal livers.[162] Levels of albumin, a product of hepatic synthesis, are frequently reduced in the older adults. Although albumin metabolism is influenced by many factors, it appears that the rate of albumin synthesis in older people is not sensitive to changes in protein intake, suggesting an altered set point in synthetic rate.[163]

The potential for changes in drug metabolism in the aging liver is of greater concern to clinicians than the apparent minor and probably insignificant changes in morphology and function.[164] The reduction of lean body mass and total body water alters the distribution of water-soluble and fat-soluble drugs (Chapter 14). The disposition and side effects of drugs in older patients are of concern.[165] Contrary to conventionally held views, impaired clearance of drugs may not be due to reduced hepatic microsomal enzyme activity. Further study is required to understand this important subject.[166] No generalizations can be made about drug disposition with respect to altered blood flow, drug distribution, and principal metabolic pathways. Nutritional factors can be important, however, as levels of vitamin C and folic acid have been associated with decreased antipyrine clearance in older people.[167]

The rate of total-body protein synthesis is decreased in older individuals; much of this decrease is presumed to be in the liver.[168] In animal studies, synthesis of nucleic acids and proteins in old liver cells is diminished.[169] There is an increase in the synthesis of faulty proteins; such "junk" proteins may account for disturbed drug disposition and function.[170]

**Liver Disease in the Older Population**

Little has been written about the influence of multisystem disease on the liver, which may be of great importance in older adults. For cardiac, renal, diabetic, stroke, and arthritic patients, among others, the poorly understood intertwining effects of disease, treatment, and complications on nutrition and hepatic function must be considered rationally.

Chronic or acute alcohol use, starvation, protein-energy malnutrition, obesity, diabetes mellitus, and hypothyroidism can alter hepatic lipoprotein metabolism and cause fatty liver. Fatty liver can be associated with some element of liver cell necrosis when alcohol or drugs are involved. Fat in liver cells results from an imbalance of oxidation, esterification, or excretion of fatty acids that accumulate from a flux of fatty acids from adipose tissue to the liver. Generally, fatty liver does not interfere with hepatic function but results only in enlargement of the liver. Advanced cases may be associated with cholestasis, portal hypertension, and ascites. Liver cell necrosis accompanying fatty liver is a precursor of a progressive fibrotic process that may lead to cirrhosis.

Nonhepatitis causes of jaundice predominate in older patients.[171] Drugs account for 20% of causes of jaundice in this group.[172] Although adverse drug reactions are more common in older subjects, and although systemic and hepatic alterations exist that can affect drug disposition, there is little evidence that the older liver is more susceptible to drug injury. There is some evidence to suggest that when injury occurs it may be more severe, as in the case of fatal anesthesia-induced liver disease. Commonly used drugs that may have an adverse effect on the liver include NSAIDs, anesthetic agents, antibiotics, antimetabolic agents, antihypertensives, cardiac drugs, and psychotropic drugs.[173,174]

Viral hepatitis is most often due to hepatitis C associated with blood transfusions before testing for hepatitis C was available. The clinical course of patients older than 60 years is not different from that of younger patients, although the illness may progress more rapidly in older adults.[175] However, acute type B hepatitis, especially when associated with other illness, has a higher risk of severe disease and hepatic failure.[176,177] In older patients with severe liver disease, age adversely affects prognosis.[178]

Primary biliary cirrhosis represents a model of cholestatic liver disease. There is chronic destruction of the bile ducts that results in cirrhosis and eventual liver failure. Although it is usually considered a disease of middle age, the age range of presentation is actually 20 to 80 years.[179] Fatigue and pruritus are the usual presenting symptoms. Since there is no specific treatment for this disease, symptomatic relief and prevention of the nutritional complications are the current treatment aims. Late in the disease, when hepatic cirrhosis and its complications develop, liver transplantation is indicated.

Older cirrhotics often are asymptomatic. The cirrhosis is caused by multiple factors and is not an inherent characteristic of aging. The peak incidence of cirrhosis due to alcoholism occurs beyond age 60. There may be few clinical indicators of this disease.[180] Patients with primary biliary cirrhosis who are survivors of early-onset disease have associated long-standing metabolic complications in old age.[181,182]

## Nutrition in Liver Disease

It is unlikely that there are unique nutritional factors in the cause or treatment of liver disease in older patients, but changes that occur in digestion, absorption, and intermediary metabolism as a result of acute or chronic liver cell injury or cholestasis do affect nutrition.

### Fatty Liver

Hepatic lipid metabolism can be disturbed at many points and can result in fat accumulation. Alcohol increases lipolysis, causing a flow of fatty acids to the liver; increases intrahepatic lipid synthesis; decreases fatty acid oxidation in the liver; increases triglyceride formation; and decreases the release of lipoprotein in the form of VLDLs. It is uncertain where alcohol exerts its greatest effect, but a direct hepatotoxic effect of alcohol is favored.[183] Nutritional deficiency is not essential for the formation of acute fatty liver, but it does seem to have some modifying effect, perhaps increasing the severity of the condition when serious levels of nutritional deficiency exist.[184] The source of fatty acids that accumulate as triglyceride in the liver cell differs depending on the fed state of the individual. Under fasting conditions, the source is adipose tissue. During the fed state, triglycerides are of intestinal origin. Stress hormones in acute alcohol intoxication may play a role.[185,186] It is unclear whether alcohol-induced hepatic fatty acid synthesis, decreased oxidation, or decreased secretion of triglycerides is most important.[183] It is generally accepted that alcohol-induced fatty liver is reversible. As many as one third of asymptomatic alcoholics may have fatty liver.[183]

Fatty liver can also have features of cholestasis with jaundice and abnormal liver-associated enzymes. Some patients with fatty liver due to alcohol ingestion actually develop hepatitis with evidence of liver cell necrosis. These patients often have anorexia, nausea, vomiting, fever, and jaundice.

The treatment of acute alcoholic fatty liver is abstinence from alcohol. Principles of general nutrition dictate a well-balanced diet, adequate protein and calorie intake without overfeeding, and supplementation with vitamins. Prolonged fasting and starvation can produce fatty liver; this is especially true when the classic adaptation to starvation, which involves the change from peripheral oxidation of glucose to oxidation of fatty acid products, is blocked by carbohydrate feeding. In the classic form of starvation disease, kwashiorkor, fatty liver is a feature. It is treated with a high-protein diet.[187] It is probable that the fat in the livers of these patients arises not from mobilization of peripheral fat stores but rather from glucose administration, resulting in intrahepatic lipid synthesis.[188] Low serum levels of albumin and of VLDLs suggest an impairment of hepatic lipoprotein and protein synthesis that is reversible with protein feeding.[189] In fatty liver associated with obesity, insulin resistance and increased levels of free fatty acids are probably secondary to increased adipose tissue mass.[190] Fatty infiltration is potentially reversible by weight reduction. Fatty liver and diabetes are often associated.[187] Obesity, occurring in about 45% of diabetics older than 60 years, may be a more important factor in type II diabetics. Recommendations for treatment include weight reduction and a low-carbohydrate, high-protein diet. Fatty liver seen with total parenteral nutrition is probably due to excessive calorie infusion.

### Acute Hepatitis

Whatever the primary cause of acute hepatitis, extensive liver cell necrosis leads to fulminant hepatic failure and impairment of nearly all hepatic functions, including carbohydrate, protein, and lipid metabolism; the catabolic rate is also increased. Hypoglycemia is a common feature of fulminant hepatic failure due to impaired hepatic gluconeogenesis and reduced liver glycogen content. These effects are exacerbated by hyperinsulinemia caused by increased insulin production and increased peripheral insulin resistance.[191]

Characteristic derangements in amino acid metabolism occur in severe liver disease with altered plasma amino acid patterns. More than 85% of the liver must be nonfunctional before these patterns develop. Increased levels of tyrosine, phenylalanine, glutamine, and methionine and decreased levels of valine, leucine, and isoleucine are seen in chronic hepatic encephalopathy; but in fulminant hepatic failure, branched-chain amino acids are either normal or slightly depressed, while there is a marked elevation of all others, probably representing amino acid release from dying liver cells.[192] The urea cycle, which is responsible for the clearance of metabolic nitrogen, is depressed in fulminant hepatic failure and leads to low urea levels and hyperammonemia.

For patients who have severe hepatic failure, hypoalbuminemia and edema are due to a substantial loss of hepatic protein synthetic activity (to less than 10% of normal). Reduced synthesis of vitamin K–dependent clotting factors can contribute to increased prothrombin time. If patients are unresponsive to vitamin K supplementation, bleeding complications are exacerbated. Low levels of total cholesterol, triglycerides, and esterified cholesterol are seen in fulminant hepatic failure.

For most patients who have acute hepatitis of various etiologies, no specific nutritional treatment measures are necessary unless anorexia, nausea, or vomiting becomes protracted. The anorexia seen in acute liver disease is best managed by a high-carbohydrate diet, with the greatest number of calories provided in the morning meal. If oral intake is poor or not possible, intravenous fluids containing glucose should be provided. In patients who have fulminant hepatic failure, continuous infusions of concentrated glucose sufficient to maintain normal serum glucose levels may be necessary. The negative nitrogen balance seen in fulminant hepatic failure makes the use of protein infusions at the rate of 0.8 to 1 g/kg of body weight rational. However, this often works out to be a practice of compromises because of limited protein tolerance and fluid overload. Lipid emulsions are not recommended in fulminant hepatic failure when hepatic encephalopathy is present. Supplemental vitamins, especially folic acid and vitamins $B_6$ and $B_{12}$, should be provided.[193]

### Cholestasis

Because of the chronic course of primary biliary cirrhosis, this cholestatic disease has the most profound nutritional consequences. The decreased secretion of conjugated bile salts into the intestine leads to steatorrhea and bone disease.[194–196] Diarrhea, weight loss, and muscle wasting occur in patients when steatorrhea is significant. Reduced intake of neutral triglycerides and substitution of medium-chain triglycerides for calories can be effective in the treatment of this condition, since bile salts are not necessary for medium-chain triglyceride absorption.[195]

Although osteomalacia has been assumed to be the principal bone disease of primary biliary cirrhosis, osteoporosis appears to be more important.[197] Nevertheless, treatment is directed toward correcting calcium and vitamin D metabolism, although the results are mixed. Despite normal 25-hydroxyvitamin $D_3$ levels achieved by monthly intramuscular injections of vitamin $D_3$, bone disease continues.[198] Vitamin K deficiency has been demonstrated, and vitamin E deficiency is common in primary biliary cirrhosis.[199] Vitamin A levels are low in primary biliary cirrhosis, but symptoms are not commonly noted. Zinc deficiency has also been reported in association with symptomatic vitamin A deficiency.[200] Cholestyramine, which is used to bind and increase the elimination of bile salts in cholestatic liver disease, contributes to steatorrhea and the malabsorption of fat-soluble vitamins, as well as vitamin C.[201]

### Cirrhosis

Inadequate dietary intake is the most likely principal cause of malnutrition in patients with liver disease.[201] Decreased sensitivity to taste and smell may contribute to decreased or altered oral intake in the cirrhotic patient.[202] Factors that contribute to malnutrition include anorexia, nausea, poor palatability of special diets, and the indirect effects of chronic alcohol use and its social consequences.[201] The alcoholic cirrhotic may have both pancreatic insufficiency and injury to the small intestinal mucosa.[203,204] These changes are probably mediated to some extent by nutritional deficiency.[205–207] Steatorrhea, usually of mild extent, is also seen in cirrhotics; whether it is due to the effects of portal hypertension on gut congestion and lymphatic drainage or to diminished bile salt secretion is unclear.[208,209]

Changes in glucose, amino acid, and fat metabolism that occur in cirrhosis resemble those of normal adaptation to prolonged starvation. Calorie requirements of stable alcoholic cirrhotics are no different from those of normal subjects. Ketogenesis and gluconeogenesis are increased, probably reflecting the mobilization of peripheral fats and amino acids and resulting in the typical wasted appearance of patients with advanced cirrhosis.[210] Abnormally high insulin levels due to hypersecretion and reduced hepatic clearance are not associated with the usual inverse relationship and peripheral branched-chain amino acid levels in cirrhotics. Peripheral insulin resistance may account for this abnormality.[211] A protein intake of 0.8 to 1 g/kg of body weight with branched-chain or branched-chain–enriched formulas by oral or parenteral means is appropriate. Lipoprotein metabolism is disturbed in severe hepatic insufficiency. The major defects appear to be due to impaired triglyceride release by the liver rather than to disturbances of peripheral fat oxidation; lipid emulsions therefore are probably contraindicated in patients who have advanced, severe, acute liver disease. Supplementation with folic acid, vitamins $B_6$ and

$B_{12}$, and multivitamins is rational. A trial of parenteral vitamin K administration when low prothrombin levels exist is common.

Clinically significant vitamin B deficiency has been demonstrated in alcoholic patients with macrocytosis, megaloblastic changes, or microcytic anemia associated with low serum folate levels, and peripheral neuropathy is often associated with low thiamine levels; nicotinic acid and riboflavin deficiencies are often seen.[212] Septicemia frequently may accompany end-stage cirrhosis, resulting in metabolic stress.[213]

### Hepatic Encephalopathy

Hepatic encephalopathy occurs as a syndrome of impaired mental function in the setting of severe, acute, or chronic liver disease. Factors that contribute to it are multiple, and they differ depending on the clinical circumstances. The diagnosis is based on clinical features, including disturbed consciousness, which ranges from sleepiness to coma and occasionally delirium. Personality changes are most remarkable in patients who have chronic liver disease. It may be difficult to differentiate the effects of alcohol from those of hepatic encephalopathy. Specialized testing may be needed in mild cases. With advanced disease, there is gross confusion, disturbed speech, and a flapping tremor. Hepatic coma is graded on a scale of 1 through 5: grade 1, confused state with altered mood and behavior with psychometric defects; grade 2, drowsiness and inappropriate behavior; grade 3, stupor, ability to obey simple commands, inarticulate speech, marked confusion; grade 4, coma; grade 5, deep coma, no response to painful stimuli. In fulminant hepatic failure, the syndrome is due to liver cell necrosis. In cirrhosis, it is due to portosystemic shunting with other precipitating factors. In fulminant hepatic failure, the finding of hepatic encephalopathy indicates a very poor prognosis, although the symptoms are reversible if the liver recovers. In cirrhosis, the reversibility depends on the inciting factors. These findings suggest that a metabolic agent or agents interfere with normal cerebral activity. The specific nature and mechanism of action is unknown.

Current theories of hepatic encephalopathy are based on the hypotheses that the agent is nitrogenous; arises from the colon as a result of intestinal bacterial action; is present in the portal venous system; normally would be metabolized by the liver; and, under the clinical circumstances of hepatic encephalopathy, is able to enter the brain and impair function. In fulminant hepatic failure, the liver cells are unable to metabolize the agent. In cirrhotic liver, blood bypasses the liver by portal-systemic shunting. Candidate toxins include amino acids (eg, methionine), aromatic amino acids, and gamma-aminobutyric acid. The production of these agents and their transport to and into the brain, as well as brain function, can be modified by serum amino acid imbalance, alkalosis, and hypoxemia.[178]

Treatment of hepatic encephalopathy is pragmatic. Medical measures are directed at precipitating factors and at identifying and treating sources of infection, gastrointestinal bleeding, and electrolyte disturbances. Toxic medications and alcohol are withdrawn. Sources of nitrogen load are eliminated or reduced. If excess nitrogen is suspected in the intestines, they are purged; diuretics are discontinued, and antibiotics may be administered to decrease bacterial ammonia production. The synthetic disaccharide lactulose is not digested by the human intestinal mucosa but is broken down by colonic bacteria to produce fatty acids, yielding a low fecal pH; it alters colonic bacterial populations to reduce ammonia production. Although the mechanism of action is uncertain, total fecal output is increased, as well as fecal nitrogen.

While these measures are undertaken, dietary protein is discontinued, and calories are provided in carbohydrate form intravenously or by enteral feeding tube. As the patient improves, protein is added in 20-g increments on alternate days in divided doses of four meals. In chronic encephalopathic patients, it may be necessary to restrict protein intake.[214] The appropriateness of vegetable instead of meat protein diets is controversial, but some authors have demonstrated advantages.[214-216] The ratio of branched-chain to aromatic amino acids is reduced in hepatic encephalopathy, and infusions of branched-chain acids have been used in its treatment, but it is difficult to justify their use except in patients with encephalopathy refractory to all other forms of treatment, given their high cost.[217]

### Ascites

The formation of cirrhotic ascites is another serious manifestation of liver failure. The accumulation of a protein-rich fluid in the peritoneal cavity occurs as a result of venous outflow obstruction in the liver. This results in an elevated hydrostatic pressure of the liver sinusoid, transudation of plasma into the space of disse, and increased liver lymph flow. When the capacity of the lymphatic system is exceeded, fluid begins to accumulate in the peritoneal cavity. Factors contributing to the shift of fluid include low levels of plasma albumin, resulting in a low plasma oncotic pressure. In response to baroreceptors in the liver, the kidney is less able to excrete a salt load, which results in a net retention of sodium. A second alteration in renal function is impaired excretion of water loads. This multiple organ system dysfunction in patients with advanced cirrhotic ascites makes patient management and dietary treatment complex.

Although the presence of ascites dictates the need to determine its exact cause and to exclude other treatable disorders, the presence of ascites per se does not demand treatment. When ascites is massive or tense, it can interfere with respiration, can cause discomfort, and (when extreme) can contribute to herniation and necrosis of the umbilicus, resulting in spontaneous rupture and death. A traditional approach to the treatment of ascites involves a therapeutic trial of bed rest and sodium restriction. When a careful history reveals a recent substantial increase in salt intake or exacerbation of a reversible liver disease, the prognosis for response is quite good. However, patients with cirrhotic ascites require a more substantial restriction of sodium intake than do typical patients with heart disease. Restrictions as low as 250 to 500 mg of sodium per day are often required. This represents a significant challenge to meeting other dietary goals.

If diuresis is not evident within several days, the diuretic spironolactone may be effective in nonazotemic patients. In addition to azotemia, hyperkalemia may limit the usefulness of spironolactone, and often furosemide is given as well to decrease hyperkalemia and promote diuresis. Patients taking spironolactone should not use potassium-containing salt substitutes because of this potential complication. Weight loss should be limited to 1 kg/d. Patients with peripheral edema can tolerate a large volume. In addition to the dietary restriction of salt, at least 50 g of high-biologic protein and a 2000-kcal/d diet are usually recommended. Fluid restriction is not required unless serum sodium levels are below 130 mmol/L.[218]

One treatment that is regaining popularity is large-volume paracentesis. A volume of 4 to 6 L of fluid (and perhaps much more) can be withdrawn safely with fewer complications than occur with standard diuretic programs. In patients without peripheral edema, albumin infusions are necessary to prevent volume contraction and azotemia. Fluid is withdrawn over 20 to 30 minutes and is followed by an infusion of 6 to 8 g of salt-poor albumin per liter of ascites fluid removed.[219]

The advantages of this approach are that it can be accomplished in an outpatient setting with less utilization of hospital resources. The goals of nutritional management are to ensure adequate dietary intake with salt restriction to avoid recurrence, although some patients are able to eliminate salt and water loads more effectively as treatment progresses.

## COLON

Like the gallbladder and the appendix, the colon is not essential for health and well-being. However, for many older people, the colon is a major source of symptoms and disease. The most important function of the colon is its role as a reservoir and final processor of fecal residue. Water, electrolytes, bile salts, and short-chain fatty acids are absorbed. Of the physiologic processes of motility, secretion, and absorption, movement disorders predominate.

Little is known about age-related alterations in structure and function of the colon. Biopsy specimens from healthy older subjects have demonstrated mucosal atrophy, alteration of mucosal glands, muscularis mucosa hypertrophy, increased connective tissue, and changes of atherosclerosis.[220] Electron microscopic cytologic changes in nuclei, cytoplasm, and cell organelles have also been noted but are of questionable significance. The most significant functional change that occurs with aging is constipation; the most important morphologic change is diverticular disease.

### Constipation

Two mechanisms of chronic constipation are known: colon dysmotility and disordered defecation. Contributing causes include drug effects, neurologic disease, structural abnor-malities, and systemic disease. Although constipation often is attributed to diet, behavior, and inactivity, it is a condition of multiple causes. It is a symptomatic disease with decreased frequency of bowel movements, difficult passage, passage of hard stools, or a sensation of incomplete evacuation. In nonconstipated adults, intestinal transit time does not appear to be increased with advancing age.[221] However, colonic transit times may be increased in older adults.[222] Normal bowel habits range from three per week to two per day.[223] Overall bowel habits and stool outputs of older adults are not significantly different than in the young.[224] About 30% of aged women use laxatives regularly. Frequent laxative use has been attributed to social attitudes brought about by popular misconceptions in the early part of the 20th century.[225] Older people who chronically consume laxatives have demonstrated prolonged transit time as well as electromyographic and physiologic changes in colorectal and anal function.[219,226,227]

Postprandial sigmoid, rectosigmoid, and rectal motility in healthy older people is not altered.[228] Abnormalities of anorectal function in older persons include decreased maximal basal and squeeze pressures of the anal canal; higher rectal pressures with distention; reduced tolerance for rectal distention; and progressive neuropathic damage to the nerves of the anal sphincters, which occurs most frequently in women and is probably related to childbirth. Many of these factors also contribute to the risk of incontinence in older people.[229]

A strategy for the effective treatment of chronic constipation involves a careful diagnostic classification and search for underlying and complicating factors. Patients with slow-transit constipation, established by a prolonged colonic transit study, and normal colonic anatomy have either colonic atonia with retention of markers in the right colon or outlet dysfunction with delay of rectosigmoid emptying.[230] Some of these patients may actually suffer from a neuropathic disorder similar to the functional abnormalities found in the esophagus, proximal gastrointestinal tract, and bladder.[231] Patients with outlet dysfunction due to impaired sensory perception or disturbances of anatomy that cause impaired expulsion do not respond to laxatives. These patients may respond to biofeedback or surgical procedures. If transit studies suggest outlet obstruction, further diagnostic evaluation of anorectal physiology is necessary. Patients with normal-transit constipation have either a defecatory disorder or a misperception of what normal bowel function should be.[232,233]

Dietary treatment of constipation invariably involves the addition of dietary or supplemental fiber.[234] An increase of 25% to 40% in fiber intake is accompanied by prevention or elimination of constipation in up to 60% of patients; transit time is also reduced.[235] An intake of 10 to 20 g of bran daily usually is required; initially this almost invariably causes altered bowel habits, distention, and occasional discomfort. Stool bulking is contraindicated in patients who are severely debilitated or who have obstruction as an element of their disease. Coarse bran has a greater laxative effect than fine bran. The concept that the water-holding capacity of bran is the mechanism by which it works may not be true, as similar modifications of stool consistency, weight, and ease of passage were experienced by subjects taking indigestible plastic particles.[236] For older patients who have taken laxatives for years, it is not reasonable to adhere slavishly to a concept of fiber supplementation without laxatives when results of therapeutic efforts dictate otherwise.

When bran supplementation is impractical, preparations containing psyllium seed at a dosage of 1 teaspoon twice daily as a hydrophilic agent are effective when accompanied by generous amounts of fluid. The dosage may be slowly increased and titrated to the desired effect. Since these agents can obstruct the esophagus, they should be avoided in patients with dysphagia or known esophageal strictures. Sugar-containing supplements may alter diabetic control. Many other laxatives commonly used may lead to a cathartic colon or toxic systemic effects. Lactulose may be used, but mineral oil is not recommended because of its interference with fat-soluble vitamin absorption and its potential for pulmonary aspiration. Anthracine purgatives are known to cause degeneration of the myoneural chains of the colon.[225] Nonabsorbable osmotic agents such as lactulose are preferable agents to use if a laxative is needed.

## Diverticulosis

Diverticulosis is a common disorder of older individuals, occurring in 30% of those older than 60 years and 60% of those older than 80 years.[237] The disease is usually asymptomatic. Symptomatic uncomplicated diverticulosis is thought to be essentially the same as irritable bowel syndrome. Diverticulitis is an inflammatory disease that causes obstruction, abdominal pain, and/or bleeding. Most pathophysiologic concepts have included the idea of a specific motility disorder resulting in increased intraluminal pressure. Although diverticulosis increases in frequency with age, among active older people there is no difference in fecal output.[238] There has been no demonstrated increased sigmoid colon pressure with age.[239] Although muscular layers are greatly thickened in diverticular disease, the morphology of muscle cells is normal. There is no evidence that intrinsic changes in muscle cells account for the thickening associated with diverticulosis. There is a progressive elastosis of the taeniae coli compared with normal structures, which supports the concept of a shortening or contracture of the colon as an initiating factor in the development of diverticulosis. This results in a greater cross-section mass of both longitudinal and circular muscle fibers of the muscularis propria. The luminal dimensions are decreased, and therefore higher pressures can be developed with contraction of these circular muscle folds. The length of the taeniae do respond to fecal bulk. Rural Africans consuming a high-fiber diet have a redundant sigmoid colon with a generous lumen.[240]

The usual dietary measures prescribed in diverticulosis are identical with those used in the treatment of irritable bowel syndrome or chronic constipation. Small, undigestable foods such as seeds or nuts are not recommended, as they may obstruct the orifice of a diverticulum and contribute to diverticulitis. Patients with high levels of sigmoid colon obstruction or stenoses, like their constipated cohorts, may be intolerant of usual amounts of dietary or supplementary fibers, so that symptoms of constipation may need to be treated somewhat independently.

## CONCLUSION

Although changes in structure and function of the gastrointestinal tract do occur with aging, they do not seem to be clinically significant in the healthy older population. Enzyme and bicarbonate secretions by the pancreas are diminished; whether this is a result of lessened or faulty enteral stimulation or intrinsic age-related pancreatic insufficiency is not clinically relevant because of the huge pancreatic secretory reserve. Mucosal regeneration of the small bowel is accompanied by functional enzyme-related differentiation, which has been noted to be reduced in laboratory animals, but it does not approach clinical significance, nor has it been demonstrated to be important in human studies. Alteration in motility could have far-reaching effects, but to date clinical problems appear to be caused by disease rather than aging. Alterations resulting from disease have to be the focus for the diagnosis and treatment of malnutrition in the setting of gastrointestinal dysfunction in the older adult.

Chewing and swallowing problems are the most easily recognized causes of nutritional failure because of poor intake, notwithstanding the frequent drug-induced alterations of taste, nausea, or disturbed mood or attention, which also reduce intake. Simple clinical observations can identify these disorders and lead to appropriate diagnostic studies to enable treatment plans. Disturbances of digestion and absorption in the midgut are more occult and difficult to differentiate. A knowledgeable diagnostic approach based on pathophysiologic principles often requires treatment by trial and error when multiple problems exist. Here the collaboration of the dietitian and physician is most important.

The effects of functional gastrointestinal disorders, such as constipation, on dietary intake are difficult to quantify. A lifetime of learned behavior can exasperate attempts at a very scientific approach and necessitate a practical and compromising plan for successful management to include good nutrition goals. In the care of the very old, ethical and spiritual issues may come to dominate the theme of respectful care.

## REFERENCES

1. Pelemans W, Vantrappen G. Oesophageal diseases in the elderly. *Clin Gastroenterol.* 1985;14:635–656.

2. Shaker R, Ren J, Zamir Z, Sarna A, Liu J, Sui Z. Effect of aging, position, and temperature on the threshold volume triggering pharyngeal swallows. *Gastroenterology.* 1994;107:396–402.

3. Siebens H, Trupe MA, Hilary A, et al. Correlates and consequences of eating dependency in institutionalized elderly. *J Am Geriatr Soc.* 1986;34:192–198.

4. Dorff GL, Rytel MW, Farmer SG, et al. Etiologies and characteristic features of pneumonias in a municipal hospital. *Am J Med Sci.* 1973;266:349–358.

5. Ebright JR, Rytel MW. Bacterial pneumonia in the elderly. *J Am Geriatr Soc.* 1980;28:220.

6. Miller RM. Evaluation of swallowing disorders. In: Groher ME, ed. *Dysphagia: Diagnosis and Management.* Stoneham, Mass: Butterworth Publishers; 1984.

7. Dobie RA. Rehabilitation of swallowing disorders. *Am Fam Phys.* 1978;17(5):84–95.

8. Castell DO. Dysphagia in the elderly: likely causes of oropharyngeal dysphagia in elderly patients. *J Am Geriatr Soc.* 1986;34:248.

9. Ravich WJ. Classification of dysphagia on the basis of the clinical examination. In: *Second Symposium on Dysphagia.* Baltimore, Md: Johns Hopkins Swallowing Center; March 1988.

10. Robbins J. Approaches to rehabilitation of neurogenic dysphagia. In: *Second Symposium on Dysphagia.* Baltimore, Md: Johns Hopkins Swallowing Center, March 1988.

11. Ekberg O, Feinberg MJ. Altered swallowing function in elderly patients without dysphagia. *Am J Roentgenol.* 1991;156:1181–1184.

12. Hollis JB, Castell DO. Esophageal function in elderly men. *Ann Intern Med.* 1974;80:371–374.

13. Mold JW, Rankin RA. Symptomatic gastroesophageal reflux in the elderly. *J Am Geriatr Soc.* 1987;35:649–659.

14. Kekki M, Sipponen P, Siurala M. Age behavior of gastric acid secretion in males and females with a normal antral body and body mucosa. *Scand J Gastroenterol.* 1983;18:1009–1016.

15. Bock OA, Arapakis G, Witts LJ, et al. The serum pepsinogen level with special reference to the histology of the gastric mucosa. *Gut.* 1963;4:106–111.

16. Hurwitz A, Brady DA, Schaal E, Samloff IM, Dedon J, Ruhl CE. Gastric acidity in older adults. *JAMA.* 1997;278:659–662.

17. Saltzman JR. Epidemiology and natural history of atrophic gastritis. In: Holt PR, Russell RM, eds. *Chronic Gastritis and Hypochlorhydria in the Elderly.* Boca Raton, La: CRC Press; 1993:31–47.

18. Strickland R, Mackay I. A reappraisal of the nature and significance of chronic atrophic gastritis. *Dig Dis Sci.* 1973;18:426–437.

19. Krasinski SD, Russell RM, Samloff IM, et al. Fundic atrophic gastritis in an elderly population: effect on hemoglobin and several serum nutritional indicators. *J Am Geriatr Soc.* 1986;34(11):800–806.

20. Stricklin RG, Mackay IR. A reappraisal of the nature and significance of chronic atrophic gastritis. *Am J Dig Dis.* 1973;18:426–440.

21. Siurala M, Isokoski M, Varis K, et al. Prevalence of gastritis in a rural population: bioptic study of subjects selected at random. *Scand J Gastroenterol.* 1968;3:211–223.

22. Saltzman JR, Kowdley KV. The consequences of *Helicobacter pylori* infection and gastritis. *Contemp Intern Med.* 1994;6:7–16.

23. Elashoff JD, Grossman MI. Trends in hospital admissions and death rates for peptic ulcer in the United States from 1970 to 1978. *Gastroenterology.* 1980;78:28–285.

24. Sonneberg A. Changes in physician visits for gastric and duodenal ulcer in the United States during 1958–1984 as shown by National Disease and Therapeutic Index. *Dig Dis Sci.* 1987;32:1–7.

25. Walt R, Katschinski B, Logan R, et al. Rising frequency of ulcer perforation in elderly people in the United Kingdom. *Lancet.* 1986;1:489–492.

26. Myren J. The natural history of peptic ulcer views in the 1980s. *Scand J Gastroenterol.* 1983;18:993–997.

27. Stewart RB, Hale WE, Marks RG. Antacid use in an ambulatory elderly population: a report from Dunedin program. *Dig Dis Sci.* 1983;28:1062–1069.

28. Gerbino PP, Gans JA. Antacids and laxatives for symptomatic relief in the elderly. *J Am Geriatr Soc.* 1982;30:581–585.

29. Girotti MJ, Ruddan J, Cohanim M. Amphojeloma: antacid impaction in critically ill patients. *Can J Surg.* 1984;27(4):379–380.

30. Godsall JW, Baron R, Insogna KL, et al. Vitamin D metabolism in bone histomorphometry in a patient with antacid induced osteomalacia. *Am J Med.* 1984;77:747–750.

31. Baum C, Kennedy DL, Forbes MB, et al. Drug utilization in the geriatric age group. In: Moore SR, Teal TW, eds. *Geriatric Drug Use: Clinical and Social Perspectives.* New York, NY: Pergamon Press; 1985:63–69.

32. Baum C, Kennedy DL, Forbes MB. Utilization of nonsteroidal anti-inflammatory drugs. *Arthritis Rheum.* 1985;28:686–692.

33. Coles LS, Fries JK, Kraines RG, et al. From experiment to experience: side effects of nonsteroidal anti-inflammatory drugs. *Am J Med.* 1983;74:820–828.

34. Silvoso GR, Ivey KJ, Butt JH, et al. Incidence of gastric lesions in patients with rheumatic disease on chronic aspirin therapy. *Ann Intern Med.* 1979;91:517–520.

35. Bartle WR, Gupta AK, Lazor J. Nonsteroidal anti-inflammatory drugs and gastrointestinal bleeding: a case-control study. *Arch Intern Med.* 1986;146:2365–2367.

36. Minami H, McCallum RW. The physiology and pathophysiology of gastric emptying in humans. *Gastroenterology.* 1984;86:1592–1610.

37. Moore JG, Tweedy C, Christian PE, et al. Effect of age on gastric emptying of liquid solid meals in man. *Dig Dis Sci.* 1983;28:340–344.

38. Frank EB, Lange R, McCallum RW. Abnormal gastric emptying in patients with atrophic gastritis with or without pernicious anemia. *Gastroenterology.* 1981;80:1151.

39. Kupfer RM, Heppell M, Haggith JW, et al. Gastric emptying and small bowel transit rate in the elderly. *J Am Geriatr Soc.* 1985;33:340–343.

40. Laugier R, Sarles H. The pancreas. *Clin Gastroenterol.* 1985;14:749–756.

41. Kreel L, Scandin B. Changes in pancreatic morphology associated with aging. *Gut.* 1973;14:962–970.

42. Schmitz-Moorman P, Himmelmann GW, Brandes JW, et al. Comparative radiological and morphological study of the human pancreas: pancreatitis-like changes in post-mortem ductograms and their morphological pattern. *Gut.* 1985;26:406–414.

43. Snook JT. Effect of age and long-term diet on exocrine pancreas of the rat. *Am J Physiol.* 1975;228:262–268.

44. Kim SK, Weinhold PA, Calkins DW, et al. Comparative studies of the age-related changes in protein synthesis in the rat pancreas and parotid gland. *Exp Gerontol.* 1981;16:91–99.

45. Greenberg RE, Holt PR. Influence of aging upon pancreatic digestive enzymes. *Dig Dis Sci.* 1986;31:970–977.

46. Greenberg RE, McCann PP, Holt PR. Trophic responses of the pancreas differ in aging rats. *Pancreas.* 1988;3:311–316.

47. Fenyo G. Acute abdominal diseases in the elderly: experience from two series in Stockholm. *Am J Surg.* 1982;143:751–754.

48. Bourke JB, Mead GM, McIllmurray MB, et al. Drug associated primary acute pancreatitis. *Lancet.* 1978;1:706–708.

49. Ranson JH, Pasternack BS. Statistical methods for quantifying for severity of clinical acute pancreatitis. *J Surg Res.* 1977;22:79–91.

50. Corfield AP, Cooper MJ, Williamson RCN. Acute pancreatitis: a lethal disease of increasing incidence. *Gut.* 1985;26:724–729.

51. Blamey SL, Imrie CW, O'Neill J, Gilmour WH, Cater DC. Prognostic factors in acute pancreatitis. *Gut.* 1984;25:1340–1346.

52. Walsh TN, Rode J, Theis BA, Russell RC. Minimal change chronic pancreatitis. *Gut.* 1992;33:1566–1571.

53. DiMagno EP, Malagelada JR, Go VL. Relationship between alcoholism and pancreatic insufficiency. *Ann NY Acad Sci.* 1975;252:200–207.

54. Mackie RD, Levine AS, Levitt MD. Malabsorption of starch in pancreatic insufficiency. *Gastroenterology.* 1981;80:1220. Abstract.

55. Toskes PP, Greenberger NJ. Acute and chronic pancreatitis. *Dis Mon.* 1983;29:1–81.

56. Russell RM, Dutta SK, Oaks EV, et al. Impairment of folic acid absorption by oral pancreatic extracts. *Dig Dis Sci.* 1980;25:369–373.

57. Dutta SK, Bustin MP, Russell RM, et al. Deficiency of fat-soluble vitamins in treated patients with pancreatic insufficiency. *Ann Intern Med.* 1982;97:549–552.

58. Toskes PP, Hansell J, Creda J, et al. Vitamin $B_{12}$ malabsorption in chronic pancreatic insufficiency. *N Engl J Med.* 1971;284:627–632.

59. Lankisch PG, Creutzfeldt W. Therapy of exocrine and endocrine pancreatic insufficiency. *Clin Gastroenterol.* 1984;13:985–999.

60. Lipski PS, Bennett MK, Kelly PJ, James OFW. Aging and duodenal morphometry. *J Clin Pathol.* 1992;45:450–452.

61. Holt PR, Kotler DP, Pascal RR. Delayed enterocyte differentiation: a defect in aging rat jejunum. *Clin Res.* 1982;30:496A.

62. Saltzman JR, Kowdley KV, Perrone G, Russell RM. Changes in small-intestine permeability with aging. *J Am Geriatr Soc.* 1995;43:160–164.

63. Saltzman JR, Russell RM. The aging gut: nutritional issues. *Gastrol Clin N Am.* 1998;27:309–324.

64. Klimas JE. Intestinal glucose absorption during the life-span of a colony of rats. *J Gerontol.* 1968;23:529–532.

65. Calingaert A, Zorzoli A. The influence of age on 6-deoxy-D-glucose by mouse intestine. *J Gerontol.* 1965;20:211–214.

66. Feibusch JM, Holt PR. Impaired absorptive capacity for carbohydrate in the aging human. *Dig Dis Sci.* 1982;27:1095–1100.

67. Arora S, Kassarjian Z, Krasinski S, Croffey B, Kaplan MM, Russell RM. Effect of age on tests of intestinal and hepatic function in healthy humans. *Gastroenterology.* 1989;96:1560–1565.

68. Hollander D, Ruble PE Jr. Beta-carotene intestinal absorption: bile, fatty acid, pH and flow rate effects on transport. *Am J Physiol.* 1978;235:E686–E691.

69. Holt PR, Dominguez AA. Intestinal absorption of triglyceride and vitamin $D_3$ in aged and young rats. *Dig Dis Sci.* 1981;26:1104–1115.

70. Geokas MC, Conteas CN, Majumdar AP. The aging gastrointestinal tract, liver and pancreas. *Clin Geriatr Med.* 1985;1:177–205.

71. Werner I, Hambraeus L. The digestive capacity of elderly people. In: Carlson LA, ed. *Nutrition in Old Age.* Uppsala, Sweden: Almquist & Wiksell. 1972:55.

72. Southgate DAT, Durnin JVGA. Calorie conversion factors: an experimental reassessment of the factors used in the calculation of the energy value of human diets. *Br J Nutr.* 1970;24:517–535.

73. Pelz KS, Gottfried SP, Soos E. Intestinal absorption studies in the aged. *Geriatrics.* 1968;23:149.

74. Simko C, Michael S. Absorptive capacity for dietary fat in elderly patients with debilitating disorders. *Arch Intern Med.* 1989;149:557–560.

75. Wegener M, Borsch G, Schaffstein J, Luth I, Rickels R, Ricken D. Effect of aging on the gastrointestinal transit of a lactulose-supplemented solid-liquid meal in humans. *Digestion.* 1988;39:40–46.

76. Cheng AHR, Gomez A, Bergan JG, et al. Comparative nitrogen balance study between young and aged adults using three levels of protein intake from a combination wheat-soy-milk mixture. *Am J Clin Nutr.* 1978;31:12–22.

77. Gersovitz M, Motil D, Munro HN, et al. Human protein requirements: assessment of the adequacy of the current recommended dietary allowance for dietary protein in elderly men and woman. *Am J Clin Nutr.* 1982;35:6–14.

78. Munro HN, McGandy RB, Hartz SC, Russell RM, Jacob RA, Otradovec CL. Protein nutriture of a group of free-living elderly. *Am J Clin Nutr.* 1987;46:586–592.

79. Sklar M, Krisner JB, Palmer WL. Gastrointestinal disease in the aged. *Med Clin North Am.* 1956;40:223–337.

80. Suter PM, Russell RM. Vitamin requirements of the elderly. *Am J Clin Nutr.* 1987;45:501–512.

81. Russell RM. New views on the RDAs for older adults. *J Am Diet Assoc.* 1997;97:515–518.

82. Hollander D, Morgan D. Increase in cholesterol intestinal absorption with aging in the rat. *Exp Gerontol.* 1979;14:301–305.

83. Hollander D, Morgan D. Aging: its influence on vitamin A intestinal absorption *in vivo* by the rat. *Exp Gerontol.* 1979;14:301–305.

84. Hollander D, Dadufalza VD, Sletten EG. Does essential fatty acid absorption change in aging? *J Lipid Res.* 1984;25:129–134.

85. Krasinski DS, Cohn JS, Schaefer EJ, Russell RM. Postprandial plasma retinyl ester response is greater in older subjects compared with younger subjects. *J Clin Invest.* 1990;85:883–892.

86. Webb AR, Kline L, Holick MF. Influence of season and latitude on the cutaneous synthesis of vitamin $D_3$: exposure to winter sunlight in Boston and Edmonton will not promote vitamin $D_3$ synthesis in human skin. *J Clin Endocrinol Metab.* 1988;67:373–378.

87. McLaughlin J, Holick MF. Aging decreases the capacity of human skin to produce vitamin $D_3$. *J Clin Invest.* 1985;76:1536–1538.

88. Webb AR, Pilbeam C, Hanafin N, Holick MF. An evaluation of the relative contributions of exposure to sunlight and of diet to the circulating concentrations of 25-hydroxyvitamin D in an elderly nursing home population in Boston. *Am J Clin Nutr*. 1990;51:1075–1081.

89. Sadowski JA, Hood SJ, Dallal GE, Garry PJ. Phylloquinone in plasma from elderly and young adults: factors influencing its concentration. *Am J Clin Nutr*. 1989;50:100–108.

90. Paiva SAR, Sepe TE, Booth SL, et al. The interaction between vitamin K nutriture and bacterial overgrowth in hypochlorhydria induced by omeprazole. *Am J Clin Nutr*. 1998;68:699–704.

91. Russell RM, Dhar GJ, Dutta SK, Rosenberg I. Influence of intraluminal pH on folate absorption: studies in control subjects and in patients with pancreatic insufficiency. *J Lab Clin Med*. 1979;93:428–436.

92. Russell RM, Krasinski SD, Samloff IM, Jacob RA, Hartz SC, Brovender SR. Folic acid malabsorption in atrophic gastritis: possible compensation by bacterial folate synthesis. *Gastroenterology*. 1986;91:1476–1482.

93. Camilo E, Zimmerman J, Mason JB, et al. Folate synthesized by bacteria in the upper intestine is assimilated by the host. *Gastroenterology*. 1996;110:991–998.

94. Selhub J, Jacques PF, Wilson PWF, Rush D, Rosenberg IH. Vitamin status and intake as primary determinants of homocysteinemia in an elderly population. *JAMA*. 1993;270:2693–2698.

95. Kirsh A, Bidlack WR. Nutrition and the elderly: vitamin status and efficiency of supplementation. *Nutrition*. 1987;3:305.

96. Ribaya-Mercado JD, Russell RM, Sahyoun N, et al. Vitamin B$_6$ requirements of elderly men and women. *J Nutr*. 1991;121:1062–1074.

97. Verhoef P, Stamfer MJ, Buring JE, et al. Homocysteine metabolism and risk of myocardial infarction: relation with vitamin B$_6$, B$_{12}$ and folate. *Am J Epidemiol*. 1996;143:845–859.

98. Carmel R, Sinow R, Siegel M, Samloff M. Food cobalamin malabsorption occurs infrequently in patients with unexplained low serum cobalamin levels. *Arch Intern Med*. 1988;148:1715–1719.

99. King C, Leibach J, Toskes P. Clinically significant vitamin B$_{12}$ deficiency secondary to malabsorption of protein-bound vitamin B$_{12}$. *Dig Dis Sci*. 1979;24:397–402.

100. Saltzman JR, Kemp JA, Golner BB, Pedrosa MC, Dallal GE, Russell RM. Effect of hypochlorhydria due to omeprazole treatment or atrophic gastritis on protein-bound vitamin B$_{12}$ absorption. *J Am Coll Nutr*. 1994;13:584–491.

101. Suter PM, Golner BB, Goldin BR, et al. Reversal of protein-bound vitamin B$_{12}$ malabsorption with antibiotics in atrophic gastritis. *Gastroenterology*. 1991;101:1039–1045.

102. Selhub J, Jacques PF, Wilson PWF, Rush D, Rosenberg IH. Vitamin status and intake as primary determinants of homocysteinemia in an elderly population. *JAMA*. 1993;270:2693–2698.

103. Nelson, JB, Casteli DO. Effects of aging on gastrointestinal physiology. *Pract Gastroenterol*. 1988;12:28–35.

104. Marx JJM. Normal iron absorption and decreased cell iron uptake in the aged. *Blood*. 1979;53:204–211.

105. Jacobs P, Bothwell T, Charlton RW. Role of hydrochloric acid in iron absorption. *J Appl Physiol*. 1964;19:187–188.

106. Gallagher JC, Riggs BL, Eisman J, Hamstra A, Arnaud SB, DeLuca HF. Intestinal calcium absorption and serum vitamin D metabolites in normal subjects and osteoporotic patients. *J Clin Invest*. 1979;64:729–736.

107. Dawson-Hughes B, Jacques P, Shipp S. Dietary calcium intake and bone loss from the spine in healthy postmenopausal woman. *Am J Clin Nutr*. 1987;46:685–687.

108. Dawson-Hughes B, Dallal GE, Krall EA, Sadowski L, Sahyoun N, Tannenbaum S. A controlled trial of the effect of calcium supplementation of bone density on postmenopausal women. *N Engl J Med*. 1990;323:878–883.

109. Knox TA, Kassarjian Z, Dawson-Hughes B, et al. Calcium absorption in elderly subjects on high and low fiber diets: effect of gastric acidity. *Am J Clin Nutr*. 1991;53:1480–1486.

110. Serfaty-Lacrosniere CS, Wood RJ, Voytko,D, et al. Hypochlorhydria from short-term omeprazole treatment does not inhibit intestinal absorption of calcium, phosphorus, magnesium or zinc from food in humans. *J Am Coll Nutr*. 1995;14;364–368.

111. Husebye E, Engedal K. The patterns of motility are maintained in the human small intestine throughout the process of aging. *Scand J Gastroenterol*. 1992;27:397.

112. Madsen J. Effects of gender, age, and body mass index on gastrointestinal transit times. *Dig Dis Sci.* 1992;37:1548.

113. Anuras S, Sutherland J. Jejunal manometry in healthy elderly subjects. *Gastroenterology.* 1986;86:1016.

114. Pelz KS, Gottfried SP, Soos E. Intestinal absorption studies in the aged. *Geriatrics.* 1968;23:149–153.

115. Montgomery RD, Hainey MR, Ross IN, et al. The aging gut: a study of intestinal absorption in relation to nutrition in the elderly. *Q J Med.* 1978;47:197–211.

116. Price HL, Gazzard BG, Dawson AM. Steatorrhea in the elderly. *Br Med J.* 1977;1:1582–1584.

117. Scrimshaw N, Murray E. Prevalence of lactose maldigestion. *Am J Clin Nutr.* 1988;48:1086–1098.

118. Bayless TM, Rothfeld B, Massa C, et al. Lactose and milk intolerance: clinical implications. *N Engl J Med.* 1975;292:1156–1159.

119. Bond JH, Levitt MD. Use of breath hydrogen ($H_2$) in the study of carbohydrate absorption. *Am J Dig Dis.* 1977;22:379–382.

120. Lindi C, Marciani P, Faelli A, Esposito G. Intestinal sugar transport during aging. *Biochim Biophys Acta.* 1985;816:411–414.

121. Vincenzini MT, Iantomasi T, Stio M, et al. Glucose transport during aging in human intestinal brush-border membrane vesicles. *Mech Aging Dev.* 1989;48:33–41.

122. Trier JS. Celiac sprue. *N Engl J Med.* 1991;325:1709–1719.

123. Swinson CM, Levi AJ. Is coeliac disease underdiagnosed? *Br Med J.* 1980;281:1258–1260.

124. Kirby J, Fielding JF. Very adult coeliac disease, the need for jejunal biopsy in the middle aged and elderly. *Ir Med J.* 1984;77:35–36.

125. Harkey GL, Holmes GK. Celiac disease in the elderly. *Gut.* 1994;35:65–67.

126. Hallert C, Gothard R, Norrby K, et al. On the prevalence of adult coeliac disease in Sweden. *Scand J Gastroenterol.* 1981;16:257–261.

127. Robertson DAF, Dixon MF, Scott BB, et al. Small intestinal ulceration: diagnostic difficulties in relation to coeliac disease. *Gut.* 1983;24:565–574.

128. Matuchansky C, Collin R, Helmet J et al. Cavitation of mesenteric lymph nodes, splenic atrophy and a flat small intestinal mucosa: report of six cases. *Gastroenterology.* 1984;87:606–614.

129. Dawson DJ, Sciberras CM, Whitwell H Coeliac disease presenting with intestinal pseudo-obstruction. *Gut.* 1984;25:1003–1008.

130. Fine KD. The prevalence of occult gastrointestinal bleeding in celiac sprue. *N Engl J Med.* 1996;334:1163–1167.

131. Friis SU, Gudmand-Hoyer E. Screening for coeliac disease in adults by simultaneous determination of IgA and IgG antibodies. *Scand J Gastroenterol.* 1986;21:1058–1062.

132. Vogelsang M, Genser D, Wyatt J, et al. Screening for celiac disease: a prospective study on the value of noninvasive tests. *Am J Gastroenterol.* 1994;90:394–398.

133. Corazza GR, Strocchi A, Gasbarrini G. Breath hydrogen and celiac disease. *Gastroenterology.* 1987;93:53–58.

134. Pena AS, Truelove SC, Whitehead R. Disaccharidase activity and jejunal morphology in coeliac disease. *Q J Med.* 1972;41:457–476.

135. McEvoy A, Dutton J, James OFW. Bacterial contamination of the small intestine is an important part of the occult malabsorption in the elderly. *Br Med J.* 1983;287:289–293.

136. Saltzman JR, Kowdley KV, Pedrosa MC, et al. Bacterial overgrowth without clinical malabsorption in elderly hypochlorhydric subjects. *Gastroenterology.* 1994;106:615–623.

137. Haboubi NY, Montgomery RD. Small-bowel bacterial overgrowth in elderly people: clinical significance and response to treatment. *Age Ageing.* 1992;21:13–19.

138. Isaacs PET, Kim YS. The contaminated small bowel syndrome. *Am J Med.* 1979;67:1049–1057.

139. Mayberry JF, Ballantyne KC, Hardcastle JD, et al. Epidemiologic study of asymptomatic inflammatory bowel disease: the identification of cases during a screening programme for colorectal cancer. *Gut.* 1989;30:481–483.

140. Brandt LJ, Boley S, Goldberg L, et al. Colitis in the elderly: a reappraisal. *Am J Gastroenterol.* 1981;76:239–245.

141. Tedesco FJ, Hardin RD, Harper RN, et al. Infectious colitis endoscopically simulating inflamma-

tory bowel disease: a prospective evaluation. *Gastrointest Endosc.* 1983;29:195–197.

142. France MJ, Vuletic JC, Koelmeyer TD. Does advancing age modify the presentation of disease? *Am J Forensic Med Pathol.* 1992;13:120–123.

143. Zimmerman J, Gavish D, Rachmilewitz D. Early and late onset ulcerative colitis: distinct clinical features. *J Clin Gastroenterol.* 1985;7:492–498.

144. Brocklehurst JC. Colonic disease in the elderly: aging and bowel habits. *Clin Gastroenterol.* 1985;14:725–747.

145. Brandt LJ, Boley SJ, Mitsudo S. Clinical characteristics and natural history of colitis in the elderly. *Am J Gastroenterol.* 1982;77:382–386.

146. Joslin CA, Smith CW, Malik A. The treatment of cervix cancer using high activity cobalt-60 sources. *Br J Radiol.* 1972;45:247–270.

147. Yeoh EK, Horowitz M. Radiation enteritis. *Surg Gynecol Obstet.* 1987;165:373–379.

148. O'Brien PH, Jenrette JM III, Garvin AJ. Radiation enteritis. *Am Surg.* 1987;53:501–504.

149. Cox JD, Byhardt RW, Wilson F, et al. Complications of radiation therapy and factors in their prevention. *World J Surg.* 1986;10:171–188.

150. Galland RB, Spencer J. Surgical management of radiation enteritis. *Surgery.* 1986;99:133–138.

151. Harling H, Balslev IB. Radical surgical approach to radiation injury of the small bowel. *Dis Colon Rectum.* 1986;29:371–372.

152. Arlow FL, Dekovich AA, Priest RJ, et al. Bile acids in radiation-induced diarrhea. *South Med J.* 1987;80:1259–1261.

153. McArdle AH, Reid EC, Laplante MP, et al. Prophylaxis against radiation injury. *Arch Surg.* 1986;121:879–885.

154. Miller DH, Ivey M, Young J. Home parenteral nutrition in treatment of severe radiation enteritis. *Ann Intern Med.* 1979;91:858–860.

155. Calloway NO, Foley CF, Lagerbloom P. Uncertainties in geriatric data, II: organ size. *J Am Geriatr Soc.* 1965;13:20–28.

156. Thomas FB, Clausen KP, Geenberger NJ. Liver disease in multiple myeloma. *Arch Intern Med.* 1973;132:195–202.

157. Tauchi H, Sato T. Effective environmental conditions upon age changes in the human liver. *Mech Aging Dev.* 1975;4:71–80.

158. Schaffner F, Popper H. Nonspecific reactive hepatitis in aged and infirm people. *Am J Dig Dis.* 1959;4:389–399.

159. Schmucker DL. Age-related changes in hepatic fine structure: a quantitative analysis. *J Gerontol.* 1976;31:135–143.

160. Landowne M, Stanley J. Aging of the cardiovascular system. In: Shock NW, ed. *Aging: Some Social and Biological Aspects.* Washington, DC: American Association for the Advancement of Science; 1960.

161. Bender AD. The effect of increasing age on distribution of peripheral blood flow in man. *J Am Geriatr Soc.* 1965;13:192–198.

162. Kampmann JP, Sinding J, Moller-Jorgensen I. Effect of age on liver function. *Geriatrics.* 1975;30(8):91–95.

163. Gersovitz M, Munro HN, Udall J, et al. Albumin synthesis in young and elderly subjects using a new stable isotope methodology: response to level of protein intake. *Metabolism.* 1980;29:1076–1086.

164. Kitani K. Hepatic drug metabolism in the elderly. *Hepatology.* 1986;6:316–319. Editorial.

165. Crooks J, O'Malley K, Stevenson IH. Pharmacokinetics in the elderly. *Clin Pharmacokinet.* 1976;1:280–296.

166. Woodhouse KW, Mutch E, Williams FM, et al. The effect of age on pathways of drug metabolism in human liver. *Age Ageing.* 1984;13:328–334.

167. Smithard DJ, Langman MJ. The effect of vitamin supplementation upon antipyrine metabolism in the elderly. *Br J Clin Pharmacol.* 1978;5:181–185.

168. Young VR, Steffee WP, Pencharz PB, et al. Total human body protein synthesis in relation to protein requirements at various ages. *Nature.* 1975;253:192–194.

169. Geokas MC, Conteas CN, Majumdar AP. The aging gastrointestinal tract, liver, and pancreas. *Clin Geriatr Med.* 1985;1:177–205.

170. James OFW. Gastrointestinal and liver function in old age. *Clin Gastroenterol.* 1983;12:671–691.

171. Mooney H, Roberts R, Cooksley WGE, et al. Alternations in the liver with aging. *Clin Gastroenterol.* 1985;14:757–771.

172. Gibinski K, Fajt E, Suchan L. Hepatitis in the aged. *Digestion.* 1973;8:254–260.

173. Ludwig J, Baggenstoss AH. Cirrhosis of the aged and senile cirrhosis: are there two conditions? *J Gerontol.* 1970;25:244–248.

174. Ludwig J, Axelsen R. Drug effects on the liver: an updated tabular compilation of drugs and drug-related hepatic disease. *Dig Dis Sci.* 1983;28:651–666.

175. Goodson JD, Taylor PA, Campion EW, et al. The clinical course of acute hepatitis in elderly patients. *Arch Intern Med.* 1982;142:1485–1488.

176. Fenster LF. Viral hepatitis in the elderly: an analysis of 23 patients over 65 years of age. *Gastroenterology.* 1965;49:262–271.

177. Saint EG. Infectious hepatitis in older age groups. *Med J Aust.* 1952;2:613–619.

178. Sherlock S. Acute hepatic failure. In: *Diseases of the Liver Biliary System.* 8th ed. Boston, Mass: Blackwell Scientific Publications, Inc; 1989.

179. Kaplan M. Primary biliary cirrhosis. *N Engl J Med.* 1987;316:521–528.

180. James OFW. Gastrointestinal and liver function in the old age. *Clin Gastroenterol.* 1983;12:671–691.

181. Hislop WS, Hopwood D, Bouchier IA. Primary biliary cirrhosis in elderly females. *Age Ageing.* 1982;11:153–159.

182. Lehman AB, Bussendine MF, James OF. Primary biliary cirrhosis: a different disease in the elderly? *Gerontology.* 1985;31:186–194.

183. Alpers DH, Sabesin SM. Fatty liver: biochemical and clinical aspects. In: Schiff L, Schiff ER, eds. *Diseases of the Liver.* 6th ed. Philadelphia, Pa: JB Lippincott Co: 1987.

184. Lieber CS. Alcohol-nutrition interaction: 1984 update. *Alcohol.* 1984;1:151–157.

185. Lieber CS, Spritz N. Effects of prolonged ethanol intake in man: role of dietary, adipose, and endogenously synthesized fatty acids in the pathogenesis of the alcoholic fatty liver. *J Clin Invest.* 1966;45:1400–1411.

186. Reboucas G, Isselbacher JJ. Studies on pathogenesis of ethanol induced fatty liver. 1: synthesis and oxidation of fatty acids by the liver. *J Clin Invest.* 1961;40:1355.

187. Alpers DH, Sabesin SM. Fatty liver: biochemical and clinical aspects. In: Schiff L, Schiff ER, eds. *Diseases of the Liver.* 6th ed. Philadelphia, Pa: JB Lippincott Co: 1987.

188. Katz J, McGarry JD. The glucose paradox: is glucose a substrate for liver metabolism? *J Clin Invest.* 1984;74:1901–1909.

189. Flores H, Pak N, Maccioni A, et al. Lipid transport in kwashiorkor. *Br J Nutr.* 1970;24:1005–1011.

190. Flatt JP. Role of increased adipose tissue mass in the apparent insulin insensitivity of obesity. *Am J Clin Nutr.* 1972;25:1189.

191. Chase R, Sullivan SR, Bloom DB. Insulin, glucagon, and amino acid imbalance in fulminant hepatic failure. *Gut.* 1977;18:A953.

192. Rosen HM, Yoshimura N, Hodgman JM, et al. Plasma amino acid patterns in hepatic encephalopathy of differing etiology. *Gastroenterology.* 1977;72:483–487.

193. Fiaccadori F, Magnani G, Pedretti G. Nutritional status in acute liver damage. In: Barbara L, ed. *Nutrition and Gastrointestinal Disease.* New York, NY: Raven Press; 1987:241–251.

194. Atkinson M, Nordin BE, Sherlock S. Malabsorption and bone disease in prolonged obstructive jaundice. *Q J Med.* 1956;25:299–312.

195. Ros E, Garcia-Puges A, Reixach M, et al. Fat digestion and exocrine pancreatic function in primary biliary cirrhosis. *Gastroenterology.* 1984;87:180–187.

196. Lanspa SJ, Chan AT, Bell JS III, et al. Pathogenesis of steatorrhea in primary biliary cirrhosis. *Hepatology.* 1985;5:837–842.

197. Hodgeson SF, Dickson ER, Wahner HW, et al. Bone loss and reduced osteoblast function in primary biliary cirrhosis. *Ann Intern Med.* 1985;103:855–860.

198. Skinner RK, Long RG, Sherlock S, et al. 25-Hydroxylation of vitamin D in primary biliary cirrhosis. *Lancet.* 1977;1:720–721.

199. Epstein O. Nutritional therapy in women with primary biliary cirrhosis. *Geriatr Med Today.* 1983;2(10):48–60.

200. Herlong MF, Russell RM, Maddrey WC. Vitamin A and zinc therapy in primary biliary cirrhosis. *Hepatology.* 1981;1:348–351.

201. Mezey E. Progress in hepatology: liver disease and nutrition. *Gastroenterology.* 1978;74:770–783.

202. Burch RE, Sackin DA, Ursick JA, et al. Decreased taste and smell acuity in cirrhosis. *Arch Intern Med.* 1978;138:743–746.

203. Baraona E, Pirola RC, Lieber CS. Small intestinal damage and changes in cell population produced by ethanol ingestion in the rat. *Gastroenterology.* 1974;66:226–234.

204. Rubin E, Rybak BJ, Lindenbaum J, et al. Ultrastructural changes in the small intestine induced by ethanol. *Gastroenterology.* 1972;63:801–814.

205. Mezey E, Jow E, Slavin RE, et al. Pancreatic function and intestinal absorption in chronic alcoholism. *Gastroenterology.* 1970;59:657–664.

206. Mezey E, Potter JJ. Changes in endocrine pancreatic function produced by altered dietary protein intake in drinking alcoholics. *Johns Hopkins Med J.* 1976;138(1):7–12.

207. Mezey E. Intestinal function in chronic alcoholism. *Ann NY Acad Sci.* 1975;252:215–227.

208. Malagelada JR, Pihl O, Linscheer WG. Impaired absorption of micellar long-chain fatty acid in patients with alcoholic cirrhosis. *Am J Dig Dis.* 1974;19:1016–1020.

209. Vlahcevic ZR, Buhac I, Farrar JT, et al. Bile acid metabolism in patients with cirrhosis: kinetic aspects of cholic acid metabolism. *Gastroenterology.* 1971;60:491–498.

210. Owen OE, Trapp VE, Reichard GA Jr, et al. Nature and quantity of fuels consumed in patients with alcoholic cirrhosis. *J Clin Invest.* 1983; 72:1821–1832.

211. Marchesini G, Bianchi G, Zoli M, et al. Plasma amino acid response to protein ingestion in patients with liver cirrhosis. *Gastroenterology.* 1983;85:283–290.

212. Leevy CM, Baker H, TenHove W, et al. B complex vitamins in liver disease of the alcoholic. *Am J Clin Nutr.* 1965;16:339–346.

213. Gradual N, Milman N, Kirkegaard E, et al. Bacteremia in cirrhosis of the liver. *Liver.* 1986; 6(5):297–301.

214. Greenberger NJ, Carley J, Schenker S, et al. Effect of vegetable and animal protein diets in chronic hepatic encephalopathy. *Dig Dis.* 1977; 22:845–855.

215. Uribe M, Marquez MA, Ramos GG, et al. Treatment of chronic portal systemic encephalopathy with vegetable and animal protein diets: a controlled crossover study. *Dig Dis Sci.* 1982;27: 1109–1116.

216. Jonung T, Jeppsson B, Ashlund U, et al. A comparison between meat and vegan protein diet in patients with mild chronic hepatic encephalopathy. *Clin Nutr.* 1987;6:169–174.

217. Rossi-Fanelli F, Cascino A, Cagiano C. Branched chain amino acids in the management of hepatic encephalopathy. *J Clin Nutr Gastroenterol.* 1987; 2:44.

218. Rocco VK, Ware AJ. Cirrhotic ascites: pathophysiology, diagnosis and management. *Ann Intern Med.* 1986;105:573–585.

219. Quintero E, Geines P, Arroyo V, et al. Paracentesis versus diuretics in the treatment of cirrhosis with tense ascites. *Lancet.* 1985;1:611–612.

220. Yamajata A. Histopathological studies of the colon due to age. *Jpn J Gastroenterol.* 1965; 62:224–235.

221. Melkerson M, Anderson H, Bosaeus I, et al. Intestinal transit time in constipation and nonconstipated geriatric patients. *Scand J Gastroenterol.* 1983;18:593–597.

222. Madsen JL. Effects of gender, age and body mass index on gastrointestinal transit times. *Dig Dis Sci.* 1992;37:1548–1553.

223. Connell AM, Hilton C, Irvin C. Variations in bowel habit in two population samples. *Br Med J.* 1965;2:1095–1099.

224. Milne JS, Williamson J. Bowel habit in older people. *Gerontologia Clin.* 1972;14:55–60.

225. Brocklehurst JC. Colonic disease in the elderly. *Clin Gastroenterol.* 1985:14:725–747.

226. Frieri G, Parisi F, Corazziari E, et al. Colonic electromyography in chronic constipation. *Gastroenterology.* 1983;84:737–740.

227. Shoulder P, Keighley MRB. Changes in colorectal function in severe idiopathic chronic constipation. *Gastroenterology.* 1986;90: 414–420.

228. Loening-Baucke V, Apuras S. Sigmoidal and rectal motility in healthy elderly. *J Am Gerontol Soc.* 1984;32:887–891.

229. Bannister JJ, Abouzekry L, Read NW. Effect of aging on anorectal function. *Gut.* 1987;28:353–357.

230. Martelli H, Devroede G, Arhan P, et al. Mechanisms of idiopathic constipation: outlet obstruction. *Gastroenterology.* 1978;75:623–631.

231. Watier A, Devroede G, Duranceau A, et al. Constipation with colonic inertia: a manifestation of systemic disease? *Dig Dis Sci.* 1983;28:1025–1033.

232. Read MW, Timms JM. Defecation in the patho-physiology of constipation. *Clin Gastroenterol.* 1986;15:937–965.

233. Wald A, Stoney B, Hinds JP. Physiological profiles in patients with constipation associated with normal and slow colonic transit. *Gastroenterology.* 1988;95:892. Abstract.

234. Hull C, Greco RS, Brooks DL, et al. Alleviation of constipation in the elderly by dietary fibre supplementation. *J Am Geriatr Soc.* 1988;28(9): 41–44.

235. Anderson H, Bosaens I, Falkheden T, et al. Transit time in constipated geriatric patients during treatment with a bulk laxative and bran: a comparison. *Scand J Gastroenterol.* 1979;14:821–826.

236. Tomlin J, Read NW. Laxative properties of indigestible plastic particles. *Br Med J.* 1988; 297:1175–1176.

237. Parks TG. Natural history of diverticular disease of the colon. *Clin Gastroenterol.* 1975;4:53–69.

238. Eastwood MA, Watters DAK, Smith AN. Diverticular disease: is it a motility disorder? *Clin Gastroenterol.* 1982;11:545–561.

239. Weinreich J, Anderson D. Intraluminal pressure in the sigmoid colon, II: patients with sigmoid diverticula and related conditions. *Scand J Gastroenterol.* 1976;11:581–586.

240. Burkitt DP. Epidemiology of cancer of the colon and rectum. *Cancer.* 1971;28:3–13.

# CHAPTER 9

# Aging and the Cardiovascular System

*Jeanne P. Goldberg and Jennifer P. Hellwig*

The maximal life span of humans, about 114 years, has remained unchanged over time, while life expectancy in the United States has increased dramatically over the past several decades, reaching a high of 75.8 years in 1995.[1] By 2030, it is expected that the percentage of those living to age 65 years and beyond will double, accounting for 25% of the total population. Given the fixed upper limit of the human life span, the objective of chronic disease prevention in the growing population of elderly people should be to delay the onset of diseases, and the resulting disabilities, to that limit.[2]

Diseases of the heart and blood vessels are by far the most important cause of morbidity and mortality among elderly individuals, rising logarithmically with age. Elderly people, who account for 68% of all deaths in the United States annually, make up 78% of all deaths attributed to coronary heart disease (CHD). Among those individuals who reach age 65 years, more than half will suffer a cardiovascular catastrophe. Morbidity is similarly prevalent in this age group. In 1990, 17.6% of persons 65 years or older suffered an acute fatal myocardial infarction.[3]

It is widely agreed that primary efforts to prevent cardiovascular disease should begin with altering lifestyle habits during middle age; many experts believe that these efforts should begin considerably earlier. Prevention activities include maintaining ideal body weight, detecting and treating hypertension, maintaining a blood lipid profile consistent with minimizing risk, stopping smoking, and increasing physical activity. Most of these risk factors are closely linked to dietary factors (Table 9–1).[4] However, the relevance of risk factor modification among older populations remains a matter of conjecture, based to a great extent on extrapolation of findings from studies conducted on younger populations.

Although no controlled intervention trials have focused specifically on the elderly, the fact that the dramatic decline in the cardiovascular mortality rate has included them argues in favor of risk reduction efforts in this group.[5] Dietary recommendations for elderly people must be based on our knowledge of the benefits of risk factor modification in older populations and on appropriate modifications for individuals with frank disease. Recommendations must be made within a framework that acknowledges the universal importance of a nutritionally adequate diet and the unique constellation of constraints that might make it difficult to achieve that goal. Moreover, interventions that will reduce risk should take into account the potential for diminishing morbidity and disability that result from cardiovascular disease.[6]

**Table 9–1** Risk Factors for Atherosclerosis

Not reversible
  Aging
  Male sex
  Genetic traits—positive family history of premature atherosclerosis
Reversible
  Cigarette smoking
  Hypertension
  Obesity
Potentially or partially reversible
  Hyperlipidemia-hypercholesterolemia and/or hypertriglyceridemia
  Hyperglycemia and diabetes mellitus
  Low levels of high-density lipoprotein
Other possible factors
  Physical inactivity
  Emotional stress or personality type

*Source:* Reprinted with permission from E.C. Bierman, Aging and Atherosclerosis, in *Principles of Geriatric Medicine and Gerontology,* 2nd ed., W.R. Hazzard et al., eds., p. 459, © 1990, McGraw-Hill, Inc.

## THE DISEASE PROCESSES

Decline in cardiovascular function is a major physical impairment associated with aging from middle age onward. Loss of cardiovascular reserve capacity can be attributed to three factors: age-associated changes, physical deconditioning associated with an increasingly sedentary lifestyle, and changes associated with atherosclerotic cardiovascular disease. The relative contribution of each of these factors is unclear.[7] It is clear, however, that environmentally induced atherosclerotic changes play a major role in this process.

Atherosclerosis, thickening and hardening of the intima (the lining of the coronary arteries), underlies most cardiovascular disease in elderly individuals; hypertension and diabetes act as important contributing factors. The development of atherosclerosis is believed to result from years of interaction between intrinsic aging processes and environmental factors—including diet—superimposed on unknown, predisposing genetic factors (Figure 9–1).[8] At least two lines of evidence suggest that atherosclerosis is not simply the result of unmodified biologic aging processes. The first line of evidence is that some mammalian species age without developing atherosclerosis; second, there are populations that realize the human life span without clinical evidence of the disease.[9]

Changes do occur in the arteries during normal aging. A slow, apparently continuous, symmetric increase in the thickness of the interior walls of the arteries results from the gradual accumulation of smooth muscle cells from the middle layer of the vessels, surrounded by additional connective tissue. In addition, there is a progressive accumulation of both sphingomyelin and cholesterol ester. These age-associated changes result in a gradual increase in the rigidity of the vessels. Larger arteries may become dilated, elongated, and tortuous. Aneurysms (balloonings of the arterial wall) may form in areas of

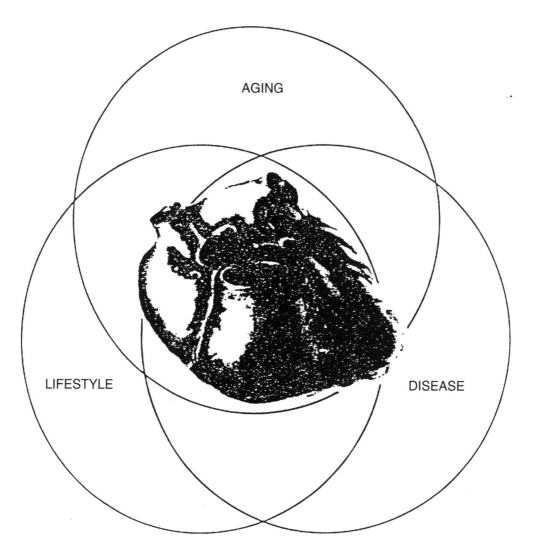

**Figure 9–1** Age-related changes in cardiac structure and function interact to alter the presentation of cardiovascular disease in the elderly. *Source:* Reprinted with permission from *Cardiovascular Medicine* (1985; March: 38), Copyright © 1985, Physicians' World.

expanding arteriosclerotic plaques. These wear-and-tear changes often depend on the diameter of the vessel and tend to occur where vessels branch and curve and at anatomic attachment points.[9]

Although these structural changes are considered to be a normal part of the aging process, atherosclerotic changes are believed to be strongly influenced by environmental factors, especially diet. The lesions of atherosclerosis are generally classified into three categories: fatty streaks, fibrous plaques, and complicated lesions. Fatty streaks are characterized by an accumulation of lipid-filled smooth muscle cells and are surrounded by lipid in the lining of the vessels. Whether they are the earliest lesions is a matter of debate. They are universal, appearing in the aorta by age 10 years, and occupying as much as 50% of the aortic surface by age 25 years. The age-related increase in the surface area of coronary arteries involved with fatty streaks is believed to be readily reversible.[10]

Fibrous plaques, which are not ubiquitous among populations, are elevated areas of thickening in the lining of the arteries. They represent the most characteristic lesions of progressive atherosclerosis, appearing first in the intima of the abdominal aorta, coronary arteries, and carotid arteries during the third decade and gradually increasing with advancing age. A fibrous plaque is firm, elevated, and dome shaped, with an opaque, glistening surface that bulges into the lumen of the affected artery. It consists of an accumulation in the arterial intima of smooth muscle cells rather heavily laden with cholesterol and surrounded by other lipids, collagen, elastic fibers, and other substances. The protrusion of fibrous plaques into the lumina of arteries reduces their diameter. The cholesterol in plaques closely resembles that in plasma lipoproteins. Raised lesions are thought to develop in the setting of a disruption of the endothelial cell continuity overlying fatty streaks. Evidence suggests that the progression of raised lesions continues into very old age.[11]

Complicated lesions are calcified fibrous plaques exhibiting various degrees of necrosis, thrombosis, and ulceration. Increasing necrosis, accumulation of cell debris, and weakening of the arterial wall increase the likelihood of rupture of the interior wall, causing hemorrhage. Arterial emboli may occur when fragments of plaque dislodge into the lumen. The thickening of plaque and the formation of thrombi (clots) lead to narrowing of blood vessels, reduced blood flow, and impaired organ function.[9] Arteries narrowed by raised lesions are more vulnerable to occlusion or blockage than are normal arteries.

The extent of the surface area of coronary arteries involved with fatty streaks increases in men during the second and third decades of life and remains constant through the remainder of their lives. However, the development of raised lesions, which gradually impair blood flow, continues. In women, the extent of fatty streaks increases to about age 50 years, but the development of raised lesions lags nearly 20 years behind that for men.

Interventions designed to prevent clinical complications of raised, atherosclerotic lesions have focused on men aged 40 to 50 years for several reasons. First, raised lesions generally appear earlier in men than in women. Second, associated with the first observation, risk of death from CHD increases in men at an earlier age than in women. Finally, the greatest likelihood of reversing the atherosclerotic process focuses on the smaller, less mature plaques.[12] However, several studies have demonstrated significant regression of larger fatty lesions.[13–16] Fibrous, calcified lesions may be prevented from further progression, but they probably do not regress. To date, there have been no clinical intervention trials with elderly subjects.

## RISK FACTORS AND THEIR MODIFICATION IN ELDERLY SUBJECTS

Coincidentally with the increased publicity focused on CHD as a cause of death, death rates from CHD began to decline. This decline began in 1950, with dramatic decreases observed in the 1960s and 1970s and slower declines during the 1980s and 1990s.[17] Between 1968 and 1976, CHD death rates in the adult population declined 20%. Among individuals over age 65 years, there was a decline of between 13% and 27%. Even among men and women aged 85 years and older, the death rate dropped 17% and 21%, respectively.[18] The most recent figures show a decline in CHD death rates from 505,592 in 1988 to 489,171 in 1990.[3] A key question is whether this decline is associated only with better survival rates attributable to improved medical management or whether a decline in incidence also is a contributing factor. For example, a large decline in age-specific incidence rate between the early 1960s and mid-1970s has been demonstrated in a prospective study of both blue-collar and white-collar workers. However, the rate of decline was steeper among the white-collar workers.[19] Among the subjects in the oldest age group, the decline was 22%.

A number of risk factors predict the likelihood of developing a clinical atherosclerotic event, but only some of them can be altered (Table 9–1). Research conducted over several decades has identified a series of diet-related factors associated with the incidence of cardiovascular disease and the development and progression of the underlying atherosclerosis. The role of dietary fats (particularly saturated and *trans*-fatty acids) in regulating circulating lipoprotein levels is of particular importance, as is the role of body weight in affecting both blood lipoprotein levels and blood pressure. Dietary sodium also has a role in hypertension.[20] Recent research has elucidated possible roles of other micronutrients in CHD: vitamin E, with its antioxidant function, has been shown to have protective effects on risk for CHD,[21] and vitamin $B_6$, vitamin $B_{12}$, and folate may act to lower levels of plasma homocysteine.[22,23] Elevated homocysteine levels have been associated with increased risk of myocardial infarction[24] and mortality in patients with CHD.[25]

## Blood Lipids

Patterns of atherogenic blood lipid levels and their relationship to risk of CHD differ among older men and women. Data from the Third National Health and Nutrition Examination Survey (NHANES III, 1988–1991) show that total serum cholesterol and low-density lipoprotein (LDL) cholesterol fractions tend to peak in men at 55 to 64 years of age and then decrease; in women, serum cholesterol levels also peak at 55 to 64 years of age and actually exceed those seen in men (Figures 9–2 and 9–3).[26] High-density lipoprotein (HDL) cholesterol levels are substantially higher in women and remain higher than HDL cholesterol levels in men. HDL cholesterol is inversely correlated with weight and is likely to be lower in individuals with impaired glucose tolerance.[27] It is also lower among individuals who have suffered a coronary event.[27]

In the Framingham study, the relative predictive power of the major cardiovascular risk factors weakened with age for both men and women.[28] Among 35-year-old men with total cholesterol levels of 310 mg/dL, the risk of suffering a coronary event was 5.2 times greater than among those with total cholesterol levels of 185 mg/dL. However, by age 65 years the relative risk at the higher cholesterol level was only 1.1. Among 45-year-old women with total cholesterol levels of 310 mg/dL, the risk of a coronary event was 2.5 times that of women with total cholesterol levels of 185 mg/dL. However, by age 65 years that risk diminished to 1.1. Barrett-Connor and colleagues[29] found a significant predictive effect of total cholesterol in groups of men and women aged 65 to 79 years who were followed for 9 years. More recent data from the Framingham study confirm the long-term predictive power of serum cholesterol levels in individuals aged 65 years and older. For each 1% increase in total cholesterol, there is a 2% increase in the incidence of CHD among those 60 to 70 years old.[30]

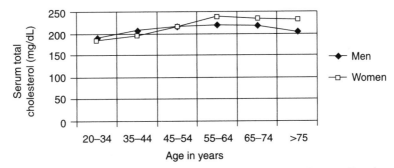

**Figure 9–2** Mean serum total cholesterol, U.S. population 1988–1991. *Source:* Reprinted with permission from C.L. Johnson et al., Declining Serum Total Cholesterol Levels Among U.S. Adults: The National Health and Nutrition Examination Surveys, *Journal of the American Medical Association*, Vol. 269, pp. 3002–3008, Copyright 1993, American Medical Association.

Elevated LDL-cholesterol concentrations and decreased HDL-cholesterol concentrations are independent risk factors for CHD, and recent studies indicate a benefit in CHD risk reduction from both lowering LDL cholesterol and increasing HDL cholesterol.[31] In the Framingham study, fractioning serum cholesterol into atherogenic LDL and protective HDL cholesterol restores the predictive power of total cholesterol demonstrated at younger ages.[27] A ratio of either LDL cholesterol to HDL cholesterol or total cholesterol to HDL cholesterol is highly predictive of CHD in elderly people. In men, this atherogenic lipid ratio plateaus at age 54 years; in women, it continues to rise until age 80 years but still remains lower than that for men. These observations still do not provide clear evidence that modifying lipoprotein levels at older ages will prevent further progression of atherosclerotic disease among elderly people.

A number of factors affect blood lipid levels. Total serum cholesterol and LDL cholesterol are elevated by saturated fat, excess calories, and dietary cholesterol. Recent evidence suggests that *trans*-fatty acids may also

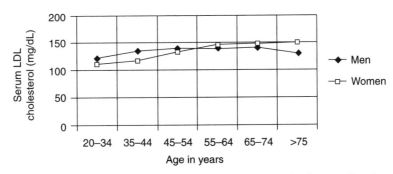

**Figure 9–3** Mean serum LDL cholesterol, U.S. population 1988–1991. *Source:* Reprinted with permission from C.L. Johnson et al., Declining Serum Total Cholesterol Levels Among U.S. Adults: The National Health and Nutrition Examination Surveys, *Journal of the American Medical Association*, Vol. 269, pp. 3002–3008, Copyright 1993, American Medical Association.

**Table 9–2** Initial Classification Based on Total Cholesterol and HDL-Cholesterol Levels

| Cholesterol Level | Initial Classification |
| --- | --- |
| Total cholesterol | |
| <200 mg/dL (5.2 mmol/L) | Desirable blood cholesterol |
| 200–239 mg/dL (5.2–6.2 mmol/L) | Borderline-high blood cholesterol |
| >240 mg/dL (6.2 mmol/L) | High blood cholesterol |
| HDL cholesterol | |
| <35 mg/dL (0.9 mmol/L) | Low HDL cholesterol |

*Source:* Reprinted with permission from Summary of the Second Report of the National Cholesterol Education Program Expert Panel on Detection, Evaluation, and Treatment of High Blood Cholesterol in Adults (Adult Treatment Panel II). *Journal of the American Medical Association,* Vol. 269, pp. 3015–3023, Copyright 1993, American Medical Association.

influence blood lipid levels and cardiovascular disease risk.[32,33] Blood lipids can be lowered by weight reduction, replacing saturated and *trans*-fatty acids with unsaturated fats[34] and complex carbohydrates,[31] and increasing water-soluble dietary fiber.[35]

The National Cholesterol Education Program (NCEP) was developed by the National Heart, Lung, and Blood Institute in 1985[36] as a means to reduce coronary morbidity and mortality related to elevated blood cholesterol levels. The NCEP Expert Panel on Detection, Evaluation, and Treatment of High Blood Cholesterol was charged with responsibility for developing population-based strategies to shift the distribution of cholesterol levels of the entire population to a lower range.[37] It was also asked to develop guidelines for patient-centered approaches that would identify individuals at high risk who would benefit from intervention efforts. The second report of the panel was released in 1993.[38] The panel recommended that total cholesterol cutoff points for relative risk for CHD be uniform for men and women of all ages. The panel acknowledged that there was limited clinical trial data available for the elderly population but stated that extrapolation

of data from trials showing reduction in CHD risk in middle-aged patients seems reasonable. The panel's report pointed out that since older age increases the risk of CHD, lowering total cholesterol levels in elderly individuals could result in substantial reductions in morbidity and mortality rates. Modifications of this general approach may be warranted, especially in extreme old age.[35]

The panel also developed a set of recommendations based on total cholesterol and HDL cholesterol levels (Table 9–2).[38] A second set of criteria for classification and treatment has been developed based on LDL cholesterol (Table 9–3). The outline for dietary modifications is presented in Table 9–4.[38] Modifications in the Step One diet are similar to the dietary modifications recommended by the American Heart Association as part of a population-based strategy for lowering serum cholesterol:

1. A total of no more than 30% of calories is provided by fat, less than 10% of calories from saturated fat. Polyunsaturated fats provide up to 10% of the calories; monounsaturates provide the remainder.

**Table 9–3** Treatment Decisions Based on LDL-Cholesterol Levels

| Patient Category | Initiation Level | LDL Goal |
|---|---|---|
| **Dietary Therapy** | | |
| Without CHD and with fewer than two risk factors | ≥160 mg/dL (4.1 mmol/L) | <160 mg/dL (4.1 mmol/L) |
| Without CHD and with two or more risk factors | ≥130 mg/dL (3.4 mmol/L) | <130 mg/dL (3.4 mmol/L) |
| With CHD | >100 mg/dL (2.6 mmol/L) | ≤100 mg/dL (2.6 mmol/L) |
| **Drug Therapy** | | |
| Without CHD and with fewer than two risk factors | ≥190 mg/dL (4.9 mmol/L) | <160 mg/dL (4.1 mmol/L) |
| Without CHD and with two or more risk factors | ≥160 mg/dL (4.1 mmol/L) | <130 mg/dL (3.4 mmol/L) |
| With CHD | ≥130 mg/dL (3.4 mmol/L) | ≤100 mg/dL (2.6 mmol/L) |

*Source:* Reprinted with permission fron Summary of the Second Report of the National Cholesterol Education Program Expert Panel on Detection, Evaluation, and Treatment of High Blood Cholesterol in Adults (Adult Treatment Panel II).*Journal of the American Medical Association*, Vol. 269, pp. 3015–3023, Copyright 1993, American Medical Association.

2. Between 50% and 60% of calories should come from carbohydrates.
3. Between 10% and 20% of calories should come from protein.
4. Cholesterol should be limited to less than 300 mg/d.
5. Calories should be adjusted to achieve and maintain ideal weight.

Specific dietary modifications are presented in Table 9–5. The goal of dietary therapy is to reduce elevated cholesterol levels while maintaining a nutritionally adequate diet. Serum cholesterol measurement, and an assessment of adherence to the diet, should be conducted at 4 to 6 weeks and at 3 months. If the total serum cholesterol goal is achieved, the LDL-cholesterol level should be measured as confirmation that it has dropped to the desired level. If this occurs, long-term monitoring should include quarterly evaluation for 1 year and twice-yearly visits after

that. At each visit, total serum cholesterol should be measured and diet and behavior modifications reviewed.

If the goal on the Step One diet is not met, a second trial on the same diet or progression to the Step Two diet with a referral to a dietitian is indicated, with measurement at similar intervals for monitoring and maintenance as for Step One. On the Step Two diet, total fat remains at 30% of total calories, but saturated fat is reduced further, to 7%, and cholesterol is reduced to 200 mg. Recent evidence indicates that a marked reduction in total fat is not necessary to lower LDL levels satisfactorily if saturated fat is reduced.[39] Whether diets with fat levels as low as 20% of total calories facilitate weight reduction is a matter of debate, but it is clear that they have a low satiety value and are not well accepted. A minimum of 6 months of intensive dietary therapy and counseling usually should precede the use of drugs, except where levels of LDL choles-

**Table 9–4** Dietary Therapy of High Blood Cholesterol Level

| Nutrient | Recommended Intake | |
| --- | --- | --- |
| | *Step One Diet* | *Step Two Diet* |
| Total fat | Less than 30% of total kcal | Less than 30% of total kcal |
| Saturated fatty acids | 8–10% of total kcal | Less than 7% of total kcal |
| Polyunsaturated fatty acids | Up to 10% of total kcal | Up to 10% of total kcal |
| Monounsaturated fatty acids | 10–15% of total kcal | 10–15% of total kcal |
| Carbohydrates | 50–60% of total kcal | 50–60% of total kcal |
| Protein | 10–20% of total kcal | 10–20% of total kcal |
| Cholesterol | <300 mg | <200 mg |
| Total calories | To achieve and maintain a desirable weight | To achieve and maintain a desirable weight |

*Source:* Reprinted with permission from *Archives of Internal Medicine* Vol. 148, Table 4, pp. 36–39, Copyright 1989, American Medical Association.

terol exceed 225 mg/dL or where CHD exists. Drug therapy should be added to dietary therapy, not substituted for it.[38]

Other dietary modifications targeted toward risk reduction of cardiovascular disease have gained widespread attention in the popular press. They include water-soluble fibers (particularly oat bran), fish oils, and, more recently, antioxidants and B vitamins.

Water-soluble fibers found in oat products and beans, if consumed in large amounts (as much as 15 to 25 g/d), have been reported to lower plasma cholesterol by 5% to 15%.[40,41] The U.S. Food and Drug Administration recently approved the use of health claims on the labels of foods containing soluble fiber from whole oats (rolled oats, oat bran, and oat flour) noting that these foods, as part of a diet low in saturated fat and cholesterol, may reduce the risk of heart disease.[42] However, the panel does not make specific recommendations for increasing fiber consumption as a component of the Step One diet. Similarly, no specific recommendations are made for alcohol, which has been shown to raise HDL-cholesterol levels.[43]

The highly polyunsaturated omega-3 fatty acids, found mainly in fish oils, have been shown to lower both triglyceride and LDL-cholesterol levels when given in high doses and substituted for saturated fats.[44] High doses (>3g/d) may also reduce blood pressure.[45] However, there is no evidence that they reduce the risk for CHD, and whether long-term use will lead to undesirable side effects is unknown.[46,47] Therefore, use of dietary fish oil supplements is not recommended.[44] However, increased consumption of fish, including those with omega-3 fatty acids, is recommended as substitutions for other sources of protein that are high in saturated fat. Evidence from epidemiologic studies suggests an association of reduced risk from consumption of fish of any type, independent of omega-3 fatty acid levels.[47]

Epidemiologic evidence has shown a protective effect of antioxidant nutrients (vitamin E, vitamin C, and beta carotene) on CHD risk.[48–50] Antioxidants decrease the formation of atherosclerosis by preventing oxidation of LDL cholesterol. The effect of vitamin E supplementation on CHD has garnered particular interest. The secondary prevention of CHD with doses of 400 to 800 IU/d of vitamin E is well established. Few studies have focused on the elderly, though some have

**Table 9–5** Recommended Dietary Modifications To Lower Blood Cholesterol

*Step One Diet*

| Foods | Choose | Decrease |
|---|---|---|
| Fish, chicken, turkey, lean meats* | Fish, poultry without skin, lean cuts of beef, lamb, pork, veal, shellfish | Fatty cuts of beef, lamb, pork; spareribs, organ meats, regular cold cuts, sausage, hot dogs, bacon, sardines, roe |
| Skim milk and low-fat milk, cheese, yogurt,* dairy substitutes | Skim or 1% fat milk (liquid, powdered, evaporated), buttermilk | Whole milk (4% fat) or (regular, evaporated, condensed), cream, half-and-half, 2% fat milk, imitation milk products, most nondairy creamers, whipped toppings |
| | Nonfat (0% fat) or low-fat yogurt | Whole-milk yogurt |
| | Low-fat cottage cheese (1% or 2% fat) | Whole-milk cottage cheese (4%) |
| | Low-fat cheeses, farmer or pot cheeses (all of these should be labeled no more than 2–6 g of fat per ounce) | All natural cheese (eg, blue, Roquefort, Camembert, Cheddar, Swiss), low-fat or "light" cream cheese, low-fat or "light" sour cream, cream cheeses, sour cream |
| | Sherbet, sorbet | Ice cream |
| Eggs* | Egg whites (2 whites equal 1 whole egg in recipes), cholesterol-free egg substitutes | Egg yolks |
| Fruits and vegetables* | Fresh, frozen, canned, or dried fruits and vegetables | Vegetables prepared in butter, cream, or other sauces |
| Breads and cereals | Home-baked goods using unsaturated oils sparingly, angel food cake, low-fat crackers, low-fat cookies | Commercial baked goods; pies, cakes, doughnuts, croissants, pastries, muffins, biscuits, high-fat crackers, high-fat cookies |
| | Rice, pasta | Egg noodles |

*continues*

**Table 9–5** continued

*Step One Diet*

| Foods | Choose | Decrease |
|---|---|---|
| | Whole-grain breads and cereals (oatmeal, whole wheat, rye, bran, multigrain) | Breads in which eggs are a major ingredient |
| Fats and oils* | Baking cocoa | Chocolate |
| | Unsaturated vegetable oils: corn, olive, rapeseed (canola oil), safflower, sesame, soybean, sunflower Margarine and shortenings made from one of the unsaturated oils listed above, light margarine | Butter, coconut oil, palm oil, palm kernel oil, lard, bacon fat |
| | Mayonnaise, salad dressings made with unsaturated oils listed above, low-fat dressings | Dressings made with egg yolks |
| | Seeds and nuts | Coconut |

*Limit lean meat, chicken, turkey, and fish to 6 oz/d. Have at least 2 servings of low-fat dairy products per day. Include fruits and/or vegetables at every meal. Up to 6 to 8 teaspoons of unsaturated vegetable oil is acceptable. Limit nuts and peanut butter, which are high in fat and calories.

found a protective effect of vitamin E supplementation in the elderly, consistent with that observed in younger populations.[21,51] The use of vitamin E supplements for primary prevention of CHD has not been definitively demonstrated. Large-scale randomized intervention trials currently under way will contribute to clarifying specific recommendations regarding vitamin E supplementation.

The association between plasma homocysteine concentration and CHD has been the subject of a number of recent studies.[22–25] Plasma homocysteine concentration may be inversely associated with vitamin $B_6$, vitamin $B_{12}$, and folate status, suggesting that adequate intakes of these nutrients may be protective against CHD risk.[22] It has been estimated that the recent decision of the federal government to fortify the food supply with folate at the level of 140 g per 100 g of cereal grain product[52] in an effort to prevent neural tube birth defects, would reduce the percentage of the elderly population with folate intake below the recommended 400 µg/d from 66% to 49%.[53]

## Blood Pressure

Hypertension in elderly individuals is generally classified in three ways.[9] Isolated hypertension is defined as systolic blood pressure greater than 160 mm Hg with an accompanying diastolic pressure less than 95 mm Hg. Predominant systolic hypertension is characterized by a disproportionate elevation in systolic pressure compared with a slightly elevated diastolic pressure. Two formulas are used to express the expected relationship:

expected systolic pressure =
3/2 × diastolic pressure

or

expected systolic pressure =
(diastolic Pressure – 15) × 2

Combined systolic and diastolic hypertension, characteristic of essential hypertension, consists of a proportional increase in both systolic and diastolic pressures continuing into old age. For diagnostic purposes, hypertension has been variously defined as systolic pressure exceeding 130 mm Hg to 200 mm Hg, or diastolic pressure between 90 and 120 mm Hg. The National Heart, Lung, and Blood Institute Advisory Committee defines it as systolic blood pressure greater than or equal to 160 mmHg and diastolic blood pressure less than 90 mm Hg.[54]

Hypertension is the most powerful predictor of stroke and the risk factor most readily amenable to treatment. It accelerates atherogenesis and imparts a two- to threefold increased risk of cardiovascular disease events, including CHD.[55] Multiple U.S. prospective population studies demonstrate that systolic blood pressure and diastolic blood pressure relate strongly and independently to risk of cardiovascular events.[56] Hypertension is also extremely common among elderly people,

doubling the overall mortality and tripling cardiovascular mortality.[57] Over a period of 38 years of follow-up in Framingham study subjects aged 75 to 94, increasing cardiovascular morbidity and mortality rates with increasing blood pressure levels were observed in both men and women initially free of cardiovascular disease.[58] An age-adjusted increased risk of death from all causes and from cardiovascular causes during 24 years of follow-up in the Framingham study was at least twice that of subjects with blood pressure at or below 140/95 mm Hg.

Longitudinal observations from the Framingham study show different patterns for systolic and diastolic pressures in men and women. Among women, there is an almost linear rise in systolic pressure, with obesity acting as a significant contributing factor. Diastolic pressure rises until the early 60s and then declines. In men, systolic pressure peaks in middle age and then levels off, whereas diastolic pressure rises until the mid-50s and then declines.[59]

The rise in blood pressure with age that is observed in most countries does not occur among some primitive populations, which may indicate that hypertension is not an inevitable consequence of aging.[9] Until recently, however, isolated systolic hypertension (ISH) was widely viewed as a benign disease of older persons and was thought to be a physiologic adaptation necessary for the perfusion of aging organ systems. Antihypertensive therapy was commonly believed by practicing physicians to be of little value and too dangerous in individuals older than 65 years.

ISH, usually a reflection of diminished distensibility of the aorta, accounts for 65% to 75% of hypertension in the elderly in the Framingham study, occurring as the endpoint of several contributing factors.[55,57] These include the effects of systolic hypertension on arterial wall compliance, inducing a gradual reduction in diastolic pressure and increased pulse pressure. The disproportionate rise in systolic pressure is consistent with a progressive loss of elasticity. The fact that it is predominantly systolic pressure that rises does not make it less dangerous. In fact, evidence from the Framingham study indicates that no measure is superior to systolic pressure in predicting cardiovascular events in general and stroke in particular—the hypertensive event most closely related to blood pressure elevation.[9]

The National High Blood Pressure Education Program (NHBPEP) Working Group report on hypertension in the elderly[60] outlines a diagnostic and treatment program for the management of elevated blood pressure in elderly individuals. The rationale for the program is based on findings from both observational and intervention studies. The Medical Research Council trial found that patients treated for diastolic hypertension experienced a 17% reduction in all cardiovascular events, as compared with a placebo-treated control group.[60]

The Systolic Hypertension in the Elderly Program (SHEP) was the first intervention trial to show that antihypertensive therapy could reduce cardiovascular events in individuals with ISH.[60] SHEP, which was a double-blind, placebo-controlled, randomized clinical trial of antihypertensive therapy in subjects with ISH, observed a significant 36% reduction in the combined incidence of fatal and nonfatal stroke, a 27% reduction in nonfatal myocardial infarction or coronary death, and a 32% reduction in all major cardiovascular events.[60]

On the basis of available evidence, the NHBPEP Working Group has made several recommendations for the detection and treatment of hypertension of elderly people, with the objective of reducing the cardiovascular risk associated with high blood pressure.[60]

Lifestyle modification, including weight loss, dietary sodium restriction, alcohol reduction, nutrition therapy, and exercise, is recommended. Weight loss has been shown to have an independent antihypertensive effect on blood pressure.[61,62] Unfortunately, the success rate for long-term weight maintenance is limited. Not all individuals with hypertension experience a drop in blood pressure on reduced sodium intake.

If diet is not effective, drug therapy should be initiated. The choice of medication is based on the coexistence of both risk factors and disease.[63] Diuretics are often the drugs of choice for elderly patients. They were evaluated during the feasibility trial for the SHEP and were found to be both effective and acceptable. The possibility of particular sensitivity to the hypokalemic effects of diuretics among elderly people suggests that serum potassium should be monitored closely and that extra emphasis should be placed on including generous amounts of potassium-rich foods in the diet. Although potassium supplements reportedly can help offset the effects of a high sodium intake, cost and the potential hazards associated with their use make them impractical.[19] Sodium restriction, used in conjunction with diuretics, has been shown to reduce dependence on antihypertensive medications.[59]

Alcohol is associated with increased blood pressure; caffeine, however, is not.[19] Evidence for relationships between blood pressure and other nutrients is more sparse, and their relationship to hypertension in elderly people is unclear. The long-term effects of increased calcium and magnesium, modification of food intake, and vegetarian diets on hypertension in older subjects remain to be explored.[19]

The recent Dietary Approaches to Stop Hypertension (DASH) trial[64] studied the effect of dietary patterns on blood pressure. Subjects were placed on one of three diets:

(1) a control diet similar to the typical American diet; (2) a diet providing more fruits and vegetables and fewer snacks and sweets, but otherwise similar to the control diet; and (3) a combination diet rich in fruits, vegetables, and low-fat dairy foods, with reduced amounts of saturated fat, total fat, and cholesterol. The sodium content of each diet was similar (approximately 3 g/d). Those on the combination diet experienced the greatest drop in blood pressure: systolic blood pressure was reduced by 5.5 mm Hg more than in the control group, and diastolic blood pressure was reduced by 3.0 mm Hg more. The authors suggest that adoption of the DASH combination diet could potentially shift the population distribution of blood pressure downward, reducing the occurrence of blood pressure–related cardiovascular disease.[64] They also state that it has been estimated that a populationwide reduction in systolic or diastolic blood pressure of the magnitude observed with the DASH combination diet would reduce incident CHD by approximately 15% and stroke by approximately 27%.

While subjects in the DASH study were younger, it is reasonable to extrapolate the findings to the elderly, given the high prevalence of hypertension in older cohorts, and to recommend modification of the Step One diet described earlier to reflect the DASH combination diet. Other recommendations to reduce blood pressure include reducing weight when indicated, restricting sodium intake to 2 g/d (88 mmol/d), and restricting alcohol to 2 oz/d.

## Obesity

The relationship of obesity to increased risk for cardiovascular disease in elderly individuals remains controversial, with some studies indicating increased risk at both extremes of the weight distribution curve.[65] Much of the controversy is explained by the confounding effects of smoking, coexisting disease, and inadequate follow-up.[59] However, the preponderance of evidence suggests that obesity heightens other atherogenic risk factors[66] and thereby contributes to increased risk. The relationships between weight and cardiovascular risk are presented in Figure 9–4.[67]

Data from the Framingham study at 30-year follow-up demonstrate a continuous relationship between obesity and coronary morbidity and mortality (stronger in men than in women). Obesity is associated with both blood pressure and serum lipoprotein levels. In the Framingham study,[68] correlation between relative weight and either systolic or diastolic pressure declined steadily over adult life. Havlik and colleagues,[69] using the body mass index (weight/height$^2$) (BMI) and blood pressure, reported similar declines in men over the age range of 30 to 70 years. Harlan and associates[70] showed a reduction in association between BMI and systolic blood pressure in older women. The weaker association at older ages remains significant for men but not for women.

In the Framingham study, the correlation between relative body weight and total plasma cholesterol is not significant in men older than 50 years; in women, it is significant only among 35- to 39-year-olds.[71] After age 50 years, BMI is no longer significantly associated with LDL cholesterol in either sex. However, the strong inverse relationship between HDL cholesterol and BMI remains statistically significant, even among subjects aged 70 to 79 years.[71,72] Therefore, the benefits of maintaining optimal weight for height are associated with a positive effect on HDL-cholesterol levels.[7]

Lamon-Fava et al[73] found that BMI increased with age in men until the age of 50

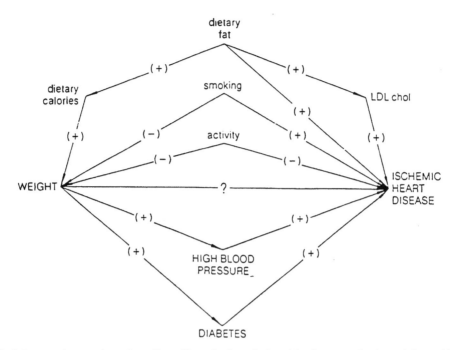

**Figure 9–4** Interactions and confounding effects in the relationships between body weight and ischemic heart disease. LDL chol, low-density lipoprotein cholesterol. *Source:* Reprinted with permission from *Annals of Internal Medicine* (1985;103:1003–1005), Copyright © 1985, American College of Physicians.

and then plateaued, while in women it increased with age through the seventh decade of life. BMI was significantly associated with systolic blood pressure, fasting glucose levels, total cholesterol, and LDL cholesterol and was inversely associated with HDL cholesterol, leading the authors to conclude that "elevated BMI is associated with adverse effects on all major CHD risk factors."

National surveys have found that the incidence of overweight among U.S. adults has increased. Overweight prevalence increased 8% between 1976–1980 and 1988–1991 surveys.[74] During this period, mean BMI increased from 25.3 to 26.3 for adult men and women aged 20 to 74 years, and mean body weight increased 3.6 kg. This suggests that weight reduction does not explain the observed decline in serum cholesterol levels in men and that increased fatness may even

have blunted the trend. Among women, relative weights decreased at young and middle ages, but no trend has emerged among the older cohort.[7]

A small but significant drop in age-specific blood pressure over the past 22 years has been observed,[75] despite increased relative weight. More effective control of obesity, and especially the prevention of weight gain in middle adult life, is of potentially great value in further reducing CHD mortality. Direct evidence for long-term benefits of weight reduction is lacking and is likely to remain so. The inability to achieve and maintain sustained weight loss is widely documented.[76] Moreover, it is impractical to conduct a controlled trial with random assignment of subjects to a weight reduction program. Few data compare the relative risks associated with weight fluctuation and sustained obesity. In the Framingham study, weight at younger ages has been found to be an important predictor of cardiovascular disease.[77,78] Relative weights at the time of initial examination predicted a 26-year incidence of CHD and cardiac failure in men, independent of risk factors associated with increased fatness. In women, there was an independent association between relative weight and CHD, stroke, cardiac failure, and cardiovascular mortality. The relative risk of CHD 25 years later in a group of men ranging in age from 45 to 57 years at time of entry into the study who reported weight fluctuation during young adulthood was double that of men whose weight remained stable or increased.[79]

Weight reduction has been shown to confer substantial improvement in the cardiovascular risk profile. Therefore, it is recommended for elderly individuals who are 20% or more above desirable weight as defined by BMIs of 27.2 for men and 26.9 for women. In individuals with diabetes, hypertension, dyslipidemia, and gout, lesser degrees of overweight should be reversed.[59]

## Dietary Modification for Cardiovascular Risk Reduction

The decline in CHD mortality that began in the 1960s coincided with considerable changes in the American diet. Between 1960 and 1974, milk and cream consumption declined by 25%, butter by 50%, and animal fat by 39%. Per capita use of poultry increased by 50% and use of fish by 30%.[80–82] Between 1980 and 1995 per capita egg consumption decreased by approximately 13%—from 271 to 234 per year.[83] And while consumption of whole milk has decreased over the last 20 years, the amount of 1% and skim milk as a percentage of total milk consumed has been increasing and recently replacing 2% milk as the reduced-fat alternative to whole milk.[83]

A comparative analysis of dietary data obtained over more than 20 years from epidemiologic studies of middle-aged Americans shows the impact of these altered food habits on fat intake. Energy derived from total and saturated fat declined by 2% to 3%, and dietary cholesterol consumption declined between 100 and 200 mg/d. The decline in saturated (S) fat intake and the increase in polyunsaturated (P) fats raised the dietary P:S ratio from 0.25 to 0.5 by the mid-1970s.[84]

Information about changes in dietary intake in elderly people is limited. However, elderly individuals (aged 60 and over) surveyed in the NHANES III were found to have fat intakes of 31% to 34% of total calories and cholesterol intakes of 200 to 225 mg for men and 132 to 150 mg for women.[85] A study of free-living elderly subjects aged 60 to 100 found higher values: men consumed 35% of calories from fat, 16.5% of calories from saturated fat, and 350 mg/d of cholesterol; women consumed 35.4% of calories from fat, 16.3% of calories from saturated fat, and 265 mg/d of cholesterol.[86]

Studies of secular trends in blood lipid levels have shown that serum total cholesterol began to decline in the late 1950s across the broad age span from 20 to 74 years. Data from the large national health surveys and from the Framingham study have shown substantial decreases among individuals of both sexes.[7] Data from the Baltimore Longitudinal Study extend this observation to men in their 70s and 80s. Therefore, the decline in blood total cholesterol over the past 25 years is consistent with dietary changes, even among older age groups.[7]

Consideration of further dietary modifications for elderly persons must address two questions. First, are the dietary modifications of value for older people? Second, are the proposed changes feasible? A consistent observation in elderly people has been their extremely low energy intakes. Since intake of essential nutrients is closely related to calorie intake, the risk of nutrient deficiencies rises in older groups. Further calorie restriction carries with it the potential danger of increasing the risk of nutrient deficiencies. For weight reduction and maintenance, it is perhaps more reasonable to suggest increased physical activity rather than further decreases in calorie intake.

Any dietary modification in older individuals should begin with a careful assessment to determine both the nutritional adequacy of the diet and the level of intake of nutrients to be modified. In particular, current and usual levels of sodium intake should be assessed before dietary modifications are made. To succeed, the diet plan should be developed in cooperation with the patient, allowing for differences in cultural patterns and taste preferences. The concept that only 30% of calories should come from fat and no more than 10% from saturated fat is difficult for many individuals to apply to their diets. To be effective, the nutrition counselor must develop unique methods of communicating simple concepts to older individuals who are expected to modify their diets. A nutrition counselor who prescribes diets modified in calories, fat, and sodium to older subjects and neglects to teach them how to select and prepare the diets is likely to see failure and noncompliance.

## CONCLUSION

Recommendations for cardiovascular disease prevention for older people are extensions of recommendations for younger age groups; they focus primarily on functional ability or the full spectrum of conditions associated with advancing age, largely because the efficacy of prevention in elderly people is undetermined.[6] The model for consideration of intervention strategies for the management of hypertension can be applied to other cardiovascular risk factors as well. The development of more effective nutritional interventions for elderly people requires a series of steps. It is essential, first, to define appropriate risk factors and effective modifiers for the natural history of disease; second, to define outcomes meaningful to elderly individuals in terms of the burden of illness; and third, to identify critical points of intervention to prevent disability.

## REFERENCES

1. National Center for Health Statistics. Report of final mortality statistics: 1995. *Mon Vital Stat Rep.* 1995;45(2 suppl).

2. Bierman EL, Hazzard WR. Preventive gerontology: strategies for attenuation of the chronic diseases of aging. In: Hazzard WR, Andres R, Bierman EL, Blass JP, eds. *Principles of Geriatric Medicine and Gerontology.* 2nd ed. New York, NY: McGraw-Hill, Inc; 1990.

3. Gillum RF. Trends in acute myocardial infarction and coronary heart disease death in the United States. *J Am Coll Cardiol.* 1993;23:1273–1277.

4. Bierman EL. Aging and atherosclerosis. In: Hazzard WR, Andres R, Bierman EL, Blass JP, eds. *Principles of Geriatric Medicine and Gerontology.* 2nd ed. New York, NY: McGraw-Hill, Inc; 1990.

5. *Technology and Aging in America.* Washington, DC: US Office of Technological Assessment; 1985. US Congress, Office of Technology Assessment, OTA NS-264.

6. Fried LP, Bush TL. Morbidity as a focus of preventive health care in the elderly. *Epidemiol Rev.* 1988;10:48–64.

7. McGandy RB. Nutrition and the aging cardiovascular system. In: Hutchinson ML, Munro HN, eds.

*Nutrition and Aging*. Orlando, Fla: Academic Press Inc; 1986.

8. Lakatta EG. Health, disease and cardiovascular aging. *Cardiovasc Med*. March 1985;38.

9. Lakatta EG. Heart and circulation. In: Schneider EL, Rowe JN, eds. *Handbook of the Biology of Aging*. San Diego, Calif: Academic Press; 1990.

10. McGandy RB. Atherogenesis and aging. In: Chernoff R, Lipschitz DA, eds. *Health Promotion and Disease Prevention in the Elderly*. New York, NY: Raven Press; 1988.

11. Waller BF, Roberts WC. Cardiovascular disease in the very elderly. *Am J Cardiol*. 1983;51:403–421.

12. Hennerici M, Rautenberg W, Trockel U, et al. Spontaneous progression and regression of small carotid atheromata. *Lancet*. 1985;1:1415–1419.

13. Blankenhorn DH. Prevention or reversal of atherosclerosis: review of current evidence. *Am J Cardiol*. 1989;63:38H–41H.

14. Cashin-Hemphill L, Sanmarco ME, Blankenhorn DH. Augmented beneficial effects of colestipol-niacin therapy at four years in the CLAS trial. Presented at the American Heart Association Annual Meeting; New Orleans, La; November 1989.

15. Ornish D, Scherwitz W, Brown SE, et al. Adherence to lifestyle changes and reversal of coronary atherosclerosis. Presented at the American Heart Association Annual Meeting; New Orleans, La; November 1989.

16. Gould KL, Ornish D, Scherwitz L, et al. Changes in myocardial perfusion abnormalities by positron emission tomography after long-term, intense risk factor modification. *JAMA*. 1995;274:894–901.

17. *CDC Fact Sheet: Facts about Cardiovascular Disease*. Atlanta, Ga: Centers for Disease Control and Prevention, Office of Communication, Division of Media Relations; June 27, 1997.

18. Rosenberg HM, Klebba AJ. Trends in cardiovascular mortality with a focus on ischemic heart disease: United States 1950-1976. In: Havlik RJ, Feinleib M, eds. *Proceedings of the Conference on the Decline in Coronary Heart Disease Mortality*. Washington, DC: Conference on Decline in Coronary Heart Disease Mortality; 1979. US Dept of Health, Education, and Welfare publication NIH 79-1610.

19. Pell S, Fayerweather WE. Trends in the incidence of myocardial infarction and in associated mortality and morbidity in a large employed population. *N Engl J Med*. 1985;312:1005–1011.

20. Corry DB, Tuck ML. Nutritional interventions as antihypertensive therapy in the elderly. In: Morley JE, Glick Z, Rubenstein LZ, eds. *Geriatric Nutrition: A Comprehensive Review*. 2nd ed. New York, NY: Raven Press; 1995.

21. Losonczy KG, Harris TB, Havlik RJ. Vitamin E and vitamin C supplement use and risk of all-cause and coronary heart disease mortality in older persons: the Established Populations for Epidemiologic Studies of the Elderly. *Am J Clin Nutr*. 1996; 64:190–196.

22. Selhub J, Jacques PF, Wilson PF, et al. Vitamin status and intake as primary determinants of homocysteinemia in an elderly population. *JAMA*. 1993;270:2693–2698.

23. Tucker KL, Selhub J, Wilson PWF, et al. Dietary intake pattern relates to plasma folate and homocysteine concentrations in the Framingham Heart Study. *J Nutr*. 1996;126:3025–3031.

24. Stampfer MJ, Malinow MR, Willett WC, et al. A prospective study of plasma homocyst(e)ine and risk of myocardial infarction in US physicians. *JAMA*. 1992;268:877–881.

25. Nygård O, Nordrehaug JE, Refsum H, et al. Plasma homocysteine levels and mortality in patients with coronary artery disease. *N Engl J Med*. 1997; 337:230–236.

26. Johnson CL, Rifkind BM, Sempos CT, et al. Declining serum total cholesterol levels among US adults: the National Health and Nutrition Examination Surveys. *JAMA*. 1993;269:3002–3008.

27. Castelli WP, Doyle JT, Gordon T, et al. HDL cholesterol and other lipids in coronary heart disease. *Circulation*. 1977;55:767–772.

28. Kannel WB, Gordon T, eds. *The Framingham Study: An Epidemiological Investigation of Cardiovascular Disease*. Washington, DC: US Public Health Service; 1971. US Dept of Health, Education, and Welfare publication NIH 1740-0320.

29. Barrett-Connor E, Suarez L, Kjaw K, et al. Ischemic heart disease risk factors after 50. *J Chronic Dis*. 1984;27:103–114.

30. Castelli WP, Wilson PWF, Levy D, et al. Cardiovascular risk factors in the elderly. *Am J Cardiol*. 1989;63:12H–19H.

31. Schaefer EJ, Lichtenstein AH, Lamon-Fava S, et al. Lipoproteins, nutrition, aging, and atherosclerosis. *Am J Clin Nutr*. 1995;61(suppl):726S–740S.

32. Willett WC, Stampfer MJ, Manson JE, et al. *Trans*-fatty acid intake in relation to risk of coronary heart disease among women. *Lancet*. 1993;341:581–585.

33. Ascherio A, Hennekens CH, Buring JE, et al. *Trans*-fatty acid intake and risk of myocardial infarction. *Circulation*. 1994;89:94–101.

34. Hu FB, Stampfer MJ, Manson JE, et al. Dietary fat intake and the risk of coronary heart disease in women. *N Engl J Med*. 1997;337:1391–1399.

35. Blum CB, Levy R. Current therapy for hypercholesterolemia. *JAMA*. 1989;261:3582–3587.

36. Lenfant C. New national cholesterol education program. *Cardiovasc Med*. 1985;10:39–40.

37. Expert Panel: report of the National Cholesterol Education Program Expert Panel on Detection, Evaluation, and Treatment of High Blood Cholesterol in Adults. *Arch Intern Med*. 1989;148:36–69.

38. Expert Panel on Detection, Evaluation, and Treatment of High Blood Cholesterol in Adults. Summary of the second report of the National Cholesterol Education Program (NCEP) Expert Panel on Detection, Evaluation, and Treatment of High Blood Cholesterol in Adults (Adult Treatment Panel II). *JAMA*. 1993;269:3015–3023.

39. Knopp RH, Walden CE, Retzlaff BM, et al. Long-term cholesterol-lowering effects of 4 fat-restricted diets in hypercholesterolemic and combined hyperlipidemic men: the Dietary Alternatives Study. *JAMA*. 1997;278:1509–1515.

40. Anderson JW, Story L, Sieling B, et al. Hypocholesterolemic effects of oat-bran or bean intake for hypercholesterolemic men. *Am J Clin Nutr*. 1984;40:1146–1155.

41. VanHorn L, Liu K, Parker D, et al. Serum lipid response to oat product intake with a fat-modified diet. *J Am Diet Assoc*. 1986;86:759–764.

42. Food and Drug Administration, Dept of Health and Human Services. Food labeling: health claims; oats and coronary heart disease. 21 CFR, Part 101. January 23, 1997, Docket No. 959-0197.

43. Marques-Vidal P, Ducimetiere P, Evans A, et al. Alcohol consumption and myocardial infarction: a case-control study in France and Northern Ireland. *Am J Epidemiol*. 1996;143:1089–1093.

44. Stone NJ. Fish consumption, fish oil, lipids, and coronary heart disease. *Am J Clin Nutr*. 1997;65:1083–1086.

45. Appel LJ, Miller ER, Seidler AJ, Whelton PK. Does supplementation of diet with "fish oil" reduce blood pressure? A meta-analysis of controlled clinical trials. *Arch Int Med*. 1993;153:1429–1438.

46. Committee on Diet and Health, National Research Council. *Diet and Health: Implications for Reducing Chronic Disease Risk*. Washington, DC: National Academy Press; 1989.

47. Daviglus ML, Stamler J, Orencia AJ, et al. Fish consumption and the 30-year risk of fatal myocardial infarction. *N Engl J Med*. 1997;336:1046–1053.

48. Manson JE, Gaziano JM, Jonas MA, Hennekens CH. Antioxidants and cardiovascular disease: a review. *J Am Coll Nutr*. 1993;12:426–432.

49. Rimm EB, Stampfer MJ. The role of antioxidants in preventive cardiology. *Curr Opin Cardiol*. 1997;12:188–194.

50. Gaziano JM. Antioxidant vitamins and coronary artery disease risk. *Am J Med*. 1994;97(3A):18S–21S.

51. Paolisso G, Gambardella A, Giugliano D, et al. Chronic intake of pharmacological doses of vitamin E might be useful in the therapy of elderly patients with coronary heart disease. *Am J Clin Nutr*. 1995;61:848–852.

52. Food standards: amendment of standards of identity for enriched grain products to require addition of folic acid. *Federal Register*. March 5, 1996;61:8781–8797.

53. Tucker KL, Mahnken B, Wilson PWF, et al. Folic acid fortification of the food supply: potential benefits and risks for the elderly population. *JAMA*. 1996;276:1879–1885.

54. Applegate WB. Hypertension. In: Hazzard WR, Andres R, Bierman EL, Blass JP, eds. *Principles of Geriatric Medicine and Gerontology*. 2nd ed. New York, NY: McGraw-Hill; 1990.

55. Kannell WB. Blood pressure as a cardiovascular risk factor. *JAMA*. 1996;275:1571–1576.

56. Stamler J, Stamler R, Neaton JD. Blood pressure, systolic and diastolic, and cardiovascular risks. *Arch Int Med*. 1993;153:598–615.

57. Wilking SVB, Belanger A, Kannell WB, et al. Determinants of isolated systolic hypertension. *JAMA*. 1988;260:3451–3455.

58. Kannel WB, D'Agostino RB, Silbershatz H. Blood pressure and cardiovascular morbidity and mortality rates in the elderly. *Am Heart J*. 1997;134;758–763.

59. Kannel WB. Nutrition and the occurrence and prevention of cardiovascular disease in the elderly. *Nutr Rev*. 1988;46:68–78.

60. National High Blood Pressure Education Program Working Group. National High Blood Pressure Education Program Working Group report on hypertension in the elderly. *Hypertension*. 1994; 23:275–285.

61. Reisen E, Frohlich EG, Messerli FH, et al. Cardiovascular changes after weight reduction in obesity hypertension. *Ann Intern Med*. 1983;98:315–319.

62. Maxwell MH, Kushiro T, Dornfeld LP, et al. Blood pressure changes in obese hypertensive subjects during rapid weight loss: comparison of restricted versus unchanged salt intake. *Arch Intern Med*. 1984;144:1581–1584.

63. Weber MA, Neutel JM, Chung DG. Hypertension in the aged: a pathologic basis for treatment. *Am J Cardiol*. 1989;63:25H–32H.

64. Appel LJ, Moore TJ, Obarzanek E, et al. A clinical trial of the effects of dietary patterns on blood pressure. *N Engl J Med*. 1997;336:1117–1124.

65. Manson JE, Willett WC, Stampfer MJ, et al. Body weight and mortality among women. *N Engl J Med*. 1995;333:677–685.

66. Willett WC, Manson JE, Stampfer MJ, et al. Weight, weight change, and coronary heart disease in women: risk within the "normal" weight range. *JAMA*. 1995;273:461–465.

67. Stallones R. Epidemiologic studies of obesity. *Ann Intern Med*. 1985;103:1003–1005.

68. Kannel WB, Gordon T. *An Epidemiologic Investigation of Cardiovascular Disease*. Washington, DC: US Public Health Service; 1968. US Dept of Health, Education, and Welfare publication.

69. Havlik RJ, Hubert HB, Fabsitz RR, et al. Weight and hypertension. *Ann Intern Med*. 1983;98:855–859.

70. Harlan WR, Hull AL, Schmouder RL, et al. High blood pressure in older Americans: the first national health and nutrition examination survey. *Hypertension*. 1984;6:802–809.

71. Kannel WB, Gordon T, Castelli WP. Obesity, lipids, and glucose intolerance: the Framingham study. *Am J Clin Nutr*. 1979;32:1238–1245.

72. Wilson PWF, Garrison RJ, Abbott RD, et al. Factors associated with lipoprotein cholesterol levels: the Framingham study. *Arteriosclerosis*. 1983; 3:273–281.

73. Lamon-Fava S, Wilson PW, Schaefer EJ. Impact of body mass index on coronary heart disease risk factors in men and women: the Framingham Offspring Study. *Arterioscler Thromb Vasc Biol*. 1996; 16:1509–1515.

74. Kuczmarski RJ, Flegal KM, Campbell SM, Johnson CL. Increasing prevalence of overweight among US adults: the National Health and Nutrition Examination Surveys, 1960 to 1991. *JAMA*. 1994; 272:205–211.

75. Drizd T, Dannenberg AL Engel A. Blood pressure levels in persons 18-74 years of age in 1976-80, and trends in blood pressure from 1960 to 1980 in the United States. *Vital Health Stat*. 1986;234(11):1–68.

76. Brownell KD. Public health approaches to obesity and its management. In: Breslow L, Fielding JE, Lave LB, eds. *Annual Review of Public Health*. Palo Alto, Calif: Annual Reviews Inc; 1986.

77. Dannenberg A, Drizd T, Horan M, et al. CVD. *Epidemiol Newslett*. January 1985;68. Abstract.

78. Higgins M, Kannel WB, Garrison R, et al. Hazards of obesity: the Framingham experience. *Acta Med Scand*. 1987;723(suppl):23–26.

79. Hubert HB, Feinleib M, McNamara PM, et al. Obesity as an independent risk factor for cardiovascular disease: a 26-year follow-up of participants in the Framingham Heart Study. *Circulation*. 1983; 67:968–977.

80. Hamm P, Shekelle RB, Steinler J. Large fluctuations in body weight during young adulthood and twenty-five year risk of coronary death in men. *Am J Epidemiol*. 1989;29:312–318.

81. Stamler J. Hypertension, blood lipids and cigarette smoking as co-risk factors for coronary heart disease: discussion. *Ann NY Acad Sci*. 1978;304:140–146.

82. Slattery ML, Randall DE. Trends in coronary heart disease mortality and food consumption in the United States between 1909 and 1980. *Am J Clin Nutr*. 1988;47:1060–1067.

83. Allshouse J, Putnam J. *Food Consumption, Prices, and Expenditures, 1970–95*. Washington, DC: US Dept of Agriculture; 1997.

84. Walker WJ. Changing U.S. lifestyle and declining vascular mortality: a retrospective. *N Engl J Med*. 1983;308:649–651.

85. Marwick C. NHANES III health data relevant for aging nation. *JAMA*. 1997;277:100–102.

86. Lamon-Fava S, Jenner JL, Jacques PF, Schaefer EJ. Effects of dietary intakes on plasma lipids, lipoproteins, and apolipoproteins in free-living elderly men and women. *Am J Clin Nutr*. 1994;59:32–41.

# CHAPTER 10

# The Aging Renal System

*Robert D. Lindeman*

The accuracy and simplicity with which renal clearance studies can be performed, requiring only timed urine samples and blood samples drawn at the midpoints of these collection periods, make the kidney an ideal organ for studying the physiologic changes that occur with aging. Many descriptive studies performed in the 1950s and 1960s on cross-sectional populations show mean changes in renal function in each age group. In 1958, the Baltimore Longitudinal Study of Aging was initiated at what is now the Gerontology Research Center of the National Institute of Aging, and up to 30 years of information are available to add substantially to our knowledge of the normal aging process.

Controversy still remains as to the pathophysiology of the decline in renal function observed with age. Cross-sectional and longitudinal studies show a mean loss approximating 1 mL/min per year in glomerular filtration rates (GFR), and other physiologic renal functions parallel this change. Is this all due to superimposed, often undetectable, pathologic processes, or is there a progressive involutional loss of function that is inevitable? Do hyperperfusion and hyperfiltration develop in residual nephrons of aging persons, leading to development of glomerulosclerosis as seen in rats and in humans with diabetes mellitus? Does vasoconstriction or a decrease in protein intake in elderly persons account for a portion of the loss in kidney function?

## CHANGES IN RENAL MORPHOLOGY WITH AGE

The weight of both kidneys, about 50 g at birth, increases to 270 g in the third and fourth decades and thereafter decreases to 185 g in the ninth decade.[1] The loss of renal mass is principally from the cortex and is primarily vascular in origin, with the most significant changes occurring at the capillary level. The number of glomerular tufts per unit area and the number of glomerular and tubular cells decrease, while the size of individual cells increases with age.[2]

A detailed description of the course of ischemic obsolescence of glomeruli has been provided by several investigators.[3,4] Initially, there is progressive collapse of the glomerular tuft with wrinkling of the basement membranes, followed by a simplification and reduction in the vascular channels. Hyaline is deposited within both the residual glomerular tuft and the space of Bowman's capsule. Identifiable structures rapidly disappear. The obsolete glomerulus may be resorbed and disappear entirely; resorption is suggested because of the scantiness of the cellular response and residual scar. This process can leave a single vessel in place of the glomerular capillary, thus producing a shunt between the afferent and efferent arterioles. Ljungvist[5] and Takazakura and colleagues[6] confirmed the presence of these shunts in the juxtamedullary glomeruli. In the cortical area, atrophy resulted in an abrupt termination of the arteriole (Figure 10–1).

Kasiske[7] has shown that a direct correlation does exist between the number of obsolete glomeruli observed and the severity of atherosclerosis elsewhere in the body, but some sclerotic glomeruli were observed in virtually all kidneys studied. For example, in his 60-year-old subjects with the least atherosclerotic disease, the mean percentage of glomeruli that were sclerotic was approximately

5%. The functional loss associated with this would be hard to detect, and functional adjustments in the remaining kidney nephrons might compensate for such an anatomic loss without being reflected by changes in physiologic function.

## CHANGES IN RENAL FUNCTION WITH AGE

### Glomerular Filtration Rate

A number of studies have been reported that show an age-related decline in renal function after age 30 years (Figure 10–2).[8,9] All of these cross-sectional studies indicate that the rate of decline in the GFR approxi-

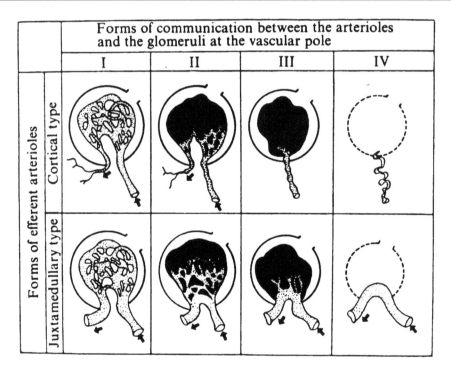

**Figure 10–1** The arteriole-glomerular units are classified into two basic types, cortical and juxtamedullary. Cortical glomeruli are shown in various stages of degeneration, terminating in complete atrophy of the arteriolar-glomerular units. The vasculature in the juxtamedullary glomeruli shows a shunt forming between the afferent and efferent arterioles. *Source:* Reprinted with permission from *Kidney International*, Vol. 2, pp. 224–230, © 1972, International Society for Nephrology.

mates 1 mL/min per year. Rowe and colleagues[10] reported a 10-year analysis of the first large-scale longitudinal study of renal function. Serial true creatinine clearances were obtained on 884 community-dwelling volunteers at 12- and 18-month intervals (Baltimore Longitudinal Study on Aging). The cross-sectional analysis provided data similar to those observed in other studies. An analysis of the serial creatinine clearances (longitudinal analysis) showed an accelerating decline in creatinine clearances similar to that observed in cross-sectional studies, indicating that selective mortality and cohort differences had no significant impact on the cross-sectional results.

Although mean creatinine clearance rates fell from 140 mL/min per 1.73 $m^2$ at age 25 to 34 years to 97 mL/min per 1.73$m^2$ at age 75 to 84 years, mean serum creatinine concentrations rose insignificantly from 72 to 74 μmol/L (0.81 to 0.84 mg/100 mL). The reduction in creatinine clearance with age is accompanied by a reduction in daily urinary creatinine ex-

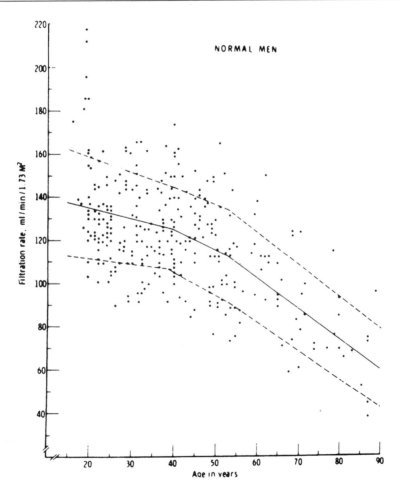

**Figure 10–2** Glomerular filtration rates (inulin clearances) per 1.73 $m^2$ in normal men versus age in 38 studies. The solid and broken lines represent 1 standard deviation. *Source:* Reprinted with permission from L.G. Wesson, *Physiology of the Human Kidney,* © 1969, Grune & Stratton.

cretion, reflecting the decreased creatinine production from decreased muscle mass. The net effect is a near constancy of mean serum creatinine concentrations with GFR reductions. The practical implication of these observations is that serum creatinine concentrations in older persons must be interpreted with this effect in mind when these data are used to determine or modify dosages of drugs cleared completely or partially by the kidneys, such as digoxin and aminoglycoside antibiotics.

As recently demonstrated by Malmose et al[11] and reviewed by Epstein,[9] no currently available method of estimating GFR from easily obtainable variables, such as age, sex, weight, and serum creatinine concentration, is very accurate. When a precise estimate of GFR is needed, a timed creatinine clearance should be obtained. Nevertheless, in everyday clinical practice, use of an estimate, such as the Cockcroft-Gault formula, may provide a prompt and reasonable guide for clinical decision making. The Cockcroft-Gault formula is used to estimate creatinine clearance from serum creatinine concentration:

men $C_{cr}$ = (140 − age) (weight in kilograms)/72 × serum creatinine (mg/100mL)

women $C_{cr}$ = men $C_{cr}$ × 0.85

A number of subjects, even some in the older age categories, show no decrease in their creatinine clearance when studied serially at 12- to 18-month intervals.[12] The mean decrease in creatinine clearance for 254 normal subjects (free of renal and urinary tract disease and untreated with diuretics or antihypertensives) was 0.75 mL/min per year. Figure 10–3 shows the serial plots of creatinine clearances of six representative subjects followed for 15 to 21 years who showed no decreases in the slopes of the creatinine clearances plotted over time (against

age of subject) (positive $B_{cr}$). One third of the subjects followed had a positive $B_{cr}$, indicating that creatinine clearance actually was increasing over the time span covered. These observations may have important implications in understanding the pathophysiology of the decrease in renal function with age, as discussed later in this chapter.

### Renal Blood (Plasma) Flow

The quantity of blood perfusing the kidney, generally estimated by measuring p-aminohippuric acid (PAH) clearances, decreases with age at a rate greater than that of the inulin clearances.[13] The PAH clearance at low serum PAH concentrations measures effective renal plasma flow (ERPF). All PAH that reaches renal tubular cells is secreted into the tubular fluid (urine) in a single pass through the kidney. The percentage of PAH cleared, compared with renal plasma flow as measured by direct-flow techniques (extraction ratio), is 92%; this percentage is similar in young and old subjects. The PAH clearances fall from a mean of 649 mL/min during the fourth decade to a mean of 289 mL/min during the ninth decade.[13]

The decrease in renal blood flow with age without a proportionate decrease in blood pressure is indicative of either vascular impedance due to intraluminal pathology (atheromata, sclerosis) or an increase in renal vascular resistance due to vasoconstriction. Since renal blood flow can be increased transiently by administration of vasodilators or pyrogens in both young and old subjects, a vasoconstrictive or reversible component must be implicated in the regulation of renal circulation in both age groups. Administration of a pyrogen produced a greater vasodilation of the arteriolar system in the kidneys of older subjects than in the kidneys of young subjects, suggesting that a greater vasocon-

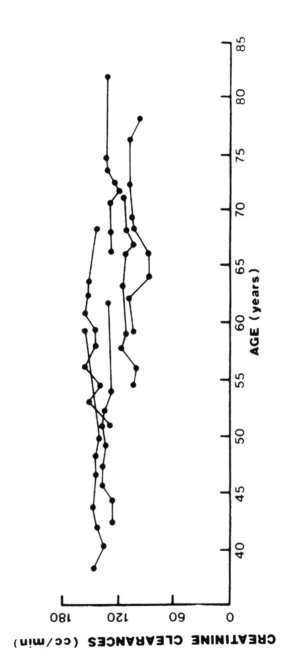

**Figure 10–3** Individual displays of serial creatinine clearances plotted against age in years for six representative subjects from the Baltimore Longitudinal Study of Aging. These six subjects were followed from 15 to 21 years and showed no decrease in creatinine clearances over this period of time (positive slope of creatinine clearance plotted against time in years). This was representative of the one third of the 254 normal subjects followed who showed no decline in renal function over the 23 years that the study was being conducted. *Source:* Reprinted with permission from R.D. Lindeman et al. Longitudinal Studies on the Rate of Decline in Renal Function with Age, *Journal of the American Geriatric Society* Vol. 23, p. 281, © 1985, Williams and Wilkins.

striction exists in the resting state.[14]

Hollenberg and colleagues[15] provided conflicting information in their xenon washout studies; they found that the perfusion of the outer cortical nephrons decreased more with age than did perfusion of the cortico-medullary nephrons. Whether this selective decrease in cortical nephron perfusion was due to sclerotic changes in the small arcuate arterioles or represented a selective vasoconstriction of the peripheral vasculature was investigated. Acetylcholine increased renal blood flow in both young and old subjects, but the effect was much more striking in the young subjects. In contrast, the vasoconstrictor responses to angiotensin were similar in the young and old subjects. These studies, in contrast to the studies conducted by McDonald and associates,[14] suggest that the renal vasculature in the aged subject is in a relatively greater state of baseline vasodilation compared with the renal vasculature of the young subjects.

Because the cortical component of blood flow decreases more rapidly than does mean flow rate, it has been thought that cortical nephrons are more severely affected by age than are juxtamedullary nephrons. Since the juxtamedullary nephrons have a higher filtration fraction than do cortical nephrons, a selective loss of the latter would explain the increase in the mean filtration fraction (GFR/ERPF) observed with age. An alternative, but less likely, explanation for the increase in filtration observed with age is that the efferent arteriole is disproportionately vasoconstricted compared with the afferent arteriole, thereby increasing the filtration pressure in the glomerular capillary bed.

## Maximal Tubular Transport Capacity

The tubular maximum for iodopyracet (Diodrast) or PAH secretory transport decreases with age at a rate nearly parallel to the decrease in inulin clearance.[13] The tubular maximum for secretion of PAH is measured by determining PAH clearances and subtracting inulin clearances at increasingly high serum PAH concentrations until a maximal clearance of PAH is obtained. This gives a measure of the maximal amount of PAH that the tubules can secrete. The tubular maximal rate for glucose resorption also decreases at a rate closely paralleling the decrease in inulin clearance.

Although the reduction in the secretory and resorptive tubular maximums with age could be explained by a progressive loss of whole functioning nephrons, animal experiments also have shown fewer energy-producing mitochondria,[16] lower enzyme concentrations,[16,17] lower concentrations of total or sodium-potassium-activated adenosine triphosphatase (ATPase),[18] decreased sodium extrusion and oxygen consumption,[19] and decreased tubular transport in the tubular cells[16] in old as compared with young kidneys. Therefore, aging not only reduces the population of functioning nephrons but also produces changes in the basic biochemistry of the tubular cell, even though no changes in tubular function per se can be detected by using available clearance techniques in human studies.

## Concentrating and Diluting Ability

A decrease in the kidneys' concentrating ability with age has been well documented.[8,9] In the Baltimore Longitudinal Study of Aging analysis,[20] 12 hours of water deprivation increased urine osmolality to a mean 1109 mOsm/L in young subjects, 1051 mOsm/L in middle-aged subjects, and 882 mOsm/L in old subjects.

Attempts to relate the decrease in concentrating ability to a more rapid decrease in GFR than in solute load, resulting in an osmotic or solute diuresis per residual nephron (which would impair concentrating ability), were not successful. Rowe and associates[20] suggested that the development of a continuity between juxtamedullary afferent and efferent arterioles[5,6] would increase medullary blood flow, and this is supported by the observations of Hollenberg and colleagues.[15] This relative increase with age in medullary blood flow per nephron would result in an enhanced removal of solute (washout) from the medullary interstitium, thereby decreasing concentrating ability.

Maximum urine osmolality after infusion of large amounts of vasopressin was significantly decreased in older subjects undergoing water diuresis.[21] This decrease appears most likely to be the result of diminished medullary tonicity rather than a defect in the ability of the kidney tubule to respond to vasopressin; elderly persons responded normally to graded doses of vasopressin insufficient for the kidney to concentrate urine maximally.[22] Elderly persons were better able to achieve urine isotonicity with a lower dose of vasopressin than were younger subjects.

Maximum diluting ability, as measured by minimum urine osmolality achieved with water loading, also decreases with age.[22] A comparison of free water clearance per unit of nephron mass (GFR) reveals little difference between young and old, suggesting that there is no basic defect in the ability to produce a dilute urine.

### Urine Acidification

Despite the decrease in renal function with age, blood pH, $pCO_2$, and bicarbonate values of aged persons without renal disease do not differ from the values observed in young subjects under basal conditions.[23] The decreases in blood pH and bicarbonate concentrations after ingestion of an acid load are prolonged in elderly persons. The minimum urine pH values achieved after an acid load are similar in young and old subjects. A much larger percentage of the ingested acid load as measured by total acid excretion (ammonium plus titratable acid [TA] minus bicarbonate) was excreted over an 8-hour period by the young subjects, compared with the older subjects. However, if total acid excretion in 8 hours is factored by GFR, similar rates of excretion are obtained. The young subjects excreted a greater percentage of their total acid as ammonium, compared with older subjects, presumably because there was an increase in urinary buffers responsible for titratable acid (eg, phosphate, creatinine) per unit of GFR in older subjects. This varies with dietary protein, and although dietary protein generally decreases in older subjects, it does not decrease as rapidly as GFR; therefore, TA/GFR increases. Agarwal and Cabebe[24] subsequently reported that elderly subjects showed a small pH gradient defect and that ammonium excretion was reduced significantly in elderly subjects even after correction for GFR. These investigators attempted to select older patients who had GFRs more similar to those observed in the young.

### Glomerular Permeability

Little information exists to indicate that glomerular permeability changes with age in humans. VanZonneveld[25] found an increasing incidence of proteinuria in a population survey of persons older than 65 years. Nevertheless, by age 85 years, only a minority of patients had evidence of clinical proteinuria. Glomerular permeability to free hemoglobin, determined by factoring free hemoglobin clearances by inulin clearances in healthy young and old subjects, did not change with age.[26] Furthermore, there was no difference between young and old subjects in glomerular permeability to a spectrum of dextrans of different molecular weights.[27]

## AGE-RELATED CHANGES IN RENAL RESPONSE TO ENVIRONMENTAL ALTERATIONS

The factors responsible for the age-related changes in renal sodium handling remain incompletely defined. GFR, physical factors determined in part by hemodynamics, the renin-angiotensin-aldosterone system, and atrial natriuretic peptide (ANP) are recognized as determinants of renal sodium handling, and each has been shown to vary significantly with age. Epstein and Hollenberg[28] found that older subjects failed to conserve sodium as rapidly or efficiently as did younger subjects. The half-lives of urinary sodium excretions when old patients were placed on a restricted dietary salt intake were much longer than those of young subjects in the same circumstance. Elderly persons have lower plasma renin activities and urinary aldosterone excretions both on an unrestricted salt diet and after 3 to 6 days of salt restriction.[29,30] However, the mechanism explaining this decreased plasma renin activity and aldosterone excretion in elderly individuals remains unknown; is it a renal or an extrarenal defect? This unexplained phenomenon probably accounts for the decreased ability of elderly subjects to conserve sodium when challenged with a low-salt diet. It may also account for the propensity of elderly subjects to develop hyperkalemia when given potassium supplements, as discussed in Chapter 4. The elderly also appear prone to develop extracellular fluid volume expansion when challenged with increased sodium intake or an intravenous sodium load.[9]

Similarly, there is a marked decrease in the ability of elderly people to convert 25-hydroxyvitamin $D_3$ to 1,25-dihydroxyvitamin $D_3$.[31] This appears to be related to a deficiency of 1 α-hydroxylase enzyme activity in old kidneys as compared to young kidneys.

Again, whether this is related to renal or extrarenal influences remains unclear. This is just one of the factors that may contribute to deficient vitamin D activity in older persons, which, in turn, may contribute to the development of senile osteoporosis.

## PATHOPHYSIOLOGY OF AGE-RELATED DECLINE IN RENAL FUNCTION

As discussed earlier, cross-sectional studies of normal subjects over a wide age range indicate that there is a mean decrease in renal function with age that accelerates in the oldest age groups. It remains unclear whether this decrease is due to a progressive involutional change with loss of nephron units and a decline in cellular function throughout the life of the individual or whether renal function remains stable until intermittent pathologic processes produce acute or chronic injuries and impairments. For example, undetected glomerulonephritis caused by immunologic injury after an infection, pyelonephritis due to bacterial or viral infection, acute tubular injury or interstitial nephritis due to a drug reaction, and vascular occlusion with resultant ischemic injury are pathologic processes that lead to impairment of renal function.

Normal cells (eg, fibroblasts), when placed in culture medium, have a finite life span in that the population-doubling potential of these cells is inversely related to the age of the donor.[32] Normal cells cannot be maintained in a state of active proliferation or even in a functional state in culture medium for a period of time in excess of the specific age of the species from which the cells were obtained. As cultured normal cells approach the end of their life spans, a number of biochemical decrements occur that indicate the approaching loss of divisional capacity, much like those observed in tubular cells: fewer energy-producing mitochondria, lower enzyme concentrations, lower concentrations of sodium-potassium-activated ATPase activity, decreased sodium transport and oxygen consumption, and diminished tubular transport in old kidneys compared with young kidneys. These sequences of glomerular loss in the absence of overt lesions in the large or small vessels, as described by Ljungvist[5] and Takazakura and colleagues,[6] suggest that nephron loss occurs normally without an overt vascular lesion.

On the other hand, the studies reported earlier[12] from the Baltimore Longitudinal Study of Aging, on a cohort of male volunteers followed between 1958 and 1981, provide evidence that the decrease in renal function observed with age may be the result of intervening pathologic processes rather than a relentless involutional process. One third of the normal subjects showed no decrease in renal function (positive slope of creatinine clearance plotted against time).

Friedman and associates,[33] for example, used scintillation scanning techniques to localize defects in kidney function in elderly persons with no past history of renal disease. They found abnormal scans in 25 of 35 elderly patients with a mean age of 75 years and mean creatinine clearance of 53 mL/min; 16 patients showed focal areas of diminished uptake that were thought to represent ischemic lesions.

Asymptomatic bacteriuria may be another contributor to decreased renal function in the aged. Dontas and colleagues[34] found that 27% of clinically healthy residents of the Athens House for the Aged had persistent bacteriuria, and the mean inulin clearances (70 versus 81 mL/min) were lower in this group. These are just two representative studies that indicate that pathologic changes must contribute, at least in part, to the observed decline in renal function with age. In a longitudinal study in which subjects were followed for periods up to 24 years, the failure of all subjects to show some decline in renal function indicates that a decline in renal function with age is not inevitable—that is, it is not the result of an involutional aging process.

This has led to the concept of "successful" versus "usual" aging, where the former is what is seen in subjects who weather aging well and the latter is obtained using physiologic measures in any "normal" aging population.[35] The decrease in function normally seen in cross-sectional or even longitudinal studies is probably due to the superimposition of asymptomatic, or at least undocumented, pathology.

## ROLE OF HYPERPERFUSION, HYPERFILTRATION, AND RENAL RESERVE

When the population of normal glomeruli is reduced by surgical ablation or renal disease in the rat model, the remaining glomeruli react with an "adaptive" hyperperfusion and hyperfiltration.[36] This glomerular hyperfiltration disrupts the integrity of the capillary membrane, resulting in proteinuria, accumulation of mesangial deposits, and initiation or acceleration of the loss of renal function through a process of developing glomerular sclerosis. This phenomenon of hyperfiltration also is seen in humans in the remaining kidney after uninephrectomy, in uncontrolled diabetes mellitus, and acutely after the ingestion of protein or infusion of amino acids. Restriction of protein, calories, or phosphate delays the renal progression. The earlier the underfeeding starts, the more the renal problems are delayed. Brenner and colleagues[37] proposed that the progressive decline in renal function in persons with primary renal disease, with hypertension, with diabetes mellitus, and with age could be related to this hyperperfusion and hyperfiltration, resulting in glomerular sclerosis. The mechanisms are illustrated in Figure 10–4. Neuringer and Brenner[38] reviewed additional evidence published over the subsequent 20 years supporting and refining this hypothesis.

Both GFR and kidney size are increased in early diabetes mellitus, producing changes in humans similar to those observed in animal models with remnant kidney or renal disease.[39] The state of glomerular hyperperfusion and hyperfiltration created by abnormal carbohydrate metabolism is corrected when the carbohydrate metabolism is normalized. Glomerulosclerosis with impaired glomerular filtration develops in diabetes with hyperperfusion and hyperfiltration of long duration.

Hypertension in diabetic animal models hastens the development of glomerulosclerosis. When hypertension is experimentally induced using the kidney Goldblatt model (clipped and unclipped renal arteries), asymmetry of the renal lesions is seen.[40] In the unclipped kidneys exposed to elevated systemic pressures, more severe glomerulosclerosis is seen than in the clipped kidney, where

reduced systemic pressure occurs. Similarly, normotensive diabetic rats have less severe lesions compared with hypertensive diabetic animals.[41]

Not all evidence favors the theory that hyperfiltration leads to glomerulosclerosis in humans. Uninephrectomy does not lead to impairment in renal function in transplant donors followed for a mean duration of 6 years.[42] Hyperperfusion and hyperfiltration in humans does not necessarily lead to glomerulosclerosis and progression of renal insufficiency. Fine[43] has proposed the concept that "glomerular tolerance" to injury as well as perfusion pressure determines whether glomerulosclerosis will develop.

Bosch and associates[44] quantified the increase in GFR and ERPF after an oral protein load and termed this increase "renal functional reserve capacity." In four normal subjects, they showed a mean increase in GFR (creatinine clearance) from 105 to 171 mL/min after an 80-g protein meal. They theorized that this represented the ability of the kidney under periods of stress to increase flow and filtration. If the kidney reaches the point where it is hyperperfusing and hyperfiltering at all times, it seems likely that it is susceptible to damage resulting from

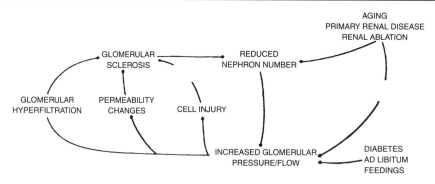

**Figure 10–4** Role of increased glomerular pressures and flows leading to the development of glomerular sclerosis. *Source:* Reprinted from S. Anderson and B.M. Brenner, *American Journal of Medicine*, Vol. 80, p. 435, © 1986, Cahners Publishing Company.

*Correction of impaired CHO metabolism can reduce hyperperfusion & hyperfiltration.*

glomerular sclerosis. Using low (40-g/d), normal (70-g/d), and high (90-g/d) protein diets, they also showed that GFR varied directly with protein intake from a mean of 101 mL/min on the low-protein diet to a mean of 127 mL/min on the high-protein diet.

Since the GFR increases more than the ERPF, the mechanisms for the GFR increase would appear to be due to a vasodilatation of the afferent arteriole. One might suspect that this would increase the filtration pressure in the glomerulus more than would other vasodilator agents, especially the converting enzyme inhibitors, which act by vasodilating the efferent arteriole, thereby subjecting the kidney to greater damage (glomerulosclerosis).

The same investigators[45] further showed that patients with underlying renal disease lost some to all of this ability to increase their GFR after an oral protein load and suggested that loss of this ability meant that they were already hyperfiltering. Since others[46] have demonstrated that limitation of protein intake in patients with chronic renal disease reduces the rate of progression of renal insufficiency, it has been speculated that a low-protein diet might restore renal functional reserve and thereby provide protection to the kidneys. Rodriguez-Iturbe and colleagues[47] compared creatinine clearances before and after a high-protein meal in 25 kidney donors and 35 patients with poststreptococcal glomerulonephritis with those of 44 normal control subjects. The mean increase in GFR in the postacute nephritis and nephrectomy patients was 18% compared with 58% in the control subjects, suggesting that the first two groups had a diminished renal reserve capacity. Infusions of amino acids and dopamine to increase GFR also have been used to quantify renal reserve[48] but offer no advantages other than a more rapid onset of action.

Older persons, or at least some older persons, may have lost their "renal reserve," indicating that they already are hyperperfusing and hyperfiltering. The studies of Hollenberg and associates[15] suggest that older patients are in a relative state of renal vascular vasodilatation. Such individuals might be at risk for development of glomerulosclerosis and might benefit from protein restriction, particularly if this allows a renal reserve to be reestablished. Studies by Fliser et al[49] compared hemodynamics before and after an amino acid infusion in healthy normotensive young (median age 26 years) and elderly subjects (median age 70 years) without evidence of renal disease. Glomerular filtration rates increased significantly and similarly in both young and old subjects. These studies suggest that the renal reserve or residual vasodilatory capacity of the kidney is not impaired in normal elderly subjects.

## CONCLUSION

Most renal functions decline with age at a rate similar to those observed for the GFR and ERPF. Cross-sectional and longitudinal population studies have suggested that this progressive decline in renal function results from an inevitable (involutional) loss of cellular function ending ultimately in cell death, and this suggestion is supported by studies of cell culture and tubular function in aging rats. Longitudinal studies of individual patients indicate that many patients, some of whom are old, go for decades with no evidence of a decline in renal function. This suggests that the decline in renal function observed with age is related to the superimposition of pathologic processes, often asymptomatic or at least undetected. The concept of "ideal" or "successful" aging as opposed to "usual" aging has emerged as a result of similar findings in other organ systems.[35]

## REFERENCES

1. Roessle R, Roulet F. *Mass and Zahl in der Pathologie*. Berlin, Germany: F Springer; 1932.

2. Goyal VK. Changes with age in the human kidney. *Exp Gerontol*. 1982;17:321–331.

3. MacCallum DB. The bearing of degenerating glomeruli on the problem of the vascular supply of the mammalian kidney. *Am J Anat*. 1939;65:69–103.

4. McManus JFA, Lupton CH Jr. Ischemic obsolescence of renal glomeruli. *Lab Invest*. 1960;9:413–434.

5. Ljungvist A. Structure of the arteriole-glomerular units in different zones of the kidney. *Nephron*. 1964;1:329–337.

6. Takazakura E, Wasabu N, Handa A, et al. Intrarenal vascular changes with age and disease. *Kidney Int*. 1972;2:224–230.

7. Kasiske BL. Relationship between vascular disease and age-associated changes in the human kidney. *Kidney Int*. 1987;31:1153–1159.

8. Lindeman RD. Overview: renal physiology and pathophysiology of aging. *Am J Kidney Dis*. 1990;16:275–282.

9. Epstein M. Aging and the kidney. *J Am Soc Nephrol*. 1996;7:1106–1122.

10. Rowe JW, Andres R, Tobin J, et al. The effect of age on creatinine clearance in men: a cross-sectional and longitudinal study. *J Gerontol*. 1976;31:155–163.

11. Malmose LC, Gray SL, Pieper CF, et al. Measured versus estimated creatinine clearance in a high-functioning elderly sample: MacArthur Foundation Study of Successful Aging. *J Am Geriatr Soc*. 1993;41:715–721.

12. Lindeman RD, Tobin JD, Shock NW. Longitudinal studies on the rate of decline in renal function with age. *J Am Geriatr Soc*. 1985;33:278–285.

13. Davies DF, Shock NW. Age changes in glomerular filtration rate, effective renal plasma flow, and tubular excretory capacity in adult males. *J Clin Invest*. 1950;29:496–507.

14. McDonald RF, Solomon DH, Shock NW. Aging as a factor in the renal hemodynamic changes induced by a standardized pyrogen. *J Clin Invest*. 1951;5:457–462.

15. Hollenberg NK, Adams DF, Solomon HS, et al. Senescence and the renal vasculature in normal man. *Circ Res*. 1974;34:309–316.

16. Barrows CH Jr, Falzone JA Jr, Shock NW. Age differences in the succinoxidase activity of homogenates and mitochondria from the livers and kidneys of rats. *J Gerontol*. 1960;15:130–133.

17. Burich RJ. Effects of age on renal function and enzyme activity in make C57 BL/6 mice. *J Gerontol*. 1975;30:539–545.

18. Beauchene RE, Fanestil DD, Barrows CH Jr. The effect of age on active transport and sodium-potassium activated ATPase activity in renal tissue of rats. *J. Gerontol*. 1965;20:306–310.

19. Proverbio F, Proverbio T, Marin R. Ion transport and oxygen consumption in kidney cortex slices from young and old rats. *Gerontology*. 1985;32:166–173.

20. Rowe JW, Shock NW, De Fronzo RA. The influence of age on the renal response to water deprivation in man. *Nephron*. 1976;17:270–278.

21. Rowe JW, Shock NW. Age differences in the renal tubular response to antidiuretic hormone. *J Gerontol*. 1953;8:446–450.

22. Lindeman RD, Lee TD Jr, Yiengst MJ, et al. Influence of age, renal disease, hypertension, diuretics, and calcium on the antidiuretic response to suboptimal infusions of vasopressin. *J Lab Clin Med*. 1966;68:206–223.

23. Adler S, Lindeman RD, Yiengst MJ, et al. Effect of acute acid loading on urinary acid excretion by the aging human kidney. *J Lab Clin Med*. 1968;72:278–289.

24. Agarwal BN, Cabebe FG. Renal acidification in elderly subjects. *Nephron*. 1980;26:291–293.

25. VanZonneveld RJ. Some data on the genito-urinary system as found in old-age surveys in the Netherlands. *Gerontol Clin*. 1959;1:167–173.

26. Lowenstein J, Faulstick DA, Yiengst MJ, et al. The glomerular clearance and renal transport of hemoglobin in adult males. *J Clin Invest*. 1961;40:1172–1177.

27. Faulstick D, Yiengst MJ, Ourster DA, et al. Glomerular permeability in young and old subjects. *J Gerontol*. 1962;17:40–44.

28. Epstein M, Hollenberg NK. Age as a determinant of renal sodium conservation in normal man. *J Lab Clin Med*. 1976;87:411–417.

29. Crane MG, Harris JJ. Effect of aging on renin activity and aldosterone excretion. *J Lab Clin Med*. 1976;87:947–959.

30. Weidman P, DeMyttenaere-Burzstein S, Maxwell MH, et al. Effect of aging on plasma renin and aldosterone in normal man. *Kidney Int*. 1975;8:325–333.

31. Armbrecht HJ, Zenser RV, Davis BB. Effect of age on the conversion of 25-hydroxyvitamin $D_3$ to 1,25-dihydroxyvitamin $D_3$ by kidney of rats. *J Clin Invest*. 1980;66:1118–1123.

32. Hayflick L. The cell biology of human aging. *N Engl J Med*. 1976;295:1302–1308.

33. Friedman SA, Raizner AE, Rosen H, et al. Functional defects in the aging kidney. *Ann Intern Med*. 1972;76:41–45.

34. Dontas AS, Papanayiotou P, Marketos SG, et al. The effects of bacteriuria on renal functional patterns in old age. *Clin Sci*. 1968;34:73–81.

35. Rowe JW, Kahn RL. Human aging: usual and successful. *Science*. 1987;237:143–149.

36. Hostetter TH, Olson JL, Rennke HG, et al. Hyperfiltration in remnant nephrons: a potentially adverse response to renal ablation. *Am J Physiol*. 1981;9:F85–F93.

37. Brenner MM, Meyer TW, Hostetter TH. Dietary protein intake and the progressive nature of kidney disease: the role of hemodynamically mediated glomerular injury in the pathogenesis of progressive glomerular sclerosis in aging, renal ablation and intrinsic renal disease. *N Engl J Med*. 1973;307:652–712.

38. Neuringer JR, Brenner BM. Hemodynamic theory of progressive renal disease: a 10-year update in brief review. *Am J Kidney Dis*. 1993;22:98–104.

39. Mogensen CE, Andersen MJF. Increased kidney size and glomerular filtration rate in early juvenile diabetes. *Diabetes*. 1973;22:706–712.

40. Mauer SM, Steffes MW, Azar S, et al. The effects of Goldblatt hypertension on development of the glomerular lesions of diabetes mellitus in the rat. *Diabetes*. 1978;27:738–744.

41. Bank N, Klose R, Aynedjian HS, et al. Evidence against increased glomerular pressure initiating diabetic nephropathy. *Kidney Int*. 1987;31:898–905.

42. Miller IJ, Suthanthiran M, Riggio RR, et al. Impact of renal donation: long term clinical and biochemical follow-up of living donors in a single center. *Am J Med*. 1985;79:201–208.

43. Fine LG. Preventing the progression of human renal disease: have rational therapeutic principles emerged? *Kidney Int*. 1988;33:116–128.

44. Bosch JP, Saccaggi A, Lauer A, et al. Renal functional reserve in humans: effect of protein intake on glomerular filtration rate. *Am J Med*. 1983;75:943–950.

45. Bosch JP, Lauer A, Glabman S. Short-term protein loading in assessment of patients with renal disease. *Am J Med*. 1984;77:873–879.

46. Barsoni G, Morelli E, Giannoni A, et al. Restricted phosphorus and nitrogen intake to slow the progression of chronic renal failure: a controlled trial. *Kidney Int*. 1984;24(suppl 16):278–284.

47. Rodriguez-Iturbe B, Herrera J, Garcia R. Response to acute protein load in kidney donors and in apparently normal postacute glomerulonephritis patients: evidence for glomerular hyperfiltration. *Lancet*. 1985;2:461–464.

48. Ter Wee PM, Rosman JB, VanDerGiest S, et al. Renal hemodialysis during separate and combined infusion of amino acids and dopamine. *Kidney Int*. 1986;29:870–874.

49. Fliser D, Zeier M, Nowack R, et al. Renal functional reserve in healthy elderly people. *J Am Soc Nephrol*. 1993;3:1371–1377.

# CHAPTER 11

# Impact of Nutrition on the Age-Related Declines in Hematopoiesis

*Manish Kohli, David A. Lipschitz, and Gurkamal S. Chatta*

The production of hematopoietic cells involves a complex interaction between proliferating marrow stem cells, a unique stroma, and a series of diffusible molecules that regulate the production of erythroid, myeloid, and megakaryocytic elements. The high cellular turnover makes the bone marrow particularly susceptible to nutritional deprivation, leading to significantly compromised function. The aging hematopoietic system is characterized by a decline in reserve capacity that makes it particularly susceptible to environmental insults that are known to affect the bone marrow adversely. This review discusses the effects of age on the hematopoietic system and the role of nutrition in the common hematologic problems seen in elderly people.

## EFFECT OF AGE ON THE HEMATOPOIETIC SYSTEM

### Pluripotent Stem Cells

All immunohematopoietic elements are derived from a small pool of pluripotent stem cells that are characterized by a unique self-renewal capacity.[1] They have the ability to divide and yield a progenitor cell committed to differentiating into a specific cell lineage, and an identical daughter cell, thus maintaining the pluripotent stem cell pool size. These morphologically unidentifiable cells are referred to as colony-forming unit—spleen (CFU-S) because they form colonies when marrow is injected into lethally irradiated mice recipients. One of the major questions about the aging of the hematopoietic system is whether or not CFU-S have a finite replicative capacity. Studies using serial transplantation to assess finite replicative capacity have yielded conflicting results. When cells are subjected to in vivo serial transfer by repeated injection into lethally irradiated recipients, they gradually lose their ability to replicate.[2,3] Recent evidence has suggested that results of serial transplantation may well be the result of methodologic artifact.[4,5] Even if their life span is finite, it is clear that CFU-S have a vastly redundant reserve capacity, enabling production of hematopoietic cells in numbers that far exceed the maximal life expectancy of the animal.[6] This point is further highlighted by the observation that as few as 20 CFU-S are able to reconstitute the bone marrow of lethally irradiated mice.[7]

The effect of age on CFU-S senescence has been studied in long-term bone marrow culture. Several studies have shown an inverse relationship between donor age and maintenance of hematopoiesis in this long-term bone marrow culture system.[8,9] Additional studies using this in vitro culture system have shown that CFU-S with high replicative histories are more likely to be recruited into the committed cell compartments than are CFU-S that have divided fewer times. Additional evidence for a finite life span comes from a series of elegant studies that examined stem cell kinetics in long-term marrow culture subjected to various doses of irradiation.[10–12]

## Effect of Age on Normal Marrow Function

The CFU-S divide into an identical daughter cell and progenitor cells committed to differentiation, and, in the case of hematopoiesis, into myeloid, erythroid, megakaryocytic, and macrophage precursors (Figure 11–1). There are two forms of erythroid progenitor cells. The first is a more primitive precursor, which requires high concentrations of erythropoietin and is referred to as a burst-forming unit—erythroid (BFU-E). This precursor is thought to give rise to a more mature progenitor cell that requires lower erythropoietin concentrations. It is referred to as a colony-forming unit—erythroid (CFU-E) and is the immediate precursor of the proerythroblast, which is the first morphologically identifiable erythroid element. Committed myeloid progenitors include the colony-forming unit—culture (CFU-C), which is the immediate precursor of the myeloblast. A primitive progenitor cell that gives rise to megakaryocytes (CFU-MEGG) and to macrophages (CFU-M) can also be identified under appropriate culture conditions. Morphologically recognizable hematopoietic cells proliferate and mature in a transit or amplification compartment, eventually giving rise to terminally differentiated cells that continually enter the peripheral blood.

Recent studies have examined the effect of age on committed hematopoietic progenitor cell number and on the number of differentiated cells in the various marrow compartments. In both animals and humans, no age-related declines in any bone marrow element can be demonstrated when carefully selected subjects are examined in the basal state.[13,14] These observations strongly suggest that marrow function can be adequately maintained, and that no measurable declines occur as a consequence of age per se. The aging process is characterized, however, by a significant reduction in reserve capacity, so that abnormalities not present in the basal state become apparent when the response to maximal stimulation is examined. Udupa and Lipschitz [15,16] have undertaken a number of studies in which they examined hematopoietic function in animals exposed to increased stimulation. Both in vivo and in vitro studies have shown that the hematopoietic response to increased stimulation in old mice is blunted and more variable. Furthermore, greater pathologic abnormalities are noted in response to infection or protein deficiency.

## DOES ANEMIA OCCUR AS A CONSEQUENCE OF NORMAL AGING?

It is generally recognized that anemia is a common clinical problem in the elderly. Studies have shown a high prevalence in hospitalized older subjects, patients attending geriatric clinics, and institutionalized older individuals. A series of epidemiologic studies from the United States, Canada, and Europe[17–19] demonstrated a high prevalence of anemia in the elderly. In women above age 59, anemia occurs as frequently as in women of childbearing age. In men, a definite increase in the prevalence of anemia is found in older age groups. Studies from Great Britain are important, as they have determined the prevalence of anemia in large numbers of

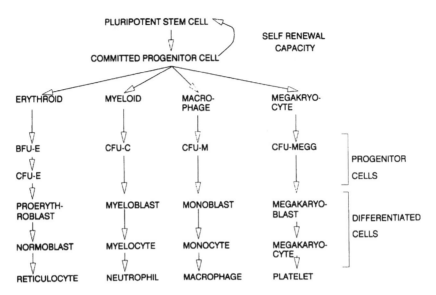

**Figure 11–1** The production of terminally differentiated cells of various lineages is derived from a small pool of pluripotent stem cells (CFU-S) with a unique self-renewal capacity. They give rise to progenitor cells of specific lineages that divide and differentiate, resulting in the daily production of the required amounts of hematopoietic elements. *Source:*

subjects above age 60. In both men and women, the prevalence of anemia increased significantly with each successive decade.

An analysis of the second National Health and Nutrition Education Survey (NHANES II) demonstrated a significant reduction in hemoglobin levels with advancing age in apparently healthy males and a minimal although significant decrease in elderly females.[20] Based upon a lower normal limit of 14 g/dL for hemoglobin concentration, a very large percentage of elderly males would be found to be anemic. This study proposed that the reduction in hemoglobin in males was a consequence of aging, and most likely secondary to a decline in the serum testosterone. Hence, age-specific reference standards for hemoglobin concentration should be adopted and used for diagnosing anemia in the elderly.

There are few reports on the incidence of new cases of anemia in the elderly popula-

tion. In the general population, the annual incidence of anemia is estimated to be 1% to 2%.[21,22] Compared to this, the incidence of anemia in a well-defined population of elderly (over 65 years of age) Caucasians attending the Mayo Clinic[23] was reported to be four- to sixfold higher; the incidence of anemia was 13% per year in the "oldest-old" (over 85 years of age). Anemia was diagnosed in accordance with World Health Organization (WHO) criteria, if the hemoglobin concentration was less than 13 g/dL in men and less than 12 g/dL in women. In this study, in every age group over 65 years, the incidence of anemia in men was higher than that in women. At the time of diagnosis, less than 50% of the men had a hemoglobin concentration lower than 12 g percent. Significantly, despite an exhaustive workup, in 16% of the elderly the etiology of the anemia was uncertain.

The above data are consistent with an evaluation of apparently healthy elderly subjects with mild anemia, which also failed to uncover an obvious cause of the anemia.[24] A careful assessment of hematopoiesis in these individuals revealed mild marrow failure, as evidenced by reductions in bone marrow progenitor cell numbers and modest decreases in peripheral leukocyte counts.[25] A major unanswered question is whether this decline in hemoglobin with advancing age is a consequence of the normal aging process or reflects some yet to be defined abnormality. Of particular importance in this regard is the finding that anemia is extremely rare in an affluent, healthy elderly population examined in New Mexico.[26] None of the elderly males and females in this group were anemic. Furthermore, longitudinal monitoring of these subjects over a 5-year period failed to demonstrate an increased prevalence of anemia. Based upon this observation and the animal studies of hematopoiesis, it seems highly likely that the decrease in hemoglobin seen commonly with advancing age is not a consequence of the normal aging process and is related to some extrinsic variable that remains to be determined.

Inflammation or chronic disease is one likely etiology of apparent age-related anemia.[27] A second possibility is that the anemia has a nutritional basis. This is suggested by a closer examination of data obtained in epidemiologic surveys in which anemia has been shown to be most prevalent in populations that are at a low socioeconomic level, where the prevalence of nutritional deficiencies is high.

We have performed a comprehensive nutritional and hematologic evaluation of a group of 73 elderly veterans living in a domiciliary facility. A high prevalence of anemia was present in this population. A close evaluation demonstrated that iron deficiency, folate deficiency, and other commonly described causes of anemia were rare. We then performed a multivariate analysis of the data using age, hematopoietic indices, and nutritional factors as covariants. We demonstrated that while age appeared to be the major variable accounting for the decline in immunologic measurements observed in this elderly population, age did not appear to be an important factor in the prevalence of anemia. In contrast, serum albumin, transferrin, and prealbumin, which assess nutritional status, appeared to be excellent predictors of anemia. This information provides indirect evidence that a nutritional variable may contribute to the anemia seen in these elderly populations. Further evidence suggesting that a nutritional factor may contribute to the anemia comes from the observation that there is a marked similarity between the alterations in immunologic and hematopoietic function that occur with aging and those that occur with protein deprivation. This raises the possibility that protein deprivation in some form may contribute to the hematopoietic changes normally ascribed to aging.

There is evidence that correction of protein-energy malnutrition in the hospitalized elderly can markedly improve hematopoietic function.[28] In these subjects, interpretation of improvements in hematologic status is extremely difficult. Any hospitalized elderly individual has coexisting diseases that can affect hematopoietic function. Thus the overall improvement seen with nutritional rehabilitation may reflect an overall improvement of the patient's medical status. The effect of increased feeding on hematopoietic status has been examined in relatively healthy elderly individuals who lived at home, who were ambulatory but were underweight, and who had marginal evidence of protein-energy deprivation. By providing polymeric dietary supplements to these subjects between meals, it was possible to correct nutritional deficiencies and obtain weight gain. Despite a positive impact on nutritional status, however, the anemia, invariably present in this population, did not improve.

Some conclusions can be drawn from these observations. It is clear that significant nutritional deficiencies reversibly aggravate the hematologic abnormalities in the elderly. Even in apparently healthy older individuals, it is possible that nutritional factors contribute to hematopoietic changes, but alternative mechanisms other than simple nutritional deficiency must be considered. Marginal reductions of one or more nutrients acting alone or in combination over a prolonged period of time may modulate hematopoietic change usually ascribed to aging. Alternatively, nutrient delivery to the target organ may be altered with aging or changes in nutrient target interaction may occur. These possibilities could account for the higher prevalence of anemia reported in epidemiologic studies. They remain no more than potential hypotheses that will require further research.

In contrast to healthy older persons, in whom the prevalence of anemia is relatively low, the disorder is extremely common in hospitalized patients in both acute and chronic care settings. In a recent survey of hospitalized patients in a Department of Veterans Affairs hospital, 56% of patients over the age of 75 had a significant anemia (Rothstein et al., personal communication) (Table 11–1).

## HEMATOLOGIC MANIFESTATIONS OF PROTEIN ENERGY MALNUTRITION IN THE ELDERLY

A high incidence of protein-energy malnutrition (PEM) has been reported in hospitalized elderly patients. The incidence is also very high in nursing homes and in other long-term care settings.[29] The disorder is characterized by hypoalbuminemia, increased pro-

**Table 11–1** Anemia in Patients over Age 75 in an Acute Care Veterans Hospital

| Diagnosis | Percentage |
|---|---|
| Multiple diagnoses | 53 |
| No diagnosis | 17 |
| Single diagnosis | 30 |
| Anemia of chronic disease | 10 |
| Malnutrition | 9 |
| Infection | 4 |
| Post-op bleeding | 3 |
| Alcohol | 1 |
| Iron deficiency | 1 |

*Source:*

tein and energy requirements, and declines in immune and hematologic function. Anemia is invariably present in patients with PEM, the features being identical to those that occur as the "anemia of chronic disease," and with inflammatory processes.[28] In both men and women the hemoglobin concentration ranges from 100 to 120 g/L. The disorder is associated with an impaired ability of the reticuloendothelial system to recycle iron from senescent red cells. As a result, serum iron concentrations are low and the transferrin saturation is less than 20%. These findings indicate the presence of iron-deficient erythropoiesis, which also occurs in iron deficiency anemia that most commonly results from blood loss. In this disorder, iron stores are absent and, as a result, the serum ferritin level, which is a relatively accurate measure of iron stores, is reduced (usually less than 50 mg/L) and total iron-binding capacity (TIBC) is increased.

In contrast, iron stores are normal or increased in the anemia associated with chronic disease and in the anemia associated with PEM. This is reflected in a normal to elevated serum ferritin level (<60 mg/L) and a low TIBC (<45 mmol/L). In elderly people the immunohematopoietic sequelae of PEM tend to be more severe than they are in younger individuals. This may well relate to the diminished reserve capacity that is believed to exist in elderly individuals. Furthermore, the effects of age on the immune and hematologic systems are remarkably similar to the declines in function noted in PEM. The effects of age and PEM on declines in function may well be additive, resulting in more severe abnormalities in older individuals.

An example of this additive effect is provided by the observations made of the effect of age and protein deficiency on neutrophil function in mice. Lipschitz and Udupa[30] showed that, although neutrophil function was compromised in aged mice and in young mice fed a low-protein diet, the reduction was not sufficient in either case to compromise the neutrophil's ability to phagocytose or kill bacteria. In contrast, the reserve capacity of the neutrophil was markedly compromised when aged mice were fed a low-protein diet. Neutrophils obtained from these animals had a marked impairment of their ability to phagocytose and kill bacteria. These results may explain the high prevalence of severe bacterial infections in hospitalized, malnourished elderly people. They also emphasize that the reduced reserve in cellular function as a consequence of aging results in increased susceptibility to external stress.

The most appropriate definition of PEM is that it is a metabolic response to stress associated with increased requirements for calories and protein.[31] It may be that elderly people are more susceptible to PEM and develop pathologic conditions more rapidly and with less stress than do younger subjects. The stresses that result in this disorder include trauma, infection, and other acute or chronic inflammatory conditions. Considering these pathophysiologic facts, it is likely that the hematologic changes noted in these patients re-

flect the underlying disease and only indirectly relate to a nutritional problem.

Clinical studies have shown that the initial responses to stress that characterize PEM are beneficial and assist the patient in developing an optimal response to the underlying primary pathology. Since acute stress is associated with severe anorexia, patients rarely if ever consume sufficient calories or protein to meet their daily needs. In young subjects, inadequate nutrient intake for a period of up to 10 days usually does not affect outcome adversely. Thereafter, inadequate protein and calorie intake results in further lowering of serum albumin and worsening of hematologic, immunologic, and hepatic function, which can affect outcome adversely. In elderly subjects, the time period before PEM exerts a negative effect is likely to be much shorter than that observed in younger subjects. In elderly individuals, failure to meet nutrient needs after a period as brief as 2 to 3 days can lead to further lowering of the serum albumin, worsening immunohematologic function, and increased morbidity. It is essential, therefore, that the presence of PEM be appropriately diagnosed and managed in elderly people.

Lipschitz and Mitchell[28] have studied the effects of nutritional rehabilitation on the hematologic system in elderly subjects with PEM who did not have terminal disease. They confirmed previous reports that adequate nutritional support improved delayed cutaneous hypersensitivity and increased lymphocyte count. In addition, marked improvements in the hematologic system were demonstrated. Correction of the nutritional deficits resulted in a highly significant increase in the hemoglobin concentration, which was accompanied by a return of both serum iron levels and TIBC to normal ranges. Simultaneously, serum ferritin levels fell, presumably as a result of redistribution of iron from stores to the circulating erythrocyte mass (Figure 11–2).

In selected individuals, Lipschitz and Mitchell also demonstrated that improved nutritional status was accompanied by significant increases in the number of bone marrow-differentiated cells and immature stem cells. The observation that delivery of adequate nutrition resulted in a prompt rise in both serum iron level and TIBC is of great interest, particularly since these changes occurred long before any other improvement in the clinical status was noted. This observation provides the strongest evidence for a nutritional role in the hematopoietic alterations occurring in PEM.

The overall interpretation of the improved immunohematopoietic function in malnourished elderly subjects is extremely difficult. Any hospitalized elderly patient who has PEM also has coexisting medical conditions (including infection, dehydration, and psycho-

neurologic changes) that will affect immune and hematologic function. Therefore, the overall improvement seen with nutritional rehabilitation may reflect an overall improvement of the medical status of the patient.

To examine this possibility more closely, Lipschitz et al.[32] studied the effects of increased feeding on the immune and hematologic status of mildly malnourished, elderly, homebound subjects. These individuals were underweight, had evidence of inadequate food intake, were invariably anemic, and had diminished immune function. By providing polymeric dietary supplements between meals, it was possible to increase total calorie and protein intake by 50% for a total of 16 weeks. A significant improvement in nutritional status occurred: weight gain, increased serum albumin and transferrin, and significant increases in selected vitamins and minerals were seen. Despite this improved nutritional profile, immune function or hematologic sta-

## QUANTITATION OF HEMATOPOIESIS IN ELDERLY SUBJECTS WITH UNEXPLAINED ANEMIA

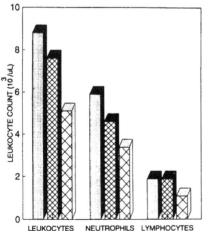
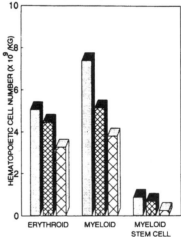

**Figure 11–2** Peripheral blood counts (left panel) and hematopoietic precursor number (right panel) in groups of healthy young subjects and groups of carefully selected elderly subjects with or without an unexplained anemia. *Source:* Reprinted with permission from Lipschitz et al., *Blood*, Vol. 63, p. 502, © 1984, Grune & Stratton, Inc.

tus remained unchanged. No anergic subject demonstrated improved delayed cutaneous hypersensitivity. T and B cell function remained abnormal, and the hemoglobin concentration did not increase.

This study, and one on more severely malnourished elderly, suggested that nutritional deficiencies aggravated immune and hematopoietic function in elderly subjects. Correction of coexisting disease and nutritional rehabilitation in the severely malnourished was associated with measurable improvements in host defense parameters. Mildly malnourished elderly individuals who had changes in immune and hematopoietic function similar to those seen in healthy elderly did not show an improvement in their function despite an obviously improved nutritional status. A reasonable conclusion from these studies is that neither protein nor calorie deprivation entirely accounts for the immune and hematologic changes seen in elderly people.

## IRON DEFICIENCY ANEMIA

Throughout the world, iron deficiency as a result of blood loss is the most common nutritional problem and accounts for significant morbidity in Third World countries. In both men and women, a progressive increase in iron stores occurs with advancing age. This has been demonstrated in numerous studies that have shown an age-associated increase in serum ferritin in both men and women (Figure 11–2). In older men, tissue iron stores average 1,200 mg. In older women, iron stores increase from an average of 300 mg to 800 mg in the decade after menopause. The rise in iron stores clearly relates to improved iron balance because of cessation of menstruation.[33] Consequently, in contrast to younger women, iron deficiency is not the most common cause of anemia in ambulatory, healthy elderly people.[24,25]

In the hospital setting, however, iron deficiency anemia is more common in elderly patients. In a number of studies of elderly hospitalized subjects, the prevalence of anemia ranged from 6.4% to 41%.[34–36] In 21% to 90% of the patients, the etiology of the anemia was thought to be caused by iron deficiency. This information must be interpreted with a lot of caution, as the criteria for the diagnosis of anemia varied and in many cases only serum iron concentration and TIBC were used to make the diagnosis. Factors such as co-morbid conditions and different cut-off values in the above studies for diagnosing anemia contribute to the significant variation of these prevalence rates. However, it is apparent that iron deficiency is a common problem in hospitalized people.

In the United States, the prevalence rates for iron deficiency anemia were recently reported in the third National Health and Nutrition Examination Survey (NHANES III; 1988–1994).[37] In this large, nationally representative survey, the prevalence rates of iron deficiency state and iron deficiency anemia were relatively higher in toddlers, adolescent girls, and women of childbearing age. The prevalence rates of iron deficiency state and iron deficiency anemia in the 50- to 69-year age group for females was reported to be 5% and 2% of the U.S. population, while in the age group older than 70 years it was 7% and 2%, respectively. For males the reported figures in the 50 to 69 years' group were 2% and 1%, while in the older than 70 years' group it was 4% and 2%, respectively. While this points to relatively low prevalence rates in the elderly U.S. population, emerging aging trends in the U.S. population would translate relatively low rates to high numbers over the next few years. Screening strategies, therefore, should be evolved to pursue work-up for preventable etiologies of iron deficiency states in the elderly (Table 11–2), which will translate into early diagnosis and treatment, as well as low health care costs for the elderly.

Epidemiological studies have in general focused on the prevalence of anemia and few data exist regarding the frequency or etiology of newly diagnosed anemia in the elderly. Ania et al.[22,23] assessed the incidence and clinical spectrum of anemia in the elderly in a predominantly Caucasian, affluent community with excellent access to health care facilities. In this community-based survey, the incidence of anemia among older people was 4 to 6 times greater than that suspected clinically and rose higher with age, with the highest incidence being recorded in elderly males. In half of the cases, the apparent cause of newly diagnosed anemia in this population base survey was blood loss. Even mild anemia was associated with reduced survival.

The role of nutrition in contributing to iron deficiency anemia and other nutritional deficiencies in the elderly depends on cultural, regional, and socioeconomic factors. There is no strong evidence to suggest that poor diet and/or poor bioavailability of dietary iron is a cause for iron deficiency anemia in large segments of the population in industrialized nations. Small cross-sectional and longitudinal studies have attempted to underscore the role of diet in developing iron deficiency states along with deficiencies of elements such as zinc and copper. In a small longitudinal study of healthy elderly vegetarians, the long-term consequences of ovo-lacto or lacto-vegetarianism were assessed.[38] The results indicated that in comparison to omnivorous elderly, the vegetarian elderly population is at a higher risk for a marginal iron, zinc, and vitamin $B_{12}$ status.

Recently, Fleming et al.[39] reported on the role of dietary factors modulating iron bioavailability in the elderly population. Based on the elderly cohort from the Framingham Heart Study, five significant dietary factors were found to be associated with iron stores. Heme iron, supplemental iron, dietary vitamin C, and alcohol were positively associated with serum ferritin after correcting for other causes of raised ferritin. On the other hand, coffee consumption was found to have a negative association.

When iron deficiency does occur in elderly individuals, it is almost always secondary to

---

**Table 11–2** Major Causes of Iron Deficiency in the Elderly

*Gastrointestinal Blood Loss*
Tumors
Polyps
Carcinoma of the colon
Carcinoma of the stomach

*Peptic Ulcer Disease*
Gastric
Duodenal

*Drugs*
Nonsteroidal anti-inflammatory drugs
Aspirin
Indomethacin
Anticoagulants

*Miscellaneous Causes*
Angiodysplasia of the large bowel
Hiatal hernia
Hemorrhoids
Diverticulosis

*Other Sources of Blood Loss*
Genitourinary blood loss
Carcinoma of the uterus and cervix
Hematuria (rare)

*Miscellaneous*
Frequent blood drawings in hospitalized patients
Thrombocytopenia
Coagulopathies

gastrointestinal blood loss. The common causes of blood loss anemia in elderly patients are listed in Table 11–2. The etiology of this blood loss in both elderly men and elderly women must be assumed to be gastrointestinal malignancy until proved otherwise. Depending on the patient's medical condition, an aggressive attempt to define the cause of the anemia should be undertaken, whether or not occult blood is detected in the stool. Comprehensive evaluation of the gastrointestinal tract, including radiography and endoscopy, frequently will identify a malignancy or the presence of polyps that accounts for the blood loss. Other common causes of blood loss from the gastrointestinal tract include atrophic gastritis and angiodysplasia of the large bowel.

Iron deficiency anemia primarily must be distinguished from other disorders that are characterized by the presence of iron-deficient erythropoiesis. These include the anemia of chronic disease, the anemia associated with inflammation, and, as described above, protein-energy malnutrition.[40] The major defect in these disorders appears to be an impaired ability of the reticulo-endothelial cells to recruit the iron derived from previously phagocytosed erythrocytes. Therefore, serum iron levels are low, iron supply to the marrow is inadequate, and iron deficient erythropoiesis develops. In contrast to iron deficiency, tissue iron stores are normal or increased rather than absent. The mechanism accounting for the reticuloendothelial abnormality is not well understood. Other factors contributing to this anemia include a modest reduction in erythrocyte survival. The erythropoietin response to the level of the anemia is frequently reduced, but in some circumstances has been shown to be normal or increased.

Figure 11–3 lists an approach to distinguishing whether iron deficiency is caused by iron deficiency anemia, chronic disease, or inflammation. In both, there is evidence of iron-deficient erythropoiesis characterized by a low serum iron level and low transferrin saturation. Transferrin saturation is the percentage of circulating transferrin that is saturated with iron; it is calculated by dividing the serum iron value by the TIBC and expressing the result as a percentage. The free erythrocyte protoporphyrin is also elevated in iron-deficient erythropoiesis. However, a saturation below 15% favors iron deficiency. Although microcytosis does occur in the anemia of chronic disease, a mean corpuscular volume below 75 fL is very unusual.

The major distinguishing feature between the two disorders is the absence of iron stores in iron deficiency and its presence in chronic disease or inflammation. In classic iron deficiency anemia, the serum ferritin level is less than 20 µg/L and the TIBC is greater than 72 µmol/L. In the anemia of inflammation, serum ferritin is usually greater than 100 µg/L provided that iron stores are adequate. In this circumstance, TIBC is usually less than 45 µmol/L. Frequently the serum ferritin and the TIBC yield equivocal results. This is particularly likely in patients with inflammatory disorders complicated by iron deficiency. For example, a patient with active rheumatoid disease and iron deficiency caused by drug-induced gastrointestinal blood loss may demonstrate confusing blood chemistries. In a patient like this, the serum ferritin level is usually above 12 µg/L but less than 100 µg/L. Despite the presence of inflammation, this type of patient will respond to oral iron therapy with a significant increase in hemoglobin.

A reasonable recommendation for subjects with anemia and inflammatory disorders is to consider a trial of oral iron when the ferritin level is less than 100 µg/L. Alternatively, the diagnosis of iron deficiency can be made definitively by demonstrating absent hemosid-

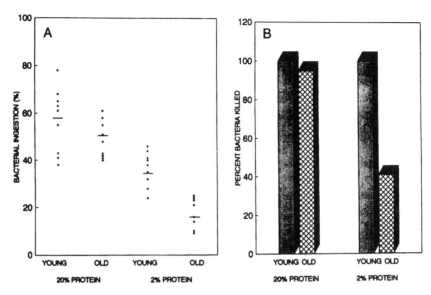

**Figure 11–3** Bacterial ingestion (panel A) and percentage bacteria killed (panel B) in neutrophils obtained from the peritoneal cavity of young (aged 6 months) or old mice (aged 24 months) fed a 20% (normal) or 2% protein diet for 3 weeks. The results demonstrate that phagocytosis and bacterial killing are significantly compromised only in the old animals fed the low-protein diet. *Source:* Reprinted with permission from *Journal of Gerontology*, Vol. 41, p. 690, © 1986, The Gerontology Society of North America.

erin iron in a bone marrow aspirate. In the anemia of chronic disease, sideroblasts are absent but hemosiderin iron is readily seen in marrow macrophages.

Once the diagnosis has been made, initial therapy should be directed at correcting the underlying pathologic process that resulted in the iron deficiency. In most cases, the iron deficiency can be corrected by oral administration of an iron salt. Ferrous sulfate in either tablet form or as an elixir should be given 3 times per day with meals[41]; the usual dose contains 60 mg of elemental iron. An adequate response to iron therapy is an increase in the hemoglobin concentration of approximately 0.5 g weekly. Elderly patients appear to respond as rapidly to oral iron as do younger individuals.[42]

Side effects, which include nausea, vomiting, epigastric discomfort, constipation, and diarrhea, are common causes for cessation of medication. The best approach to minimize these complications is to reduce the dose and assure that iron therapy is administered with meals. In some elderly subjects there may be value in prescribing one tablet daily to diminish polypharmacy and aid with compliance. A slow-release iron preparation may be more appropriate when prescribing iron on a daily basis.

Failure to respond is not uncommon and usually results from noncompliance or continued bleeding. Once these possibilities have been excluded, an incorrect diagnosis or a contributing condition such as renal impairment, infection, or neoplasia should be considered. In the rare patient who does not respond to oral iron, parenteral iron therapy may be considered. This should be reserved for those individuals proven to have iron malabsorption or when noncompliance is a serious problem. The importance of treating with oral iron only when indicated cannot be overemphasized. There is evidence that as many as 83% of elderly subjects have received oral iron therapy unnecessarily.[43]

## FOLIC ACID AND VITAMIN B$_{12}$

Folic acid deficiency in elderly people can result from inadequate intake. As a general rule, however, pathologic deficiencies occur only when decreased intake is accompanied by increased requirements, as in alcoholics or in patients with gastrointestinal malabsorption. Epidemiological studies conducted in Great Britain indicate that significant folate deficiency is relatively common, with significantly low erythrocyte folate levels as well as low serum B$_{12}$ levels occurring in 8% to 14% of subjects examined.[44] Low B$_{12}$ and folate levels reported in this sample population were not associated with any clinical manifestations of their deficiencies.

In another survey of folate intake among adults in the Netherlands, only 4% of elderly males were found to be deficient per the daily recommended allowance.[45] Physiological and lifestyle variables such as alcohol and tobacco use were also important determinants of folate levels. Again, no clear association was found between low folate levels and the clinical manifestations of its deficiency. Potatoes, vegetables, and fruit provided 36% of the folate in diet along with bread (18%) and dairy products (16%).

In general, other than special requirements for additional folate—such as pregnancy, hemolysis, or ongoing alcohol abuse—the adult diet in most industrialized countries is adequate in meeting daily recommended folate consumption. Dietary recall information suggests that a large fraction of older in-

dividuals consume well below the recommended dietary allowance of 400 μg/d. In three separate studies, intakes ranging from 129 to 300 μg/d have been reported.[46–48] In a Canadian study of elderly men, intake averaged 150 μg daily. The inadequate intake, coupled with the relatively uncommon incidence of biochemical deficiency, probably relates to the unrealistically high recommended daily intake. It must be emphasized, however, that folate balance in older individuals is marginal and that significant deficiencies are likely to develop rapidly if intake is further compromised by illness or if demand for the vitamin is increased.

Megaloblastic anemia due to folate deficiency in elderly people usually occurs in association with other medical problems. Of these, chronic alcoholism is the most important. In alcoholics, significant folate deficiency results from a combination of inadequate dietary intake combined with decreased absorption and altered folate metabolism.[49,50] Intestinal malabsorption is rare in the elderly but can present or manifest with isolated megaloblastic anemia caused by folate deficiency.

Drugs are another common cause of folate deficiency. Phenytoin (Dilantin) causes folate deficiency by a direct effect on the ability of cells to incorporate thymidine into DNA.[49] The common use of combinations of sulfamethoxazole with trimethoprim in elderly individuals with chronic urinary tract infections can also result in folate deficiency. Trimethoprim inhibits dihydrofolate reductase and hence prevents the formation of the active tetrahydrofolate. Although macrocytosis is common in patients consuming drugs that interfere with folate metabolism, frank anemia is rare. Finally, folate deficiency has been reported in elderly individuals who have hemolytic anemia. The presence of increased erythrocyte production results in increased folate requirements that frequently cannot be met from diet alone.

Significant folate deficiency results in ineffective erythropoiesis and a classic megaloblastic anemia. The disorder should be diagnosed by the detection of features of ineffective erythropoiesis, which include a low absolute reticulocyte count and evidence of intramedullary hemolysis, suggested by an indirect bilirubin level of greater than 0.6 mg/dL and an elevated lactic acid dehydrogenase level. The presence of macrocytosis (mean corpuscular volume greater than 100 fL) suggests either vitamin $B_{12}$ or folate deficiency. The diagnosis is confirmed by the presence of pathologically low serum (less than 2 nmol/L) and erythrocyte (less than 227 nmol/L) folate concentrations. Oral folate is the treatment of choice.

As with iron and folate deficiencies in the elderly, nutritional intake of $B_{12}$ appears to have an association with regional, cultural, and socioeconomic factors. Long-term vegetarian dietary patterns may predispose to a marginal risk of vitamin $B_{12}$ deficiency.[38] Other causes of vitamin $B_{12}$ deficiency in the elderly include malabsorption, gastric surgeries such as stapling procedures performed in the past for treatment of obesity, pernicious anemia, intestinal overgrowth (stasis syndrome), Crohn's disease, resection of terminal ileum, tropical sprue, pancreatic insufficiency, drugs (e.g., biguanides, neomycin, cholestyramine, ethanol), fish tapeworm, and acquired abnormality of $B_{12}$ metabolism.[51–53]

An overwhelming majority of cases of vitamin $B_{12}$ deficiency in elderly individuals are due to pernicious anemia, in which impaired secretion of intrinsic factor by gastric parietal cells results in reduction of active vitamin $B_{12}$ absorption in the terminal ileum. The initial diagnostic work-up should include a Schilling test, which helps to distinguish vitamin $B_{12}$ deficiency due to lack of intrinsic factor from other causes of $B_{12}$ malabsorption.[54] The presence of serum intrinsic factor and parietal cell antibodies may point toward a diagnosis of pernicious anemia, but the latter are also reported in healthy elderly people. Further investigation of pernicious anemia should include a screen for other auto-immune disorders, especially hypothyroidism. In view of the increased incidence of gastric carcinoma and carcinoid tumors in pernicious anemia, endoscopy should also be considered.

Serum $B_{12}$ levels have been reported in some studies to fall with aging.[51–55] Numerous clinical manifestations of $B_{12}$ deficiency have been well documented in the literature. These include hematological defects such as megaloblastic anemia; neuro-psychiatric disorders such as dementia, psychosis, peripheral neuropathies, subacute degeneration of the spinal cord; and gastrointestinal manifestations such as glossitis and malabsorption. Threshold levels of $B_{12}$ below which clinically important manifestations of deficiency are seen are controversial. Patients with pernicious anemia usually have a level less than 90 pmol/L and a megaloblastic marrow is generally found in patients with a serum $B_{12}$ level of less than 115 pmol/L. Patients with neuropsychiatric manifestations of $B_{12}$ deficiency commonly have a level of less than 175 pmol/L. These patients may thus have a normal blood count.

Stott et al.[51] recently reported the prevalence and hematopoietic effects of low $B_{12}$ levels in both an outpatient as well as an inpatient elderly population. Thirteen percent of the population sampled prospectively were found to have serum $B_{12}$ levels less than 175 pmol/L, without any significant reduction of the hemoglobin values. Interestingly, one-third of these vitamin $B_{12}$ deficient patients also were iron deficient, perhaps resulting in normal values of their mean corpuscular volume (MCV). Therefore, some evidence exists to suggest that vitamin $B_{12}$ deficiency is more common in the elderly. However, the clinical manifestations are subtle and may not be reflected in the peripheral complete blood count (CBC). In a separate, subsequent prospective study, the same authors assessed the hematological response to intramuscular hydroxycobalamin in 34 patients with low serum $B_{12}$ levels. Treatment resulted in a significant fall in MCV and rise in hemoglobin values even in those patients who had a normal CBC prior to treatment.

The treatment of vitamin $B_{12}$ deficiency is based on the underlying cause. Replacement therapy for severe vitamin $B_{12}$ deficiency consists of intramuscular injections of hydroxycobalamin 1 mg each, initially for a total of 5 to 7 injections at weekly intervals. Once stores are replenished, the dosage frequency can be reduced to once every 3 months for life. Utmost care should be taken to follow the potassium levels during the initial weekly injections since a reduction in plasma potassium of 1 to 2 meq/dL may occur in the first 48 hours after the first injection of vitamin $B_{12}$. Although vitamin $B_{12}$ is generally replaced by intramuscular injection, oral replacement with 1 mg daily can be effective.

## CONCLUSION

There is compelling evidence that nutritional factors contribute to, or account for, age-related changes in the hematopoietic system. A clear relationship exists between the prevalence of anemia and socioeconomic status, the disorder being common in groups in whom poverty is prevalent and rare in affluent elderly people. In low socioeconomic populations a relationship exists between the prevalence of anemia and other nutritional deficiencies. Furthermore, nutritional deprivation reversibly aggravates hematologic changes in the elderly. If nutritional factors do contribute to the anemia seen in relatively healthy elderly individuals, mechanisms other than simple single-nutrient deficiencies must be considered. In older people, erythropoietic reserve is diminished, resulting in abnormalities under less stressful conditions than is likely to occur in younger subjects. A minor nutritional deficit that would cause no abnormality in young people may result in anemia in elderly individuals. Clearly, further research is required to unravel the complex nature of the interrelationships among age, nutrition, disease in general, and hematopoiesis in particular. Iron and folate are common nutritional causes of hematologic abnormalities in elderly subjects. In the case of both nutrients, deficiency that is severe enough to result in anemia occurs only in the presence of an associated pathologic process. Gastrointestinal blood loss is the major cause of iron deficiency. Increased folate requirements, altered metabolism, or decreased absorption invariably accompany the presence of significant folate deficiency.

# REFERENCES

1. Schofield R. The pluripotent stem cell. *Clin Haematol.* 1979;8:221.

2. Schofield R, Lord BI, Kyffin S, et al. Self maintenance capacity of CFU-S. *Cell Physiol.* 1980;103:355.

3. Albright JA, Makinodan T. Decline in the growth potential of spleen-colonizing bone marrow stem cells of long lived aging mice. *J Exp Med.* 1976;144:1204.

4. Harrison DE, Astle CM, Delaittre JA. Loss of proliferative capacity in immunohemopoietic stem cells caused by serial transplantation rather than aging. *J Exp Med.* 1978;147:1526.

5. Ross EAM, Anderson H, Micklem HS. Serial depletion and regeneration for the murine hematopoietic system: implication for hematopoietic organization and the study of cellular aging. *J Exp Med.* 1982;155:432.

6. Harrison DE. Normal production of erythrocytes by mouse marrow continues for 73 months. *Proc Natl Acad Sci USA.* 1972;70:3184.

7. Spangrude GJ, Heimfeld S, Weissman IL. Purification and characterization of mouse hematopoietic stem cells. *Science.* 1988;261:58.

8. Mauch P, Greenberger JS, Sotnick L, et al. Evidence of structured variation in self-renewal capacity within long-termed bone marrow cultures. *Proc Natl Acad Sci USA.* 1980;77:2927.

9. Lipschitz DA, McGinnis SK, Udupa KB. The use of long term marrow culture as a model for the aging process. *Age.* 1983;6:122.

10. Mauch P, Botnick LE, Hannon EC, et al. Decline in bone marrow proliferative capacity as a function of age. *Blood.* 1982;60:245.

11. Hellman S, Botnick L, Hannon EC, et al. Proliferative capacity of murine hematopoietic stem cells. *Proc Natl Acad Sci USA.* 1978;75:490.

12. Reincke U, Hannon EC, Rosenbalt M, et al. Proliferative capacity of murine hematopoietic stem cells in vitro. *Science.* 1982;215:1619.

13. Williams LH, Udupa KB, Lipschitz DA. An evaluation of the effect of age on hematopoiesis in the mouse. *Exp Hematol.* 1985;19:237.

14. Boggs DR, Patrene KD. Hematopoiesis and aging III. Anemia and a blunted erythropoietic response to hemorrhage in aged mice. *Am J Hematol.* 1985;19:327.

15. Udupa KB, Lipschitz DA. Erythropoiesis in the aged mouse, I. Response to stimulation in vivo. *J Lab Clin Med.* 1984;103:574.

16. Udupa KB, Lipschitz DA. Erythropoiesis in the aged mouse, II. Response to stimulation in vitro. *J Lab Clin Med.* 1984;103:581.

17. McLennan WJ, et al. Anaemia in the elderly. *Q J Med.* 1973;52:1.

18. Myers MA, et al. The hemoglobin level of fit elderly people. *Lancet.* 1968;2:261.

19. *Nutrition Canada: National Survey.* Ottawa, Canada: Information Canada; 1973.

20. Yip R, et al. Age-related changes in laboratory values used in the diagnosis of anemia and iron deficiency. *Am J Clin Nutr.* 1984;39:427.

21. McPhee SJ. The evaluation of anemia. *West J Med.* 1982;137:253.

22. Ania BJ, et al. Prevalence of anemia in medical practice: community versus referral patients. *Mayo Clin Proc.* 1994;69:730.

23. Ania BJ, et al. Incidence of anemia in older people: an epidemiologic study in a well defined population. *J Am Geriatr Soc.* 1997;45:825.

24. Lipschitz DA, et al. The anemia of senescence. *Am J Hematol.* 1981;11:47.

25. Lipschitz DA, et al. Effect of age on hematopoiesis in man. *Blood.* 1984;63:502.

26. Garry PJ, et al. Iron status and anemia in the elderly. *J Am Geriatr Soc.* 1983;31:389.

27. Sears DA. Anemia of chronic disease. *Med Clin North Am.* 1992;76:567.

28. Lipschitz DA, Mitchell CO. The correctability of the nutritional, immune and hematopoietic manifestations of protein calorie malnutrition in the elderly. *J Am Coll Nutr.* 1982;1:17.

29. Rudman D, Mattson DE, et al. Antecedents of death in the men of a Veterans Administration nursing home. *J Am Geriatr Soc.* 1987;35:496.

30. Lipschitz DA, Udupa KB. Influence of aging and protein deficiency on neutrophil function. *J Gerontol.* 1986;41:690.

31. McMahon MM, Bistrian BR. The physiology of nutritional assessment and therapy in protein calorie malnutrition. Disease of the Month.

32. Lipschitz DA, Mitchell CO, Milton KY. Nutritional evaluation and supplementation of elderly

participants in a "Wheels on Meals" program. *J Parenter Enter Nutr.* 1985;9:343.

33. Cook JD, Finch CA, Smith NJ. Evaluation of iron status of a population. *Blood.* 1976;48:449.

34. Bedford PD, Wollner L. Occult intestinal bleeding as a cause of anaemia in elderly people. *Lancet.* 1958;1:1144.

35. Kirkeby OJ, Fossum S, Risoe C. Anemia in elderly patients: Incidence and causes of low hemoglobin concentration in a city general practice. *Scand J Prim Health Care.* 1991;9:167–171.

36. Joosten E, Pelemans W, Hiele M, et al. Prevalence and causes of anemia in a geriatric hospitalized population. *Gerontology.* 1992;38:111–117.

37. Looker CA, Dallman RP, Carroll MS, Gunter WE, Johnso LC. Prevalence of iron deficiency in the United States. *JAMA.* 1997;277:

38. Chiel RL, Schrijver J, Odink J, et al. Long term effects of a vegetarian diet on the nutritional status of the elderly (Dutch nutrition study). *J Am Coll Nutr.* 1990;9:600–609.

39. Fleming DJ, et al. Dietary determinants of iron stores in the elderly population in the Framingham Heart Study. *Am J Clin Nutr.* 1998;67:722–733.

40. Hillman RS, Finch CA. *Red Cell Manual.* Philadelphia: FA Davis Co; 1985.

41. Brise H. Influence of meals on iron absorption in oral therapy. *Acta Med Scand.* 1962;171(suppl 376):39.

42. Fulcher RA, Hyland CM. Effectiveness of once daily oral iron in the elderly. *Age Ageing.* 1981;10:44.

43. Reizenstein P, Ljunggren G, Smedby B, et al. Overprescribing iron tablets to elderly people in Sweden. *Br Med J.* 1979;2:962.

44. Elwood PC, Shinton NK, Wilson CID, et al. Hae-

moglobin, vitamin B 12 and folate levels in the elderly. *Br J Haematol.* 1971;21:557.

45. Rosenberg IH, Bowman BB, Cooper BA, et al. Folate nutrition in the elderly. *Am J Clin Nutr.* 1982;36:1060.

46. Brussaard JH, et al. Folate intake and status among adults in the Netherlands. *Eur J Clin Nutr.* 1997;51 (suppl 3):S46–S50.

47. Jagerstad M, Westesson AK. Folate. In Bergstrom B, Nordin A, Akesson B, et al, eds. *Nutrition and Old Age.* Oslo: Universities Forlaget; 1979.

48. *Nutrition Canada. Food Consumption Patterns Report.* Ottawa, Ont, Canada: Department of National Health and Welfare; 1979.

49. Lindenbaum J, Roman MJ. Nutritional anemia in alcoholism. *Am J Clin Nutr.* 1980;33:2727.

50. Chanarin I. *The Megaloblastic Anaemias.* 2nd ed. Oxford, England: Blackwell Scientific Publications Ltd; 1979.

51. Stott D, Langhorne P, Hendry A, et al. Prevalence of hematological effects of low serum vitamin B12 levels in geriatric medical patients. *Br J Nutr.* 1997;78:57–63.

52. Lindenbaum J, Rosenburg IH, Wilson PWF, Stabler SP, Allen RH. Prevalence of cobalamin deficiency in the Framingham elderly population. *Am J Clin Nutr.* 1994;60:2–11.

53. Lindenbaum J, Healton EB, Svage DG, et al. Neuro-psychiatric disorders caused by cobalamin deficiency in the absence of anemia or macrocytosis. *N Engl J Med.* 1988;318:1720–1728.

54. Chanarin I. Pernicious anemia. Diagnosis should be certain before treatment is begun. *Br Med J.* 1992;304:1584–1585.

55. Murphy PT, Hutchinson RM. Identification and treatment of anemia in older patients. *Drugs Aging.* 1994;4(2):13–127.

# CHAPTER 12

# Skeletal Aging

*Robert Marcus*

At any time during the course of adult life, bone mass reflects the amount of bone gained during growth minus that which has been subsequently lost. It now appears that about 60% of final adult bone mass is acquired during the pubertal growth spurt, particularly during the 3 to 4 year period surrounding the time of maximum height velocity, with only about 5% of final bone mass accruing during the decade from age 18 to 28 years. After that time, bone balance is largely negative, reflecting the fundamentally inefficient nature of bone remodeling. The rate at which bone is lost in adults varies from one skeletal site to another and according to measurement technique and is highly influenced by an assortment of so-called "lifestyle" factors, including body weight, reproductive hormonal function, habitual physical activity, diet, tobacco and alcohol consumption, illness, and medication. Specific mechanisms that lead to severe bone loss in some people but not in others are not completely understood. However, considerable interest has been directed toward clarifying the elements that determine peak bone mass at maturity and its subsequent decline.

Osteoporosis is a condition of skeletal fragility that is associated with low bone mass and disruption of the normal bony microarchitecture. It appears clinically as fractures that are sustained with little or no trauma. These have been described most frequently for the spine, wrist, and hip, but in truth osteoporosis is a condition of global fragility, and fractures elsewhere in the skeleton are also common. Osteoporotic fractures are more commonly observed in women. This reflects the fact that women have lower bone mass than men and that there are twice as many older women as men. Nonetheless, age-specific incidence of fracture in men is about half that of women, and fracture incidence is rising substantially in older men.

## SKELETAL ORGANIZATION

The skeleton can be considered to be organized into two compartments, peripheral and axial. The peripheral (cortical) skeleton constitutes 80% of skeletal mass and is composed primarily of compact plates (lamellae) organized around central nutrient canals. The shafts of long bones consist almost entirely of cortical bone that envelopes the central marrow cavity.

The axial, or central, skeleton is composed about 70% (by volume) and about 35% (by weight) of trabecular (cancellous) bone.[1] Trabecular bone is a honeycomb of vertical and horizontal bars (trabeculae), inside which is found bone marrow (Figure 12–1). The meta-

304

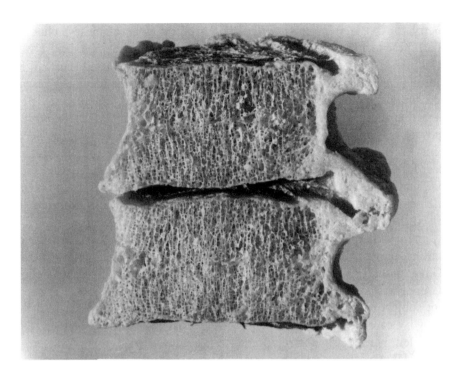

**Figure 12–1** Normal vertebral bone. Surrounded by a thin shell of cortical bone, vertebral bodies are composed of a honeycomb of vertical and horizontal struts, or trabeculae. Trabecular bone has a much higher surface-to-mass ratio than cortical bone, and its interstices represent the sole repository of red bone marrow in adult humans.

physeal ends of long bones also contain trabecular bone, but they contain no red marrow in the adult. Since marrow elements are the source of osteoclast precursors, and since bone turnover occurs on bone surfaces, the occurrence of high–surface density bone in close proximity to the cellular elements that participate in its turnover results in trabecular bone's responding earlier and more intensely to whole-body changes in bone remodeling rate.

## IN VIVO ASSESSMENT OF BONE MASS

Accurate, noninvasive measurement of bone mass emerged with the development of photon absorptiometry. Results are given as the mass of bone mineral (grams) contained within a given area (square centimeters) of scanned bone. The resulting value, called bone mineral density (BMD) is therefore an areal density, and not a true volumetric density. Single-photon absorptiometry (SPA) is based on the attenuation of a narrowly focused photon beam (usually [125]I) by bone. Measurements are accurate, precise, and suited to skeletal regions in which variations in soft tissue composition are minimal, such as the forearm or heel. Estimates of cortical bone mass at these sites correlate reasonably well with whole-body bone mineral but only poorly reflect the axial skeleton.[2]

Techniques based on the transmission of photons at two energies permit measurements of the central skeleton. Dual-energy X-ray absorptiometry (DXA) has emerged as the most useful of these techniques.[3] Subjects lie recumbent while a photomultiplier tube records transmission from an X-ray source located under the scanning table. The lumbar spine is scanned in about 4 minutes with a radiation exposure of less than 5 mrem. DXA measurements in the usual anteroposterior position record the complete mineral content of a vertebra, including the cortical shell and posterior elements, in addition to the vertebral body itself. Moreover, patients with degenerative joint disease of the spine and aortic calcifications may have falsely elevated spine BMD readings. DXA is also routinely used to measure BMD at the proximal femur, which is not subject to these latter artifacts but requires very careful attention to positioning of the leg, particularly for repeated measurements. DXA software also permits some machines to provide measurements of whole-body and regional skeletal mineral, as well as body composition assessments (lean and adipose tissue). The precision error for DXA varies from 1% to 1.5% in young and older subjects, respectively.

Quantitative computed tomography (QCT) has been used frequently to estimate trabecular bone density at the lumbar spine.[4] The subject lies on a scanning table above a set of materials of standard densities. The operator selects a region of pure trabecular bone for analysis, and the mineral density, given as milligrams per cubic centimeter of bone volume, is calculated. Although this technique can be modified for any skeletal region, most work has involved the lumbar spine, for which commercial software is available. For healthy, nonosteoporotic subjects, the precision error in experienced hands may approach that of DXA, but in routine clinical practice such performance is rarely achieved. Radiation exposure, usually 500 to 1000 mrem, is modest but substantially greater than that of DXA.

Modifications of these technologies have become available, including DXA and CT scanners that are used exclusively on the forearm or leg. Besides their research applications, these techniques may permit bone density screening of large populations at much lower cost than can be accomplished with DXA. In addition, several companies are developing methods based on the transmission of ultrasound through bones, such as the heel and patella. Results of these measurements correlate well with BMD measurements and could therefore be used as a screening modality to identify those individuals who should undergo comprehensive testing with DXA.[5]

## THE PIVOTAL ROLE OF BONE REMODELING (3 Basic Bone Activities)

Bone carries out three fundamental activities: modeling, repair, and remodeling. *Modeling* refers to the process by which the characteristic shape of a bone is achieved and maintained. *Repair* is the regenerative response to fracture. *Remodeling* is a continuous cycle of destruction and renewal of bone that occurs throughout life in humans, primates, and some other mammals.[6] This process is carried out by independent osteons, called bone remodeling units, and alterations in remodeling activity constitute the final common pathway through which diverse stimuli, such as dietary or hormonal insufficiency, affect the rate of bone loss. The characteristic features of bone remodeling are illustrated in Figure 12–2 and outlined below.

Normally, 90% of bone surfaces are at rest, covered by a thin layer of inactive lining cells. Remodeling is initiated by hormonal or physical signals that cause marrow-derived precursor cells to cluster on the bone surface, where they fuse into multinucleated osteoclasts, which in turn dig a cavity into the

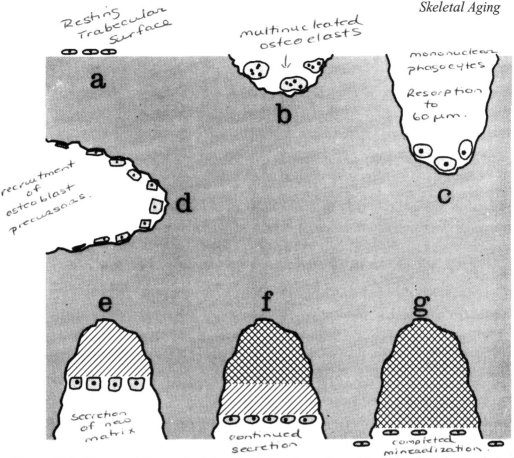

**Figure 12–2** The remodeling cycle: (a) resting trabecular surface; (b) multinucleated osteoclasts digging a cavity of approximately 20 µm; (c) completion of resorption to 60 µm by mononuclear phagocytes; (d) recruitment of osteoblast precursors to the base of the resorption cavity; (e) secretion of new matrix by osteoblasts; (f) continued secretion of matrix, with initiation of calcification; and (g) completion of mineralization of new matrix. Bone has returned to a quiescent state, but a small deficit in bone mass persists. *Source:* With permission from the *Annual Review of Medicine*, Vol. 38, © 1987, by Annual Reviews Inc.

bone. In cortical bone, this cavity appears as a resorption tunnel within a Haversian canal. On trabecular surfaces, it is a scalloped area called a Howship's lacuna. The resorption front leaves a cavity about 60 µm deep, whose deepest boundary appears as a cement line, a region of poorly organized collagen fibrils, as opposed to the surrounding lamellar bone.

Coupled to resorption, bone formation is triggered when the local release of chemical mediators embedded in the bone matrix attracts preosteoblasts into the resorption cavity. The identity of these mediators is not known with certainty, but transforming growth factor-β and insulinlike growth factors may each play a role. The preosteoblasts mature into osteoblasts and replace the missing bone by secreting new collagen and matrix constituents. Matrix production is initially rapid, with the new osteoid seam approaching 20 µm in thickness when mineral deposition begins. With time, mineralization catches up to matrix deposition, and the new bone becomes fully mineralized. A normal bone-remodeling cycle takes about 6 months to reach completion.

If the remodeling cycle were completely efficient, bone would be neither lost nor gained. Each remodeling unit would be associated with complete replacement of the packet of bone that was initially lost. However, remodeling, like most biological processes, is not entirely efficient. The amount of bone replaced by formation does not always equal the amount previously removed, so that a small bone deficit persists after each cycle. This remodeling imbalance is minuscule for any single normal bone-remodeling event. Unless remodeling dynamics are perturbed, the resulting accumulation of bone deficits may be detected only after many years. The concept of remodeling imbalance carries the profound implication that age-related bone loss is a normal, predictable phenomenon and that any increase in the overall rate of bone remodeling will increase the rate of bone loss. Another long-term consequence of remodeling is the acquisition of cement lines. These areas of woven bone are not as strong as the surrounding lamellar bone and thus form a site of least resistance to strain.[7] In fact, examination of fractured bone shows propagation of fracture from one cement line to the next.

## CHANGES IN BONE MASS WITH AGE

### Overview

Accumulation of bone during the growth years exactly mirrors linear growth. Bone mass increases linearly until the onset of puberty and then undergoes an intense and rapid increase that follows by a short interval the time of maximum height velocity. About 95% of ultimate, "peak" bone mass is acquired by age 18 in girls, perhaps a year or two later in boys.[8–10] Between the ages of 18 and 28 years, small amounts of bone continue to be accrued, but bone acquisition is essentially complete by age 28 years.[11] As measured by noninvasive techniques, bone mass then remains stable until about age 50, when progressive decrease in BMD occurs in both men and women. In women, the loss of estrogen at menopause results in an accelerated rate of loss, particularly from trabecular sites, during the first several years after menopause, but afterwards the rates of loss in women and men are fairly similar.

### Adolescent Bone Acquisition

The 2- to 3-year period corresponding to the time of peak height velocity represents a brief window of opportunity for laying down bone. Fully 60% of peak bone mass is acquired during this period. Its onset is triggered by pubertal progression, and increases in bone mass are highly correlated to body weight, height, and pubertal stage. The critical role of estrogen in this process, for both boys and girls, is evidenced by a single case report of a young man with profound osteopenia and failure of epiphyseal closure whose growth hormone and testicular function were normal but who was shown to have a mutation in the estradiol receptor that rendered him completely unresponsive to even massive amounts of estrogen.[12] The role of estrogen is probably to stimulate cartilage cells to proliferate and proceed down the bone differentiation pathway.

The greatest influence on pubertal bone acquisition is genetics, which appears to account for approximately 75% of the population variance in peak bone mass. The largest single influence of genetics on BMD is bone size, which itself is a polygenic function, reflecting at the very least the activities of the somatotrophic (growth hormone and somatomedin) and gonadotrophic axes. Recent evidence also implicates genetic polymorphisms in the vitamin D receptor as being significantly related to bone mass,[13] and it is highly likely that other genes will also be found to be related to bone mass in the future.

Environmental, or lifestyle, elements that affect bone acquisition are incompletely understood, but substantial evidence implicates the adequacy of dietary calcium and habitual physical activity as being of great importance. Slemenda et al[14] and others[15] have shown that BMD in children is significantly influenced by physical activity, particularly activities that have a weight-bearing component to them (such as running, jumping, and dancing). Moreover, studies of tennis players who started to train seriously at a very young age indicate not only that BMD is higher in the racket arm than in the nonracket arm but that overall forearm bone width is also greater in the racket arm.[16] In other words, children have the capacity to respond to mechanical loads not only by increasing bone density but also by undergoing adaptive changes in bone geometry that ultimately are favorable for bone strength.

Epidemiological data have not been consistent in defining the relationship of dietary calcium to bone acquisition by children, and the reality of such a relationship has, until recently, remained in question. However, during recent years, several well-conceived placebo-controlled clinical trials have consistently shown larger increases in bone mass by children and adolescents receiving supplemental calcium than were observed in those receiving placebo.[17,18] Remaining questions concerning these reports concern not their accuracy but the implications of the findings for peak bone mass in these individuals. Follow-up data from one of these studies[17] indicated that 2 years after termination of the calcium intervention, the difference in bone mass between the two treatment groups was no longer significant. Thus, one possibility is that to achieve permanent skeletal benefit, it will be necessary to sustain the increased calcium intake long term.

It should be noted here that habitual calcium intakes of American girls and women are seriously deficient. According to data from the U.S. Center for Health Statistics (N-HANES),[19] median calcium intake of girls decreases below recommended standards at age 11 and never recovers. Of teenage girls, about 30% consume less than 400 mg of calcium per day, reflecting a serious reduction in milk consumption over the past few decades.

I have indicated that the adolescent growth spurts represents a window of opportunity for achieving major increases in bone mass and maximizing an individual's chances for achieving full peak bone mass potential. It can also be argued that this period represents a window of vulnerability during which neglect of bone-healthy behavior may cause irretrievable deficits in bone mass at maturity, so that a person's long-term risk for osteoporotic fracture is greatly increased even if bone loss is minimal. Causes of such "acquisitional osteopenia" are legion. A partial list is shown in Table 12–1.

## ADULT BONE LOSS

The traditional model of age-related bone loss was clearly enunciated by the landmark studies of Garn et al.[20] Using careful measurements of metacarpal cortical thickness from hand radiographs, they described a characteristic trajectory of bone mass change that was similar in men and women and was observed in virtually all ethnic groups: bone is gained during adolescence, remains stable until about age 50 years, then progressively decreases. This model has been independently validated by numerous laboratories us-

**Table 12–1** Representative Examples of Low Bone Mass Due to Inadequate Bone Acquisition

Genetic
  Cystic fibrosis
  Marfan syndrome
  Galactosemia
  Osteogenesis imperfecta
Childhood Illness–Related
  Renal insufficiency
  Intestinal malabsorption
  Immobilization
  Corticosteroid use
  Anorexia nervosa

ing newer densitometric methods[21–23] and has been modified by the observation that the initial rate of loss at age 50 in women is temporarily more rapid than in men, reflecting the effects of menopausal estrogen loss.

Although the age-related decline in BMD of the radius accurately describes the trajectory of appendicular (limb) cortical bone mass, it was difficult for many years to validate its applicability to other regions of the cortical skeleton, such as the proximal femur, or to the axial or trabecular skeleton. Pioneering studies with postmortem material[25–27] clearly indicated that loss of axial bone occurred earlier than one would predict from noninvasive data. Subsequent analyses of iliac crest biopsy material confirm this view.[28–30] There is unanimous agreement, using multiple techniques, that trabecular bone is lost with age and that axial density is substantially lower in older subjects than in young people. Uncertainty remains over the timing of onset of axial bone loss.

## ONSET OF BONE LOSS

A decline in bone density has been reported to begin after the second,[31] third,[32] fourth,[33] or fifth[34] decade. Measurements of anatomic specimens and results from biopsy studies indicate that axial loss occurs as early as the third decade.[29,35,36] In particular, iliac crest biopsy data suggest that trabecular bone mass declines significantly in women before menopause. Meunier and colleagues[28] showed an age-related loss of trabecular bone that began as early as the third decade in a series of specimens obtained from sudden death accident victims. Marcus et al[29] examined trabecular bone volume in biopsy specimens taken from active women with normal menstrual function and reported that trabecular bone volume was negatively correlated with age, with an annual predicted loss of 0.7% (Figure 12–3). The cumulative effect of such loss over a span of 30 years might amount to a deficit of 25% of original trabecular bone volume before menopause is reached. Birkenhager-Frenkel et al[30] conducted iliac crest biopsies on a large group of healthy men and women and reported a correlation of trabecular bone volume with age for premenopausal women that was the same as that observed by Marcus and colleagues.[29] Trabecular vertebral specimens show the same pattern with age as iliac crest samples. Mosekilde and Mosekilde[37] examined postmortem trabecular samples of the first lumbar vertebra and found an age-related decrease in vertebral bone mass beginning in the third decade.

The development of accurate noninvasive densitometry has permitted evaluation of this issue on a much larger scale. Measurements of spine BMD in normal and osteoporotic individuals have revealed both a linear and a nonlinear loss of bone with age. A major problem with these studies is the difficulty in predicting longitudinal changes from cross-sectional analyses. Depending on the number of subjects and the measurement technique, some investigators have reported correlations

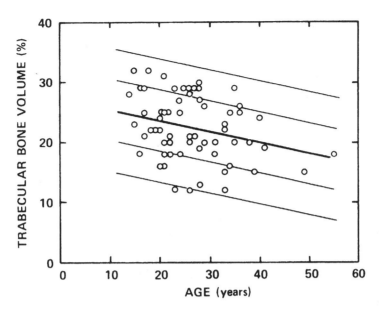

**Figure 12–3** Trabecular bone volume (iliac crest biopsies) versus age. Parallel lines indicate mean ± 1 and 2 standard deviations. *Source:* Reprinted with permission from *Calcified Tissue International* (1983; 35:406–409), Copyright 1983 Springer-Verlag.

of bone mineral density with age that fit a linear model, in which loss of lumbar BMD with age remains constant from young adulthood[31]; others have described an exponential model, in which loss is minimal or nonsignificant before age 50 years (or menopause in women), followed by significant linear declines thereafter.[38] Results with dual-energy absorptiometry and QCT have been variable. Some groups have observed significant axial bone loss before age 50,[39–42] while others have failed to confirm such a change.[32–34,43–46] Madsen[39] and Riggs et al[40] have reported linear decreases in lumbar spine BMD of 0.5% to 1.0% per year in women. Similar measurements in normal men also gave negative regressions with age, although the slopes were somewhat less than half those observed with women. Buchanan and associates[41] measured vertebral BMD by QCT in premenopausal women and found a highly significant decrease with age ($r = -.39$, $p = .0006$), con-

cluding that vertebral trabecular bone loss begins during or prior to the third decade. Other investigators who have not observed significant loss of bone before age 50 years report that major loss begins at the time of menopause. The reasons for discrepancies among reports are not clear. The principal difficulty may arise from the fact that the vast majority of these studies are cross-sectional analyses. Although such reports may provide valid insights into population changes across time, they cannot distinguish secular trends and are subject to multiple confounding factors. For example, the observation of a bone density at age 40 years that is lower than that at age 20 could reflect loss of bone over two decades, but it is also consistent with an interpretation that peak bone mass is higher today than was true 20 years ago. Therefore, a number of important geographic, ethnic, dietary, and physical activity differences within and between study populations could account for the inconsistencies observed in the literature. In addition, Sambrook et al[38] showed that the population size necessary to detect subtle changes in regression slope with certainty is far greater than that of any reported study. This is particularly relevant to detecting a menopausal acceleration of bone loss.

## CHANGES IN BONE MASS AT MENOPAUSE

Most studies confirm that trabecular bone loss accelerates at menopause.[32–34,43–46] Gallagher et al[43] measured spine BMD of almost 400 women and reported that the largest decrease occurred in the first 5 years after menopause. They found a 3.4% annual decline in the second year, a 1.7% decline in the fourth year, and a 0.8% decline in the ninth year. Cann and associates,[45] using QCT to measure spine BMD, found that values for trabecular mineral remained stable until menopause, then declined rapidly for 5 to 8 years, and then continued to decline, but more slowly. Firooznia et al[46] showed the same trend.

By contrast, some cross-sectional reports claim a linear decline in BMD from age 50 years.[33,34] However, one of these groups also reported longitudinal results in the same report[33] in which accelerated loss during the first 5 years from menopause was observed. In the recently concluded Postmenopausal Estrogen/Progestin Interventions trial (PEPI), involving almost 900 women within 10 years of menopause, bone density at the spine and hip decreased in a curvilinear fashion, supporting the concept of menopausal acceleration of bone loss.[47]

To summarize, trabecular bone loss in women begins before age 50 years and increases at menopause. The weight of evidence supports the conclusion that menopausal loss of bone is curvilinear—that is,

most rapid within the first few years. The absolute rates of menopausal bone loss are highly variable and appear to follow a normal distribution. Some investigators have developed predictive models to identify those patients who are most likely to have the most rapid loss and who therefore might be the most logical candidates to screen with densitometry and for whom to prescribe therapy. The problem with that approach is that there is no obvious relationship between rates of bone loss and the initial bone mass. Thus, a woman whose peak bone density was already low might be predicted to have a low rate of loss, but since her skeleton was already at jeopardy, it would be important to assess her and offer treatment. By contrast, another woman might have rapid bone loss, but starting with an initial bone mass that was greater than 1 standard deviation above age-related norms, she would still have a very low risk of fracture even if she were untreated.

## RELATIONSHIP OF LOSS OF BONE MASS TO BONE STRENGTH

Most patients with vertebral, wrist, and hip fractures have low bone mass. However, it is important to understand that bone's strength depends not only on its amount but on its material quality and architecture. A number of so-called qualitative abnormalities have been described in bone from older individuals that render older bone more fragile in comparison to bone of equal BMD in younger individuals. These abnormalities include the lifelong accumulation of cement lines as a consequence of remodeling events (Figure 12–4) and the presence of unremodeled fatigue damage. Other qualitative abnormalities include subtle degrees of undermineralization at critical areas of Haversian systems, loss of trabecular connectivity, and the accumulation of cortical porosity.[48]

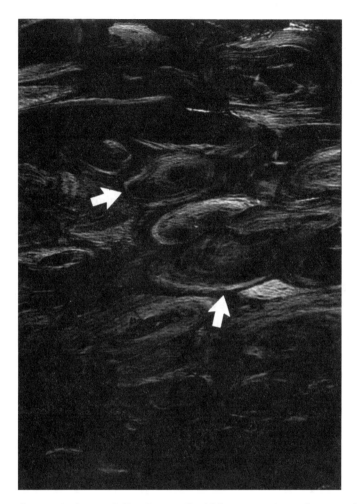

**Figure 12–4** Extensive cortical remodeling in transileal biopsy specimen from an elderly woman. Arrows point to cement lines. These are areas of woven bone that are structurally weaker than the original compact lamellar bone. Photograph courtesy of R. R. Recker, with permission of Academic Press, Inc.

Mosekilde and Mosekilde[37] demonstrated the importance of bone quality to vertebral body strength by showing 90% reductions in strength between ages 15 and 87, whereas ash density, the amount of mineral present, declined only 50% over this span. In a young person, trabecular bone is characterized by thick vertical plates and columns that are connected by thinner horizontal elements. Maximal strength is provided by the connection of all trabecular elements into a honeycomblike structure. With age, skeletal fragility is created by both the thinning of trabecular plates and the dropout of complete horizontal elements, with a corresponding increase in intertrabecular spaces.[49,50]

Another important determinant of bone strength is its geometry. The strength of a bone in compression reflects its mineral density squared times its cross-sectional area. Thus, a larger bone will be stronger than a small bone even if BMD values are equivalent. Recent attention has focused on a measurement called the hip axis length (HAL), seen on bone density printouts as the straight-line distance between the inferior surface of the greater trochanter to the inner surface of the acetabulum. Faulkner et al[51] have shown that longer HAL is independently predictive of hip fracture. It appears that shorter HAL values are characteristic of Asian women and may contribute to their lower incidence of hip fracture.

## MECHANISMS OF BONE MASS REGULATION

As stated above, alteration in remodeling activity is the final common pathway to modulating bone mass in adults. Primary regulators of this process include physical activity, calcium nutriture, and reproductive endocrine status. The relationship of these issues to bone acquisition has been discussed above. The next section will consider these relationships in adults.

### Physical Activity

The estimated loss of bone from its peak value to age 80 years is comparable to the reported 35% to 45% decline in muscle strength over the same period.[52] Since a clear relationship between muscle strength and bone mass has been established,[27,53–55] physical activity has gained attention as a strategy for improving bone mass. The mechanisms by which the skeleton responds to activity remain incompletely understood,[56] but overwhelming evidence indicates that bone mass increases in response to the cyclic administration of mechanical loads.[57–59] Data from numerous studies permit the conclusion that bone mass of athletes exceeds that of the sedentary individuals who watch them.[60–64] Not only is bone density higher in physically ac-

tive people, but the literature suggests that exercise reduces the rate of age-related bone loss.[65–67] A small group of exercise intervention trials indicates that imposing a vigorous exercise program does increase BMD, particularly at the spine, but the magnitude of increase that is achieved in these programs does not approach the large differences that distinguish athletes from controls. It is not currently known which type of exercise is optimal for improving bone mass. In intervention trials, both weight training and jogging increased spine BMD by approximately 1.3%,[68–70] with little, if any, response at the hip. Remarkably high BMD values in gymnasts[71] raises the possibility that high-impact activity, such as jumping or high-impact aerobics, may be uniquely potent stimuli for increased bone mass. However, applying such activity to older, more frail individuals may not be practical for safety reasons.

### Calcium Nutriture

The skeleton is the repository for 99.5% of total body calcium and constitutes a source of mineral that can support plasma calcium concentrations at times of need. Relationships between dietary calcium and skeletal integrity are complex and frequently ambiguous[72] and are not detailed here, although a few summary remarks are in order.

The recommended dietary calcium intake for adolescents has been discussed above, as has the fact that American women systematically underconsume calcium after the age of 11 years. During the third through fifth decades, robust compensatory mechanisms permit rapid adaptation to even severe dietary restriction. Therefore, it should not be surprising that calcium nutritional state appears to be less an influence on changes in bone mass during this period[73]; as a corollary, it is unlikely that calcium supplementation will exert important beneficial effects on bone mass for women in this age group. It is ironic to note that this population receives the greatest portion of calcium supplement advertising.

At menopause, the initial acceleration in bone loss in women reflects loss of endogenous estrogen, and it has little relationship to dietary calcium. Riis and colleagues[74] showed only modest effects on bone loss when early-menopausal women were given supplemental calcium. However, the habitual dietary calcium intake of Danish women approximates 1100 mg, considerably higher than that in the United States, so what may have been a marginal effect for Danish women might be more substantial for their American counterparts.

After age 60 years, early effects of estrogen deficiency have subsided, whereas the compensatory mechanisms for accommodating dietary deficiencies have become less efficient in both men and women. It is considered likely that disruption of these mechanisms leads to secondary hypersecretion of parathyroid hormone, leading to support of plasma calcium at the expense of aggravated bone loss.[75,76] At this time, attention to proper calcium nutriture, whether from dietary calcium or from supplementation with calcium/vitamin D, is rational and has been shown to have beneficial effects on bone mass as well as on fracture incidence.[77]

**Reproductive Endocrine Status**

Formidable evidence supports an important role for gonadal function in the acquisition and maintenance of bone mass. Hypogonadal boys and girls have substantial deficits in both cortical and trabecular bone mineral. Loss of endogenous androgen or estrogen during adult life regularly leads to accelerated loss of bone, an effect that is particularly striking when it occurs at an early age, such as after oophorectomy in a young woman.

In women, loss of estrogen has dual effects. Decreased efficiency of intestinal and renal calcium homeostasis increases the level of calcium intake necessary to maintain calcium balance. In addition, estrogen directly affects bone cell function,[78-80] an interaction thought to underlie the accelerated bone loss of early estrogen deficiency. With respect to bone remodeling, estrogen deficiency permits the recruitment of increased numbers of osteoclasts, which individually also seem to resorb bone with greater efficiency. This may lead to perforation of trabeculae, with no scaffold left for initiation of new bone formation. Therefore, entire trabecular elements may be permanently eliminated. Replacement of estrogen at menopause protects bone mass and gives significant protection against fracture.[81] Estrogen deficiency may have an overwhelming influence on bone mass even when adequate attention is given to other important influences on bone health. For example, women athletes who experience interruption of menstrual function lose bone, despite regular exercise at high intensity.

The skeletal role of androgens is less well understood. Testosterone deficiency is an important contributor to osteoporosis in men, and replacement therapy improves bone mass,[82] but the precise nature of this interaction remains unresolved. Specific receptors for testosterone do exist in bone cells in low abundance, but the major androgen influence on bone may result from its trophic effects on skeletal muscle.

**CONCLUSIONS**

Extensive evidence documents important contributions of physical activity, calcium nutriture, and reproductive endocrine status to the acquisition and maintenance of bone mass. For too long, investigators in this field have maintained parochial interests in one or another of these areas, championing its particular importance while occasionally denigrating the relevance of others. It is important to understand that proper maintenance of bone throughout life requires integrated and balanced attention to all of these several influences.

## REFERENCES

1. Nottestad SY, Baumel JJ, Kimmel D, et al. The proportion of trabecular bone in human vertebrae. *J Bone Miner Res.* 1987;2:221–229.

2. Mazess RB. The noninvasive measurement of skeletal mass. In: Peck WA, ed. *Bone and Mineral Research Annual.* New York: Elsevier Science Publishing Co, Inc; 1981:1.

3. Wahner, HW. Use of densitometry in management of osteoporosis. In: Marcus R, Feldman D, and Kelsey J, eds. *Osteoporosis.* San Diego, Calif: Academic Press; 1996:1055–1074.

4. Cann CE, Genant HK. Precise measurement of vertebral mineral content using computed tomography. *J Comput Assist Tomogr.* 1980;4:493–500.

5. Bauer DC, Glüer C-C, Genant HK, Stone K. Quantitative ultrasound and vertebral fracture in postmenopausal women. *J Bone Miner Res.* 1995;10:353–358.

6. Marcus R. Normal and abnormal bone remodeling in man. *Annu Rev Med.* 1987;38:129–141.

7. Burr DB, Martin RB, Schaffler MB, et al. Bone remodeling in response to in vivo fatigue damage. *J Biomech.* 1985;12:189–200.

8. Bonjour JP, Theintz, G, Buchs B, Slossman, D, Rizzoli R. Critical years and stages of puberty for spinal and femoral bone mass accumulation during adolescence. *J Clin Endocrinol Metab.* 1991;73:555–563.

9. Katzman DK, Bachrach LK, Carter DR, Marcus R. Clinical and anthropometric correlates of bone mineral acquisition in healthy adolescent girls. *J Clin Endocrinol Metab.* 1991;73:1332–1339.

10. Budhikanok GS, Wang M-C, Eckert K, Matkin C, Marcus R, Bachrach LK. Differences in bone density (BMD) in young Asian- and Caucasian-Americans reflects differences in bone size. *J Bone Min Res.* 1996;11:1545–1556.

11. Recker RR, Davies KM, Hinders S, Heaney RP, Stegman MR, Kimmel DB. Bone gain in young adult women. *JAMA.* 1992;268:2403–2408

12. Smith EP, Boyd J, Frank GR, et al. Estrogen resistance caused by a mutation in the estrogen-receptor in a man. *N Engl J Med.* 1994;331:1056–1061.

13. Gross C, Eccleshall TR, Feldman D. Vitamin D receptor gene alleles and osteoporosis. In: Bilezikian JP, Raisz LG, Rodan G, eds. *Principles of Bone Biology.* San Diego, Calif: Academic Press; 1996: 917–934.

14. Slemenda CW, Miller JZ, Hui SL, Resiter TK, Johnston CC Jr. Role of physical activity in the development of skeletal mass in children. *J Bone Min Res.* 1991;6:1227–1233.

15. Ruiz JC, Mandel C, Garabedian M. Influence of spontaneous calcium intake and physical exercise on the vertebral and femoral bone mineral density of children and adolescents. *J Bone Miner Res.* 1995;10:675–682.

16. Kannus P, Haapasalo H, Sankelo M, et al. Effect of starting age of physical activity on bone mass in the dominant arm of tennis and squash players. *Ann Intern Med.* 1995;123:27–31.

17. Johnston CC Jr, Miller JZ, Slemenda CW, et al. Calcium supplementation and increases in bone mineral density in children. *N Engl J Med.* 1992;327:82–87.

18. Lloyd T, Andon MB, Rollings N, et al. Calcium supplementation and bone mineral density in adolescent girls. *JAMA* 1993, 270: 841-844.

19. Eck LH, Hackett-Renner C. Calcium intake in youth: sex, age, and racial differences in NHANES II. *Prev Med.* 1992,21:473–482.

20. Garn SM, Rohman CG, Nolan P Jr. The developmental nature of bone changes during aging. In: Birren JE, ed. *Relations of Development and Aging.* Springfield Ill: Charles C Thomas Publisher; 1966.

21. Mazess RB. On aging bone loss. *Clin Orthop.* 1982;165;239–252.

22. Smith DM, Khairi MRA, Norton J, et al. Age and activity effects on rate of bone mineral loss. *J Clin Invest.* 1976;58:716–721.

23. Hui SL, Wiske PS, Norton JA, et al. A prospective study of change in bone mass with age in postmenopausal women. *J Chronic Dis.* 1982;35:715–725.

24. Slemenda C, Hui SL, Longcope C, et al. Sex steroids and bone mass: a study of changes about the time of menopause. *J Clin Invest.* 1987;80:1261–1269.

25. Arnold JS, Bartley MH, Bartley DDS, et al. Skeletal changes in aging and disease. *Clin Orthop.* 1966;49:37.

26. Trotter M, Broman GE, Peterson RP. Densities of bones of white and Negro skeletons. *J Bone Joint Surg.* 1960;42A:58.

27. Doyle F, Brown J, LaChance C. Relation between bone mass and muscle weight. *Lancet.* 1970;1:391–393.

28. Meunier P, Courpron P, Edouard C, et al. Physiological senile involution and pathological rarefaction of bone. *Clin Endocrinol Metab.* 1973;2:239–256.

29. Marcus R, Kosek J, Pfefferbaum A, et al. Age-related loss of trabecular bone in premenopausal women: a biopsy study. *Calcif Tissue Int.* 1983;35:406–409.

30. Birkenhager-Frenkel DH, Courpron P, Hupscher EA, et al. Age-related changes in cancellous bone structure. *Bone Miner.* 1988;4:197–216.

31. Riggs BL, Wahner HW, Melton JL III, et al. Rates of bone loss in the appendicular and axial skeletons of women: evidence of substantial vertebral bone loss before menopause. *J Clin Invest.* 1986;77:1487–1491.

32. Geusens P, Dequeker A, Verstraeten A, et al. Age-, sex-, and menopause-related changes of vertebral and peripheral bone population study using dual and single photon absorptiometry and radiogrammetry. *J Nucl Med.* 1986;27:1540–1549.

33. Krølner B, Pors Nielsen S. Bone mineral content of the lumbar spine in normal and osteoporotic women: cross-sectional and longitudinal studies. *Clin Sci.* 1982;62:329–336.

34. Aloia JF, Vaswani A, Ellis K, et al. A model for involutional bone loss. *J Lab Clin Med.* 1985;106:630–637.

35. Weaver JK, Chalmers J. Cancellous bone: its strength and changes with aging and in evaluation of some methods for measuring its mineral content. *J Bone Joint Surg.* 1966;48A:289–299.

36. Arnold JS. Amount and quality of trabecular bone in osteoporotic vertebral fractures. *Clin Endocrinol Metab.* 1973;2:221–238.

37. Mosekilde L, Mosekilde L. Iliac crest bone volume as a predictor for vertebral compressive strength, ash density and trabecular bone volume in normal individuals. *Bone.* 1988;9:195–199.

38. Sambrook PN, Eisman JA, Furler SM, et al. Computer modeling and analysis of cross-sectional bone density studies with respect to age and the menopause. *J Bone Miner Res.* 1987;2:109–114.

39. Madsen M. Vertebral and peripheral bone mineral content by photon absorptiometry. *Invest Radiol.* 1977;12:185–188.

40. Riggs BI, Wahner HW, Dann WL, et al. Differential changes in bone mineral density of the appendicular and axial skeleton with aging. *J Clin Invest.* 1981;67:328–335.

41. Buchanan JR, Myers C, Lloyd T, et al. Early vertebral trabecular bone loss in normal premenopausal women. *J Bone Miner Res.* 1988;3:583–587.

42. Hanson T, Roos B. Age changes in bone mineral of the lumbar spine in normal women. *Calcif Tissue Int.* 1986;38:249–251.

43. Gallagher JC, Goldgar D, Moy A. Total bone calcium in normal women: effect of age and menopause status. *J Bone Miner Res.* 1987;2:491–496.

44. Nilas L, Gotfredsen A, Hadberg A, et al. Age-related bone loss in women evaluated by the single and dual photon technique. *Bone Miner.* 1988;4:95–103.

45. Cann CE, Genant HK, Kolb FO, et al. Quantitative computed tomography for prediction of vertebral fracture risk. *Bone.* 1985;61:1–7.

46. Firooznia H, Golimbu C, Rafi M, et al. Quantitative computed tomography assessment of spinal trabecular bone, I: age-related regression in normal men and women. *J Comput Tomogr.* 1984;8:91–97.

47. Marcus R, Greendale G, Blunt B, et al. Correlates of bone mineral density in the post-menopausal estrogen/progestin interventions trial (PEPI). *J Bone Min Res.* 1994,9:1467–1476.

48. Marcus, R. The nature of osteoporosis. In: Marcus R, Feldman D, Kelsey J, eds. *Osteoporosis.* San Diego, Calif: Academic Press. 1996: 647–659.

49. Parfitt AM. Age-related structural change in trabecular and cortical bone: cellular mechanisms and biomechanical consequences. *Calcif Tissue Int.* 1984;8:137–142.

50. Weinstein RS, Hutson MS. Decreased trabecular width and increased trabecular spacing contribute to bone loss with aging. *Bone.* 1987;8:137–142.

51. Faulkner KG, Cummings SR, Black D, Palermo L, Glüer C-C, Genant HK. Simple measurement of femoral geometry predicts hip fracture: the study of osteoporotic fractures. *J Bone Miner Res.* 1993,8:1211–1218.

52. Johnson T. Age-related differences in isometric and dynamic strength and endurance. *Phys Ther.* 1982;62;985–989.

53. Aloia JF, Cohn SH, Babu T, et al. Skeletal mass and body composition in marathon runners. *Metabolism.* 1978;27:1793–1796.

54. Sinaki M, Offord K. Physical activity in postmenopausal women: effect on back muscle strength and bone mineral density of the spine. *Arch Phys Med Rehabil.* 1988;69:277–280.

55. Sinaki M, McPhee MC, Hodgson SF. Relationship between bone mineral density of spine and strength of back extensors in healthy postmenopausal women. *Mayo Clin Proc.* 1986;61:116–122.

56. Marcus R. The mechanism of exercise effects on bone. In: Bilezikian JP, Raisz LG, Rodan G, eds. *Principles of Bone Biology.* San Diego, Calif: Academic Press; 1996;1435–1445.

57. Rubin CT, Lanyon LE. Regulation of bone mass by mechanical strain magnitude. *Calcif Tissue Int.* 1985;37:411–417.

58. Rubin CT, Lanyon LE. Regulation of bone formation by applied dynamic loads. *J Bone Joint Surg.* 1984;66:397–402.

59. Carter DR, Fyhrie DP, Whalen RT. Trabecular bone density and loading history: regulation of connective tissue biology by mechanical energy. *J Biomech.* 1987;20:785–794.

60. Nilsson BE, Westlin NE. Bone density in athletes. *Clin Orthop.* 1971;77:179–182.

61. Huddleston AL, Rockwell D, Kulund DN, et al. Bone mass in lifetime tennis players. *JAMA.* 1980:244:1107–1109.

62. Dalen N, Olsson KE. Bone mineral content and physical activity. *Acta Orthop Scand.* 1974;45:170–174.

63. Marcus R, Cann C, Madvig P, et al. Menstrual function and bone mass in elite women distance runners: endocrine and metabolic features. *Ann Intern Med.* 1985;102:158-163.

64. Jacobson PC, Beaver W, Grubb SA, et al. Bone density in women: college athletes and older athletic women. *J Orthop Res.* 1984;2:328–332.

65. Talmadge RV, Stinnett SS, Landwehr JT, et al. Age-related loss of bone mineral density in nonathletic and athletic women. *Bone Miner.* 1986;1:115–125.

66. Brewer V, Meyer BM, Keele MS, et al. Role of exercise in prevention of involutional bone loss. *Med Sci Sports Exerc.* 1983;15:445–449.

67. Smith EL, Reddan W, Smith PE. Physical activity and calcium modalities for bone mineral increase in aged women. *Calcif Tissue Int.* 1981;13:60–64.

68. Snow-Harter C, Bouxsein ML, Lewis BT, Carter DR, Marcus R. Effects of resistance and endurance exercise on bone mineral status of young women: a randomized exercise intervention trial. *J Bone Min Res.* 1992;7:761–769.

69. Lohman T, Going S, Pamenter R, et al. Effects of resistance training on regional and total bone mineral density in premenopausal women: a randomized prospective study. *J Bone Miner Res.* 1995;10:1015–1024.

70. Friedlander AL, Genant HK, Sadowsky S, Byl NN, Glüer C-C. A two year program of aerobics and weight training enhances bone mineral density of young women. *J Bone Miner Res.* 1995;10:574–585.

71. Robinson TL, Snow-Harter C, Taaffe DR, Gillis D, Shaw J, Marcus R. Gymnasts exhibit higher bone mass than runners despite similar prevalence of amenorrhea. *J Bone Min Res.* 1995;10:26–35.

72. Heaney RP, Nutrition and risk for osteoporosis. In: Marcus R, Feldman D, Kelsey J, eds. *Osteoporosis.* San Diego, Calif: Academic Press. 1996:483–528.

73. Riggs BL, Wahner HW, Melton LJ III, et al. Dietary calcium intake and rates of bone loss in women. *J Clin Invest.* 1987;80:979–982.

74. Riis B, Thomsen K, Christiansen C. Does calcium supplementation prevent postmenopausal bone loss: a double-blind controlled clinical study. *N Engl J Med.* 1987;316:173–177.

75. Young G, Marcus R, Minkoff JR, et al. Age-related rise in parathyroid hormone in man: the use of intact and midmolecule antisera to distinguish hormone secretion from retention. *J Bone Miner Res.* 1987;2:367–374.

76. Eastell R, Heath H III, Kumar R, et al. Hormonal factors: PTH, vitamin D and calcitonin. In: Riggs

BL, Melton LJ, eds. *Osteoporosis: Etiology, Diagnosis, and Management.* New York, NY: Raven Press; 1988.

77. Chapuy MC, Arlot ME, Duboeuf F, Brun J, et al. Vitamin D₃ and calcium to prevent hip fractures in elderly women. *N Engl J Med.* 1992;327:1637–1642.

78. Eriksen EF, Colvard DS, Berg NJ, et al. Evidence of estrogen receptors in normal human osteoblast-like cells. *Science.* 1988;241:84.

79. Komm BS, Terpenning CM, Benz DJ, et al. Estrogen binding, receptor mRNA, and biologic response in osteoblast-like osteosarcoma cells. *Science.* 1988;241:81–83.

80. Gray TK, Flynn TC, Gray KM, et al. 17β-estradiol acts directly on the clonal osteoblast cell line UMR 106. *Proc Natl Acad Sci USA.* 1985;84:62–67.

81. Gallagher JC, Estrogen: prevention and treatment of osteoporosis. In: Marcus R, Feldman D, Kelsey J, eds. *Osteoporosis.* San Diego, Calif: Academic Press. 1996:1191–1208.

82. Orwoll ES, Klein RF. Osteoporosis in men: epidemiology, pathophysiology, and clinical characterization. In: Marcus R, Feldman D, Kelsey J, eds. *Osteoporosis.* San Diego, Calif; Academic Press. 1996: 745–784.

# CHAPTER 13

# Endocrine Aspects of Nutrition and Aging

*John E. Morley*

Hormones play a major role in the regulation of nutrient intake and utilization within an individual. Conversely, nutritional status can markedly affect circulating hormone levels. Treatment of a number of endocrine disorders (eg, diabetes mellitus and osteoporosis) involves dietary modification.

With advancing age, there are several alterations in circulating hormone levels and hormonal action. Some of these changes are related to the multiple diseases often present in older individuals, while other changes are due to aging per se. The loss of functional reserve in many endocrine organs increases the propensity for the elderly to develop deficiency diseases, such as diabetes mellitus, hypothyroidism, and hypogonadism. With advancing age, there is a tendency for endocrine disease to present with atypic or nonspecific symptoms, making diagnosis increasingly difficult. Weight loss is the classic nonspecific presentation of endocrine disease in elderly people.

In this chapter, the interactions of the endocrine system and nutrition are examined, and the impact of aging and its modulation of these interactions is described. More detailed information on the effect of aging on hormones is reported elsewhere.[1,2]

## NUTRITIONAL ASPECTS OF DIABETES MELLITUS

Diabetes mellitus occurs in approximately 18% of the population between ages 65 and 75 years.[3] Almost half of the persons with type II diabetes mellitus are older than 60 years. The diagnosis is missed in almost half of older patients with frank diabetes. In many older patients with diagnosed diabetes mellitus, the diabetes is inadequately treated.[4]

In general, older subjects tend to have an impaired glucose tolerance compared with younger subjects; however, recent data suggest that only 10% of the variance in total serum glucose response to an oral glucose load can be attributed to age.[5]

The level of body weight and physical activity appears to have a more important role in the pathogenesis of the hyperglycemia of aging. Recent data have suggested that a failure to suppress the pancreatic hormone amylin in older persons may play a role in the pathogenesis of the hyperglycemia of aging. Table 13–1 lists the major factors thought to play a role in the pathogenesis of the hyperglycemia of aging and the development of type II diabetes mellitus. It should be recognized that older persons with type II diabetes

**Table 13–1** Major Factors Involved in the Pathogenesis of the Hyperglycemia of Aging and Type II Diabetes Mellitus

1. Poor insulin secretion
2. Failure to inhibit hepatic glucose production
3. Insulin receptor and postreceptor defect
4. Obesity
5. Lack of physical activity
6. Failure to suppress amylin
7. Increased leptin

**Table 13–2** Reasons To Control Diabetes Mellitus in Elderly People

Prevention of acute complications
  Diabetic coma
  Hyperosmolar ketoacidotic lactic acidosis
  Complications related to hyperosmolality
    Diuresis leading to incontinence and nocturia
    Visual disturbances
    Falls related to above two factors
    Poor outcome following stroke
    Increased pain perception
    Cognitive dysfunction
  Complications related to altered function of circulating blood cells
    Worsening peripheral vascular disease due to decreased erythrocyte deformability
    Increased prevalence of myocardial infarction and stroke due to increased platelet stickiness
Prevention of chronic complications*
  Neuropathic complications    *— visual impair.*
  Diabetic retinopathy    *— cognitive*
  Diabetic nephropathy    *impairment*
  Amputation    *— ↑ed susceptibility*
*— ↑ed Urinary Inc.*    *to infection*
*There is some evidence that these complications occur more rapidly in late-onset diabetes.

*— Greater Risk of stroke*

tend to be less overweight than middle-aged ones and more likely to have a significant degree of insulin insufficiency.

While fasting and postprandial glucose levels increase slightly with age, the basic definition for treatable diabetes mellitus should not change. Treatment should be instituted when any individual has two fasting plasma glucose levels greater than 7.8 mmol/L. Alternatively, 2-hour postprandial values greater than 10.0 mmol/L on two or more occasions would also suggest the need for treatment.

Regardless of the causes of diabetes mellitus in the elderly, there is increasing evidence that reasonable control of glucose will improve the patient's quality of life, as well as possibly decrease morbidity and mortality rates. The major reasons for control of diabetes in elderly people are listed in Table 13–2. The special features of diabetes mellitus in elderly individuals have been the subject of a number of recent reviews.[6-8] At present, it is recommended that the blood glucose be maintained between 5.6 and 11.1 mmol/L for all diabetics older than 70 years.

**Treatment of Diabetes Mellitus**

The modalities for treatment of diabetes mellitus in elderly subjects are the same as those used in younger subjects: diet, exercise, oral medications, and insulin. In 1674, Sir Thomas Willis advised patients with diabetes mellitus to have gummy and starchy foods. Since then, diabetologists have made a variety of recommendations about what should constitute the appropriate diet for diabetic patients. The following are the current recommendations of the American Diabetes Association[9] for the dietary management of persons with type II diabetes mellitus: The approach should be individualized and based on a careful nutrition assessment. The number of calories should aim at a weight that both the patient and the health care provider believe is achievable and maintainable. Moderate weight loss (5–9 kg) can have important effects, including reducing hyperglycemia, blood pressure level, and lipid levels. Protein intake should make up about 10% to 20% of the total caloric intake (~0.8 g/kg per day). Protein restriction below this level has no clear benefit and may lead to sarcopenia. Fat intake should be limited to 30% of calories, with less than 10% of fat from polyunsaturated fat and 10% to 15% from mono-unsaturated fats. The use of omega-3 polyunsaturated fats (fish fats) should not be curtailed. The rest of the caloric content should obviously be made up of carbohydrate. There is little scientific evidence that simple sugars impair the blood glucose concentration more than complex carbohydrates, and they are therefore no longer proscribed. Some soluble fibers may delay glucose absorption. An ideal diet should contain 20 to 35 g of a mixture of soluble and insoluble fibers. It should be recognized that the modern diabetic diet does not differ from the recommended healthy diet for all Americans. Alcohol should be limited to two or fewer alcoholic beverages per day.

Finally, there are no studies on dietary intervention in ambulatory individuals older than 70 years. A study of elderly nursing home patients suggested that the "diabetic" diet resulted in no better glycemic control than did a regular diet.[10] For these reasons, it is difficult to make a firm recommendation on the ideal diet for the older diabetic. It is important that state surveyors in nursing homes recognize that an order for a "diabetic special diet" represents an order for a regular diet.

Cross-sectional studies have shown that the impaired glucose tolerance of aging is significantly related to the level of physical fitness or activity.[7] Only one prospective trial of the effects of exercise on glucose tolerance

has been carried out in men older than 60 years. While glucose levels did not change, both insulin and C peptide levels were lower.[11] In addition, high-density–lipoprotein cholesterol levels increased, and triglyceride levels decreased. Exercise trials in patients with type II diabetes mellitus have failed to show a major advantage of short-term exercise programs over diet alone.[12] However, two trials that lasted 5 and 11 months did find improvements in glucose tolerance without change in body weight.[13, 14] Besides the possible beneficial effects of exercise on glucose tolerance, exercise training may improve cardiovascular fitness, lipid profiles, hypertension, osteopenia, and psychologic function in diabetic patients. Risks of exercise in diabetics include hypoglycemia, ketosis, dehydration, myocardial ischemia, arrhythmias, acceleration of proliferative retinopathy, increased proteinuria, and trauma (particularly in patients with neuropathy). The NIH consensus panel concluded that the effect of exercise on metabolic control in non–insulin-dependent diabetes mellitus is often variable and of small magnitude.[15] Pacini and colleagues[16] have demonstrated that normal-weight, physically active older subjects have normal insulin-binding capacity, insulin sensitivity, and insulin secretory capacity in response to a glucose stimulus. An individualized 12-week exercise program in elderly African Americans with type II diabetes mellitus improved glycemic control and reduced high blood pressures.[17] Studies of long-term exercise programs need to be undertaken before a formal recommendation for an exercise prescription can be given.

The sulfonylurea oral hypoglycemic agents produce their major effect by stimulating insulin release from pancreatic B cells through a different signal recognition system than that by which glucose stimulates insulin release. Chlorpropamide should never be used in subjects older than 60 years because it produces prolonged hypoglycemia and hyponatremia. The prevalence of hypoglycemia with other sulfonylureas is less than that with chlorpropamide; nevertheless, elderly people are always at increased risk for developing hypoglycemia. The combination of insulin and sulfonylureas has not been proven to be effective. For the majority of older diabetics, Glimepiride is a third-generation sulfonylurea whose actions appear similar to those of the second-generation agents.

Metformin is a biguanide that enhances insulin action and produces anorexia. It acts, in part, through effects on nitric oxide synthase. It should not be used in persons with a serum creatinine greater than 1.4 g/dL or in those with severe heart failure or chronic acidosis. In persons older than 80 years, a normal creatinine clearance needs to be demonstrated before it should be used. Its major side effect is lactic acidosis, which occurs extremely rarely if the above prescribing precautions are followed. Older persons need to be monitored for the possibility of excessive weight loss. Metformin may decrease vitamin $B_{12}$ levels.

Troglitazone is a thiazolidinedione that enhances peripheral insulin action. It works through the activation of PPARγ. It does not produce hypoglycemia. It can be used as monotherapy or in combination with other oral antidiabetic agents or insulin. It may produce mild degrees of liver dysfunction.

Acarbose is an alpha-1-glucosidase inhibitor. It delays the absorption of complex carbohydrates, thus smoothing out the glycemic response to a meal. It also releases the incretion glucagonlike peptide 1 from the gastrointestinal tract, resulting in enhanced insulin levels in response to the meal. Its major side effects are diarrhea and gastrointestinal gas production.

Chronic insulin deficiency is similar to starvation in that both conditions are catabolic states that lead to cachexia. The catabolic state of uncontrolled diabetes mellitus is readily reversed by insulin therapy. For this reason, and those listed in Table 13–2, insulin should not be withheld from elderly patients whose glucose levels cannot be reduced below 11.1 mmol/L. At present, human insulin is recommended as the insulin of choice to decrease the formation of anti-insulin antibodies; however, polymerization of human insulin at therapeutic dosage levels does lead to some antibody formation.

Older diabetics may have up to a 20% error when drawing up their insulin into a syringe.[18] For this reason, older diabetics with visual deficiencies should use syringe magnifiers or dose gauges. Some patients also benefit from using needle guides and vial holders. Older diabetic persons with depression have poor outcomes, and depression needs to be vigorously treated in these persons.[19] Much of the diabetic care for older persons is carried out by caregivers; therefore, they should be involved in appropriate diabetic education programs if optimum outcomes are to be obtained.

## Micronutrient Status and Diabetes Mellitus

Diabetes mellitus produces a number of effects on vitamin and mineral status of patients.[20] Many of these changes are similar to those seen with aging (Table 13–3). Elderly people often have a decreased zinc intake and are at risk for developing zinc deficiency when illness occurs (Chapter 5). Diabetes mellitus is associated with decreased zinc absorption and hyperzincuria.[21] Zinc deficiency is associated with poor wound healing, poor immune function, immune dysfunction, and anorexia.[22] In addition, zinc is cosecreted from pancreatic islets and enhances insulin binding, suggesting a possible role of zinc in

**Table 13–3** Comparison of the Effects of Type II Diabetes Mellitus and Aging on Micronutrients

| Micronutrient | Changes in Type II Diabetes Mellitus | Changes with Aging |
|---|---|---|
| Vitamins | | |
| A | N | N |
| B$_1$ | N | N |
| B$_6$ | N or ↓ | ↓ |
| B$_{12}$ | N or ↓ | ↓ |
| C | ↓ | N or ↓ |
| 25-hydroxyvitamin D$_3$ | N | ↓ |
| E in serum | N | N |
| E in platelets | ↓ | ↑ |
| | | |
| Trace elements | | |
| Zinc | N or ↓ | ↓ |
| Chromium | N | ↓ |
| Copper | N or ↑ | ↑ |
| Manganese | ↑ | ? |
| Selenium | ? | N or ↓ |

*Note:* N, Normal; ↑, increased; ↓, decreased.

the pathogenesis of some forms of diabetes. Pharmacologic zinc administration has been demonstrated to improve immune function[23] and foot ulcer healing[24] in patients with deficient zinc status.

Chromium has been suggested to have a role in normal glucose homeostasis. Deficiency of chromium (Chapter 5) or its biologically active form, glucose tolerance factor, has been implicated in the glucose intolerance of aging.[25] The main sources of glucose tolerance factor include brewer's yeast, liver, and kidney.

In most double-blind studies, chromium supplementation has failed to reverse the hyperglycemia of aging. In one recent small study, the combination of chromium and nicotinamide resulted in a minor diminution of the glucose response to oral glucose, but it did not alter fasting glucose levels.[26] In chromium-deficient areas, such as parts of China, chromium replacement can have more dramatic effects on glucose tolerance.[25]

Copper and ceruloplasmin levels are elevated in type II diabetes mellitus. Copper deficiency, induced experimentally, results in elevated total cholesterol levels.[27]

Thiamine is essential for the transport of metabolized glucose from the Embden-Meyerhof pathway into the Krebs cycle. The elevated levels of erythrocyte transketolase activity (an indirect measure of thiamine status) in type II diabetes mellitus may be related to the poor availability of intracellular glucose. When malnourished patients receive glucose, they may utilize all of the available thiamine, resulting in Wernicke's syndrome. Conversely, in malnourished patients, thiamine administration may result in hypoglycemia.

Diabetes mellitus may be associated with pernicious anemia. Vitamin $B_{12}$ deficiency should be suspected in any diabetic patient with macrocytic anemia, posterior column neuropathy, or dementia. Recent studies have suggested that low vitamin $B_{12}$ levels, in the absence of macrocytic anemia, may explain the cognitive dysfunction seen in elderly individuals. Low vitamin $B_{12}$ levels are associated with increased levels of methyl malonic acid and homocysteine. Elevated homocysteine levels have been associated with coronary artery disease.

Vitamin C in large doses acts as a reducing agent and can interfere with glucose measurements in both urine and serum.

### Diabetes Mellitus in Long-term Care

The management of diabetes mellitus in the long-term care setting is steeped in mythology.[28] It should be realized that hypoglycemic reactions occur infrequently in institutionalized patients, permitting reasonable control of diabetes mellitus in this population.[29] In a study of diabetic patients in a nursing home, it was found that one in five were 20% below average body weight.[29] Weight loss often leads to improved glycemic control in nursing home patients. Awareness of weight loss in this population is important, since it may necessitate a reduction in insulin or oral hypoglycemic dosage. As previously mentioned, there is little evidence that an American Dietetic Association/American Diabetes Association diabetic diet is appropriate for diabetic patients in long-term care.

Generally, the management of diabetes mellitus in older patients is the same as that in younger patients. In elderly patients, diabetes mellitus can interact with the normal aging process to produce major changes in micronutrient requirements. In particular, older diabetics are at risk for developing minor degrees of zinc deficiency. When instituting dietary changes in older diabetics, care needs to be taken not to produce protein-calorie malnutrition. This is particularly true of patients residing in nursing homes.

### THYROID FUNCTION

With advancing age, there is no change in the circulating levels of total thyroxine or triiodothyronine or the free hormone values.[1] However, this apparent stability of the circulating thyroid hormones belies the underlying physiologic turmoil that results in the hypothalamic-pituitary-adrenal axis with advancing age. There is a decreased production of thyroid hormones with aging that is counterbalanced by a decreased thyroid hormone degradation. In addition, there is a tendency for diminished feedback of thyroid hormones, leading to a mild increase in thyrotropin (TSH) levels, particularly in women. In older men, there is an increased prevalence of failure for TSH to respond to thyrotropin-releasing hormone (TRH).

In subjects younger than 60 years, the prevalence of hypothyroidism tends to be 1% or less, whereas in those older than 60 years, the prevalence rises to 4% to 7%.[30] Between 7% and 12% of patients with hyperthyroidism are older than 60 years.[1] While there are limited changes in circulating thyroid hormones with aging, when illness supervenes, there can be major changes in thyroid hormones that can mimic the changes seen with hypothyroidism.[31] These changes are delineated in Table 13–4. Malnutrition is a particularly common cause of the euthyroid sick syndrome in elderly people.

Atypical presentations of thyroid disease become increasingly common with advancing age. One study estimated that only 10% of older patients with biochemical hypothyroidism were suspected of having thyroid dis-

**Table 13–4** Typical Changes in Thyroid Hormone Levels with Various Diseases

| Hormone | Aging | Hyperthyroid | Hypothyroid | Euthyroid Sick |
|---|---|---|---|---|
| Thyroxine | N | ↑ | ↓ | N or ↓ |
| Triiodothyronine | N | ↑ | N or ↓ | ↓ |
| Uptake | N | ↑ | ↓ | ↑ |
| Free thyroxine index | N | ↑ | ↓ | N or ↓ |
| TSH | | | | |
| Normal | N | N | ↑ | N or ↑ |
| Supersensitive | N | ↓ | ↑ | ↓, N, ↑ |
| Response to TRH | ↓ | ↓ | ↑ | ↓ |

*Note:* N, Normal; ↑, increased; ↓, decreased.

ease on clinical examination.[32] The classic hyperkinetic state, thyromegaly, and eye signs of hyperthyroidism may be replaced by heart failure, apathy, and unexplained weight loss in elderly persons—so-called apathetic hypothyroidism.[33] For these reasons, it is recommended that all patients older than 60 years who are admitted to the hospital or who have unexplained weight loss, fatigue, depression, dementia, or atrial fibrillation be screened biochemically for thyroid disease.[31]

**Nutritional Aspects of Thyroid Disease**

The classic nutritional change associated with hyperthyroidism is weight loss. Thyroid hormones produce a marked increase in the basal metabolic rate. The exact mechanism by which thyroid hormones increase the metabolic rate remains controversial.[34] There is an increase in mitochondrial size, number, and surface area, and thyroid hormone stimulates mitochondrial turnover. Thyroid hormone also increases $Na^+$, $K^+$-adenosine triphosphatase activity. Pharmacologic concentrations of thyroid hormone produce uncoupling of oxidative metabolism in vitro.

Thyroid hormone results in stimulation of both protein synthesis and degradation. In hyperthyroidism, the predominance of pro-

tein degradation leads to loss of muscle mass, muscle weakness, and a negative nitrogen balance. In younger subjects, hyperthyroidism is often associated with hyperphagia, which tends to offset the weight loss to some degree. However, anorexia occurs in up to 30% of older hyperthyroid subjects.

Hyperthyroidism is associated with an increase in glucose utilization and a depletion of liver glycogen. While fasting glucose levels are generally normal in hyperthyroidism, glucose intolerance is present in approximately half of these patients.[35] In hypothyroidism, there is decreased glucose absorption from the gastrointestinal tract and a reduction in peripheral glucose utilization. A flat glucose tolerance curve is not unusual in hypothyroidism.

In hyperthyroid subjects, there is an increase in free fatty acid and triglyceride levels and a decrease in cholesterol levels.[34] In hypothyroidism, fat cell lipolysis in response to catecholamines is reduced.[34] Free fatty acid levels are normal or slightly decreased in hypothyroidism.[34] Plasma triglyceride levels are markedly increased secondary to a marked decrease in the triglyceride removal rate.[36] Cholesterol levels are also increased in hypothyroidism; more than four fifths of hypothyroid patients have cholesterol levels greater than 250 mg/dL.[37] The increase is mostly in low-density–lipoprotein cholesterol. Cholesterol secretion in the bile is markedly decreased in hypothyroidism.

Osteopenia commonly is present in hyperthyroidism, and the development of hyperthyroidism aggravates the normal age-related bone loss. Mild hypercalcemia commonly is seen in hyperthyroidism. Calcium absorption is decreased and calcium excretion is increased in hyperthyroidism. In hypothyroidism, there is a mild decrease in the rate of calcium deposition in bone.

The alterations in vitamin status that occur in thyroid disease are outlined in Table 13–5.[38,39] Decreased dark adaptation occurs occasionally in hyperthyroidism and may be related to diminished vitamin A levels in this disorder. The characteristic yellow color of the skin of hypothyroid patients is due to increased carotene values secondary to decreased conversion of carotene to vitamin A.

### Effects of Nutritional Status on Thyroid Hormones

There is increasing evidence that vitamin status may alter thyroid function. Vitamin A deficiency in animals leads to mild increases in circulating thyroid hormones in the presence of normal TSH secretion, suggesting a resetting of the hypothalamic-pituitary axis in response to thyroid hormones.[40] Vitamin A excess lowers circulating total thyroid hormone levels, but not free hormone levels, as the dialyzable function of thyroid hormones increases.[41] In animals, thiamine administration decreases the weight loss seen when pharmacologic amounts of thyroid hormone are administered.[42] Riboflavin deficiency diminishes the hepatic deiodination of thyroxine.[43] Vitamin E may attenuate the effects of thyroid hormone on some of its target organs.[44] These findings and others suggest that

a careful study of vitamin status in elderly patients with hyperthyroidism is warranted. A recent study also suggested that some protection from thyroid cancer is afforded by vitamins C and E and that there is an inverse association between beta carotene and thyroid cancer.[45]

### ADRENAL CORTEX

Aging produces only minor changes in the hypothalamic-pituitary-adrenal axis. There are mild decreases in both cortisol production and clearance rates; as a result, plasma cortisol levels remain unchanged with aging.[1] In addition, with advancing age there is a decreased sensitivity of the anterior pituitary to negative feedback by circulating cortisol.[46] Therefore, with advancing age there is an increased prevalence of failure of dexamethasone to suppress cortisol adequately.

Less than 10% of patients with Addison disease (hypoadrenalism) are older than 60 years.[47] Nutritional and clinical manifestations are commonly seen in patients with Addison disease. These include weakness, easy fatigability, vomiting, constipation or diarrhea, abdominal pain, salt craving, weight loss, hypoglycemia, hyponatremia, and hyperkalemia. Additional manifestations include hyperpigmentation and postural hypotension.

The clustering of hypertension, hypokalemia, diabetes mellitus, and osteopenia is suggestive of Cushing's syndrome. However, in elderly people all of these conditions occur commonly, and the presence of multiple disease states represents a more likely finding. The classic appearance of patients with Cushing's syndrome is central obesity with thin arms and legs, although weight loss may occur in elderly individuals. The screening test for Cushing's syndrome is the failure of 1 mg of dexamethasone to suppress cortisol

**Table 13–5** Effects of Thyroid Diseases on Vitamin Status

| Vitamin | Hypothyroid | Hyperthyroid |
|---|---|---|
| Vitamin A | ↑ | ↓ |
| Retinol-binding protein | ↑ | ↓ |
| Thiamine | | |
|    Erythrocyte transketolase | ? | ↓ |
|    In vitro thiamin pyridinylase (thiammase) | ? | None[a] |
| Riboflavin | ? | ↑ |
| Pyridoxine | | |
|    Xanthurenic acid excretion after tryptophan administration | ? | [b] |
| Vitamin $B_{12}$ | ↓ or N[c] | ↓ |
| Folate | N | ? |
| Vitamin C | N | N |
| 25-Hydroxyvitamin $D_3$ | N | N |
| 1,25-Hydroxyvitamin $D_3$ | ↑ | ↓ |
| α-Tocopherol (vitamin E) | ↑ | ↓ |

*Note:* N, Normal; ↑, increased; ↓, decreased.

a. The decrease in erythrocyte transketolase suggests thiamine deficiency, but the failure of in vitro thiamine augmentation suggests other causes.
b. Suggests pyridoxine deficiency.
c. About 5% to 10% have pernicious anemia.

levels below 138 mmol/L. In elderly patients, failure of dexamethasone suppression may be secondary to depression, Alzheimer's disease, obesity, or alcoholism.

While Cushing's syndrome is rare in elderly individuals, ectopic corticotropin syndrome secondary to tumors, such as oat cell carcinoma of the lung, is relatively common. These patients are usually cachectic rather than obese, and have severe proximal muscle weakness, hypokalemic alkalosis, mental changes, and hyperpigmentation. Patients with ectopic corticotropin fail the dexamethasone suppression test and have relatively high circulating corticotropin levels.

In elderly people, by far the most common cause of elevated cortisol levels is exogenous cortisol administration. The use of steroids in elderly patients should be limited to situations in which they are absolutely essential, and the steroids should be tapered off as rapidly as possible. Exogenous steroid use is a major cause of osteopenia; patients receiving steroids should receive calcium prophylactically and possibly vitamin D supplementation, as steroids inhibit the conversion of 25-hydroxyvitamin $D_3$ $(25(OH)D_3)$ to 1,25-dihydroxyvitamin $D_3$ $(1,25(OH)_2D_3)$.

Nutritionally, glucosteroids promote the conversion of protein to carbohydrate (gluconeogenesis). This leads to a negative nitrogen balance, an increase in circulating glucose, and increased liver glycogen. Corticosteroids also reduce hexose transport into the cells, which further increases circulating glucose levels and produces a secondary hyperinsulinemia. Patients receiving corticosteroids who develop frank diabetes mellitus usually require insulin therapy rather than oral hypoglycemic agents.

Cortisol increases DNA synthesis in human adipose cells in vitro. Cortisol promotes hyperphagia and mobilization of free fatty acids. Pharmacologic doses of cortisol elevate triglyceride levels.

## Other Adrenal Hormones

Plasma levels and urinary excretion of aldosterone tend to fall with advancing age.[48] Active renin levels also fall with advancing age.[49] These changes increase the propensity of older subjects to develop hyperkalemia secondary to hyporeninemic hypoaldosteronism. This is particularly common in patients with diabetes mellitus and mild renal failure.

In contrast to the relative preservation of cortisol secretory dynamics, dehydroepiandrosterone (DHEA) secretion declines dramatically with advancing age.[50] In animals, DHEA administration prolongs life span, which may be related to its ability to reduce weight.[51] In men, DHEA-sulfate (DHEA-S) has been suggested to be inversely related to death from cardiovascular disease, though this has not been a universal finding.[52] Diminished levels of DHEA and DHEA-S are associated with hypercholesterolemia[53] and hypertension.[54] The mechanism by which DHEA deficiency promotes atherosclerosis is uncertain but may be related to excessive stimulation of lipogenesis by reduced nicotinamide-adenine dinucleotide phosphate (NADPH). Replacement studies with DHEA have been disappointing, though high doses (100 mg) have resulted in reduced body fat and increased muscle mass and strength.

## WATER METABOLISM

Elderly people are at increased risk for developing disturbances of water metabolism. Aging is associated with a decline in total body water and intravascular water. Both dehydration and hyponatremia occur with increasing frequency in elderly subjects. Phillips and colleagues[55] have demonstrated that even healthy elderly subjects fail to respond adequately to mild dehydration. In part, this failure to develop an appropriate thirst response may be secondary to an impaired secretion of angiotensin.[56] The mu opioid drinking drive is also severely impaired in older persons. This has led to the concept that elderly people live in a "water desert" and that hospitalized elderly patients need a prescription of at least 1 L of fluid intake per day.

There is greater argipressin release for a given osmotic stimulus in elderly subjects than in younger subjects.[57] Older subjects also have a decrease in free water clearance in response to argipressin, predominantly related to the age-related fall in glomerular filtration rate.[58] Atrial natriuretic factor (ANF) is released by volume overload and acts on the kidney to increase glomerular filtration rate and induce natriuresis. Recently, ANF levels have been demonstrated to be elevated in elderly individuals.[59] Greater elevations of ANF occur in persons with heart failure.

These hormonal changes explain why hyponatremia occurs commonly in elderly people.[60] Many institutionalized elderly persons have the syndrome of inappropriate secretion of antidiuretic hormone, which may lead to hyponatremia; tube feeding represents another major cause of hyponatremia in institutionalized elderly people.

## GROWTH HORMONE AND INSULIN GROWTH FACTORS

There is evidence that growth hormone secretion is impaired with advancing age. A single study of medically impaired elderly subjects found adequate nitrogen retention and free fatty acid increase after growth hormone administration, but impaired urinary hydroxyproline secretion.[61] This highly limited study is the basis for the claim that metabolic responses to growth hormone are impaired in elderly persons.

In contrast to the minor decreases in growth hormone with aging, plasma levels of insulinlike growth factor I (IGF I; somatomedin C) are markedly decreased with advancing age.[62] IGF I levels are also decreased by malnutrition. In malnourished, institutionalized elderly patients, the levels of IGF I are even lower than those seen in healthy elderly people, suggesting an interaction between nutrition and aging in these individuals.[63]

Rudman[64] and colleagues[65] have suggested that the growth hormone "menopause" that occurs with advancing age may explain a number of the normal changes seen with aging. These include the diminished nitrogen retention, the decrease in lean body mass, the increase in adipose tissue, and some of the osteopenia characteristically associated with aging. Overall, growth hormone replacement studies in older persons have been disappointing. At best, these studies have demonstrated an increase in muscle mass with no increase in strength. Side effects, such as carpal tunnel syndrome, appear to limit the long-term use of growth hormone.[65,66] On the other hand, severely ill older persons who are highly catabolic may benefit from short-term growth hormone treatment.[67]

## MALE HYPOGONADISM

With advancing age, sexual dysfunction occurs with increasing frequency. Kinsey and colleagues[68] reported that impotence occurred in 18.6% of 60-year-old men and 75% of 80-year-old men. Over age 50 years, one in three men who are examined by a physician is impotent.[69] The causes of impotence in older men are multifactorial.[70] The major cause for the increasing prevalence of impotence with advancing age is arteriosclerosis. Medications also have an important role in the pathogenesis of impotence. Nutritionally, it has been found that a small subset of older impotent men have low serum zinc levels and hyperzincuria.[71] Approximately half of these subjects improve after the administration of pharmacologic amounts of zinc.

Hypogonadism occurs with increasing frequency with advancing age. In older men, there is a marked decrease in testosterone and bioavailable testosterone.[72] A longitudinal study demonstrated that testosterone levels decline in all elderly men. Both luteinizing hormone and follicle-stimulating hormone levels tend to increase with advancing age in an attempt to compensate for the decreased levels of testosterone.[73] However, in a number of older individuals, the hypothalamus fails to detect the decrease in testosterone adequately, resulting in the development of hypothalamic hypogonadism.[74]

Testosterone not only plays a role in maintaining normal sexual function (libido and potency) but also has a number of effects that enhance the general well-being of the individual.[75] Testosterone promotes nitrogen retention, maintains muscle mass, protects bone from excessive calcium loss, helps to maintain erythrocyte mass, and produces a general feeling of well-being. Testosterone deficiency appears to play an important role in the development of age-related sarcopenia. Testosterone replacement in older individuals improved muscle strength and libido and decreased serum leptin levels. For these reasons, it is recommended that testosterone replacement therapy be instituted in all subjects with proven hypogonadism, regardless of whether they desire to have sexual intercourse. In patients receiving testosterone, regular rectal examinations need to be conducted to detect prostatic growth.

## CALCIUM METABOLISM

Both calcium intake and calcium absorption diminish with advancing age[1] (Chapter 4). With advancing age, there is a decrease in vitamin D synthesis in the skin[76] and decreased activity of 1-$\alpha$-hydroxylase in the kidney[77] (Chapter 3). Recent studies have clearly demonstrated that at least a proportion of older individuals have a decrease in $25(OH)D_3$ and its active metabolite, $1,25(OH)_2D_3$.[77] Lower vitamin D levels are particularly prevalent in institutionalized and housebound elderly people who are rarely exposed to sunlight and who have low calcium intakes. Our longitudinal study in healthy older persons suggests that decreased sunlight exposure is more important than aging per se in the pathogenesis of the age-related decline in serum vitamin D levels. Treatment with vitamin D and calcium has been demonstrated to decrease hip fracture in nursing home residents.[78]

These changes tend to lead to a decrease in ionized calcium, which, in turn, results in a compensatory increase in parathyroid hormone (PTH) levels.[79] Calcitonin levels may decline slightly with advancing age.[80] As already mentioned, the age-related declines in IGF I and testosterone also impinge on calcium metabolism. The changes in calcium metabolism that occur with age are summarized in Figure 13–1.

Seventeen percent of patients with hyperparathyroidism are older than 60 years.[70] Clinically, hyperparathyroidism is often characterized by vague complaints, including anorexia, weight loss, weakness, abdominal symptoms, cognitive disturbances, polyuria, and dehydration. Diagnosis is made by demonstrating elevated calcium and PTH levels.

Treatment consists of surgical removal of the parathyroid adenoma. In postmenopausal women, estrogen therapy has been shown to lower mild hyperparathyroidism. In the differential diagnosis of hypercalcemia, it should be remembered that megadoses of vitamin A activate cathepsin D, resulting in increased PTH secretion and elevated calcium levels.

A detailed discussion of osteopenia in elderly people is presented elsewhere[76] (Chapter 12). In postmenopausal (type I) osteopenia, clearly estrogen deficiency represents the major problem. The etiologic factors involved in type II osteopenia are multifactorial and include a variety of nutritional factors such as low calcium intake, a high-protein diet that produces hypercalciuria, late-onset lactase deficiency, coffee consumption, alcoholism, lack of physical exercise, and cigarette smoking. Boron supplementation has been demonstrated to reduce the urinary excretion of calcium.[81]

## HORMONAL REGULATION OF ENERGY BALANCE

The early phase of aging typically is associated with a positive energy balance and an increase in adiposity but a decrease in lean body mass.[82] While lean body mass continues to decline in the last phase—often seen beyond age 65 years—negative energy balance often is maintained.[83] Protein-energy malnutrition occurs in this age group at an alarming frequency.[22,84] In elderly people, both energy intake and output typically are reduced, but reduction in intake exceeds the reduced output, leading to the observed loss in energy stores, including lean body mass.

Control of energy intake and output involves complex autonomic, hormonal, and metabolic mechanisms that are only partially understood. It is therefore difficult to iden-

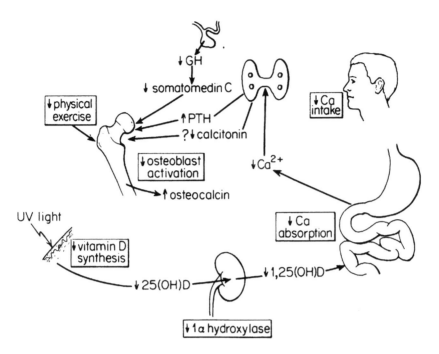

**Figure 13–1** Overview of the effects of aging on calcium metabolism. GH, Growth hormone; PTH, parathyroid hormone. *Source:* Reprinted with permission from *Journal of American Geriatrics Society* (1988;36:845–859), Copyright © 1988, American Geriatrics Society.

tify, with any level of certainty, the age-related dysfunctions responsible for the status of negative energy balance in elderly individuals.

## Hormonal Control of Energy Intake

The control mechanism of food intake has central and peripheral components. The primary central structures are in the hypothalamus and include the ventromedial hypothalamus (VMH), lateral hypothalamus (LH), and paraventricular nucleus (PVN).[85] The primary peripheral aspects are thought to include the gastrointestinal tract, liver, and adipose tissue and to involve some key hormones and metabolites.[86,87]

Whatever effect a peripheral hormone or metabolite has on feeding, its effect will be encoded into the neurotransmitter system in the hypothalamus, and a behavioral feeding response will be elicited subsequent to the specific neurotransmitter signal. Accordingly, discussion of hormone influences on feeding must include the neurotransmitter system (neurohormones), exerting a direct effect in the hypothalamus, and hormones secreted in the periphery.

### Neurohormones

*Monoamines.* Norepinephrine, dopamine, and serotonin all have important roles in determining feeding behavior.[85] Direct injection of norepinephrine into the VMH or PVN will stimulate feeding; its administration into the LH will inhibit feeding. This effect of norepinephrine is mediated through α-adrenergic receptors in the VMH and β-adrenergic receptors in the LH.[85] Brain tissue from aged rats has an impaired capacity for synthesis and regulation of α- and β-adrenergic receptors. This impairment has been demonstrated in the cortex and cerebellum,[88] but it has not been studied in the hypothalamus.

The effects of serotonin on feeding also appear to depend on the type of serotonin receptor, with a decrease in feeding induced by $1_B$ receptor agonist in the PVN and an increase in feeding with a $1_A$ receptor agonist.[89] Dopamine neurotransmitters have also been thought to have a role in controlling feeding behavior, but the effects of aging on the serotonin and the dopamine feeding systems have not been studied.

*Neuropeptides.* Several peptide neurotransmitters have been found in recent years in mammalian brain. These include cholecystokinin (CCK), bombesin, substance P, neurotensin, opioids, neuropeptide Y (NPY), and others.[90] A number of these peptides were shown to decrease feeding after central administration. However, a reduced food intake need not imply a physiologic role for these neuropeptides in modulating feeding behavior, as their effect may be secondary to nonspecific behavioral effects. The administration of either opioid peptides[91] or NPY[92] was reported to stimulate feeding, suggesting a physiologic role for these neuropeptides. Moreover, the opioid antagonist naloxone suppresses food intake.[91] Recently, it was reported that older rats display a much smaller response to opioid agonists and antagonists.[93] Older rats also have a lower concentration of opioid peptides in the hypothalamus.[91] Aging is thus associated with a decreased opiate-based feeding drive, but the relative importance of the latter in anorexia of aging is not clear. The orexigenic effect of NPY is less age dependent.[94]

*Nitric Oxide.* Nitric oxide is a gaseous neurotransmitter. It appears to play an important role in increasing food intake. It produces its effects both within the central nervous system and by increasing adaptive relaxation to food in the fundus of the stomach. Available studies suggest that nitric oxide deficiency may play a role in the anorexia of aging.[95]

### Peripheral Hormones

*Growth Hormone.* Administration of growth hormone into experimental animals stimulates food intake and growth of lean, but not adipose, tissue.[96] A similar effect has been reported in humans.[97] It is not clear to what extent small changes in growth hormone activity (within the normal range) influence food intake or whether the reduction in growth hormone activity, which is often observed in elderly subjects (see above), contributes to their anorexia.

*Insulin.* Daily single injections of insulin stimulate food intake and produce obesity.[86] Moreover, the hyperphagia and obesity that develop after placement of lesions in the ventromedial hypothalamus are contributed to by a vagally mediated insulin hypersecretion induced by the lesions.[86,87] The stimulatory effect of insulin on food intake is thought to result from its lipolytic effect, which decreases availability of endogenous substrate to the tissues and to specific glucose-sensitive hypothalamic sites.[86,87] The role of age-associated hyperglycemia (impaired glucose tolerance) in the anorexia of aging is not known.

*Glucocorticoids.* The stimulatory effect of norepinephrine administered in the PVN of the hypothalamus on food intake is absent in adrenalectomized rats; it is restored with corticosterone.[98] Also, peak hormone concentration in blood is observed before onset of feeding.[99] However, corticosterone administered into nonadrenalectomized rats has little or no effect on food intake.[100] Combined, these data suggest that glucocorticoids have an important "permissive" role in the central control mechanism of feeding. In both animals and humans, glucocorticoid hyperactivity is associated with a redistribution of body energy stores toward increased adiposity and decreased lean body mass.[101] In humans, this is known as Cushing's syndrome, which is rare in elderly persons.

*Thyroid Hormone.* Thyroid hormone stimulates food intake,[102] but this effect appears to be secondary to a stimulated metabolic rate and a compensatory replenishment of the greater energy losses.

*Gonadal Steroids.* The gonadal steroid estrogen suppresses food intake in female subjects; its site of action is thought to be in the VMH.[103] Food intake is decreased during days of estrus (high estrogen) and increased during diestrus (low estrogen).[104] Castration of female rats leads to overeating and obesity.[87] Testosterone, on the other hand, increases food intake and lean tissue growth, while decreasing body fat.[105]

Although there is little change in estrogen levels, bioavailable testosterone levels are reduced in the majority of elderly people. These sex hormone changes would be compatible with reduced ingestion with advancing age.

*Gastrointestinal Hormones.* Peripheral injections of a variety of gastrointestinal hormones and other peptides into rats reduce food intake. These peptides include CCK, bombesin, gastrin-releasing peptide, glucagon, somatostatin, substance P, and neurotensin.[91] However, the physiologic significance of these hormones in producing normal satiety is not clear.[106,107] It has been proposed that CCK exerts a weak effect on food intake, amounting to some 10% to 20% of the total intake at a single meal.[90] Higher than normal serum levels of CCK were observed in elderly men, perhaps contributing to their anorexia.[108] Silver and colleagues[109] have reported an increased ability of pharmacologically administered CCK-8 to decrease

feeding in older mice compared with younger mice.

*Leptin.* Leptin is a protein hormone that is secreted from fat cells.[110] It has been shown to decrease food intake and increase metabolic rate in rodents. It decreases food intake by decreasing nitric oxide synthase activity in the hypothalamus. In humans, leptin levels are strongly related to total adiposity, particularly visceral adiposity. With aging, leptin levels decline in females but increase in males. The increase in males is due to declining testosterone levels that occur with aging. Testosterone replacement therapy in older males causes leptin levels to decline. Elevated leptin levels in older males are related to decreased food intake.

## Hormonal Control of Energy Output

Energy output may be divided into the following components: basal metabolic rate, physical activity, and thermic effect of feeding. A brief discussion of each of these components, their hormonal mediators, and how they interact is necessary to present a complete discussion of the control of hormones on energy balance.

### Resting Metabolic Rate

Resting metabolic rate (RMR) accounts for about 1400 to 1600 kcal, constituting about 60% to 75% of total energy expenditure. It has several major metabolic origins. It is thought to reflect the energy cost of protein and, to a much smaller extent, carbohydrate and fat turnover. It reflects the activity of the sodium pump, the cost of maintaining muscle tone, and the work done by involuntary muscles (heart, respiratory, and gastrointestinal).[110–115] It originates primarily in, and therefore is highly correlated with, lean body mass; men, having a greater lean body mass, have a higher RMR than do women. RMR is governed by thyroid hormones through a mechanism that is not fully understood. The hormone stimulates activity of the sodium pump[116] as well as protein turnover[117]; protein turnover is stimulated through enhancement of protein breakdown via lysosomal proteinases[117] and through stimulation of protein synthesis in conjunction with other anabolic hormones, namely insulin and growth hormone. Triiodothyronine stimulates release of both insulin[118] and growth hormone.[95] Triiodothyronine is also required for sympathetic activation,[119] which can, in turn, stimulate metabolic rate. RMR is reduced in elderly people some 10% to 20%[120,121]; it is thought that this decline in metabolic rate reflects, by and large, the reduced lean body mass.[120] Females show a lesser decline in RMR than males do. The reduction in BMR is accompanied by a decrease in the rate of protein turnover[122] but with no clear change in activity of the sodium pump in the small number of tissues examined.[123] The metabolic origins for the age-dependent compositional changes have not been clearly identified. Activities of growth hormone and testosterone, which promote lean tissue growth, are reduced with aging; this may contribute to the shift in balance from lean to adipose tissue. A decreased trophic effect of the autonomic nervous system on muscle and a decreased capacity for muscle fiber regeneration have also been suggested.[124]

### Physical Activity

Physical activity is an important determinant of energy balance status. Muscle mass is increased and adiposity is decreased with physical training.[82] In elderly people, there is usually a decline in physical activity[82] imposed by age-related conditions such as cardiovascular disease, musculoskeletal disease, osteopenia, and obesity. In addition, there is a decline in physical working capacity (VO$_2$max), amounting to about 10% per decade between ages 25 and 65 years. The latter means that the same physical tasks require a greater physical effort in elderly people. Elderly individuals retain the ability to enjoy the benefit of training,[125] and physical training can correct these age-related changes in physical working capacity by as much as 50%. The level of physical activity is not under hormonal control but is determined by motivational factors.

### Thermic Effect of Feeding

The thermic effect of feeding[126,127] represents two components: an obligatory component and an adaptive component. In the obligatory component, heat is a byproduct of the metabolic cost of converting the ingested macronutrient into body glycogen, protein, and fat.[128] It amounts to an average of 5% to 10% of the energy value of the food. It is minimal after fat intake and maximal after protein intake.[128] In the adaptive component, heat is the primary end product. In rodents, this heat is produced exclusively in the brown adipose tissue, where substrate oxidation is uncoupled from phosphorylation.[129] In rodents, the brown fat has the potential of dissipating a large portion of the caloric intake, but in humans, the capacity for adaptive thermogenesis is relatively small, apparently because of the small quantity of brown fat in humans.[130,131] Thermogenic activity of brown adipose tissue is controlled primarily by norepinephrine released from a dense sympathetic innervation of this tissue.[130] Insulin[131] and glucagon,[132] which are released in response to feeding, stimulate thermogenesis of brown adipose tissue in rodents, whereas glucocorticoids[87] inhibit it.

In rodents, the capacity for feeding-induced thermogenesis declines rapidly after sexual maturity is reached.[133] In old rats, there is a 30% decrease in brown adipose tissue mass, a twofold decrease in β-adrenergic receptors (primarily due to receptors of the $\beta_1$ subtype) and a decrease in the activation of adenylate cyclase.[134] These biochemical abnormalities may contribute to the decreased capacity for feeding-induced thermogenesis in older animals. An analogous reduction in adaptive thermogenesis in humans would contribute to the observed age-related decrease in energy expenditure.

## CONCLUSION

Nutrition and the endocrine system are closely integrated. Nutritional status influences glandular activities, while endocrine function can have marked influences on nutrient requirements and status. With advancing age, changes occur in both endocrine and nutritional status.

Several factors enhance development of diabetes mellitus in elderly people, including weight gain, decreased physical activity, and defective mechanisms for insulin secretion and action. Although the efficacy of the American Dietetic Association/American Diabetes Association diet for glucose control in elderly diabetics is not clear, there is no better dietary recommendation for them at the present time. Long-term exercise programs are beneficial to elderly diabetics and should be encouraged.

A hypothyroid state is much more prevalent in elderly people than in young people. In elderly individuals, hypothyroidism is often contributed to by the presence of malnutrition. In the hyperthyroid elderly person, the rise in metabolic rate is not fully compensated for by a corresponding rise in voluntary food intake. Thyroid status can have profound effects on vitamin and calcium requirements, and their proper intake should be monitored in hyperthyroid elderly people.

Aging produces only minor changes in the hypothalamic-pituitary-adrenal axis. Diseases of the adrenal cortex, namely Addison disease and Cushing's syndrome, are not common in elderly people. However, ectopic corticotropin production, secondary to tumors, is relatively common. Steroid treatment should be used in elderly patients with extreme caution, as it can cause negative nitrogen and calcium balances as well as hyperglycemia and resistance to insulin.

Growth hormone secretion is mildly reduced in the elderly, but IGF I is markedly reduced. These may contribute to the diminished nitrogen retention and increased adiposity observed with aging. Another possible contributor to the decline in nitrogen retention in elderly persons is reduced serum testosterone levels. However, the main cause for impotence in elderly men is thought to be arteriosclerosis and not reduced testosterone levels.

In elderly individuals, both energy intake and output are reduced, but reduction in intake often exceeds output. In experimental animals, aging is associated with reduced opioid-based feeding drive and with a greater suppression of feeding by CCK, but the possible role of these events in the development of the anorexia of aging humans is not known. There is some evidence that leptin may play a role in the alterations in energy metabolism that occur with aging, particularly in males. The smaller energy expenditure observed in elderly people is brought about by a reduced RMR, by reduced physical activity, and possibly by a reduced thermic response to feeding.

## REFERENCES

1. Mooradian AD, Morley JE, Korenman SG. Endocrinology in aging. *Dis Mon.* 1988;34:395–461.
2. Morley JE. Geriatric endocrinology. In: Mendelsohn G, ed. *Diagnosis and Pathology of Endocrine Disease.* Philadelphia, Pa: JB Lippincott Co; 1988.
3. Harris MI, Hadden WC, Knowler WC, et al. Prevalence of diabetes and impaired glucose tolerance and plasma glucose levels in U.S. population aged 20-74 years. *Diabetes.* 1987;4:523–534.
4. Morley JE. Unusual aspects of diabetes mellitus in the elderly. *Clin Geriatr.* In press.
5. Zavaroni I, Dall'Aglio E, Bruschi F. Effect of age and environmental factors on glucose tolerance and insulin secretion in a worker population. *J Am Geriatr Soc.* 1986;34:271–278.
6. Morley JE, Mooradian AD, Rosenthal MJ, et al. Diabetes mellitus in elderly patients: is it different? *Am J Med.* 1987;83:533–544.
7. Morley JE, Perry HM III. The management of diabetes mellitus in older individuals. *Drugs.* 1991;41:548–565.
8. Meneilly GS, Tessier D. Diabetes in the elderly. *Diabetic Med.* 1995;12:949–960.
9. American Diabetes Association. Nutrition recommendations and principles for people with diabetes mellitus. *Diabetes Care.* 1998;21(suppl 1):S32–S36.
10. Coulston A, Mandelbaum D, Reaven G. Dietary management of nursing home residents with diabetes: diabetic versus regular diet. *Clin Res.* 1988;36:95A.
11. Seals DR, Hagberg JM, Hurley BF, et al. Effects of endurance training on glucose tolerance and plasma lipid levels in older men and women. *JAMA.* 1984;252:645–649.
12. Krotkiewski M, Lonnroth P, Mandroukas K, et al. The effects of physical training on glucose metabolism in obesity and type 2 (noninsulin-dependent) diabetes mellitus. *Diabetologia.* 1985;28:881–890.
13. Saltin B, Lindgarde F, Houston M, et al. Physical training and glucose tolerance in middle-aged men with chemical diabetes. *Diabetes.* 1979;28(suppl 1):30–32.
14. Bogardus C, Ravussin E, Robbins DC, et al. Effects of physical training and diet therapy on carbohydrate metabolism in patients with glucose intolerance and noninsulin-dependent diabetes mellitus. *Diabetes.* 1984;33:311–318.
15. Karam JH. Therapeutic dilemmas in type II diabetes mellitus: improving and maintaining B-cell and insulin sensitivity. *West J Med.* 1988;148:685–690.
16. Pacini G, Valerio A, Beccaro F, et al. Insulin sensitivity and beta-cell responsivity are not decreased in elderly subjects with normal OGTT. *J Am Geriatr Soc.* 1988;36:317–323.
17. Agurscollins TD, Kumanyika SK, Tenhave TR, Adamscampbell LL. A randomized controlled trial of weight reduction and exercise for diabetes management in older African-American subjects. *Diabetes Care.* 1997;20:1503–1511.
18. Puxty JAM, Hunter DM, Burr WA. Accuracy of insulin injection in elderly patients. *Br Med J.* 1983;287:1762–1763.
19. Rosenthal MJ, Fajardo M, Gilmore S, Morley JE, Naliboff BD. Hospitalization and mortality of diabetes in older adults: a 3-year prospective study. *Diabetes Care.* 1998;21:231–235.
20. Mooradian AD, Morley JE. Micronutrient status in diabetes mellitus. *Am J Clin Nutr.* 1987;45:877–895.
21. Kinlaw WB, Levine AS, Morley JE, et al. Abnormal zinc metabolism in type II diabetes mellitus. *Am J Med.* 1983;75:273–277.
22. Morley JE. Nutritional status of the elderly. *Am J Med.* 1986;81:679–695.
23. Niewoehner CB, Allen JI, Boosalis M, et al. The role of zinc supplementation in type II diabetes mellitus. *Am J Med.* 1986;81:63–68.
24. Hallbook T, Lanner E. Serum-zinc and wound healing of venous leg ulcers. *Lancet.* 1972;2:780–782.
25. Anderson RA, Cheng N, Bryden NA, et al. Elevated intakes of supplemental chromium improve glucose and insulin variables in individuals with type 2 diabetes. *Diabetes.* 1997;46:1786–1791.
26. Urberg M, Zemel MD. Evidence for synergism between chromium and nicotinic acid in the control of glucose tolerance in elderly humans. *Metabolism.* 1987;36:896–899.
27. Klevay LM. Hypercholesterolemia in rats produced by an increase in the ratio of zinc to copper ingested. *Am J Clin Nutr.* 1978;26:1060–1065.

28. Sinclair AJ, Allard I. Observations of diabetes care in long-term institutional settings with measures of cognitive function and dependency. *Diabetes Care.* 1997;20:778–784.

29. Mooradian AD, Osterweil D, Petrasek D, et al. Diabetes mellitus in elderly nursing home patients: a survey of clinical characteristics and management. *J Am Geriatr Soc.* 1988;36:391–396.

30. Robuschi G, Safran M, Braverman LE. Hypothyroidism in the elderly. *Endocr Rev.* 1987;8:142–153.

31. Morley JE, Slag MF, Elson MK, et al. The interpretation of thyroid function tests in hospitalized patients. *JAMA.* 1983;249:2377–2379.

32. Lloyd WA, Goldberg IJL. Incidence of hypothyroidism in the elderly. *Br Med J.* 1961;2:1256–1258.

33. Martin FI, Deam DR. Hyperthyroidism in elderly hospitalized patients: clinical features and treatment outcomes. *Med J Aust.* 1996;164:200–203.

34. Loeb JN. Metabolic changes in hyperthyroidism. In: Ingbar SM, Braverman LE, eds. *Werner's The Thyroid.* Philadelphia, Pa: JB Lippincott Co; 1986.

35. Kreines K, Jett M, Knowles HC. Observations in hyperthyroidism of abnormal glucose tolerance and other traits related to diabetes mellitus. *Diabetes.* 1965;14:740–744.

36. Nikkala EA, Kekki M. Plasma triglyceride metabolism in thyroid disease. *J Clin Invest.* 1972; 51:2103–2111.

37. Watanakunakom C, Hodges RE, Evans TC. Myxedema. *Arch Intern Med.* 1965;116:183–187.

38. Rivlin RS. Vitamin metabolism in hyperthyroidism. In: Ingbar SM, Braverman LE, eds. *Werner's The Thyroid.* Philadelphia, Pa: JB Lippincott Co; 1986.

39. Rivlin RS. Vitamin metabolism in hypothyroidism. In: Ingbar SM, Braverman LE, eds. *Werner's The Thyroid.* Philadelphia, Pa: JB Lippincott Co; 1986.

40. Morley JE, Damassa DA, Gordon J, et al. Thyroid function and vitamin A deficiency. *Life Sci.* 1978;22:1901–1906.

41. Morley JE, Melmed S, Reed A, et al. The effect of vitamin A on the hypothalamic-pituitarythyroid axis. *Am J Physiol.* 1980;238:E174–E179.

42. Drill VA. Interrelationships between thyroid function and vitamin metabolism. *Physiol Rev.* 1942; 23:355–372.

43. Galton VA, Ingbar SM. Effects of vitamin deficiency on the in vitro and in vivo deiodination of thyroxine in the rat. *Endocrinology.* 1965;77:169–174.

44. Postelnicu D. Action of an antioxidant substance (alpha tocopherol) on the myocardium of rats treated with thyroxine. *Stud Cercet Endocrinol.* 1972;23:175–182.

45. D'Avanzo B, Ron E, LaVecchia C, Francaschi S, Negri E, Zleglar R. Selected micronutrient intake and thyroid carcinoma risk. *Cancer.* 1997;79:2186–2192.

46. Oxenburg GF, Pomara N, Mclntyre IM. Aging and cortisol resistance to suppression by dexamethasone: a positive correlation. *Psychiatry Res.* 1983;10:125–130.

47. Irvine WJ, Barnes EW. Addison's disease, ovarian failure and hypoparathyroidism. *Clin Endocrinol Metab.* 1975;4:379–34.

48. Gregerman RL, Bierman EL. Aging and hormones. In: Williams RM, ed. *Textbook of Endocrinology.* 6th ed. Philadelphia, Pa: WB Saunders Co; 1981.

49. Tsundo K, Abe K, Goto T. Effect of age on the renin-angiotensin-aldosterone system in normal subjects: simultaneous measurement of active and inactive renin, renin substrate, and aldosterone in plasma. *J Clin Endocrinol Metab.* 1986;62:384–389.

50. Parker LN, Odell WD. Decline of adrenal androgen production as measured by radioimmunoassay of urinary conjugated dehydroepiandrosterone. *J Clin Endocrinol Metab.* 1978;47:600–602.

51. Pashko LL, Schwartz AG. Effect of food restriction, dehydroepiandrosterone or obesity on the binding of 3H-7, 12 dimethylbenz (a) anthracene to mouse skin DNA. *J Gerontol.* 1983;38:8–12.

52. Barrett-Connor E, Shaw KT, Yen SSC. A prospective study of dehydroepiandrosterone sulfate, mortality and cardiovascular disease. *N Engl J Med.* 1986;315:1519–1524.

53. Sonka J, Fassati M, Fassati P. Serum lipids and dehydroepiandrosterone excretion in normal subjects. *J Lipid Res.* 1968;9:769–772.

54. Nowaczynski W, Fragachon F, Silah J. Further evidence of altered adrenocortical function in hypertension: dehydroepianodrosterone excretion rate. *J Physiol (Lond).* 1964;56:650–651.

55. Phillips PA, Rolls BJ, Ledingham JGG. Reduced thirst after water deprivation in healthy elderly men. *N Engl J Med.* 1984;311:753–759.

56. Yamamoto T, Harada H, Fukeiyama J, et al. Impaired arginine-vasopressin secretion associated with hypoangiotensinemia in hypernatremic dehydrated elderly patients. *JAMA*. 1988;259:1039–1042.

57. Helderman JH. The impact of normal aging on the hypothalamic-neurohypophyseal-renal axis. In: Korenman SG, ed. *Endocrine Aspects of Aging*. New York, NY: Elsevier-North Holland; 1982.

58. Lindeman RD, Lee TD Jr, Yiengst MJ. Influences of age, renal diseases, hypertension, diuretics, and calcium on the antidiuretic responses to suboptimal infusions of vasopressin. *J Lab Clin Med*. 1966; 68:206–223.

59. Ohashi M, Fujia N, Nawata H. High plasma concentrations of human atrial natriuretic polypeptide in aged men. *J Clin Endocrinol Metab*. 1987; 64:81–85.

60. Miller M, Morley JE, Rubenstein LZ. Hyponatremia in nursing home population. *J Am Geriatr Soc*. 1995;43:1410–1413.

61. Manson JMK, Wilmore DW. Positive nitrogen balance with human growth hormone and hypocaloric intravenous feeding. *Surgery*. 1986;100:188–197.

62. Florini J, Prinz PN, Vitiello MV. Somatomedin-C levels in healthy young and old men: relationship to peak and 24 hours integrated levels of growth hormone. *J Gerontol*. 1985;40:2–7.

63. Rudman D, Nagraji HS, Mattson DE. Hyposomatomedinemia in the nursing home patient. *J Am Geriatr Soc*. 1986;34:427–430.

64. Rudman D. Growth hormone, body composition and aging. *J Am Geriatr Soc*. 1985;33:800–807.

65. Cohn L, Feller AG, Draper MW, Rudman IW, Rudman D. Carpal tunnel syndrome and gynaecomastia during growth hormone treatment of elderly men with low circulating IGF-I concentrations. *Clin Endocrinol*. 1993; 39:417–425.

66. Papadakis MA, Grady D, Black D, et al. Growth hormone replacement in healthy older men improves body composition but not functional ability. *Ann Intern Med*. 1996;124:708–716.

67. Kaiser FE, Silver AJ, Morley JE. The effect of recombinant human growth hormone on malnourished older individuals. *J Am Geriatr Soc*. 1991; 39:235–240.

68. Kinsey AC, Pomeroy WB, Martin CE. *Sexual Behavior in the Human Male*. Philadelphia, Pa: WB Saunders Co; 1948.

69. Slag MF, Morley JE, Elson MK, et al. Impotence in medical clinic outpatients. *JAMA*. 1983;249:1736–1740.

70. Morley JE. Impotence. *Am J Med*. 1986;80:897–905.

71. Billington CJ, Levine AS, Morley JE. Zinc status in impotent patients. *Clin Res*. 1983;31:714A. Abstract.

72. Morley JE, Kaiser F, Raum WJ, et al. Potentially predictive and manipulable blood serum correlates of aging in the healthy human male: progressive decreases in bioavailable testosterone, dehydroepiandrosterone sulfate, and the ratio of insulin-like growth factor 1 to growth hormone. *Proc Natl Acad Sci USA*. 1997;94:7537–7542.

73. Baker HWG, Berger HG, deKretser DM, et al. Changes in the pituitary testicular system with age. *Clin Endocrinol (Oxf)*. 1976;5:349–372.

74. Morley JE, Kaiser FE, Sih R, Hajjar R, Perry HM III. Testosterone and frailty. *Clin Geriatr Med*. 1997;13:685–695.

75. Mooradian AD, Morley JE, Korenman SG. Biological actions of androgens. *Endocr Rev*. 1987; 8:1–28.

76. MacLaughlin J, Holick MF. Aging decreases the capacity of human skin to produce vitamin D3. *J Clin Invest*. 1985;76:1536–1538.

77. Armbrecht HJ, Zenser TV, Davis BB. Effect of age on the conversion of 25-hydroxyvitamin D3 to 1,25-dihydroxyvitamin D3 by kidney of rat. *J Clin Invest*. 1980;66:1118–1123.

78. Chapuy MC, Arlot ME, Delmas PD, Meunier PJ. Effect of calcium and cholecalciferol treatment for three years on hip fractures in elderly women. *Brit Med J*. 1994;308:1081–1082.

79. Morley JE, Gorbien MJ, Mooradian AD, et al. UCLA geriatric grand rounds: osteoporosis. *J Am Geriatr Soc*. 1988;36:845–859.

80. Somaan NA, Anderson GD, Adam-Mayne ME. Immunoreactive calcitonin in mother, neonate, child and adult. *Am J Obstet Gynecol*. 1975;121:622–625.

81. Nielson FH, Hunt CD, Mullen LM, et al. Effect of dietary boron on mineral, estrogen, and testosterone metabolism in postmenopausal women. *FASEB J*. 1987;1:394–397.

82. Shepard JW. Interrelationships of exercise and nutrition in the elderly. In: Armbrecht HJ, Prendergast J, Coe R, eds. *Nutritional Intervention in the Aging Process*. New York, NY: Springer-Verlag; 1984.

83. Frisancho AR. New standards of weight and body composition by frame size and height for assessment of nutritional status of adults and the elderly. *Am J Clin Nutr*. 1984;40:808–819.

84. Morley JE. Anorexia of aging: physiologic and pathologic. *Am J Clin Nutr*. 1997;66:760–773.

85. Leibowitz SF. Neurochemical-neuroendocrine systems in the brain controlling macronutrient intake and metabolism. *Trends Neurosci*. 1992;15:491–497.

86. LeMagnen J. Body energy balance and food intake: a neuroendocrine regulatory mechanism. *Physiol Rev*. 1983;63:314–386.

87. Bray GA. The nutrient balance hypothesis: peptides, sympathetic activity, and food intake. *Ann NY Acad Sci*. 1993;676:223–241.

88. Greenberg LH. Regulation of brain adrenergic receptors during aging. *Fed Proc*. 1986;45:55–59.

89. Morley JE, Blundell JE. The neurobiological basis of eating disorders: some formulations. *Biol Psychiatry*. 1988;23:53–78.

90. Morley JE. Neuropeptide regulation of appetite and weight. *Endocr Rev*. 1987;8:256–287.

91. Morley JE, Levine AS, Yim GK, et al. Opioid modulation of appetite. *Neurosci Biobehav Rev*. 1983;7:281–305.

92. Morley JE, Levine AS, Gosnell BA, et al. Effect of neuropeptide Y on ingestive behaviors in the rat. *Am J Physiol*. 1987;252:R599–R609.

93. Gosnell BA, Levine AS, Morley JE. The effects of aging on opioid modulation of feeding in rats. *Life Sci*. 1983;32:2793–2799.

94. Morley JE, Hernandez EN, Flood JF. Neuropeptide Y increases food intake in mice. *Am J Physiol*. 1987;253:R516–R522.

95. Towle HC. Effects of thyroid hormones on cellular RNA metabolism. In: Oppenheimer JH, Samuels HH, eds. *Molecular Basis of Thyroid Hormone Action*. New York, NY: Academic Press; 1983.

96. York DA, Bray GA. Dependence of hypothalamic obesity on insulin, the pituitary, and the adrenal gland. *Endocrinology*. 1972;90:885–894.

97. Bray GA. *The Obese Patient*. Philadelphia, Pa: WB Saunders Co; 1976:9. Saunders Monographs on Major Problems in Internal Medicine.

98. Leibowitz SF, Roland CR, Hor L, et al. Noradrenergic feeding elicited via the paraventricular nucleus is dependent upon circulating corticosterone. *Physiol Behav*. 1984;32:857–864.

99. Dalman MF. Viewing the ventromedial hypothalamus from the adrenal gland. *Am J Physiol*. 1984;246:R1–R12.

100. Freedman MR, Castunguay TW, Stern JS. Effect of adrenalectomy and corticosterone replacement on meal patterns of Zucker rats. *Am J Physiol*. 1985;249:R584–R594.

101. Hollifield G. Glucocorticoid-induced obesity: a model and a challenge. *Am J Clin Nutr*. 1968;21:1471–1474.

102. Donhoffer SZ, Vonotzky J. The effect of thyroxine on food intake and selection. *Am J Physiol*. 1947;150:334–339.

103. Wade GH, Zucker I. Modulation of food intake and locomotor activity in female rats by diencephalic hormone implants. *J Comp Physiol Psychol*. 1978;72:328–336.

104. Wade GH, Zucker I. Development of hormonal control over food intake and body weight in female rats. *J Comp Physiol Psychol*. 1970;70:213–220.

105. Numez AA, Grundman M. Testosterone affects food intake and body weight of weanling male rats. *Pharmacol Biochem Behav*. 1982;16:933–936.

106. Glick Z. Intestinal satiety with and without upper intestinal factors. *Am J Physiol*. 1979;236:R142–R146.

107. Billington CJ, Levine AS, Morley JE. Are peptides truly satiety agents? a method for testing neurohormonal satiety effects. *Am J Physiol*. 1983;245:R920–R929.

108. Khalil T, Walker JP, Wiener J, et al. Effect of aging on gallbladder contraction and release of cholecystokinin-33 in humans. *Surgery*. 1985;98:423–429.

109. Silver AJ, Flood JF, Morley JE. Effect of gastrointestinal peptides on ingestion in young and old mice. *Peptides*. 1988;9:221–226.

110. Bray GA, York DA. Clinical review 90: leptin and clinical medicine: a new piece in the puzzle of obesity. *J Clin Endocrinol Metab*. 1997;82:2771–2776.

111. Garrow J. *Energy Balance and Obesity in Man*. New York, NY: American Elsevier; 1974.

112. Perry HM, Morley JE, Horowitz M, Kaiser FE, Miller DK, Wittert G. Body composition and age

in African-American and Caucasian women: relationship to plasma leptin levels. *Metabolism.* 1997;46:1399–1405.

113. Keynes RD. The energy cost of active transport. In: Bolis L, Manddrell HP, Schmidt-Nielsen K, eds. *Comparative Physiology: Functional Aspects of Structural Materials.* Amsterdam, Netherlands: North Holland Publishing Co; 1975.

114. Waterlow JC, Garlick PJ, Millward DJ. *Protein Turnover in Mammalian Tissues and in Whole Body.* New York, NY: Elsevier-North Holland; 1978.

115. Newsholme EA. A possible metabolic basis for the control of body weight. *N Engl J Med.* 1980;302:400–405.

116. Guernsey DL, Edelman IS. Regulation of thermogenesis by thyroid hormones. In: Oppenheimer JH, Samuels HH, eds. *Molecular Basis of Thyroid Hormone Action.* New York, NY: Academic Press; 1983.

117. Millward DJ. Human protein requirements: the physiological significance of changes in the rate of whole body protein turnover. In: Garrow JW, Holliday D, eds. *Substrate and Energy Metabolism in Man.* London, England: John Libbey; 1985.

118. Mariash CN, Oppenheimer JH. Thyroid hormone: carbohydrate interaction. In: Oppenheimer JH, Samuels HH, eds. *Molecular Basis of Thyroid Hormone Action.* New York, NY: Academic Press; 1983.

119. Rothwell NJ, Saville ME, Stock MJ. Sympathetic and thyroid influences on metabolic rate in fed, fasted, and refed rats. *Am J Physiol.* 1982;243:R339–R346.

120. Lipson LG, Bray GA. Energy. In: Chen LH, ed. *Nutritional Aspects of Aging.* Cleveland, Ohio: CRC Press; 1986.

121. Chernoff R, Lipschitz DA. Nutrition and aging. In: Shils ME, Young VR, eds. *Modern Nutrition in Health and Disease.* 7th ed. Philadelphia, Pa: Lea & Febiger; 1988.

122. Young VR. Impact of aging on protein metabolism. In: Armbrecht HJ, Prendergast JM, Coe RM, eds. *Nutritional Intervention in the Aging Process.* New York, NY: Springer-Verlag; 1984.

123. Guernsey DL, Koebbe M, Thomas JE, et al. An altered response in the induction of cell membrane (Na$^+$ K$^+$) ATPase by thyroid hormone is characteristic of senescence in cultured human fibroblasts. *Mech Ageing Dev.* 1986;33:283–293.

124. Evans WJ. Exercise and muscle metabolism in the elderly. In: Hutchinson ML, Munro HN, eds. *Nutrition and Aging.* New York, NY: Academic Press; 1986.

125. Hagberg JM. Effect of training on the decline of VO$_2$max with aging. *Fed Proc.* 1987;46:1830–1833.

126. Glick Z. The thermic effect of a meal. *J Obes Weight Regul.* 1987;6:170–178.

127. Rothwell NJ, Stock MJ. Diet-induced thermogenesis: concepts and mechanisms. *J Obes Weight Regul.* 1987;6:162–169.

128. Flatt JP. The biochemistry of energy expenditure. In: Bray GA, ed. *Recent Advances in Obesity Research: Proceedings of the 2nd International Congress on Obesity.* London, England: Newman Publishing; 1978.

129. Himms-Hagen J. Brown adipose tissue metabolism and thermogenesis. *Annu Rev Nutr.* 1985;5:69–94.

130. Astrup A, Bulow J, Madsen J, et al. Contribution of BAT and skeletal muscle to thermogenesis induced by ephedrine in man. *Am J Physiol.* 1985;248:E507–E515.

131. Glick Z, Teague RJ, Bray GA. Effect of prandial glucose on brown fat thermogenesis: possible implications in dietary obesity. *J Nutr.* 1984;114:286–291.

132. Billington CJ, Bartness TJ, Briggs J, et al. Glucagon stimulation of brown adipose tissue growth and thermogenesis. *Am J Physiol.* 1987;252:R160–R165.

133. Rothwell NJ, Stock MJ. Effects of age on diet-induced thermogenesis and brown adipose tissue metabolism in the rat. *Int J Obes.* 1983;7:583–589.

134. Scarpace PJ, Mooradian AD, Morley JE. Age-associated decrease in beta-adrenergic receptors and adenylate cyclase activity in rat brown adipose tissue. *J Gerontol.* 1988;43:B65–B70.

# CHAPTER 14

# Pharmacology, Nutrition, and the Elderly: Interactions and Implications

*Jeffrey Blumberg and Rebecca Couris*

Despite the recognition of interactions between pharmacology and nutrition, especially in the elderly population, the clinical significance of this relationship remains largely unappreciated. Although much of the early information on this topic had been based on anecdotal reports, current understanding of the interactions among pharmacotherapeutics, nutrition, and aging has been reviewed and compiled such that many adverse outcomes can now be predicted and avoided.[1–11] The adverse consequences of drug-nutrient interactions in the elderly can include nutritional deficiency, drug toxicity, loss of drug efficacy and disease control, and unwanted changes in body weight.

Adverse drug reactions are responsible for significant morbidity and mortality among the elderly. Even though the elderly constitute about 13% of the population of the United States, they consume more than 25% of all prescription drugs and experience 39% of the adverse drug reactions.[12,13] While the relative contributions of drug-drug interactions and drug-nutrient interactions to this problem among elderly people have not been established, the two situations have common ground: the presence of multiple disease states, the practice of polypharmacy, the poor nutritional status of elderly individuals, and age-related changes in pharmacokinetics and pharmacodynamics.

## EXTENT AND PATTERNS OF DRUG USE BY THE ELDERLY

The growing numbers of elderly people and the multiple pathologic processes that affect them appear, inevitably, to lead to increased use of drugs in old age. Clinicians manage most illnesses in elderly patients with prescription drugs. Moreover, conditions such as memory loss, confusion, and changed sleep patterns are also treated with drug therapy by some physicians. Four of every five individuals older than 65 years are afflicted with chronic conditions such as heart disease, hypertension, arthritis, and diabetes; 35% have three or more of these problems.[14] Many older patients living at home take 3 or more different drugs daily; in institutions, the quantity frequently increases to 10 or more different drugs per day.[15] This situation carries with it an increased likelihood of overprescribing practices, including inappropriate or excessive drug use, excessive dosage, and overlong drug use.

Cardiovascular drugs (eg, digitalis glycosides, diuretics, antiarrhythmics, antihypertensives, and anticoagulants) are the medica tion class most often prescribed for older patients, followed by psychoactive drugs (eg, neuroleptics and sedative hypnotics) and gastrointestinal drugs (eg, histamine$_2$ [H$_2$] blockers and laxatives)[15–18] (Table 14–1). More than 60% of the elderly population regularly use nonprescription drugs, especially non-narcotic analgesics such as acetaminophen, antacids, antihistamines, and nutrient supplements.[19,20] Interestingly, the 10 most common medical conditions reported by elderly people during health interviews include (by rank) arthritis, hearing problems, heart diseases, hypertension, visual handicaps, digestive diseases, chronic sinusitis, mental and nervous disorders, genitourinary tract problems, and circulatory problems.[21] Therefore, despite the patterns of illness among older adults, actual prescribing practices and use of over-the-counter drugs may differ from the incidence of diseases.

The problems associated with trying to provide rational drug treatment for older people can be categorized as extrinsic issues (ie, drug prescription and drug compliance) and intrinsic issues (ie, age-related pharmacokinetic and pharmacodynamic changes).[22] Polypharmacy prescribing patterns provide elderly patients with more drugs than they can reasonably be expected to cope with in a practical way; this situation leads to difficulty with compliance and greatly increases the risk of drug-drug and drug-nutrient interactions. In the context of multiple diseases, treatment without drugs is often insufficiently explored, although the risk-benefit ratio is higher in older adults than in young people.

It has been noted that the withdrawal of drug treatment once the initial indication has resolved often requires greater initiative and discipline than the original act of prescribing. "Inherited therapy," when drugs started in middle age are automatically continued, is common among elderly people. The need for periodic reevaluation of all drugs prescribed on a chronic basis is an essential component of rational drug therapy.[23] There is now evidence that long-term drug treatment with some compounds (eg, hypnotics, diuretics, cardiotonic glycosides, and nonsteroidal anti-inflammatory agents) is not necessary for many patients. Some drug category–specific suggestions to minimize potential adverse drug reactions in the elderly are listed in Table 14–2.

Issues concerning compliance are not unique to elderly people, although the elderly are more vulnerable to problems associated with packaging and labeling, difficult-to-fol-

**Table 14–1** Patterns of Drug Use by the Elderly

| | Percentage of Prescriptions for Patients ≥ 65 Years | | | |
|---|---|---|---|---|
| *Therapeutic Class of Drug* | *U.K.* | *Germany* | *Netherlands* | *Belgium* |
| Peripheral vasodilators | 68 | 67 | 68 | 65 |
| Cardiac drugs | 68 | 59 | 60 | 57 |
| Diuretics | 60 | 57 | 51 | 54 |
| Antihypertensives | 53 | 64 | 51 | 31 |
| Psycholeptics | 38 | 41 | 26 | 33 |
| Antirheumatics | 43 | 37 | 25 | 31 |

*Source:* Adapted from IMS International Audit of Prescribing in General European Practice, 1981.

**Table 14–2** Guidelines for Minimizing Adverse Drug Reactions in the Elderly

| Drug Category | Recommendation |
| --- | --- |
| Antihypertensives | Select peripherally acting drugs; avoid agents with high lipophilic properties |
| Antiarrhythmics | Suspect cardiosensitivity |
| Diuretics | Suspect risk for electrolyte disturbances |
| Anxiolytics/sedatives | Avoid long-acting agents with active metabolites |
| Anticoagulants | Suspect sensitivity to warfarin; monitor International Normalized Ratio |
| Antidepressants/antipsychotics | Select agents with the least amount of sedative, anticholinergic, and orthostatic hypotension side effects |
| Analgesics | Monitor use of salicylates and nonsteroidal anti-inflammatory agents; suspect central nervous system sensitivity |
| Antiulcer agents | Suspect drug interactions and adverse reactions |
| Hypoglycemic agents | Suspect altered kinetics and increased sensitivity |
| Antacids | Suspect risk for nutrient deficiencies; monitor for drug-drug interactions |
| Laxatives | Suspect risk for electrolyte disturbances and nutrient deficiencies |

low regimens, and poor physician-patient communication about drug use. Attention must also be directed to the self-prescribing practices of the older individual; ubiquitous over-the-counter drugs and worthless antiaging remedies may interfere with other drugs and nutrients. Intrinsic factors of prescribing for the geriatric patient are discussed below.

## AGE-RELATED PHARMACOKINETIC CHANGES

Aging produces changes in pharmacokinetics (absorption, disposition, excretion) such that any given maintenance dose can lead to a higher steady-state concentration during repeated drug administration[25–27] (Table 14–3). However, most studies of drug kinetics and efficacy have been conducted in young and middle-aged patients, and relatively few controlled scientific data are available from geriatric patients. Therefore, in-creased drug monitoring is essential in elderly individuals, since the clinical basis for quantitatively predicting changes in pharmacokinetics is not available for all compounds. Lower initial doses are usually indicated in treating elderly patients.

## Absorption

The age-related physiologic changes in the gastrointestinal tract that could affect drug absorption, such as decreases in gastric emptying, splanchnic blood flow, and intestinal motility, are overcome to a considerable degree by the very large capacity of the system for passive absorption of small–molecular weight compounds. Drugs absorbed via active transport may be affected by age-related decline in the efficiency of these mechanisms.[28] The presence of chronic diseases and the interference of foods can further alter drug pharmacokinetics.

**Table 14–3** Physiologic Changes Relevant to Pharmacokinetics in the Elderly

| Pharmacokinetic Step | Age-Related Changes |
|---|---|
| Absorption | ↓ Absorptive surface<br>↓ Splanchnic blood flow<br>↑ Gastric pH<br>↓ Gastrointestinal motility<br>↓ Gastric secretion<br>↓ Pancreatic trypsin<br>↓ Gastric emptying |
| Distribution | ↓ Lean body mass<br>↓ Total body water<br>↓ Serum albumin<br>↑ Body fat<br>↑ Serum α-glycoprotein<br>↓ Cardiac output<br>↓ Cerebral blood flow<br>↑/↓ Membrane permeability |
| Metabolism | ↓ Liver mass<br>↓ Hepatic blood flow<br>↑/↓ Enzyme activity/inducibility |
| Excretion | ↓ Renal blood flow<br>↓ Glomerular filtration<br>↓ Tubular secretion |

*Note:* ↑, increased; ↓, decreased; ↑/↓, change dependent on specific drug.

## Distribution

Age-related changes in body composition, such as the increase in adipose tissue and loss of skeletal muscle, can affect drug distribution. These changes are more marked in women than in men. The linear increase with age in the elimination half-life of diazepam, a fat-soluble drug, has been attributed to a larger volume of distribution.[29–30] Plasma protein binding of drugs also alters drug distribution and is affected by age-related declines in serum albumin levels. Decreased protein binding in the presence of lowered albumin levels has been demonstrated for antipyrine, meperidine, phenytoin, propranolol, salicylates, and warfarin.[31,32] Although many drugs exhibit decreased binding (increased free fraction) in elderly subjects, a few show increased binding because of a greater affinity for $\alpha_1$-acid glycoprotein, which increases with age, than for albumin.[33] Although protein-binding changes are important factors in determining dosage, concomitant alteration in the volume of distribution and in the metabolic clearance of the total drug make a direct relationship difficult to establish.

**Table 14–4** Drugs Showing Reduction in Hepatic Biotransformation in the Elderly

Alprazolam
Antipyrine
Carbenoxolone sodium
Chlordiazepoxide
Chlormethiazole
Clobazam
Desalkylfurazepam
Desmethyldiazepam
Indocyanine green
Meperidine hydrochloride
Norepinephrine
Nortriptyline hydrochloride
Phenytoin
Piroxicam
Propranolol
Quinidine
Quinine
Theophylline
Verapamil

## Metabolism

Pharmacokinetic studies suggest that diminished hepatic oxidative (phase I) metabolism reduces the clearance of many drugs in elderly patients; however, this decline is not universal, due in part to the differential effects of aging on individual cytochrome P-450 isozymes.[25,34] A decrease in the metabolic clearance of drugs such as antipyrine, barbiturates, diazepam, and phenylbutazone is indicative of reduced oxidative drug-metabolizing enzyme activity in the elderly people.[32,35,36] Such reduced biotransformation capacity accordingly reduces total drug clearance and causes higher steady-state plasma concentrations during repeated dosage (Table 14–4). Drugs principally biotransformed via phase II conjugation reactions seem to be less influenced by age.[25–37] However, recent studies with nonhuman primates indicate that conclusions drawn

from the extensive data on hepatic metabolism in rodent experiments may not be completely relevant to humans.[38–40] It has been suggested that the decline in liver size with age in humans, which does not occur in rats, may also account for the lower drug-metabolizing capacity in older adults.[38,41]

### Excretion

Most drugs and their metabolites are eliminated via urinary excretion. The reduction of renal function (ie, glomerular filtration, tubular secretion, and total renal plasma flow) and the decrease in nephrons and renal mass underlie the slower rate of drug elimination in elderly individuals.[32,42] Diminished renal function may be the most important factor responsible for altered drug levels in older people (Table 14–5). Dosages should be adjusted in older patients by taking into account their reduced creatinine clearances, not their serum creatinine levels. If such measurements cannot be obtained, nomograms exist that adjust for the expected change related to both age and sex.[43] In addition to the normal decline in renal function with aging, a variety of conditions (eg, congestive heart failure, dehydration, hypotension, and diabetes) can further reduce renal elimination of drugs.[44]

## AGE-RELATED PHARMACODYNAMIC CHANGES

Despite the various alterations in pharmacokinetics that occur with different drugs in elderly patients and the associated changes in drug efficacy with toxicity, there remains a significant residue of altered responsiveness; this can be explained by differences in sensitivity to the drugs.[27] Pharmacodynamic theories suggest that such altered pharmacologic effects result from age-related changes in drug receptors, homeostasis, or tissue sensi-

**Table 14–5** Drugs Showing a Reduction in Renal Excretion in the Elderly

Acetylprocainamide
Amikacin
Ampicillin
Atenolol
Azapropazone
Cefuroxime
Cephalothin
Cephradine
Cimetidine
Digoxin
Dihydrostreptomycin
Doxycycline
Ethambutol
Gentamicin
Kanamycin
Lithium carbonate
Methotrexate
Pancuronium bromide
Penicillin
Phenobarbital
Procainamide hydrochloride
Propicillin
Quinidine
Sotalol hydrochloride
Streptomycin
Sulfamethizole
Tetracycline
Tobramycin

in receptor number or affinity, receptor regulation, or translation of binding into a response. Elderly patients are less responsive to ß-adrenergic agonists and more responsive to ß-adrenergic antagonists as a result of alterations in the cyclic adenosine monophosphate second-messenger system;[45,46] on the other hand, α-adrenergic receptors do not appear to change with age.[47] Age-related changes have also been documented for brain benzodiazepine receptors and several hormone receptors.[48] The pharmacologic effects of cholinergic agonists increase with age, while those of parasympathetic antagonists produce less response in the heart rates of elderly patients. The beneficial effects of anticholinergics have been reported to decrease and their adverse side effects to become more hazardous to elderly subjects. The progressive depletion of brain dopamine with age enhances the risk of drug-induced extrapyramidal side effects. Baroreceptor sensitivity is responsible for the high incidence of drug-induced orthostatic hypotension.[49] Age-related alterations in receptor-drug interactions are difficult to evaluate because of the influence of confounding factors such as disease, previous drug exposure, and nonreceptor drug-binding sites.

tivity. Pharmacodynamic explanations are difficult to test in vivo, and most studies depend on comparisons of correlations of drug effects versus simultaneously measured plasma drug concentrations—that is, demonstrations of response differences between young and old subjects with similar tissue exposures to the drug.

**Receptors**

Mechanisms for age-related alterations in target tissue sensitivity could include changes

**Homeostasis**

A reduced homeostatic vitality may be the basis of some examples of increased drug sensitivity among elderly people. The ventilatory response to hypoxic challenge is affected by age, with direct consequences for hypoxic disease states and drug therapy. Elderly individuals also show a decreased response to dietary challenges to acid-base balance; for example, ammonium chloride will lower blood pH and prolong recovery time more markedly in old subjects than in young subjects, despite identical resting steady-state conditions. Older people are also less able to regulate blood glucose levels, pulse rate, blood pressure, and oxygen consumption, but to varying degrees. These variations are great enough to preclude clinically useful generalizations.[50,51]

### Tissue Sensitivity

As discussed above, mechanisms for age-related alterations in target tissue sensitivity often appear to be based on changes in receptor number, affinity, or signal translation. However, many altered drug actions can be ascribed partially to age-related changes in the cardiovascular, endocrine, and central nervous systems. With age, decreases in cellular brain mass, sensory condition time, and cerebral blood flow may contribute to a greater vulnerability to adverse drug effects such as confusion, falls, and urinary incontinence.[48] Changes with age in the cardiovascular system result in a decreased response of the heart to stress and catecholamines and altered sensitivity to the toxic effects of some drugs. Alterations in pancreatic and adrenal hormone levels result in decreased glucose tolerance with age and an increased susceptibility of older patients to drug-induced hypoglycemia.[52] With age, there is a progressive decline in pulmonary function and a greater rigidity of the lung, which may cause an exaggerated respiratory depression after administration of narcotic analgesics. Decreases in thyroid hormone levels can make elderly individuals less sensitive to ß-adrenergic sympathomimetics and more sensitive to digitalis and drug-induced hypothermia.[53] An age-related reduction in the synthesis of hepatic blood-clotting factors may underlie an increased sensitivity to oral anticoagulant drugs. Declines in immune responsiveness may alter the expected efficacy of antibiotic and antiviral medications. Physiologic losses

of vestibular and cochlear hair cells and ganglia make geriatric patients more susceptible to irreversible drug-induced hearing loss.

## FOOD CHOICE AND NUTRITIONAL STATUS OF THE ELDERLY

Economic, physical, psychosocial, and pathologic factors may significantly affect elderly people's accessibility to food (Table 14–6). These elements may result from lack of money to purchase food; physical disability; loss of spouse, affecting motivation to cook and eat; isolation from family and community; limited knowledge concerning balanced diets; and existing disease processes. Chronic conditions such as arthritis, impaired hearing and vision, and coronary heart disease, as well as other physical disabilities, may affect health such that the ability to carry out food-related activities (eg, shopping and cooking) is significantly affected. Reduced appetite and food intake due to decreases in taste sensitivity, inability to chew, or problems in swallowing make eating more difficult and less pleasurable. Age-related changes in body composition and physiologic function also alter the dietary requirement for some nutrients.

National surveys reveal that substantial numbers of elderly people are seriously lacking in adequate intake of some nutrients. The most common dietary deficiency in older adults is in intake of calories and calcium. In some studies, over half of the respondents fail to meet the recommended level of calorie intake, and two thirds have less than adequate calcium intake. Decreasing energy intake with advancing age has important implications for the diet in terms of protein, vitamins, and minerals. Allowances for these nutrients assume that elderly people actually consume levels of energy that considerably exceed the amounts of food actually consumed. Dietary quality becomes difficult to ensure when overall energy intake is low; prudent diets in elderly individuals require a careful selection of nutrient-dense foods. Energy intake decreases more rapidly in the very old because of disabilities that limit physical activity. Many elderly eat few fruits and vegetables, particularly vitamin A– and vitamin C–rich varieties. Despite the widespread use of enriched breads and cereals, low intake of the B-complex vitamins is common in the aged. Many studies demonstrate, however, that elderly people who take advantage of community services providing nutritional support, particularly those in congregate settings, show improved overall dietary intake and nutritional status.

Although the prevalence of nutrient supplementation among elderly people is high, exceeding 50% in some areas, the use of such supplements often appears irrational and inappropriate to their needs.[54] As with drug regimens, there can be serious problems in compliance with nutritional therapies for chronic disease.[55] The generally poor nutritional status of hospitalized and institutionalized elderly patients has been well documented.[56]

---

**Table 14–6** Factors Affecting Food Choices of the Elderly

*Primary Factors*
  Poverty
  Social isolation/depression
  Loss of spouse
  Physical disability
  Poor dentition
  Inadequate knowledge of nutrition
*Secondary Factors*
  Chronic drug therapy
  Gastrointestinal disorders/malabsorption
  Disease/pathologic processes
  Alcoholism

## DRUG EFFECTS ON NUTRITIONAL STATUS

Several classification schemes have been proposed to categorize the ways in which drugs affect nutritional status.[57] While many of these schemes provide a sense of coherence and organization to the topic, there are difficulties or limitations with each scheme. The reason for this situation is the lack of any comprehensive theory underlying the numerous biochemical and clinical observations that have been reported. For the purpose of this discussion, it is useful to employ the same scheme used to illustrate the interaction between aging and pharmacokinetics (Table 14–7).

### Absorption

The best described and most frequent type of drug-nutrient interaction results from drug-induced alteration of nutrient absorption.[58] Drugs cause malabsorption by exerting an effect in the intestinal lumen or by impairing the absorptive ability of the gastrointestinal mucosa. These effects can be limited and specific for a particular nutrient, or they can be general and can affect an entire class of nutrients, such as fat-soluble vitamins or trace minerals. Drugs may decrease nutrient bioavailability by a variety of mechanisms, including adsorption of the nutrient itself or of bile acids, therefore inhibiting the intraluminal phase of fat digestion and absorption. Drugs may form insoluble precipitates or chelate with a nutrient. Drugs may affect the environment of the gastrointestinal lumen through changes in pH, motility, or composition of bacterial flora.

Some drugs may damage the intestinal mucosa and destroy the structure of the villi and microvilli, resulting in an inhibition of brush border enzymes and intestinal transport systems needed for nutrient absorption. The malabsorptive effect of colchicine, neomycin, and p-aminosalicylic acid appears to be the result of such mucosal injury.[59]

Drugs may also interfere with nutrient absorption through secondary mechanisms. Drugs can impair digestion of food directly via initial adverse effects on gastric or intestinal secretion, pancreatic exocrine function, or hepatic bile secretion. Cimetidine and other $H_2$ blockers, because of their inhibitory effects on gastric acid production, reduce the liberation of vitamin $B_{12}$ from its protein-bound state, making it less available for association with intrinsic factor.[60] Furthermore, in elderly individuals who have atrophic gastritis, changes in bacterial flora result in colonies with an increased avidity for vitamin $B_{12}$, making the nutrient less bioavailable.[61] Chronic effects of hepatotoxic drugs, notably alcohol, include maldigestion with reduced absorption of fats and fat-soluble vitamins.[62] Direct systemic effects of a drug on one nutrient may have secondary consequences for another nutrient. For example, drugs such as isoniazid[63] and cimetidine,[64] which inhibit the hepatic or renal hydroxylation of vitamin D, and those such as phenytoin[65] and phenobarbital,[66] which promote the catabolism of vitamin D metabolites, produce a functional deficiency of vitamin D with a secondary impairment in calcium absorption.

Hypolipidemic drugs of the absorbable and nonabsorbable types may improve lipid status and decrease the risk of coronary artery disease, but they pose nutritional hazards.[67] Cholestryramine is a basis anion-exchange resin that binds salts and impairs the absorption of a number of nutrients, including carotene; vitamins A, $B_{12}$, D, K, and folic acid; and the minerals calcium, iron, and zinc.[68] Clofibrate and colestipol have similar, although less pronounced, effects.

Several classes of over-the-counter drugs may induce adverse nutritional effects. It has been suggested that drug-induced malnutrition in elderly people is commonly due to their excessive use of over-the-counter drugs such as antacids, laxatives, and non-narcotic analgesics.[69] Antacids formulated with aluminum and magnesium hydroxides form nonabsorbable phosphates in the gut lumen and may induce hypophosphatemia[70] with the development of proximal limb muscle weakness, malaise, paresthesias, anorexia, and secondary syndromes of hypomagnesemia/tetany,[71] and osteomalacia.[72] These antacids have also been associated with impaired absorption of riboflavin, copper, and iron. Excessive use of sodium bicarbonate can result in sodium overload and may render the pH of the jejunum sufficiently alkaline to decrease the absorption of folic acid.[73]

Laxative abuse is common among elderly individuals. Stool softeners such as mineral oil, if taken at mealtime or in the postprandial absorptive period, prevent the absorption of carotenes and fat-soluble vitamins via solubilization. Overuse of diphenylmethane derivatives, including phenolphthalein and bisacodyl, may result in severe malabsorption with steatorrhea; decreased glucose, calcium, potassium, and vitamin D absorption; and protein-losing enteropathy.[74] Osteomalacia resulting from excessive laxative use has been reported.[75] Laxatives such as diocytl sulfosuccinates, which alter electrolyte transport, have also been associated with potassium deficiency due to gastrointestinal losses and failure of colonic reabsorption.[76] Laxative-induced malabsorption may be related to the loss of structural integrity of intestinal epithelial cells and protein-losing enteropathy secondary to potassium depletion.[77] In elderly patients, the risks of hypokalemia and potassium deficiency, with the attendant hazards of cardiac arrhythmias, digitalis toxicity,

**Table 14-7** Drug-Induced Alterations in Nutrient Kinetics

| Drug Category/Medication | Kinetic Alteration | Mechanism | Affected Nutrient |
|---|---|---|---|
| *Anticoagulants* | | | |
| Warfarin (Coumadin) | Metabolism | ↓ Reductase/carboxylation | Vitamin K |
| *Anti-Infectives* | | | |
| Antibiotics (general) | Absorption | Δ Bacterial flora | Vitamins $B_1$, $B_2$, $B_6$, $B_{12}$, K, biotin |
| Cephalosporins | Metabolism | ↓ Reductase/carboxylation | Vitamin K |
| Tetracyclines | Absorption | Chelation | Ca |
| Isoniazid/INH (Isoniazid) | Metabolism | ↓ Pyridoxal kinase | Vitamin $B_6$ |
| | | ↓ Hepatic/renal vitamin D hy-droxylation | Ca |
| Neomycin | Absorption | Mucosal injury | Na, K, Ca, vitamins $B_{12}$, K |
| Trimethoprim/TMP | Metabolism | Folate antagonist | Folic acid |
| *Anticonvulsants* | | | |
| Phenobarbital | Metabolism | Δ Vitamin D metabolites | Vitamin D, Ca |
| | | ↑ Hepatic microsomal enzymes | Folic acid |
| Phenytoin (Dilantin) | Metabolism | Δ Vitamin D metabolites | Vitamin D, Ca |
| | | ↑ Hepatic microsomal enzymes | Folic acid |
| *Antihypertensives* | | | |
| Vasodilators | Metabolism | ↓ Pyridoxal kinase | Vitamin $B_6$ |
| Hydralazine (Apresoline) | | | |
| Loop diuretics | Excretion | ↑ Renal excretion | Na, K, Ca, Cr, Mg, Zn, vitamins $B_1$, $B_6$ |
| Furosemide (Lasix) | | | |
| Thiazide diuretics | Excretion | ↑ Renal excretion | Na, K, Mg, Zn |
| Hydrochlorothiazide (HCTZ) (HydroDIURIL) | | | |
| Triamterene/hydrochlorothiazide (Dyazide) | Excretion | ↑ Renal excretion | Na, Ca |
| | Metabolism | ↓ Dihydrofolate reductase | Folic acid |

| Drug | | | Nutrients |
|---|---|---|---|
| *Antihyperlipidemics* | | | |
| Cholestyramine (Questran) Colestipol HCL (Colestid) | Absorption | Adsorption to anion exchange resin | Vitamins A, D, E, K, B₁₂, beta carotene, folic acid, Ca, Fe, Zn |
| *Anti-Inflammatory Agents* | | | |
| Prednisone (Deltasone) | Metabolism | ↓ Hepatic/renal vitamin D hydroxylation | Vitamin D, Ca |
| Colchicine | Absorption | Mucosal injury | Vitamin B₁₂ |
| Sulfasalazine (Azulfidine) | Metabolism | ↓ Dihydrofolate reductase | Folic acid |
| Indomethacin (Indocin) | Absorption | Mucosal injury | Vitamin C, Fe |
| Sulindac (Clinoril) | Metabolism | ↓ Dihydrofolate reductase | Folic acid |
| Naproxen (Naprosyn) | | | |
| Ibuprofen (Motrin) | | | |
| Aspirin | Absorption Excretion | Mucosal injury Competition for binding sites | Vitamin C, Fe Folic acid |
| *Antineoplastics* | | | |
| (General) | Absorption | Mucosal injury | Most nutrients |
| Methotrexate | Metabolism | Folate antagonist | Folic acid |
| *Antiulcer Agents* | | | |
| H₂ receptor antagonists Cimetidine (Tagamet) Ranitidine (Zantac) Famotidine (Pepcid) | Absorption | ↓ Gastric acid secretion | Vitamin B₁₂, folic acid, Fe, Zn |
| | Metabolism | ↓ Hepatic/renal vitamin D hydroxylation | Vitamin D, calcium |
| Proton pump inhibitors Omeprazole (Prilosec) | Absorption | ↓ Gastric acid secretion | Vitamin B₁₂, folic acid, Fe, Zn |
| Lansoprazole (Prevacid) | Metabolism | ↓ Hepatic/renal vitamin D hydroxylation | Vitamin D, calcium |
| Antacids | | | |
| Aluminum and magnesium hydroxides (Amphogel, Maalox, Mylanta) | Absorption | Precipitation ↓ Gastric acid secretion | Phosphate Vitamin B₁₂, folic acid, Fe, Zn |

*continues*

**Table 14–7** continued

| Drug Category/Medication | Kinetic Alteration | Mechanism | Affected Nutrient |
|---|---|---|---|
| Na bicarbonate (Alka-Seltzer) | Absorption | ↓ Gastric acid secretion | Vitamin $B_{12}$, folic acid, Fe, Zn |
| *Laxatives* | | | |
| Lubricants | | | |
| Mineral oil (Haley's M-O) | Absorption | Solubilization | Vitamins A, D, E, K, beta carotene |
| Stimulant cathartics | | | |
| Phenolphthalein (Ex-Lax) | Absorption | ↑ GI motility | Ca, Vitamins D, K |
| Bisacodyl (Dulcolax) | | | |
| *Psychotherapeutics* | | | |
| Tricyclic antidepressants | Metabolism | ↓ Flavin adenine dinucleotide | Vitamin $B_2$ |
| Amitriptyline (Elavil) | | | |
| Nortriptyline (Pamelor) | | | |
| Imipramine (Tofranil) | | | |
| Desipramine (Norpramin) | | | |
| Doxepin (Sinequan) | | | |
| Neuroleptics | Metabolism | ↓ Flavin adenine dinucleotide | Vitamin $B_2$ |
| Chlorpromazine (Thorazine) | | | |
| Thioridazine (Mellaril) | | | |
| Fluphenazine (Prolixin) | | | |
| Thiothixene (Navane) | | | |

*Note:* ↑, increase/induce; ↓, decrease/inhibit; Δ, change.

and hyperglycemia, are associated with concurrent use of laxatives and thiazide diuretics.[78]

Anti-inflammatory drugs such as aspirin and indomethacin produce multiple small hemorrhages of the gastrointestinal mucosa, leading to iron-deficiency anemia and decreased absorption of vitamin C.[79] Chronic aspirin therapy is also associated with folic acid deficiency and macrocytic anemia; the greatest risk occurs in patients with a low intake of folic acid.[80] Colchicine has been noted to decrease the absorption of protein, fat, lactose, carotene, vitamin $B_{12}$, sodium, potassium, and bile acids as a result of villous damage.[81]

Physical and chemical interactions between food and drugs may also occur during enteral feeding through nasogastric tubes. For example, esophageal obstruction due to solidification of enteral feed refluxed from the stomach can occur in patients also being administered drugs, such as sucralfate, via the tube.[82]

## Metabolism

Drugs may act to inhibit the essential intermediary metabolism of a nutrient or to promote its catabolism. While these actions are sometimes put to therapeutic advantage (eg, with oral anticoagulants [vitamin K antagonists such as coumarin] and antineoplastics [folic acid antagonists such as methotrexate]), examples of unwanted interference must also be recognized. Drug interference of vitamin D metabolism with a secondary impairment of calcium absorption can result in osteomalacia. Anticonvulsants and sedatives/ hypnotics that induce hepatic microsomal drug-metabolizing enzymes may increase the demand for folic acid sufficiently to precipitate signs of deficiency.[84] Isoniazid[85] and hydralazine[86] may inhibit pyridoxal kinase suf-

ficiently to produce clinical symptoms of vitamin $B_6$ deficiency. Triamterene, for example, is a potent inhibitor of dihydrofolate reductase and may induce megaloblastosis in some patients.[87]

## Excretion

Drugs may act to increase the excretion of a nutrient by displacement from plasma protein-binding sites, chelation, or reduction of renal reabsorption. Aspirin competes for folic acid–binding sites on serum proteins and enhances the vitamin's excretion.[88] Long-term administration of penicillamine for rheumatoid arthritis results in chelation of essential minerals such as copper and zinc.[89] Although diuretic therapy effectively decreases the resorption of sodium, it also enhances the renal excretion of calcium, chromium, magnesium, potassium, and zinc.[90]

## Food Intake

In addition to their effects on absorption, metabolism, and excretion of nutrients, drugs also may affect nutritional status by altering food intake (Table 14–8). Several drugs have been noted to alter food intake, primarily through changes in appetite or the senses of taste and smell, or through their adverse gastrointestinal side effects.[91] Drugs may be hyperphagic or hypophagic, but the effects of drugs on appetite are strongly influenced by situational factors.[92] Psychotropic agents, such as the phenothiazines and benzodiazepines, improve mood and psychologic function, with a consequent increase in food intake in some individuals; however, in elderly patients, whose rate of drug metabolism is slow, these drugs may induce somnolence and lack of interest in food. Amitriptyline hydrochloride and related tricyclic antidepressants appear to stimulate appetite, but in el-

**Table 14–8** Drugs Inducing Alterations of Food Intake

| Hypophagia | Hyperphagia | Hypogeusia/Dysgeusia |
|---|---|---|
| Alcohol | Amitriptyline hydrochloride | Amydricaine |
| Amphetamine | Anabolic steroids | Amylocaine hydrochloride |
| Cisplatin | Benzodiazepines | Captopril |
| Cocaine | Buxclizine hydrochloride | Clofibrate |
| Diethylpropion hydrochloride | Chlorpropamide | d-Penicillamine |
| Hydroxyurea | Chlortetracycline | Encainide |
| Mazindol | Cyproheptadine hydrochloride | 5-Fluorouracil |
| Methotrexate | Glucocorticoids | Griseofulvin |
| Phenethylbiguanide | Phenothiazines | Lincomycin |
| Phenmetrazine hydrochloride | Reserpine | Lithium carbonate |
| | Tolbutamide | Methimazole |
| | | Methylthiouracil |
| | | Oxyfedrine |

derly subjects they can cause behavioral agitation that interferes with eating.[93] The oral hypoglycemic agents may stimulate appetite by pancreatic release of insulin.

Brief or prolonged periods of anorexia associated with drug therapy are often due to effects on the gastrointestinal tract. Antineoplastic drugs induce nausea, vomiting, and aversion to food.[94] Cardiac glycosides produce anorexia accompanied by nausea; high-dose treatment may result in digitalis cachexia.[95] Several antihypertensive drugs (eg, hydralazine, minoxidil, and diazoxide) are also associated with side effects of anorexia, nausea, vomiting, and diarrhea. Alcohol abuse can cause anorexia, but even elderly social drinkers tend to have lower food intakes than do age-matched nondrinkers. Some drugs (eg, lithium carbonate) produce an abnormal, unpleasant taste sensation (dysgeusia). A few drugs may also induce an unusual desire for certain foods, such as has been reported by patients taking diuretics who crave salt. Some drugs may induce untoward problems in the mouth that affect food intake, such as dry mouth (xerostomia), resulting from anticholinergic action of tricyclic antidepressants and tranquilizers; gingival hyperplasia, resulting from phenytoin; oral ulcerations, resulting from captopril; and parotid inflammation, resulting from guanethidine.

## FOOD EFFECTS ON DRUG THERAPY

The clinical effects of food on drug absorption and disposition, particularly in elderly patients and during chronic care, has not been well studied. Nonetheless, food and food components have been shown to interact with drugs in various ways.[96] Food may influence both the absorption and the presystemic metabolism of drugs, and these effects may be caused by food intake or by different nutrients or additives, food/fluid volume, or polycyclic hydrocarbons present in grilled foods. Whether the changes induced by food are clinically significant depends both on the type of drug and the extent of the change. Food-induced changes in drug therapy can be examined in much the same fashion as drug-induced changes in nutritional status.

## Absorption

Food and its constituents can influence drug absorption as a result of physical or chemical interactions between the food product and the drug or because of physiologic changes in the gastrointestinal tract induced by eating or drinking. The net effect of this interaction may be that drug absorption is reduced, slowed, or increased by food intake (Table 14–9).[97,98]

Food can act to alter the rate of gastric emptying and drug dissolution in the stomach. It can also increase the viscosity of the gastric medium, decreasing the rate of drug diffusion to mucosal absorption sites. Food can act as a mechanical barrier, preventing drug access to the mucosal surface. Food components can also act to complex or chelate drugs. The effect of food on drug absorption may also be dependent on the drug formulation. Generally, enteric-coated tablets appear to be most affected by foods, and drugs in solution may be least affected.[99]

Several food-related effects on gastrointestinal function that also affect drug absorption and may augment age-related changes include alteration in gastric emptying time; intestinal motility; splanchnic blood flow; and alteration in the secretion of bile, gastric acid, and digestive enzymes.[100] The ß-blocker drugs propranolol and metoprolol are better absorbed after meals because of food-related increases in splanchnic blood flow and reduced first-pass metabolism in the intestinal mucosa or liver.[101]

When the effect of food on drug absorption is related to interactions between the food and the drug in the gastrointestinal tract, then the timing of drug intake in relation to mealtime is of practical importance. Acetaminophen absorption, for example, is five times more rapid after fasting than after consumption of a high-carbohydrate meal containing large amounts of pectin.[102] Foods can also interfere with the mucosal transfer of drugs absorbed by active transport. Drugs such as levodopa and methyldopa, with structures similar to amino acids, are absorbed by the transport mechanism for amino acids.[103] Competition for transport between the drug and amino acids from protein in the diet diminishes drug uptake and appears responsible for the "on-off" phenomenon of levodopa in patients with Parkinson's disease.[104] In elderly patients, particularly those who have difficulty with mastication or who have had gastric surgery, long-term cimetidine administration, coupled with high fiber intake, may lead to the formation of phytobezoars.[105]

The effects of changes in gastric emptying time on drug absorption are dependent on the water solubility of the drug; drugs with very low solubility are better absorbed when they remain longer in the stomach, as they will do after large, hot, or high-fat meals.[106] For drugs that are weak bases (such as amitriptyline hydrochloride, diazepam, and pentazocine), gastric emptying rate is critical, as absorption occurs in the less acidic intestine. The gastric emptying time is approximately 50 minutes in young, healthy volunteers but greater than 120 minutes in subjects over age 77 years.[107] Food-induced decreases in gastric clearance can cause more of drugs such as digoxin, levodopa, and penicillin to be metabolized in the stomach and less of the unchanged drug to be available for absorption, resulting in an erratic therapeutic response.[31] Changes in gastric emptying affect mainly drugs that are rapidly absorbed or that have a short biologic half-life.

## Distribution

Nutritional influences on drug distribution appear to be limited to the large reduction of plasma albumin seen in poorly nourished ge-

**Table 14–9** The Potential Effect of Food on Drug Absorption

### Drug Absorption Reduced by Food

| | | |
|---|---|---|
| Amoxicillin | Ethanol | Penicillamine |
| Ampicillin | Hydrochlorothiazide | Penicillin |
| Aspirin | Isoniazid | Phenytoin |
| Atenolol | Ketoconazole | Rifampin |
| Captopril | Levodopa | Tetracycline |
| Cephalexin | Lincomycin | Theophylline |
| Doxycycline | Nafcillin | |

### Drug Absorption Delayed by Food

| | | |
|---|---|---|
| Amoxicillin | Digoxin | Quinidine |
| Aspirin | Furosemide | Sulfadiazine |
| Cefaclor | Glipizide | Sulfasoxazole |
| Cimetidine | Metronidazole | Theophylline |
| Diclofenac | Phenytoin | Valproic acid |

### Drug Absorption Increased by Food

| | | |
|---|---|---|
| Carbamazepine | Griseofulvin | Metoprolol |
| Chlorothiazide | Hydralazine | Nitrofurantoin |
| Diazepam | Hydrochlorothiazide | Phenytoin |
| Dicoumarol | Lithium | Propranolol |

riatric patients. However, even in well-nourished, healthy individuals, albumin concentrations have been found to be lower than those in young adults.[108] Therefore, for extensively protein-bound drugs, such as diazepam and warfarin, a reduced binding capacity in old age results in an increase in the drugs' free fractions so that lower ranges of therapeutic and toxic plasma concentrations can be anticipated.[109] Dietary fats may modify drug distribution; free fatty acids compete for anionic binding sites on plasma albumin, increasing the pharmacologic activity of displaced drugs.

## Metabolism

Diet and nutritional status may have a marked effect on the way drugs are metabolized, although studies in this area have rarely been conducted on elderly subjects.[110] As previously noted, rates of drug metabolism decrease with age, so this type of interaction is likely to be more marked in older adults.[111] In studies conducted on healthy young men given antipyrine or theophylline during sequential feeding of high-carbohydrate, high-fat, or high-protein diets, the rate of drug elimination was slowest when the high-carbohydrate diet was fed and fastest during the high protein period.[112,113] The high-fat diet produced a small decrease in the rate of antipyrine loss but did not alter theophylline pharmacokinetics. Reduced drug clearance has been demonstrated in lactovegetarians, whose diets are characterized by a low protein intake.[114] Balanced-protein diets produce an acid urine, whereas low-protein diets usually result in an alkaline urine. Many elderly patients switch to low-protein diets with advancing age, and drug elimination patterns consequently may change.

Subjects who switch between saturated and polyunsaturated dietary fats show a concurrent alteration in plasma lipids but no change in cytochrome P-450–mediated drug metabolism.[115] In cases of mild or moderate undernutrition, particularly in adults, the rate of drug metabolism has been found to be either normal or slightly increased.[116] Only in severely malnourished adults with nutritional edema is drug metabolism impaired, with significant increases in plasma half-life of the drug.

Natural non-nutrient components of the diet may exert a profound influence on the rate of drug metabolism, and these effects may occur rapidly after food ingestion. Indolic compounds in vegetables of the Brassica family such as broccoli, Brussels sprouts, cabbage, and cauliflower, stimulate the rate of drug metabolism in humans.[118–120] Flavones (flavonoids) occurring in citrus and other fruits, and polycyclic aromatic hydrocarbons generated during charcoal broiling, stimulate liver microsomal drug metabolism.[121,122] Grapefruit juice can inhibit the presystemic metabolism of drugs metabolized by the 3A4 form of cytochrome P-450 in the small intestine.[123] Concern has been expressed that this interaction may have a clinically significant impact with carbamazepine, cyclosporine, terfenadine, several dihydropyridines (eg, felodipine, nifedipine, and nisoldipine), and short-acting benzodiazepines like triazolam.[124–127] The impact of this interaction may present serious adverse effects such as hypotension and tachycardia by dihydropyridines and increased sedation by benzodiazepines. On the other hand, there is potential to employ the inhibition of cytochrome P-450 by grapefruit juice therapeutically—for example, to increase the bioavailability of poorly absorbed cyclosporine and rapidly metabolized HIV protease inhibitors like saquinavir.[128,129] However, it has not been established whether elderly people are as susceptible as younger people to this type of induction and inhibition of hepatic and intestinal enzymes. Alterations of intestinal microflora produced by changes in the dietary level or source of protein or fiber may also influence intestinal drug metabolism.

## EFFECT OF NUTRIENT SUPPLEMENTS ON DRUG THERAPY

Nutrient supplements are required by those on chronic drug regimens when a risk of progressive nutrient depletion exists as well as when a nutrient deficiency induced by the drug is present[20] (Table 14–10). Appropriate levels of vitamin supplementation have been proposed for specific drug therapies.[6] It is fairly common for drug-related depletion of nutrients in geriatric patients to be complicated by dietary inadequacy or by disease states that induce nutrient deficiencies. Despite such well-justified therapeutic needs for nutrient supplementation, it is important to recognize the extensive nature of self-prescribed supplement use among older adults. The estimated prevalence of nutrient supplementation in the elderly ranges from 30% to 70%.[54] In one survey of middle-class elderly individuals who had no known medical illnesses and who were not taking prescription medications, the prevalence of nutrient supplement use was 60%.[130] While several of the factors discussed above suggest that there may be valid reasons to recommend nutrient supplementation for older adults, current trends indicate that their supplementation regimens are not always appropriate; self-se-

**Table 14–10** Chronic Drug Therapy and Nutrient Supplementation

| *Drug* | *Supplement* |
| --- | --- |
| Antacids | Folic acid |
| Aspirin | Folic acid, iron, vitamin C |
| Chlortetracycline | Calcium, vitamin C, vitamin $B_2$ |
| Cholestyramine resin | Vitamins A, D, E, K, folic acid, calcium |
| Colestipol | Vitamins A, D, E, K, folic acid, calcium |
| Estrogens/progestin | Vitamin $B_6$, folic acid |
| Hydralazine hydrochloride | Vitamin $B_6$ |
| Phenothiazines | Vitamin $B_2$ |
| Phenytoin | Folic acid, vitamin D, vitamin K, calcium |
| Primidone | Vitamin D |
| Rifampin | Vitamin $B_6$, niacin, vitamin D |
| Sulfasalazine | Folic acid |
| Tetracycline | Calcium, vitamin $B_2$, vitamin C |
| Triamterene | Folic acid |

lected supplements are not based on the individual's actual needs.

High-dose vitamin supplementation has been noted to produce an alteration of some drug effects. Megadoses of vitamin E potentiate the action of the anticoagulant warfarin and produce hemorrhage by further depressing the levels of vitamin K-dependent coagulation factors.[131] Vitamin D supplements can induce hypercalcemia and precipitate cardiac arrhythmias in patients receiving digitalis.[116] The administration of supplemental calcium can cause recurrence of atrial fibrillation in patients maintained on verapamil.[132] Excessive doses of vitamin C acidify the urine and may alter drug pharmacokinetics; acidic drugs are more readily absorbed, and basic drugs are more rapidly excreted from acidic urine.[133] Large doses of vitamin C may also inhibit the anticoagulant response of warfarin.[134] Niacin supplements may have an additional vasodilating effect, producing postural hypotension in patients receiving hypertensive drugs of the sympathetic blocking type, such as clonidine hydrochloride.[132]

An increase in seizure frequency and a corresponding decrease in serum phenytoin levels have been reported in epileptic patients receiving high-dose folic acid supplements.[135]

## IMPLICATIONS FOR AGING

The long list of identified drug-nutrient interactions does not implicate the production of a clinically significant adverse effect whenever the specific ingredients, namely the drug prescription and low intake of a nutrient, are present. However, both the nutrition- and drug-related risk factors for adverse interactions are greatest in elderly subjects because of the concomitant presence of age-associated conditions[136] (Table 14–11). The nutrient intakes of most older people are less desirable, so they present with suboptimal nutritional status at the outset of drug therapy. Elderly individuals are often prescribed multiple drugs requiring frequent administration over long periods of time. Age-associated diseases, changes in body composition, and changes in physiologic function contribute to

**Table 14–11** Risk Factors for Drug-Induced Nutrient Deficiency in the Elderly

*Drug-Associated Factors*
  Dose
  Duration
  Frequency
  Polypharmacy
*Nutrition-Associated Factors*
  Nutritional quality of diet
  Initial nutritional status
  Use of nutrient supplements
  Temporal relation between meals and drug
    administration
*Age-Associated Factors*
  Gastrointestinal changes
  Hepatic changes
  Renal changes
  Body composition changes
  Homeostatic changes
  Receptor-mediated changes
  Tissue sensitivity changes
*Pathologic Factors*
  Cardiovascular disease
  Gastrointestinal malabsorption
  Liver disease
  Renal disease

---

substantial alterations in drug pharmacokinetics and pharmacodynamics. Therefore, it is important to recognize the multifactorial diet-drug-age-disease interrelationships in determining the benefits and risks of any specific therapeutic intervention.

The medical treatment of geriatric patients often tends to include practices that do not fully consider the risk factors that contribute to drug-nutrient interactions. Physician advice to older patients to take medication with foods to decrease gastrointestinal side effects and enhance compliance may increase the chance of adverse interactions. Drug-nutrient interactions may also occur as a result of the common practice of passing drugs down nasogastric tubes used for enteral feeding. This practice can induce blockage of the tube

or reduce bioavailability because of physical incompatibility between the enteral formula and the drug. As discussed above, drug metabolism and efficacy may also be affected simply by changing the diet (eg, the protein content) or the timing between meals and drug administration. These situations point out the importance of close and frequent communication among physicians, dietitians, and pharmacists on the health care team. The widespread use of nutrient supplements among elderly people may adversely or beneficially influence the therapeutic outcome of drug treatment. Relatively frequent and careful evaluation through drug monitoring and nutritional assessment becomes critical in the geriatric patient.[137]

**CONCLUSION**

Nutritional deficiencies have been linked to increased susceptibility to disease and behavioral changes. Drug-induced vitamin and mineral deficiencies can lead to a host of symptoms, including anorexia, bone pain, confusion, and malaise, that mimic what are frequently considered as signs of old age.[137] Prolonged nutrient deficiencies can also result in conditions such as anemia, laryngitis and bronchitis,[138] carpal tunnel syndrome,[139] and postoperative confusion.[140] As described, the interactions between drugs and diet have implications for therapeutic outcome, and unless the health care team is aware of such relationships, the problem may be wrongfully attributed to other factors such as age. Application of existing knowledge about the relationships among pharmacology, nutrition, and aging can directly contribute to minimizing the iatrogenic impact of drug-nutrient interactions.

Carefully controlled clinical trials as well as hospital- and community-based epidemiologic studies are needed to identify further the risk factors associated with drug-nutrient interactions in geriatric patients. In some cases, the effects of age on drug disposition and action are of less importance than the effects of inappropriately concurrent drug and meal intakes, unscheduled changes in dietary regimens, or ill-considered polypharmacy regimens. There is therefore a need to develop methods of communication to transfer this information to geriatric patients and to their caregivers, including physicians, nurses, pharmacists, dietitians, and home care personnel. Means of communication between caregivers and education programs within geriatric institutions must be developed further so that the potential consequences of changes in diet or drug therapies are recognized by the appropriate individuals. While more research is necessary to identify and characterize the mechanisms and symptoms of drug-nutrient interactions in the geriatric patient, much can be done now through education and communication to recognize the risks and avoid their adverse consequences.

## REFERENCES

1. Powers DE, Moore AG. *Food-Medication Interactions*. Tempe, Ariz: FMI Publishing; 1983.

2. Roe DA, ed. *Drugs and Nutrition in the Geriatric Patient*. New York, NY: Churchill Livingstone Inc; 1984.

3. Roe DA, Campbell TC, eds. *Drugs and Nutrients: The Interactive Effects*. New York, NY: Marcel Dekker; 1984.

4. Basu TK. *Drug-Nutrient Interactions*. Deckenham, England: Croom Helm; 1988.

5. Roe DA. *Drug-Induced Nutritional Deficiencies*. Westport, Conn: Avi Publishing; 1985.

6. Roe DA. *Handbook: Interactions of Selected Drugs and Nutrients in Patients*. Chicago, Ill: American Dietetic Association: 1982.

7. Roe DA. *Drug and Drug Interactions*. New York, NY: Van Nostrand Reinhold; 1989.

8. Blumberg JB. Drug-nutrient interrelationships. In: Calkins E, Davis P, Ford A, eds. *The Practice of Geriatrics*. Philadelphia, Pa: WB Saunders Co; 1986.

9. Blumberg J. Clinical significance of drug-nutrient interactions. *Trans Pharmacol Sci.* 1986;7:33–35.

10. Hershey LA. Avoiding adverse drug reactions in the elderly. *Mt Sinai J Med.* 1988;55:244–250.

11. Roe, DA. Medications and nutrition in the elderly. *Primary Care Clin Office Pract.* 1994;21:135–147.

12. Young FE. Clinical evaluation of medicine used by the elderly. *Clin Pharmacol Ther.* 1987;42:666–669.

13. Diehl M, Lago D, Ahern F, et al. Examination of priorities for therapeutic drug utilization review. *J Geriatr Drug Ther.* 1991;6:65–85.

14. Kovar MG. Health of the elderly and use of health services. *Public Health Rep.* 1977;92:9–19.

15. Chen LH, Liu S, Cook-Newell ME, et al. Survey of drug use by the elderly and possible impact of drugs on nutritional status. *Drug-Nutr Interact.* 1985;3:73–86.

16. Cusak B, Denham MJ, Kelly JG, et al, eds. *Clinical Pharmacology and Drug Treatment in the Elderly*. Edinburgh, Scotland: Churchill Livingstone; 1984.

17. Shapiro S, Avery KT, Carpenter RD. Drug utilization by a non-institutionalized ambulatory elderly population. *Gerodontics.* 1986;2:99–102.

18. Hyans DE. Drug usage by the elderly. In: Roe DA, ed. *Drugs and Nutrition in the Geriatric Patient*. New York; NY: Churchill Livingstone; 1984; pp. 1–26.

19. Rikans LE. Drugs and nutrition in old age. *Life Sci.* 1986;39:1027–1036.

20. Lamy PP. Nonprescription drugs and the elderly. *Am Fam Physician.* 1989;39:175–179.

21. Lofholm P. Self-medication by the elderly. In: Kayne KC, ed. *Drugs and the Elderly*. Los Angeles, Calif: University of Southern California Press; 1979.

22. Swift CG. Prescribing in old age. *Br Med J.* 1988;296:913–915.

23. Lamy P. The elderly and drug interactions. *J Am Geriatr Soc.* 1986;34:586–592.

24. Long-term care of elderly patients: chronic disease co-morbidity and other considerations. *Consult Pharm.* 1995;10:583–595.

25. Greenblatt DJ, Sellers EM, Shader RI. Drug disposition in old age. *N Engl J Med.* 1982;306:1081–1088.

26. Schmucker DL. Drug disposition in the elderly: a review of the critical factors. *J Am Geriatr Soc.* 1984;32:144–149.

27. Blumberg JB. A discussion of drug metabolism and actions in the aged. *Drug-Nutr Interact.* 1985;4:99–106.

28. Robertson D. Drug handling in old age. In: Brocklehurst JC, ed. *Geriatric Pharmacology and Therapeutics.* Oxford, England: Blackwell Scientific Publications Ltd; 1984.

29. Klotz U, Avant GR, Hoyumpa A, et al. The effects of age and liver disease on the disposition and elimination of diazepam in adult man. *J Clin Invest.* 1975;55:347–359.

30. Greenblatt DJ, Allen MD, Harmatz JS. Diazepam disposition determinants. *Clin Pharmacol Ther.* 1980;27:301–312.

31. Lamy PP. Nutrition, drugs, and the elderly. *Clin Nutr (Phila).* 1983;2:9–14.

32. Cohen JL. Pharmacokinetic changes in aging. *Am J Med.* 1986;80:31–38.

33. Wallace SM, Verbeeck RK. Plasma protein binding of drugs in the elderly. *Clin Pharmacokinet.* 1987;12:41–72.

34. Kamataki T, Maeda K, Shimada M, et al. Age-related alteration in the activities of drug-metabolizing enzymes and contents of sex-specific forms of cytochrome P-450 in liver microsomes from male and female rats. *J Pharmacol Exp Ther.* 1985;233:222–228.

35. Greenblatt DJ, Allen MD, Harmatz JS, et al. The effects of age and liver disease on the disposition and elimination of diazepam in adult man. *J Clin Invest.* 1975;55:347–359.

36. Crooks J, O'Malley K, Stevenson IH. Pharmacokinetics in the elderly. *Clin Pharmacokinet.* 1976;1:280–285.

37. Vestal RE, Woods JA, Branch RA, et al. Studies of drug disposition in the elderly using model compounds. In: Kitani K, ed. *Liver and Aging.* Amsterdam, Netherlands: Elsevier-North Holland; 1978.

38. Kitani K. Hepatic drug metabolism in the elderly. *Hepatology.* 1986;6:316–319.

39. Sutter MA, Gibson G, Williamson LS, et al. Comparison of the hepatic mixed function oxidase systems of young, adult and old non-human primates (*Macaca nemiestrina*). *Biochem Pharmacol.* 1985;34:2983–2987.

40. Maloney AG, Schmucker DL, Vessey DS, et al. The effects of aging on the hepatic microsomal mixed-function oxidase system of male and female monkeys. *Hepatology.* 1986;6:282–287.

41. Kitani K. The role of the liver in the pharmacokinetic and pharmacodynamic alterations in the elderly. In: Waddington JL, O'Malley K, eds. *Therapeutics in the Elderly.* Amsterdam, Netherlands: Elsevier Scientific Publishers BV; 1985.

42. Davies DF, Shock NW. Age changes in glomerular filtration rate, effective renal plasma flow, and tubular excretory capacity in adult males. *J Clin Invest.* 1950;29:496–507.

43. Rowe JW, Andres R, Tobin JD, et al. Age-adjusted standards for creatinine clearance. *Ann Intern Med.* 1976;84:567–569.

44. Chan GL, Matzke GR. Effects of renal insufficiency on the pharmacokinetics and pharmacodynamics of opioid analgesics. *Drug Intell Clin Pharm.* 1987;21:773–783.

45. Roth GS. Hormone receptor changes during adulthood and senescence: significance for aging research. *Fed Proc.* 1979;38:1910–1914.

46. Feldman RD, Limbird RE, Nadeau J, et al. Alterations in leukocyte beta-receptor affinity with aging: a potential explanation for altered beta-adrenergic sensitivity in the elderly. *N Engl J Med.* 1984;310:815–819.

47. Scott PJ, Reid JL. The effect of age on the response of human isolated arteries to noradrenaline. *Br J Clin Pharmacol.* 1982;13:237–239.

48. Lamy PP. Age-associated pharmacodynamic changes. *Methods Find Exp Clin Pharmacol.* 1987;9:153–159.

49. Gribbin B, Pickering TG, Sleight P, et al. Effect of age and high blood pressure on baroreflex sensitivity in man. *Circ Res.* 1971;29:424–431.

50. Kohn RR. Human aging and disease. *J Chronic Dis.* 1983;16:5–21.

51. Vestal RE. Drug use in the elderly: a review of problems and special considerations. *Drugs.* 1978;16:358–382.

52. Lamy PP. *Prescribing for the Elderly.* Littleton, Mass: PSG Publishing Co Inc; 1980.

53. Orlander P, Johnson DG. Endocrinologic problems in the aged. *Otolaryngol Clin North Am.* 1982;15:439–449.

54. Hartz SC, Blumberg JB. Use of vitamin and mineral supplements by the elderly. *Clin Nutr (Phila.)* 1986;5:130–136.

55. Glanz K. Compliance with dietary regimens. *Prevent Med.* 1980;9:787–791.

56. Colucci RA, Bell SJ, Blackburn GL. Nutritional problems of institutionalized and free-living elderly. *Compr Ther.* 1987;13:20–28.

57. Roe DA. Concurrent interactions of drugs with nutrients. In: Linder MC, ed. *Nutritional Biochemistry and Metabolism with Clinical Applications.* New York, NY: Elsevier Science Publishing Co Inc; 1985.

58. Roe DA. Nutrient and drug interactions. *Nutr Rev.* 1984;42:141–154.

59. Roe DA. Pathological changes associated with drug-induced malnutrition. In: Sidransky H, ed. *Nutritional Pathology.* New York, NY: Marcel Dekker Inc; 1985.

60. Streeter AM, Goldston KJ, Bathur FA, et al. Cimetidine and malabsorption of cobalamine. *Dig Dis Sci.* 1982;27:13–16.

61. Kassarjian Z, Russell RM. Hypochlorhydria: a factor in nutrition. *Annu Rev Nutr.* 1989;9:271–285.

62. Liber CS. Alcohol, protein nutrition and liver injury. In: Winick M, ed. *Nutrition and Drugs.* New York, NY: John Wiley & Sons; 1983.

63. Brodie MJ, Boobis AR, Hillyard CJ, et al. Effect of isoniazid on vitamin D metabolism and hepatic monooxygenase activity. *Clin Pharmacol Ther.* 1981;30:363–367.

64. Bengoa JM, Bolt MJG, Rosenberg IH. Hepatic vitamin D-25-hydroxylase inhibition by cimetidine and isoniazid. *J Clin Med.* 1984;104:546–552.

65. Robbro OT, Christiansen C, Lund M. Development of anticonvulsant osteomalacia in epileptic patients on phenytoin treatment. *Acta Neurol Scand.* 1974;50:527–532.

66. Hahn TJ, Birge SJ, Sharp CR, et al. Phenobarbital-induced alterations in vitamin D metabolism. *J Clin Invest.* 1972;51:741–748.

67. Miettinen TA. Effects of hypolipidemic drugs on bile acid in man. *Adv Lipid Res.* 1981;18:65–97.

68. West RJ, Lloyd JK. The effect of cholestyramine on intestinal absorption. *Gut.* 1975;16:93–98.

69. Roe DA. Adverse nutritional effects of OTC drug use in the elderly. In: Roe DA, ed. *Drugs and Nutrition in the Geriatric Patient.* New York, NY: Churchill Livingstone Inc; 1984.

70. Lotz M, Zisman E, Bartter C. Evidence for phosphorus depletion syndrome in man. *N Engl J Med.* 1968;278:409–415.

71. Rud Rk, Singer FR. Magnesium deficiency and excess. Annu Rev Med. 1981;32:245–259.

72. Insogna KL, Bordley DR, Caro JF, et al. Osteomalacia and weakness from excessive antacids. *JAMA.* 1980;244:2544–2546.

73. Benn A, Swan CJH, Cooke WT, et al. Effect of intraluminal pH on the absorption of pteroylmonoglutamic acid. *Br Med J.* 1971;16:148–150.

74. Fleming BJ, Genuth SM, Gould AB, et al. Laxative-induced hypokalemia, sodium depletion and hyperreninemia: effects of potassium and sodium replacement on the renin-angiotensinaldosterone system. *Ann Intern Med.* 1975;83:60–62.

75. Frame B, Guiang HL, Frost HN, et al. Osteomalacia induced by laxative (phenolphthalein) ingestion. *Arch Intern Med.* 1971;128:794–796.

76. Donowitz M, Binder HJ. Effect of dioctylsulfosuccinate on colonic fluid and electrolyte movement. *Gastroenterology.* 1975;69:941–950.

77. Heiser WD, Warshaw AL, Waldeman TA, et al. Protein losing gastroenteropathy and malabsorption associated with factitious diarrhea. *Arch Intern Med.* 1968;68:839–851.

78. Roe DA. Drug interference with the assessment of nutritional status. *J Clin Lab Med.* 1981;1:647–664.

79. Leonards JH, Levy G. Gastrointestinal blood loss during prolonged aspirin administration. *N Engl J Med.* 1973;289:1020.

80. Gouf KR, McCarthy C, Read AE, et al. Folic acid deficiency in rheumatoid arthritis. *Br Med J.* 1964;1:212–216.

81. Race TF, Paes IC, Faloon WW. Intestinal malabsorption induced by oral colchicine: comparison with neomycin and cathartic agents. *Am J Med Sci.* 1970;259:32–41.

82. Garcia-Luna P, Garcia E, Pereira JL, et al. Esophageal obstruction by solidification of the enteral feed: a complication. *Intensive Care Med.* 1997;23:790–792.

83. Keith DA, Gundberg CM, Japour A, et al. Vitamin K-dependent proteins and anticonvulsant medication. *Clin Pharmacol Ther.* 1983;34:529–532.

84. Maxwell JD, Hunter J, Stewart DA, et al. Folate deficiency after anticonvulsant drugs: an effect of hepatic enzyme induction? *Br Med J.* 1972;1:297–299.

85. Vilter RW. The vitamin $B_6$-hydrazide relationship. In: Harris RS, Loraine JA, Wool IG, eds. *Vitamins and Hormones.* New York, NY: Academic Press; 1964.

86. Kirkendall WM, Page EB. Polyneuritis occurring during hydralazine therapy: report of two cases and discussions of adverse reactions to hydralazine. *JAMA.* 1958;167:427–432.

87. Corcino J, Waxman S, Herbert V. Mechanism of triamterene-induced megaloblastosis. *Ann Intern Med.* 1970;73:419–424.

88. Lawrence VA, Lowenstein JE, Eichner ER. Aspirin and folate binding: in vivo and in vitro studies of serum binding and urinary excretion of endogenous folate. *J Lab Clin Med.* 1984;103:944–948.

89. Day AT, Golding JR, Lee PN, et al. Penicillamine in rheumatoid disease: a long term study. *Br Med J.* 1974;1:180–183.

90. Wester PO. Zinc curing diuretic treatment. *Lancet.* 1975;1:578.

91. Pawan GLS. Drugs and appetite. *Proc Nutr Soc.* 1974;33:239–244.

92. Syiel JN, Liddle GW, Lacey WW. Studies of the mechanism of cyproheptadine-induced weight gain in human subjects. *Metabolism.* 1970;19:192–200.

93. Paybel PS, Mueller PS, DeLa Vergne PM. Amitriptyline weight gain and carbohydrate craving; a side effect. *Br J Psychiatry.* 1973;123:501–507.

94. Morrison SD. Origins of anorexia in neoplastic disease. *Am J Clin Nutr.* 1978;31:1104–1107.

95. Banks T, Ali N. Digitalis cachexia. *N Engl J Med.* 1974;290:746.

96. Roe DA. Food, formula and drug effects on the disposition of nutrients. *World Rev Nutr Diet.* 1984;43:80–94.

97. Toothaker RD, Welling PG. The effect of food on drug bioavailability. *Annu Rev Pharmacol Toxicol.* 1980;20:173–199.

98. Welling P. Nutrient effects on drug metabolism and action in the elderly. *Drug Nutr Interact.* 1985;4;183-193.

99. Rosenberg HA, Bates TR. The influence of food on nitrofurantoin bioavailability. *Clin Pharmacol Ther.* 1976;20:227–232.

100. Gibaldi M. *Biopharmaceutics and Clinical Pharmacokinetics.* Philadelphia, Pa; Lea & Febiger; 1977.

101. McLean AJ, Isbister C, Bobik A, et al. Reduction of first-pass hepatic clearance of propranolol by food. *Clin Pharmacol Ther.* 1983;30:31–34.

102. Lamy PP. *Prescribing for the Elderly.* Littleton, Mass: PSG Publishing Co Inc; 1980.

103. Gillespie NG, Mena I, Cotzias GS, et al. Diets affecting treatment of parkinsonism with levodopa. *J Am Diet Assoc.* 1973;62:525–532.

104. Nutt JG, Woodward WR, Hammerstad JP, et al. The "on-off" phenomenon in Parkinson's disease: relation to levodopa absorption and transport. *N Engl J Med.* 1984;310:483–488.

105. Nichols TW. Phytobezoar formation: a new complication of cimetidine therapy. *Ann Intern Med.* 1981;95:70–73.

106. Welling PG. Influence of food and diet on gastrointestinal drug absorption: a review. *J Pharmacokinet Biopharm.* 1977;5:291–315.

107. Evans MA, Triggs EJ. Cheung M. Gastric emptying in the elderly: implications for drug therapy. *J Am Geriatr Soc.* 1981;29:201–207.

108. McLennan EJ, Martin P, Mason BJ. Protein intake and serum albumin levels in the elderly. *Gerontology.* 1977;27:360–367.

109. Richey DP, Bender AD. Pharmacokinetic consequences of aging. *Annu Rev Pharmacol Toxicol.* 1977;17:49–65.

110. McDannell RE, McLean AEM. Role of nutrition status in drug metabolism and toxicity. In: Sidransky H, ed. *Nutritional Pathology.* New York, NY: Marcel Dekker Inc; 1985.

111. O'Malley K, Crooks J, Duke E, et al. Effect of age and sex on human drug metabolism. *Br Med J.* 1971;3:607–609.

112. Conney AH, Pantuck EJ, Juntzman R, et al. Nutrition and the chemical biotransformation in man. *Clin Pharmacol Ther.* 1977;22:707–716.

113. Alvares AP, Anderson KE, Conney AH, et al. Interactions between nutritional factors and drug biotransformations in man. *Proc Natl Acad Sci USA.* 1976;73:2501–2504.

114. Mucklow JC, Caraher MT, Henderson DB, et al. Relationship between individual dietary constitu-

ents and antipyrine metabolism in Indo-Pakistani immigrants to Britain. *Br J Clin Pharmacol.* 1982;13:481–486.

115. Anderson KE, Conney AH, Kappas A. Nutrition and oxidative drug metabolism in man: relative influence of dietary lipids, carbohydrate and protein. *Clin Pharmacol Ther.* 1979;26:493–501.

116. Krishnaswamy K. Drug metabolism and pharmacokinetics in malnutrition. *Trans Pharmacol Sci.* 1983;4:295–297.

117. Krishnaswamy K, Naidu AN. Microsomal enzymes and malnutrition as determined by plasma half-life of antipyrine. *Br Med J.* 1977;1:538–542.

118. Pantuck EJ, Pantuck CB, Garland WA, et al. Stimulatory effect of Brussels sprouts and cabbage on human drug metabolism. *Clin Pharmacol Ther.* 1979;25:88–95.

119. Williams D, Hill DP, Davis JA, et al. The influence of food on the absorption and metabolism of foods: an update. *Eur J Metab Pharmacokinet.* 1996;21:201–211.

120. Kall M, Vang O, Clausen J. Effects of dietary broccoli on human drug metabolizing activity. *Cancer Lett.* 1997;114:169–170.

121. Lasker JM, Wuang MT, Conney AH. In vivo activation of zoxazolamine metabolism by flavone. *Science.* 1982;216:1419–1421.

122. Slaughter DL, Edwards DJ. Recent advances, the cytochrome P450 enzymes. *Ann Pharmacother.* 1995;29:619–624.

123. Edwards DJ, Bernier SM. Naringin and naringenin are not the primary CYP3A inhibitors in grapefruit juice. *Life Sci.* 1996;13:1025–1030.

124. Grapefruit juice interactions with drugs. *Med Lett Drug Ther.* 1995;37:73–74.

125. Josefesson M, Zackrisson AL, Ahlner J. Effect of grapefruit on the pharmacokinetics of amlodipine in health volunteers. *Eur J Clin Pharm.* 1996;51:189–193.

126. Rau SE, Bend JR, Arnold MO, et al. Grapefruit juice-terfenadine single-dose interaction: magnitude, mechanism and relevance. *Clin Pharmacol Ther.* 1997;61:401–409.

127. Hukkinen SK, Varke A, Olkkaol KT, et al. Plasma concentrations of triazolam are increased by concomitant ingestion of grapefruit juice. *Clin Pharmacol Ther.* 1995;58:127–131.

128. Min DI, Hu YM, Perry PJ, et al. Effect of grapefruit juice on cyclosporine pharmacokinetics in renal transplant patients. *Transplantation.* 1996;62:123–125.

129. VanCleef GF, Fisher EJ, Polk RE. Drug interaction potential with inhibitors of HIV protease. *Pharmacotherapy.* 1997;17:774–778.

130. Garry PJ, Goodwin JS, Hunt MA, et al. Nutritional status in a healthy elderly population: dietary supplemental intakes. *Am J Clin Nutr.* 1982;36:319–331.

131. Megavitamin E supplementation and vitamin K-dependent carboxylation. *Nutr Rev.* 1983;41:268–270.

132. Garvadian-Ruffalo SM. Alterations in drug effects secondary to vitamin supplementation. *Intern Med.* 1984;5:129–137.

133. Levy G, Leonards JR. Urine pH and salicylate therapy. *JAMA.* 1971;217:81.

134. Rosenthal G. Interaction of ascorbic acid with warfarin. *JAMA.* 1971;215:1671–1672.

135. Rall TN, Schleifer LS. Drugs effective in the therapy of the epilepsies. In: Gilman AG, Goodman LS, Gilman A, eds. *The Pharmacological Basis of Therapeutics.* New York, NY: Macmillan Publishing Co; 1980.

136. Roe DA. Drug-nutrient interactions in the elderly. *Geriatrics.* 1986;41:57–74.

137. Lamy PP. Effects of diet and nutrition on drug therapy. *J Am Geriatr Soc.* 1982;30:S99.

138. Nauss KM. Vitamin A and human response. *Nutr MD.* 1982;8:1–5.

139. Ellis J, Folgers K, Levy M, et al. Therapy with vitamin B$_6$ with and without surgery for treatment of patient's idiopathic carpal tunnel syndrome. *Res Commun Chem Pathol Pharmacol.* 1981;33:331–335.

140. Older MWJ, Dickerson JWT. Thiamin and the elderly orthopaedic patient. *Age Ageing.* 1982;11:101–106.

# CHAPTER 15

# The Geriatric Exercise Prescription: Nutritional Implications

*Maria A. Fiatarone Singh*

## IMPORTANCE OF EXERCISE IN GERIATRICS AND GERIATRIC NUTRITION

At all ages, physical activity and exercise capacity play an important role in health promotion and disease prevention. Nowhere is this dual role more in evidence than in the care of geriatric patients. It is in this cohort that genetic susceptibility, lifestyle choices, accumulated burden of disease, accidents, and iatrogenic misfortunes intersect to weave an intricate tapestry that represents both current health status as well as prognosis for the coming years. As will be outlined in this chapter, the potent ability of physical activity and exercise patterns to influence this pathway at all levels beyond genetic susceptibility defines its importance. Physical fitness levels in old age have been shown to be directly related to functional limitations, as well as indirectly related through diseases associated with inactivity.[1] Thus, health care practitioners in all disciplines will be better able to serve their elderly clientele if they understand the theoretical basis for, and the practical implementation of, an exercise prescription for this population.

Physical activity exerts benefit at multiple levels, including amelioration of the biological changes of aging; prevention or delay in the development of risk factors for chronic diseases such as ischemic heart disease, stroke, diabetes, and osteoarthritis; primary prevention of some of the most common chronic diseases in the elderly; treatment for disabling geriatric syndromes not well addressed by standard medical practice; and adjunctive treatment for established disease (Table 15–1).

In addition, the pharmacotherapy offered for chronic disease may carry with it a burden of side effects, including often unrecognized nutritional consequences in the elderly patient. In these situations (Table 15–2), a novel combination of exercise and standard care may shift the risk/benefit ratio of treatment significantly. For example, some common yet unheeded side effects of long-term corticosteroid treatment for chronic obstructive pulmonary disease or inflammatory arthritis are severe osteopenia and osteoporotic fractures, proximal myopathy, and wasting. Progressive resistance training has been shown in both animals and humans to reverse losses of both muscle and bone mass associated with corticosteroid therapy alone.[2] Loss of lean tissue secondary to hypocaloric dieting, low protein diets in chronic renal failure, or disuse accompanying bedrest or decreased

**Table 15–1** Benefits of Exercise in the Elderly

I. Minimizing Physiologic Changes of
Aging
Atrophy of tendons and ligaments
Decreased aerobic and glycolytic
enzyme capacity
Decreased bone mass and fracture
threshold
Decreased capillary density
Decreased glycogen storage, insulin
sensitivity, glucose tolerance
Decreased maximal aerobic capacity
and cardiovascular efficiency
Decreased muscle mass and strength
Decreased tissue elasticity, joint
flexibility
Immunosenescence
Increased fat mass
Increased visceral adiposity
II. Decreasing Risk Factors for Chronic
Disease
Hyperglycemia/glucose intolerance
Hyperinsulinemia/insulin resistance
Hyperlipidemia
Hypertension
Obesity
III. Preventing or Delaying Onset of
Chronic Diseases
Breast cancer
Colon cancer
Coronary artery disease
Hypertension
Osteoporosis
Stroke
Type II diabetes mellitus

IV. Providing Adjunctive Treatment for
Established Diseases
Chronic obstructive pulmonary disease
Congestive heart failure
Coronary artery disease
Depression
Diabetes mellitus
Hypertension
Inflammatory arthritis
Obesity
Osteoarthritis
Parkinson's disease
Peripheral vascular disease
Stroke
Varicose veins
V. Preventing and/or Treating Common
Geriatric Syndromes
Anorexia/nutrient deficiencies
Constipation
Functional decline
Gait and balance disorders/falls
Incontinence
Insomnia
Low back pain
Low self-efficacy/low self-esteem
Social isolation/loneliness/low morale
Weakness

mobility with any acute or chronic illness may all be similarly attenuated by an appropriate prescription of resistive exercises in these situations.

Many diseases and medications are associated with anorexia and weight loss. It is often difficult to treat such patients with nutritional interventions alone, as their energy requirements are markedly blunted by both low muscle mass, and thereby basal metabolic rate, and restricted energy expenditure in physical activity. Attempts at nutritional supplementation with additional energy are often not successful in these situations, whereas individuals who begin an exercise regimen along with supplementation have been shown to be able to augment their total energy intake significantly.[3]

**Table 15–2** Counteracting Adverse Consequences of Chronic Disease Treatment with Exercise

| Disease Treatment | Adverse Consequence | Effective Exercise Modalities |
|---|---|---|
| Anorexia secondary to drug therapy (digoxin, serotonin reuptake inhibitors, theophylline, multiple drug regimens) | Weight loss, sarcopenia | Progressive resistance exercise* |
| Corticosteroid treatment for chronic pulmonary disease or inflammatory arthritis | Myopathy<br>Osteopenia, osteoporotic fracture | Progressive resistance exercise<br>Progressive resistance exercise and endurance exercise |
| Hypocaloric dieting for obesity | Loss of lean body mass (muscle and bone) | Progressive resistance exercise |
| Low-protein diet for chronic renal failure or liver failure | Weight loss, sarcopenia | Progressive resistance exercise* |
| Postural hypotension secondary to drug therapy (diuretics, antihypertensives, Parkinsonian drugs, antidepressants) | Postural symptoms, falls, fractures | Endurance exercise |
| Slowed gastrointestinal motility secondary to anticholinergics, narcotics, calcium channel blockers, iron therapy | Constipation, fecal impaction, reduced food intake | Progressive resistance exercise and endurance training* |
| Thyroid replacement for hypothyroidism | Osteopenia | Progressive resistance exercise and endurance exercise |
| Treatment with beta blockers or alpha-methyl dopa for hypertension or heart disease | Depression | Progressive resistance training or endurance training* |

*For these conditions, the benefit of exercise remains to be tested in controlled trials in patients receiving the indicated treatment. For example, exercise has been shown to speed gastrointestinal transit time and theoretically would counteract the constipating effect of listed medications.

Overall, the concept should be to implement, whenever possible, a multidisciplinary approach to the management of medical and nutritional disorders in the elderly, recognizing the vital interdependence of the elements of nutritional requirements, energy expenditure in physical activity, body composition, and the health and medication profile in geriatric practice.

## PHYSIOLOGIC CHANGES OF AGING THAT AFFECT EXERCISE CAPACITY

The important physiologic alterations in the elderly that affect exercise capacity are listed in Table 15–3. Although these changes affect peak athletic performance, they do not prevent physiologic adaptation to an appropriate exercise stimulus, even in individuals of very advanced age. The ability of exercise training to moderate or even reverse some of these changes suggests that a proportion of what we know as "aging" is not inevitable biologic progression but is attributable to disuse of organ systems over time. Unquestionably, certain age-related phenomena would persist despite athletic training, such as the decline in maximal heart rate or perhaps motor neuron death. However, the impact of such "unavoidable" physiologic aging is primarily limited to performance in athletic competitions and will cause little disability in daily functional activities for the otherwise healthy older adult.

## NUTRITIONAL DISORDERS IN THE ELDERLY AND THEIR IMPACT ON EXERCISE CAPACITY

Physiologic aging and chronic disease are not the only factors that limit functional capacity in the elderly. If nutritional deficiencies exist as well, the potential for clinically overt consequences for functional capacity is even greater (Table 15–4). Protein-calorie malnutrition, alone or in combination with catabolic diseases, will lead to loss of lean body mass. Loss of muscle mass may result in weakness, gait and balance disorders, falls and fractures, functional decline, and insulin

insensitivity and is thus one of the most important sequelae of malnutrition in the elderly.[4]

Micronutrient status is also important for physical function. Skeletal muscle expresses receptors for 1,25 dihydroxyvitamin D, which appears to be necessary for the rapid intracellular reuptake of calcium into the sarcoplasmic reticulum in the relaxation phase of myofilament contraction.[5] Muscle that cannot fully relax in this way cannot subsequently produce maximal force during the contractile phase, and this cycle results in clinical muscle weakness, particularly of the proximal muscles of the lower extremities. The proximal myopathy of osteomalacia is also associated with pain and atrophy in the affected muscle groups but is reversible with vitamin D repletion. High-risk individuals for this condition include homebound or institutionalized elders; those chronically receiving corticosteroids, dilantin, or phenytoin; those living in countries where dairy products are not fortified with vitamin D; or individuals abstaining from dairy products due to lactose intolerance or other reasons.

Other nutritional deficiencies that impair muscle contractile activity and result in clinical weakness include deficiencies of the minerals calcium, magnesium, and potassium. Thus, patients administered long-term or high-dose diuretic therapy are at highest risk. Furosemide will cause losses of all three minerals; thiazide-type diuretics will spare calcium but not the other two. Magnesium replacement is usually not offered even when potassium is replaced, and it should be remembered that intracellular stores of potassium cannot be repleted in the face of inadequate magnesium. Because serum levels of these minerals remain normal even when tissue stores are quite low, they are an insensitive index of deficiency states and should not be relied upon to determine the need for supplementation. Patents with no other defin-

**Table 15–3** Physiologic Changes of Aging That Impair Exercise Capacity

| Physiologic Change | Habitual Exercise Minimizes Change |
|---|---|
| Decreased glucose transport and glycogen storage capacity in skeletal muscle | Yes |
| Decreased capillary density in skeletal muscle | Yes |
| Decreased ligament and tendon strength | Yes |
| Decreased maximal aerobic capacity | Yes |
| Decreased maximal heart rate | No |
| Decreased maximal muscle strength | Yes |
| Decreased muscle endurance | Yes |
| Decreased muscle mass | Yes |
| Decreased muscle power | Yes |
| Decreased nerve conduction velocity | Yes |
| Decreased oxidative and glycolytic enzyme capacity in skeletal muscle | Yes |
| Decreased pulmonary flow rates | No |
| Decreased stroke volume | yes |
| Decreased tissue elasticity and joint range of motion | Yes |
| Degeneration of cartilage | Yes* |
| Increased fat mass and percent body fat | Yes |
| Increased heart rate and blood pressure response to submaximal exercise | Yes |
| Loss of motor neurons and motor units | Unknown |
| Prolonged neural reaction time | Yes |

*Although exercise-related injuries may result in chronic damage and degeneration of cartilage, habitual weight-bearing exercise without injury is protective to cartilage viability.

able cause for muscle weakness and fatigue who have risk factors for these mineral losses should be considered candidates for replacement or alternative drug therapy. Sometimes in the elderly, fatigue may be a more prominent complaint than actual muscle weakness in these conditions, so a thorough history and a high index of suspicion are essential to early diagnosis and treatment.

## ASSESSING THE ELDERLY PATIENT FOR EXERCISE CAPACITY AND NEEDS

With rare exceptions in the United States, the majority of elderly patients in any geriatric clinical setting will not have optimized their physical fitness level and physical activity habits when they present to their health care professional. Therefore, it is critical to assess the current fitness deficits in order to set appropriate goals and develop a rational and feasible exercise prescription for each individual. The stages necessary for the adequate assessment and recommendation of exercise modalities for the elderly are outlined in Table 15–5.

The first step is to take a current exercise history, much as one would gather dietary intake information before administering any nutritional counseling. The patient should be questioned about previous involvement in sport, recreational, and competitive activities, and information about any remote or chronic

**Table 15–4** Nutritional Deficiencies That Impair Exercise Tolerance

| Deficiency | Physiologic Consequence | Primary Exercise Capacity Affected |
|---|---|---|
| B$_{12}$ | Central and peripheral nervous system dysfunction | Muscle strength and power |
| Calcium | Muscle contractile dysfunction, cardiac conduction disturbance | Aerobic capacity; muscle strength, power, and endurance |
| Carbohydrate | Reduced glycogen storage | Aerobic capacity, musculoskeletal endurance |
| Energy | Sarcopenia, osteopenia | Aerobic capacity; muscle strength, power, and endurance |
| Iron | Decreased oxygen carrying capacity | Aerobic capacity |
| Magnesium | Muscle contractile dysfunction, cardiac conduction disturbance | Aerobic capacity; muscle strength, power, and endurance |
| Potassium | Muscle contractile dysfunction, cardiac conduction disturbance | Aerobic capacity; muscle strength, power, and endurance |
| Protein | Sarcopenia, osteopenia | Aerobic capacity; muscle strength, power |
| Thiamin | Nerve conduction impairment, myopathy, cardiac dysfunction | Aerobic capacity; muscle strength, power, and endurance |
| Vitamin D | Muscle contractile dysfunction and atrophy | Aerobic capacity; muscle strength, power, and endurance |

exercise-related injuries should be gathered. Current household, work-related, and recreational activities should be solicited and quantified in terms of days per week, weeks per year, average length of each session or activity, and how long this pattern has been followed. In addition, specific questions about distances walked per week (in miles or blocks) and number of flights of stairs climbed per week will provide useful information on which to build the prescription, as well as an index of current capacity. Scales such as the Harvard Alumni Questionnaire can be used to score this information in standardized formats, which have been linked to chronic disease outcomes and longevity itself.[6] Questions about the need for human or mechanical assistance with activities of daily living and household tasks will also point out where the greatest deficits in physiologic capacity lie. Individuals should also be asked about their preferred modes of exercise, specific dislikes or fears, preferences for lone or group activity, and potential limitations to increased activity levels imposed by spousal care, transportation, finances, and so forth.

**Table 15–5** Stages of the Exercise Prescription

1. Assess exercise needs/goals on the basis of history and physical and individual preferences.
2. Identify behavioral readiness to change; provide appropriate counseling for current stage.
3. Identify potential risk factors for exercise-related adverse events.
4. Prioritize physical activity needs in relation to risks.
5. Prescribe the specific exercise modality and dose desired.
6. Provide or refer for specific training, equipment advice, facility options, safety precautions.
7. Set up behavioral program for adoption, adherence, relapse prevention.
8. Monitor compliance, benefits, adverse events over time.
9. Modify exercise prescription as health status/goals/behavioral stage changes.

---

The physical exam will augment the above exercise history by highlighting physiologic deficits amenable to an exercise prescription. Although formal exercise testing, including maximal oxygen consumption, strength and power tests, range of motion and flexibility, and balance, would be ideal before the offering of advice, the time, equipment, and expertise for such testing are outside the realm of possibility for most health care practitioners who are not exercise physiologists or physical therapists. A simplified observational approach in the clinical setting will, however, guide the examiner quite adequately in conjunction with the history of health conditions and functional status.

First, ask the patient to sit in a straight-backed chair with the arms folded across the chest and the feet on the floor. Ask the patient to stand up as quickly as possible without using the arms to assist, and observe the result closely. If the patient takes more than 1 to 2 seconds to stand or cannot do so without using his or her arms to assist, lower extremity power (hip and knee extensors) is compromised, and strengthening is indicated. If the patient complains of pain in the knees with this maneuver, quadriceps strengthening will be able to improve function and mobility and reduce pain. If the individual stands up quickly but appears unsteady and wavering in the upright position, balance or postural hypotension may be a problem. Test the balance further at this point while the patient is in the standing position by asking him or her to stand for 15 seconds in each of the following positions: feet together, one foot halfway in front of the other (semitandem stand), with the heel of one foot directly in front of the toe of the other (tandem stand), on one leg only, and finally on one leg with the eyes closed. Most elderly people, even in the absence of disease, will not be able to hold the final two postures for 15 seconds without practice, but very early failures in this sequence indicate the need for specific balance training. Next, ask the patient to walk around a circular hallway or path that you have previously measured the distance of for 6 minutes without stopping, trying to cover as much distance as possible. Walk behind the patient and offer encouragement continuously while timing and observing closely for symptoms of dizziness, gait instability, claudication, angina, shortness of breath or wheezing, muscle weakness, joint pain, or overall fatigue. Patients with reduced aerobic capacity from any cause will walk only a few hundred feet to a thousand feet during this test, whereas fit adults may cover 3 to 4 times that distance. This 6-minute walk test has the advantage of being more tolerable than a treadmill test for frail elders, providing a quantitative outcome that can be remeasured over time as an index of improvement, being able to point out the specific physical symptom that is most limiting for the patient, being possible to complete even for those using ambulatory assistive devices or wheelchairs, and requiring only a stopwatch to perform.

The combination of history and physical tests outlined above will provide the necessary information to prioritize the components of the exercise prescription shown in Table 15–6. In general, if major deficits in strength and balance are identified, along with a history of mobility difficulties, functional decline, and falls, for example, resistance training and balance training should be undertaken before attempts to increase aerobic capacity. For completely sedentary adults and novices at regular exercise, compliance will be enhanced by suggesting only one type of new physical activity at a time. Giving back the capacity to lift one's body weight out of a chair and remain upright should always precede endurance activities such as walking to maximize function safely.

Simply identifying the appropriate exercise goals is not sufficient, however. It is equally important to identify what stage of behavioral change the person is in currently if the counseling is to have any effect. In the transtheoretical model of behavior, individuals advance through stages of precontemplation, contemplation, action, regular activity, and maintenance with regard to any behavioral choice.[7] Offering a "precontemplator" a free membership to a gym will be unlikely to induce exercise adoption, for example, whereas the same incentive given to someone who has advanced to contemplation or action stages may be just the motivation needed to start a regular new habit of physical activity. Once someone is in a regular pattern, behavioral incentives such as positive reinforcement, record keeping, external reminders of the desired behavior, goal setting, and

relapse prevention all work to keep the behavior continuous. Maintenance is a phase indicating at least 6 months of continuous adherence to the new behavior, whether it is exercise, dietary change, smoking cessation, or other lifestyle habits, and evidence indicates that recidivism is quite low if you can get patients to this point.[8] Most failures in any new behavior occur long before the 6-month interval has passed, so it makes sense to put in place rigorous behavioral programs in this critical initial period. These may take the form of supervised classes, logs to send in, rewards, telephone calls, financial incentives, or group support mechanisms.

To help patients advance through the behavioral stages or prevent relapse, it is important to identify the specific barriers to changing or maintaining the behavior in that individual. Many of the most often cited barriers to appropriate physical activity in the older adult are listed in Table 15–7. Some of these barriers are at a societal level (expectations, grandparent roles), others involve local regulations or geographical features, and others are personal (fear of injury, boredom, time constraints). In all cases, it is important not to assume that all old people are alike or function with similar reasoning as regards exercise participation. For some, offering exercise in a group setting may relieve fears and provide social support; for others, embarrassment over disabilities or skill level may make exercising at home a much more appealing option. Creativity in exercise planning is a key factor. If transportation is a major barrier, then exercise classes at a meal site where elderly vans are already in service can efficiently overcome this barrier. Perceived lack of time is a barrier frequently cited even by nursing home residents when asked why they do not exercise. It is helpful to go through a daily schedule, pointing out times when watching television or other sedentary activities can be

**Table 15–6** Exercise Recommendations for Older Adults

| Modality | Resistance Training | Cardiovascular Endurance Training | Flexibility Training | Balance Training |
|---|---|---|---|---|
| Dose | | | | |
| Frequency | 2–3 days/wk | 3–5 days/wk | 2–7 days/wk | 1–7 days/wk |
| Volume | 1–3 sets of 8–12 repetitions, 6–10 major muscle groups | 20–60 minutes | 4 repetitions, 30 s/ stretch, 6–10 major muscle groups | 1–2 sets of 4–10 different exercises, including static and dynamic postures* |
| Intensity | 15–17 on Borg Scale (80% 1RM), 10 s/ repetition | 12–13 on Borg Scale (45–80% maximal heart rate reserve) | Stretch to maximal pain-free distance and hold | Progressive difficulty as tolerated** |
| Requirements | Slow speed Good form No breath holding Increase weight progressively | Low-impact activity Weight bearing if possible | Nonballistic move-ments | Safe environment or monitoring Gradual increase in difficulty |

*Examples of balance-enhancing activities include t'ai chi movements, standing yoga postures, tandem standing and walking, standing on one leg, stepping over objects, climbing up and down steps, turning, and standing on heels and toes.

**Intensity is increased by decreasing the base of support (eg, progressing from standing on two feet while holding onto the back of a chair to standing on one foot with no hand support); by decreasing other sensory input (eg, closing eyes or standing on a foam pillow); or by perturbing the center of mass (eg, holding a heavy object out to one side while maintaining balance, standing on one leg while lifting other leg out behind body, or leaning forward as far as possible without falling or moving feet).

**Table 15–7** Barriers to Appropriate Physical Activity in the Elderly

* Acute and chronic medical problems and disabilities
* Caregiving role for sick spouse or family member
* Lack of interest
* Exaggerated perception of risk
* Financial limitations
* Geographical constraints and environmental design features
* Institutional/residential policies
* Lack of advocacy by family and health care community
* Lack of appropriately designed exercise equipment
* Lack of health care professional/caregiver/family education about exercise
* Perceived lack of time
* Psychological issues (depression, dementia, bereavement, self-efficacy, fear of falling, low self-esteem, social isolation)
* Reduced appreciation of benefit
* Societal norms/expectations of sedentariness
* Transportation difficulties

---

combined with flexibility, resistive, or even stationary aerobic exercise or when stairs can be substituted for elevators and escalators, for example. Balance exercises, such as standing on one leg, can be practiced whenever one is standing in line at a bank or supermarket. Breaking down the exercise prescription into such small pieces throughout the day will encourage the integration of a more active lifestyle into the daily routine most effectively for long-term adherence.

Some elderly patients will have medical problems that place them at higher risk for exercise-related adverse events. Examples include visual impairment, balance disorders, osteoarthritis of the shoulder or weight-bearing joints, low thresholds for ischemia or bronchospasm, peripheral vascular disease, and peripheral neuropathy. In general, problems can be avoided by providing monitoring if needed, exercising in adequate lighting, strengthening muscles around arthritic joints before weight-bearing exercise, and keeping intensity levels below those that produce cardiopulmonary symptoms. If the risk of ischemia is very high with aerobic exercise, then prescribing resistance exercises may offer similar benefits in terms of health and functioning with far less potential to provoke cardiac symptoms. If an older runner who likes competition is getting into difficulty with knee and ankle injuries, substituting a lower impact yet intense activity such as race walking can provide all of the physical and psychological benefits desired without the risk of musculoskeletal trauma. In all cases, it is important to balance the pleasurable components of exercise for the individual with the health-maintaining aspects important to the practitioner, or the prescription is likely to be unheeded in the long term.

Exercise prescriptions sometimes fail because they are too vague to be useful. The exercise prescription should be thought of like a medication—the patient needs to know the indication, type, dose, frequency, potential side effects, alternatives, and interactions with other nutritional or pharmaceutical preparations that he or she is already taking. The recommendations in Table 15–6 are consistent with the most recent guidelines of the American College of Sports Medicine for healthy and older adults[9,10] and represent dose ranges of exercise that have been shown to have benefit in terms of disease prevention and treatment as well as maintenance of cardiovascular and musculoskeletal fitness. Higher intensities or greater amounts of exercise may be undertaken for competitive purposes or in highly athletic individuals but are not required for general health in the elderly and are associated with greater risk of injury and higher dropout rates. Thus, a total of about 3 to 4 hours per week is sufficient to meet the requirements for all four modes of exercise, which is feasible for most individuals of retirement age.

Most geriatric patients will require more training than can be provided by the average health care professional without special exercise knowledge. Therefore, a referral to a qualified fitness instructor or physical therapist is often needed, along with explicit graphic instructions or videotapes. Such materials provide both knowledge and motivation for the novice exerciser, and having them on hand in the waiting room or office setting reinforces the power of the prescription and emphasizes the commitment of the practitioner to healthy lifestyle principles. Set up the behavioral program at the same time that the prescription is generated by giving the client an exercise calendar or diary to fill out each week, motivational tokens, and a plan for feedback on his or her progress at frequent intervals. If relapse is likely because of intercurrent illness, caregiving responsibilities, travel, or other identified problems, address these concerns early, and outline plans to anticipate and avoid such pitfalls. Ask about the compliance with the exercise prescription at every health care visit, as well as perceived benefits and adverse events that have occurred. Repeating the physical function testing that was used to generate the initial prescription can be very motivating, as the patient can be given direct feedback on the specific physical benefits attributable to his or her new physical activity pattern. As functional status improves, modify the exercise goals to emphasize new areas of fitness once the routine of regular physical activity has been firmly established. Shaping behavior in small increments is more likely to be successful than overwhelming an adult who has been

sedentary for 50 years with an overly ambitious plan of physical activity.

## MEDICAL SCREENING FOR THE EXERCISE PRESCRIPTION

Many sets of recommendations have been created in an attempt to make exercise as safe as possible for adults, especially those at risk for cardiovascular events.[11] Indeed, exercise carries with it the possibility of complications and adverse events, the most important of which are outlined in Table 15–8. The most feared events are the cardiovascular ones, although they are relatively rare even in cardiac rehabilitation settings, whereas the most common occurrences are minor musculoskeletal injuries. Most such injuries can be prevented by paying attention to proper technique, slowly progressing in intensity as tolerated, avoiding ambulatory activities until strength and balance are adequate to support the body weight safely, and abstaining from exercise during acute illness, extremes of temperature or humidity, or the appearance of new, unidentified medical symptoms.

A broader use and definition of medical screening for exercise for the geriatric patient is suggested. Rather than asking yourself "Is this patient safe to exercise?" you might pose the question "Is this patient safe to be sedentary?" It is important to keep in mind that sedentariness is the lethal condition and that habitual exercise protects against many major chronic diseases, as well as being indicated in their treatment. In this broader concept of screening, therefore, the practitioner should be alert to the presence of sedentariness itself as a risk factor for disease and disability, to chronic diseases that are amenable to physical activity, to readiness to change behavior, and finally to exacerbations of chronic diseases that should be brought to the attention of a physician, regardless of whether an exer-

**Table 15–8** The Risks of Exercise in the Elderly

| Musculoskeletal | Cardiovascular | Metabolic |
|---|---|---|
| Falls | Arrhythmia | Dehydration |
| Foot ulceration or laceration | Cardiac failure | Electrolyte imbalance |
| Fracture, osteoporotic or traumatic | Hypertension | Energy imbalance |
| Hemorrhoids | Hypotension | Heat stroke |
| Hernia | Ischemia | Hyperglycemia |
| Joint or bursa inflammation, exacerbation of arthritis | Pulmonary embolism | Hypoglycemia |
| Ligament or tendon strain or rupture | Retinal hemorrhage or detachment, lens detachment | Hypothermia |
| Muscle soreness or tear | Ruptured aneurysm | Seizures |
| | Syncope or postural symptoms | |

cise prescription is about to be given. In general, hypertension, angina, diabetes, pulmonary disease, obesity, neurologic disease, and arthritis are indications for exercise as long as they are in control, rather than contraindications to more activity.

Some specific areas of concern in the older adult include cardiopulmonary status, musculoskeletal integrity, mental status, podiatric problems, and vision. It is important to know an individual's pattern of angina or shortness of breath and the level of exertion that produces it. Any change in chronic patterns warrants referral to a medical practitioner. For most cardiopulmonary symptoms, activity should be stopped at their onset. The notable exception to this is claudication; evidence indicates that walking a little further once the pain begins is the most effective way to extend the time to claudication and improve pain-free walking distances. Cardiac stress testing should be done for standard medical indications in consultation with the patient's physician, and not simply because an asymptomatic older adult wants to begin a moderate exercise regimen. Requiring such testing before any exercise could be undertaken would

pose an enormous psychological and financial disincentive to physical activity and would be likely to result in positive tests in many asymptomatic individuals, which would then require further medical testing such as thallium stress testing or angiography to resolve.

For patients with pulmonary disease, symptoms at rest and with exertion should be elicited, as well as determination of the need for supplemental oxygen during exercise. Plan the use of inhalers if needed for 15 to 30 minutes before exercise to allow maximum effect, and keep them on hand during all sessions. During febrile episodes or acute flares of disease, exercise should be avoided, as the risk of cardiac arrhythmias and pulmonary edema is high during this time in the elderly. Some patients may not tolerate aerobic activity at all but are able to perform resistance, balance, and flexibility exercises, which are much less consumptive of oxygen, without any difficulty. It is important to remember that the catabolic effects of chronic pulmonary disease, often accompanied by anorexia, malnutrition, and corticosteroid treatment, produce severe losses of lean tissue (muscle and bone). Such losses cannot be counter-acted by cardiovascular endurance training alone but require the adaptive response to re-sistive exercise to reverse this wasting pro-cess. Therefore, patients with the most severe lung disease, who are least likely to be able tolerate aerobic activities, in fact are more likely to benefit in terms of body composition and function from weight-lifting exercise.

Identification of depression, anxiety, or in-somnia on screening is important, as these conditions all benefit from both resistive and aerobic exercise. Severe withdrawal or leth-argy may require additional treatment and make an unsupervised exercise prescription unlikely to succeed. Cognitive impairment is not a contraindication to exercise but may ne-cessitate close supervision, group exercise, and safety precautions. Often a nonimpaired spouse or home care worker can be helpful as a walking partner or exercise trainer for those living at home. In an institutional setting, de-mented patients can successfully participate in all kinds of exercise with adequate staff-to-patient ratios. Aggressive or disruptive be-havior, poor safety awareness and judgment, or uncontrolled alcohol intake should be screened for, as these will dictate the feasibil-ity of group or isolated activity.

Many exercise-related injuries are related to the foot and ankle, although most are pre-ventable with proper foot care, shoes, socks, orthotics, assistive devices, and avoidance of high-impact activities. Look for ulcers, fun-gal infections, peripheral neuropathy, infec-tions, edema, ischemic changes, skin rashes or breakdown, calluses, bunions, ingrown or long toenails, and painful points on the ankle, heel, and foot. Those patients with peripheral vascular disease or neuropathy should be par-ticularly careful about sudden increases in weight-bearing activities. If ulcers develop on the foot or ankle and ambulation is re-stricted temporarily, advise the patient to sub-stitute seated weight-lifting exercises to pre-vent disuse atrophy from occurring during this period of reduced activity. It is wise to have a family member check the feet, particu-larly in diabetics who may also have visual impairment that prevents them from seeing early problems as they develop. Shoes with the lowest comfortable heel and nonslip soles are important, particularly in those with bal-ance impairment at risk for falls.

Visual problems are common in the geriat-ric patient, and optimal lighting, exercise in the daylight hours, and use of corrective lenses at all times will minimize safety prob-lems. Those with active or newly treated pro-liferative retinopathy, retinal detachment, or cataract surgery should not perform any exer-cise that raises the blood pressure or lift weights until cleared by their ophthalmolo-gist. Substitution of stationary bikes, rowers, and steppers for other aerobic activities al-lows even completely blind individuals to ex-ercise vigorously without supervision, and these patients should not therefore be auto-matically denied an exercise prescription, as many such alternatives are now available.

## USE OF EXERCISE IN THE PREVENTION AND TREATMENT OF COMMON GERIATRIC SYNDROMES

The exercise prescription for general health addresses the four major components of fitness: strength, endurance, flexibility, and balance (Table 15–6). Therefore, the idea is to gradually get individuals to incorporate most or all of these modalities into their weekly routine, regardless of their specific medical history. Most chronic diseases and their associated disabilities in fact benefit from both resistance training and aerobic training at the dosages indicated in the table, so there is no need to develop a specific exercise prescription for every medical condition that someone has. This is particularly important for individuals who cannot participate in one mode of exercise at all. For example, the depressed, obese elderly woman with severe degenerative disease of the knees who cannot ambulate without severe pain will benefit in terms of mood, arthritis pain, mobility, and weight loss from resistive exercises, which can be performed without standing.

In addition to isolated diseases, there are many multifactorial syndromes with which geriatric patients commonly present and for which standard medical treatment often has little to offer. For these syndromes, exercise may be very therapeutic and have far fewer side effects than attempts at pharmacological management. Some of the most commonly encountered scenarios and suggested approaches to exercise management are listed in Table 15–9.

## PRACTICAL IMPLEMENTATION OF EXERCISE PROGRAMS IN THE CLINICAL SETTING

Ideally, the exercise prescription should be integrated with all other components of the individual's care plan, since it will affect functional capacity, health status, nutritional requirements, psychological status, and other lifestyle changes that may be addressed by other members of the health care team. Physicians should be aware of any new exercise prescription that may affect medication requirements or cause exacerbations of underlying conditions. Many individuals will start an exercise regimen when they are advised to lose weight, so the incorporation of nutri-

tional recommendations with activity suggestions is critical to the success of such attempts. Often, patients will have questions about what to eat when exercising or the need for special drinks, supplements, or protein sources. Guidelines for commonly encountered exercise-nutrition interactions are outlined in Table 15–10. In general, food sources are preferable to packaged supplements, and education regarding the often overstated advertising claims for many of these expensive products should be given to patients who might better spend their money on good athletic shoes or home exercise equipment.

Include discussions of physical activity patterns in team conferences and planning meetings. Make available easily completed forms for patient assessment in terms of exercise history, physical performance, exercise prescription, and activity logs. Add to the health library references on major exercise techniques and videotapes that can be viewed in the waiting room or even borrowed from the library for home use. Consider replacing several chairs in the waiting room or lobby with stationary exercise equipment along with tables of educational materials to read. Make sure that stairways are accessible and well lighted, have sturdy handrails, and are marked clearly to encourage use. Provide incentives for exercise adherence in the form of reduced fees, free exercise equipment, lottery tickets, or whatever is meaningful to the clientele in a particular setting. Practice good exercise habits yourself, as your prescription will carry a lot more credibility if your patient sees you following it yourself in the workplace. Most environments can be creatively modified to encourage rather than restrict activity; this is as true of the doctor's or nutritionist's office as it is of the nursing home. Many small spaces in such settings can be converted to "mini-gyms" with little capi-

**Table 15–9** Choice of Exercise for Common Geriatric Syndromes

| Syndrome | Therapeutic Exercise Recommendation |
|---|---|
| Anorexia | Endurance or resistance training before meals |
| Constipation | Endurance or resistance exercise |
| Depression, anxiety, low self-efficacy | Individual or group exercises, including endurance, resistive, and calisthenic activities as preferred |
| Fatigue | Endurance training in the morning hours; increase duration and intensity as tolerated |
| Functional dependency | Walking, stair climbing for endurance; resistance training of upper and lower extremities |
| Incontinence (stress) | Pelvic muscle strengthening (Kegel exercises); mobility improvement with endurance, balance, and resistance training as needed |
| Insomnia | Endurance or resistance exercise in midafternoon |
| Low back pain, spinal stenosis | Resistance training to strengthen the back extensor muscles, rectus abdominus, and hip and knee extensor muscle groups |
| Recurrent falls, gait and balance disorders | Lower extremity resistance training for hip, knee and ankle; balance training, t'ai chi, yoga, ballet; walking in safe or supported environment; training in use of ambulatory device as needed |
| Weakness | Moderate- to high-intensity resistance training for all major muscle groups |

tal investment and may be the seed from which much larger programs develop.

Physical fitness is not merely a medical prescription or treatment; it is a right of individuals, both fit and frail, and thus caregivers, family members, and volunteers are responsible for providing education, opportunity, and access in this domain to the eldest members of our communities. Health care practices and policies for the elderly should be enlarged to promote fitness, activity, and independence to the fullest extent possible for each individual as an important component of overall quality of life.

**Table 15–10** Nutritional Recommendations for the Physically Active Older Adult

1. Encourage extra water intake (500–1000 mL) on exercise days, especially in those on diuretics or very low-sodium diets, during high ambient temperatures or humid conditions, and after recovery from dehydrating illnesses or fevers; sport drink formulations are unnecessary for fluid replacement under normal conditions and in noncompetitive athletes.

2. If a goal is fat/weight loss, combine exercise with a balanced hypocaloric diet, and supplement with multivitamin at RDA levels.

3. If goal is weight maintenance, counsel on increased energy intake (with normal ratios of fat/carbohydrate/protein) as food rather than supplements; encourage dietary diversity to fulfill energy requirements and supply micronutrient needs.

4. If goal is weight gain, add nutrient- and calorically dense food snacks between meals and after exercise sessions.

5. There is no need to supplement protein beyond 1.0 to 1.2 g/kg/per day, which can be achieved with diverse dietary sources rather than amino acid or protein supplements.

6. In diabetics, time exercise sessions for the postprandial peaks in blood glucose (1.5 to 2 hours after a meal); keep high carbohydrate and concentrated sugar snacks available during exercise sessions for brittle or insulin-dependent diabetics; advise against exercise after prolonged fasting or skipping meals.

7. Increase dietary or pharmacological sources of potassium and magnesium if levels are marginal or low, particularly in high-risk coronary artery disease or arrhythmia-prone patients on diuretics or digoxin.

## REFERENCES

1. Morey M, Pieper C, Cornoni-Huntley J. Physical fitness and functional limitations in community-dwelling older adults. *Med Sci Sports Exerc.* 1998;31:715–723.

2. Braith R, Welsch M, Mills R, Keller J, Pollock M. Resistance exercise prevents glucocorticoid-induced myopathy in heart transplant recipients. *Med Sci Sports Exerc.* 1998;30:483–489.

3. Fiatarone MA, O'Neill EF, Ryan ND, et al. Exercise training and nutritional supplementation for physical frailty in very elderly people. *New Engl J Med.* 1994;330:1769–1775.

4. Fiatarone M, Evans W. The etiology and reversibility of muscle dysfunction in the elderly. *J Gerontol.* 1993;48:77–83.

5. Jeejeebhoy KN. Muscle function and nutrition. *Gut.* 1986;27:25–39.

6. Paffenbarger RS, Wing AL, Hyde TR. Physical activity as an index of heart attack risk in college alumni. *Am J Epidemiol.* 1978;108:161–165.

7. Taylor C, Miller N, Flora J. Principles of health behavior change. *American College of Sports Medicine: Resource Manual. Guidelines for Exercise Testing and Prescription.* Philadelphia, Pa: Lea & Febiger; 1988:323–326.

8. King A, Taylor C, Haskell W, Debusk R. Strategies for increasing early adherence to and long-term maintenance of home-based exercise training in healthy middle-aged men and women. *Am J Cardiol.* 1988;61:628–632.

9. Pollock M, Gaesser G, Butcher J, et al. The recommended quantity and quality of exercise for developing and maintaining cardiorespiratory and muscular fitness, and flexibility in healthy adults. *Med Sci Sports Exerc.* 1998;30:975–991.

10. Mazzeo R, Cavanaugh P, Evans W, et al. Exercise and physical activity for older adults. *Med Sci Sports Exerc.* 1998;30:992–1008.

11. Balady G, Chaitman B, Driscoll D, et al. Recommendations for cardiovascular screening, staffing, and emergency policies at health/fitness facilities. *Med Sci Sports Exerc.* 1998;30:1009–1018.

# CHAPTER 16

# Nutritional Assessment of the Elderly

*Carol O. Mitchell and Ronni Chernoff*

One of the more challenging aspects of providing nutrition to elderly individuals is the determination of their nutritional status. Aging has an effect on many of the anthropometric, biochemical, and hematologic parameters commonly used to assess nutritional status in younger adults. Adding to the difficulty of evaluating the results of these measures is the fact that people age at individual rates, thus contributing to the heterogeneity of the older group. To make a considered judgment about the need for nutritional interventions or the possibility of nutritional depletion that may have an impact on health, it is necessary to conduct a thorough, multifaceted nutritional assessment that examines many aspects of the individual to present the most complete picture possible. To evaluate the individual adequately, a thorough nutritional assessment should be made, including appraisal of physical appearance; oral health; social and environmental situation; potential physical and psychologic disabilities; medical and drug history; performance of anthropometric measurements; evaluation of biochemical, hematologic, and immune function; functional competence; and a comprehensive dietary history.

Conducting a comprehensive nutritional assessment is an important component of providing quality health care to elderly people; malnutrition may contribute to the depletion of reserve capacity or the ability to respond rapidly and appropriately to a physiologic insult. Malnutrition may be unrecognized in elderly subjects because many of the changes that are seen with inadequate nutrition are often associated with changes that occur with aging. Severely malnourished individuals are easier to identify than those who are mildly or moderately malnourished because the latter will not manifest overt signs of malnutrition. Many health care professionals are not attuned to the important role that nutrition has in the maintenance of health throughout life; therefore, subclinical or marginal nutritional deficits may go unnoticed and undocumented.[1]

## CLINICAL ASSESSMENT

### Physical Assessment

Malnutrition is the consequence of chronically inadequate intake of essential nutrients.[2] Replenishment of normal tissue requires protein, energy, vitamins, and minerals in amounts adequate to replace old cells with new ones, to repair damaged cells and tissues, and to make substrate for protein compounds such as antigens, hormones, and enzymes. For many anabolic processes, vitamins and miner-

*Oral Health*

*GI ROS: Diarrhea*
*Constipation*

**Table 16–4** Activities of Daily Living

**Toileting**
1. Cares for self; no incontinence
2. Needs to be reminded, or needs help with cleanliness; accidents rare
3. Soiling or wetting at least once a week
4. No control of bladder or bowels

**Feeding**
1. Eats without assistance
2. Eats with minor assistance or with help in cleanliness
3. Feeds self with assistance and is messy
4. Requires extensive assistance with feeding
5. Relies on being fed

**Dressing**
1. Is independent in dressing and selecting clothing
2. Dresses and undresses with minor assistance
3. Requires moderate assistance with dressing and undressing
4. Needs major assistance in dressing but is helpful
5. Completely unable to dress or undress oneself

**Grooming**
1. Always neatly dressed and well groomed
2. Grooming adequate; may need minor assistance
3. Requires assistance in grooming
4. Needs grooming care but is able to maintain groomed state
5. Resists grooming

**Ambulation**
1. Totally independent
2. Ambulates in limited geographical area
3. Ambulates with assistance (needs cane, wheelchair, walker, railing)
4. Sits unsupported in chair or wheelchair but needs help with motion
5. Bedridden

**Bathing**
1. Bathes self independently
2. Bathes self with help getting into bath or shower
3. Washes hands and face but needs help with bathing
4. Can be bathed with cooperation
5. Does not bathe and is combative with those trying to help

*Source:* Adapted with permission from M.P. Lawton, The Functional Assessment of Elderly People, *Journal of American Geriatric Society*, Vol. 19, p. 4465, © 1971, Williams & Wilkins.

## Cognitive and Psychologic Function

It is very difficult to demonstrate a relationship between cognitive function and nutritional status, but tests with standardized instruments designed to measure abstract thinking and problem-solving ability suggest a correlation.[36] There is some evidence that there is a relationship between cognitive functioning and vitamin deficiencies.[37] Depressed nutritional status may have some effect on cognitive measures, but a causal relationship between these variables has not been determined. It is well recognized that weight loss occurs in patients with senile dementia, such as Alzheimer's disease, but it is difficult to define the etiology of the weight loss.[38–40] Poor memory, loss of feeding skills, hyperactive behavior, anorexia associated with polypharmacy, and depression may contribute to poor dietary intake. Depression occurs commonly in institutionalized people and is recognized as a treatable cause of weight loss.[41] Changes in cognitive or psychologic function must be elicited from family members or caregivers and should be considered as possible etiologies in a chronically malnourished elderly patient.

**Table 16–5** Instrumental Activities of Daily Living

*Ability to use telephone*
1. Uses telephone without help
2. Uses telephone only with familiar telephone numbers
3. Answers phone but does not initiate calls
4. Does not use telephone at all

*Shopping*
1. Shops independently for all needs
2. Shops independently for minor purchases
3. Needs accompaniment on shopping trip
4. Completely unable to shop

*Food preparation*
1. Plans, prepares, and serves adequate meals independently
2. Prepares adequate meals if foods are provided
3. Heats and serves prepared meals *or* prepares meals that are not adequate
4. Needs to have meals prepared and served

*Housekeeping*
1. Maintains house alone or with occasional help with heavy work
2. Performs light daily housework
3. Performs light daily tasks incompletely
4. Needs help with all home maintenance tasks
5. Does not participate in any housekeeping tasks

*Laundry*
1. Does personal laundry completely
2. Launders small items independently
3. All laundry must be done by others

*Mode of transportation*
1. Travels independently on public transportation or drives car
2. Arranges own travel by taxi but does not use public transportation
3. Travels on public transportation with assistance
4. Travels by private transport with assistance
5. Does not travel at all

*Responsibility for own medications*
1. Is totally independent in managing medications
2. Takes own medications if prepared in advance
3. Is not capable of dispensing or managing medications

*Ability to handle finances*
1. Manages financial matters independently
2. Manages day-to-day finances but needs help with more complex tasks
3. Incapable of handling money

*Source:* Adapted with permission from M.P. Lawton, The Functional Assessment of Elderly People, *Journal of American Geriatric Society*, Vol. 19, p. 4465, © 1971, Williams & Wilkins.

## Socioeconomic Factors

Exploring the environment in which elderly people live is important to an understanding of their nutrition and health status. Financial resources, living situation, degree of independence, level of education, and social support systems are all factors that may influence nutritional intake. Many elderly people live on a fixed income, which limits their purchasing power when the cost of living increases. Of course, there is a large population of older people who have financial resources to meet their needs, but many do not. The ability to purchase fruits and vegetables in season and fresh meats may be limited, and this limitation may contribute to reliance on high-calorie, low–nutrient-density foods such as those high in carbohydrates and fats. Dietary supplements (eg, vitamin and mineral preparations), however, are used by some older individuals who probably do not require nutritional supplementation.[42]

Financial resources are a factor that determines living arrangements. Individuals who have adequate incomes may still live in their own homes. Many alternatives to housing are available for those who cannot afford to live alone or who need support in their activities of daily living, including group or foster homes, congregate living situations, retirement homes, and minimum to skilled care facilities. For elderly individuals who choose to live at home or alone, there are congregate meal programs, home meal programs, and home health aides. Access to these services has been shown to contribute to a more successful maintenance of health status and a more rapid recovery from an episodic illness.[43] Several studies indicate that elderly people who live alone or in institutions have dietary intakes below recommended levels.[44,45]

Educational level is linked to both income and nutritional status. Several studies have indicated that level (years) of education is associated with the dietary intake of several nutrients, such as protein, iron, calcium, and several of the B vitamins.[44,46,47]

Health and nutritional status have also been linked with accessibility of social support systems. There appears to be a relationship between health status and social and community support systems, such as senior citizens' centers, churches, and other community groups.[48] This type of extended support system contributes to a sense of extended family and belonging to a caring group.

Examination of as many of these factors as possible in a nutritional assessment will contribute to a clearer picture of an individual's functional ability, lifestyle, and health problems that may interfere with adequate nutritional intake. A clinical assessment will add another dimension to the commonly used tools of nutritional assessment: anthropometric measurements; biochemical, hematologic, and immune evaluations; and dietary histories.

## ANTHROPOMETRIC ASSESSMENT

The major physiologic effect of malnutrition, either undernutrition or overnutrition, is a detrimental alteration of body composition. Protein-energy malnutrition (PEM) is first evidenced by loss of lean body mass and fat tissue. If the loss of available energy reserve (undernutrition) is severe enough, it can result in a significantly increased incidence of morbidity or mortality. Obesity (overnutrition) is characterized by an abnormal increase in body fat tissue, contributing to an increased risk for many chronic diseases.

Anthropometry is the technique by which the severity and composition of these morphologic changes can be evaluated. It also provides a method of monitoring the appropriateness of nutritional therapy. The anthropometric measurements most commonly used for assessing nutritional status are height, body weight, circumferences, and skinfold thicknesses.[49] For various reasons, the usefulness of these measures as predictors of nutritional status in the elderly is questionable. Major benefits of anthropometry over other nutritional assessment procedures are the ease with which the measurements can be accomplished, their relatively low cost, and their noninvasive nature, all of which make anthropometry particularly desirable for use in an aged population. However, the ability to obtain adequate and reproducible data is dependent on being able to obtain accurate measurements, and many elderly individuals have physical impairments that make this difficult and often impossible. Another significant limitation of anthropometry is the lack of appropriate standards with which to compare results; standards are derived from measurements compiled on younger adults and do not adjust for age-related physiologic changes.

Well-known physiologic changes in stature and body composition that occur with normal aging must be considered when using anthropometric measurements to assess nutritional status in older adults.[50] A progressive decrease in height with age is well documented and has been attributed to changes in the integrity of the vertebral column, with postural changes due to generalized osteoporosis.[51–53] An average decrease in height of 1.2 cm/20 y post maturity for whites and blacks of both sexes has been reported[54,55]; other cross-sectional studies have estimated the rate of loss in stature to be between 0.5 and 1.5 cm per decade.[52,56–58] Another longitudinal study observed a decrease in stature of 0.5 cm/y in white, healthy, middle-class, elderly men and women.[59]

Weight and body composition have also been shown to change with age[60–65] (Figure 16–1). Weight tends to increase until the early 40s in men and the early 50s in women, to hold relatively steady for the next 15 to 20 years, and to decrease thereafter.[61,63–65] A decrease in lean body mass is characteristic of aging, regardless of energy intake.[62] Along with the loss of protein mass, there is an increase in the proportion of body weight as adipose tissue. There is approximately a 10% increase in total body fat in an elderly subject above that carried as a young adult. This increase in fat is not always visually evident because of the higher proportion of fat deposited around internal organs, particularly in women.[62] Subcutaneous fat on the extremities decreases with age, while fat tends to increase on the trunk.[66–68] This shift in body composition can complicate the interpretation of skinfold and circumference measurement data as predictors of total body fat.[69]

A major objective of anthropometry in nutritional assessment is to establish an individual's protein-energy reserve compared with normal ranges.[70] This presents a perplexing problem when one is using anthropometric measures to assess nutritional status in elderly subjects because of the lack of appropriate standards with which to compare the obtained data.[69] Therefore, extreme care must be used when interpreting results of anthropometric measures; anthropometry must be used in conjunction with clinical, laboratory, dietary, and psychosocial data.

## Weight for Height

Almost all of the currently used indicators of appropriate body weight, as well as other measures of lean body mass, require knowledge of the individual's height. Accurate measurements of stature are particularly difficult to obtain from most aged subjects because the physical changes that occur with aging make it difficult or even impossible for many elderly people to stand erect. Chronic diseases, such as arthritis, osteoporosis, and Parkinson-like disorders, which affect the neuromuscular systems, contribute to this problem. Individuals who have severe kyphosis (curvature of the spine) and bowing of the legs present major problems in obtaining accurate measures of height.[49]

Additional problems are related to the fact that these same diseases may result in an actual decrease in height due to a compression of the vertebral disc space.[53] Since height is used as a constant reference point in many weight/height-related measurements, it is difficult to know whether to use actual height as "best measured" or maximal height of the individual as a young adult.[71]

To measure stature in elderly subjects who are able to stand unaided in an erect position, the following standardized procedure, as described in the *Anthropometric Standardization Reference Manual*[72] and adapted for elderly subjects,[73] is recommended:

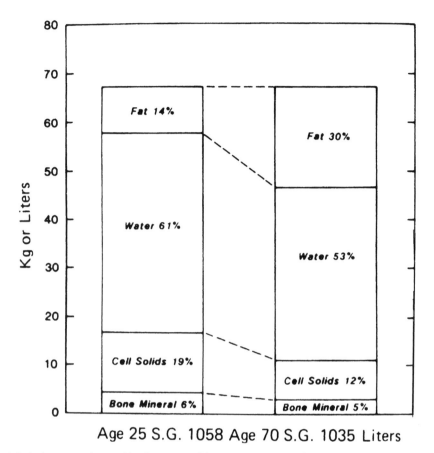

**Figure 16–1** A comparison of body composition compartments in a 25-year-old man and a 70-year-old man. *Source:* Reprinted with permission from N.W. Shock, *Biological Aspects of Aging,* pp. 59–78, © 1962, Columbia University Press.

1. The subject should be measured without shoes and in little or light clothing to allow viewing of the position of the body.
2. He or she should stand on a flat surface—that is, at a right angle to the vertical board of a stadiometer.
3. The subject should stand up straight, with heels close together, legs as straight as possible, arms at the sides, and shoulders relaxed.
4. The head should be in the Frankfort horizontal plane: that is, the line of vision should be perpendicular to the body. The headboard is then lowered onto the crown of the head.
5. The subject should then take a deep breath; the stature measurement is recorded to the nearest 0.1 cm or 1/8 in at maximal inspiration.
6. A repeated measurement should be taken to ensure reliability and should agree within 1 cm or 1/2 in of the first measurement.
7. The degree of kyphosis or bowing of the legs should be noted.
8. A sliding bar attached to a beam balance may also be used to measure

height; however, this device is generally less accurate.[69]

Because of the problems described, alternative methods for estimating stature in the
elderly have been investigated.[74,75] Arm span
is highly correlated with stature when an individual reaches his or her maximal height, before age-associated changes occur in the vertebral column.[50,76] Studies indicate that racial
differences between American blacks and
whites occur in the relationship between arm
span and stature.[54] Arm span includes both
arms and the breadth of the shoulders and is
measured with the subject's arms out-
stretched maximally. Problems similar to
those encountered in measuring stature due to
kyphosis, osteoporosis, and arthritis can prevent the use of arm span measurement in this
group. As a result, total arm length (TAL) has
been evaluated as an alternative measure.[74]
TAL is measured from the tip of the acromial
process of the scapula to the end of the styloid
process of the ulna. This study[74] indicates that
although height decreases with age, arm measurements do not change to the same degree.
Therefore, it seems likely that TAL could be
a useful value for the development of anthropometric standards for the elderly; however,
arm length varies among individuals of the
same height, so additional validation and further studies are required to determine the reliability and interpretation of this measurement
before its routine clinical use can be advocated.[74]

For those elderly individuals who cannot
stand erect, recumbent anthropometric techniques have been developed that can be used
to estimate stature from knee height measurements[75]; weight can be estimated by using recumbent measurements of arm and calf circumferences, subscapular skinfold thickness,
and knee height.[77] The clinical application of
these and other recumbent measures, along
with detailed descriptions of the measuring
techniques, have been reported elsewhere.[73]
For elderly individuals who have severe neuromuscular deformities, the best measurement of height may be obtained by measurement of individual body segments. Segment
lengths should be measured between specific
bony landmarks and as vertical distances between a flat surface and a bony landmark, but
they should not be measured from joint
creases[78] (Figure 16–2).

## Weight

Body weight is one of the simplest and
most routinely collected anthropometric indices used to monitor individuals[79] and is used
as a rough estimate of body energy stores.
Body weight is a composite measure of total
body size, reflecting everything inside the
personal envelope,[80] but it provides no information relating to body composition. Absolute weight may stay constant over time, but
the proportions of lean muscle mass and fat
may change, as seen in many elderly individuals.[55]

To increase the reliability and reproducibility of repeated measures, standardized
procedures should be followed.[81] The subject
should always be weighed in the same type
of clothing, preferably in a lightweight gown
or underclothing. Because of diurnal variations in weight, it is best to weigh at the same
time of day, before eating and after voiding.
These conditions should be recorded each
time to help to understand extreme variations
in the measurement. For ambulatory persons
who can stand unaided, an upright beam
scale with movable weights is the most accurate and reliable. One with a wide base and a
hand support is best because most elderly individuals are unsteady and need this support
to position themselves before accurate measurements can be taken. Subjects should

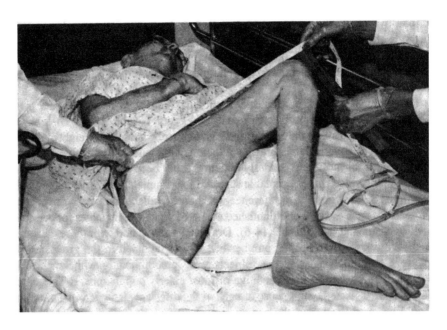

**Figure 16–2** An example of segmental measurements in an elderly, cachectic, contracted patient. Measurement points are from one bony prominence to another bony landmark. Courtesy of the John L. McClellan Memorial Veterans' Hospital.

stand with their feet over the center of the platform. Measurements should be recorded to the nearest 0.1 kg or 1/4 lb. A chair scale may be needed for persons who are unable to stand unaided. For the nonambulatory, bedfast patient, it is necessary to use a bed scale; recumbent measures developed to estimate weight can be used.[77] Every scale should be calibrated periodically against a set of standard weights.

As with most nutritional assessment parameters, it is useful to be able to compare a given weight of an individual with that of an ideal weight for a healthy subject of the same sex, age, and stature. This presents a problem, however, since there are no universally accepted standards available for evaluation of weight in very old persons.[49] The Metropolitan Life Insurance Company height and weight tables for 1959[82] and 1983[83] are commonly used standards (Table 16–6). These

tables represent weights associated with the lowest mortality rate for persons of various height and body frames. These data were compiled to represent persons up to age 59 years; however, the 1983 tables have been shown to be appropriate for older individuals.[84] Body frame is determined by measuring elbow breadth as described by Frisancho and Flegel.[85] A recent study comparing several reported methods of determining frame size showed that elbow breadth was not the most acceptable measure on the basis of assumptions inherent in use of frame size determinations.[86] No data exist on the reliability of determining frame size in very old people.

The National Center for Health Statistics has published reference data that include weights for older subjects up to age 74 years[87] (Table 16–7). These data make it possible to locate the 5th- through 95th-percentile values for weight of an elderly person of any given

**Table 16–6** Metropolitan Life Insurance Company Height and Weight Tables, 1983

| Height | | Men | | |
|---|---|---|---|---|
| Feet | Inches | Small Frame | Medium Frame | Large Frame |
| 5 | 2 | 128–134 | 131–141 | 138–150 |
| 5 | 3 | 130–136 | 133–143 | 140–153 |
| 5 | 4 | 132–138 | 135–145 | 142–156 |
| 5 | 5 | 134–140 | 137–148 | 144–160 |
| 5 | 6 | 136–142 | 139–151 | 146–164 |
| 5 | 7 | 138–145 | 142–154 | 149–168 |
| 5 | 8 | 140–148 | 145–157 | 152–172 |
| 5 | 9 | 142–151 | 148–160 | 155–176 |
| 5 | 10 | 144–154 | 151–163 | 158–180 |
| 5 | 11 | 146–157 | 154–166 | 161–184 |
| 6 | 0 | 149–160 | 157–170 | 164–188 |
| 6 | 1 | 152–164 | 160–174 | 168–192 |
| 6 | 2 | 155–168 | 164–178 | 172–197 |
| 6 | 3 | 158–172 | 167–182 | 176–202 |
| 6 | 4 | 162–176 | 171–187 | 181–207 |

| Height | | Women | | |
|---|---|---|---|---|
| Feet | Inches | Small Frame | Medium Frame | Large Frame |
| 4 | 10 | 102–111 | 109–121 | 118–131 |
| 4 | 11 | 103–113 | 111–123 | 120–134 |
| 5 | 0 | 104–115 | 113–126 | 122–137 |
| 5 | 1 | 106–118 | 115–129 | 124–140 |
| 5 | 2 | 108–121 | 118–132 | 128–143 |
| 5 | 3 | 111–124 | 121–135 | 131–147 |
| 5 | 4 | 114–127 | 124–138 | 134–151 |
| 5 | 5 | 117–130 | 127–141 | 137–155 |
| 5 | 6 | 120–133 | 130–144 | 140–159 |
| 5 | 7 | 123–136 | 133–147 | 143–163 |
| 5 | 8 | 126–139 | 136–150 | 146–167 |
| 5 | 9 | 129–142 | 139–153 | 149–170 |
| 5 | 10 | 132–145 | 142–156 | 152–173 |
| 5 | 11 | 135–148 | 145–159 | 155–176 |
| 6 | 0 | 138–151 | 148–162 | 158–179 |

*Note:* Weights at ages 25 to 59 years based on lowest mortality. Weight in pounds according to frame (in indoor clothing weighing 5 lb, shoes with 1-in heels).

*Source:* Reprinted with permission from *Statistical Bulletin* Vol. 62, p. 2, Copyright © 1983, Metropolitan Life Insurance Company.

**Table 16–7**    Average Weights for U.S. Men and Women, 1971–1974

| Sex and Height | Weight (lb) | | | |
| --- | --- | --- | --- | --- |
| | 35–44 y | 45–54 y | 55–64 y | 65–74 y |
| Men | | | | |
| 62 in | 143 | 147 | 143 | 143 |
| 63 in | 148 | 152 | 147 | 147 |
| 64 in | 153 | 156 | 153 | 151 |
| 65 in | 158 | 160 | 158 | 156 |
| 66 in | 163 | 164 | 163 | 160 |
| 67 in | 169 | 169 | 168 | 164 |
| 68 in | 174 | 173 | 173 | 169 |
| 69 in | 179 | 177 | 178 | 173 |
| 70 in | 184 | 182 | 183 | 177 |
| 71 in | 190 | 187 | 189 | 182 |
| 72 in | 194 | 191 | 193 | 186 |
| 73 in | 200 | 196 | 197 | 190 |
| 74 in | 205 | 200 | 203 | 194 |
| Women | | | | |
| 57 in | 125 | 129 | 132 | 130 |
| 58 in | 129 | 133 | 136 | 134 |
| 59 in | 133 | 136 | 140 | 137 |
| 60 in | 137 | 140 | 143 | 140 |
| 61 in | 141 | 143 | 147 | 144 |
| 62 in | 144 | 147 | 150 | 147 |
| 63 in | 148 | 150 | 153 | 151 |
| 64 in | 152 | 154 | 157 | 154 |
| 65 in | 156 | 158 | 160 | 158 |
| 66 in | 159 | 161 | 164 | 161 |
| 67 in | 163 | 165 | 167 | 165 |
| 68 in | 167 | 168 | 171 | 169 |

Note: Weights at ages 25 to 59 years based on lowest mortality. Weight in pounds according to frame (in indoor clothing weighing 5 lb, shoes with 1-in heels). Estimated values from regression equations of weight on height for specified age groups. Examined persons were measured without shoes; clothing weight ranged from 0.20 to 0.62 lb, which was not deducted from weights shown.

*Source:* Adapted from Weight by Height and Age for Adults 18-74 Years: United States, 1971-1974, Office of Health Research, Statistics and Technology, National Center for Health Statistics, U.S. Department of Health and Human Services.

height. The 50th-percentile value is probably a reasonable standard for most active elderly patients. It has been recommended that the 5th-percentile value be the acceptable standard for completely inactive patients.[88]

Limited data on average or reference weight are available on persons over age 74 years. Master and Lasser[89] published average height-weight tables for persons aged 64 years and older (Table 16–8). Limitations associated with these data are that only a limited number of subjects were included in the groups aged 85 years and older and that the subjects were predominantly white men and women and may not be representative of most elderly populations.[49] More recently, data are available from the National Health and Nutrition Examination Survey (NHANES) III, which contains data collected over the period from 1988 to 1991 (phase 1) on a sample of 600 elderly individuals 60 years of age and older, with no upper age limits. Included in this survey were equal numbers of whites, blacks, and Hispanics.[90] Concerns have been expressed regarding the use of these data as reference standards due to the limited sample size.[91] More reliable data will be available when results of the entire NHANES III data is published. This data will represent approximately 5,300 people ages 60 years and older. There are limitations associated with the use of each of the different standards. All of the standards should be considered, and the one most representative of the population being evaluated should be selected. It is important that the standards selected be recorded and used consistently by all members of the health care team, according to frame (in indoor clothing weighing 3 lb, shoes with 1-in heels).

A more clinically useful and predictive factor than relative body weight is the evaluation of changes in weight over a given period of time[92]; therefore, a careful history of previous weight gain or loss should be obtained. For a very old individual or an acutely ill, elderly patient, one must usually seek the help of a close family member or care provider to ascertain this information. Extreme differences in either weight gain or loss over very short durations are most probably related to shifts in fluid balance rather than to alterations in nutritional status.[92] Recommendations for evaluating the significance of weight change

over time have been published.[70] Similar recommendations specifically for evaluating the anorexia of aging were made at a conference on nutrition in the elderly.[93]

### Body Mass Index

Body mass index (BMI), calculated by dividing the individual's weight in kilograms by the square of the height in meters, is being used with more frequency to evaluate nutritional status in the elderly. The BMI has been shown to be a good estimate of body fat. Low levels of BMI are associated with decreases in functional abilities and increased mortality in the elderly.[94] The Nutrition Screening Initiative (NSI) includes the use of BMI and states that elderly individuals with a BMI of greater than 27 or less than 24 may be at increased risk for poor nutritional status.[95] Nomograms for calculating BMI are widely available, as well as tables for the direct conversion of height and weight into BMI.[26,96,97] The reliability of the use of BMI in the elderly has been questioned because of concerns related to changes in height and body composition in the elderly. There is some evidence that BMI in elderly individuals may not be as predictive of health outcomes as has been promoted.[98]

### Skinfold and Circumference Measures

Body weight is one indication of available energy stores; however, it is desirable to evaluate the composition of these stores and the severity of loss of lean muscle tissue versus adipose tissue. Depletion of lean muscle mass is more critical because of the role that protein plays in body function. The loss of lean muscle with aging has been referred to as sarcopenia.[99,100] More recently, the term *sarcopenia* is being used to designate abnormal losses of lean muscle, losses greater than

**Table 16–8** Average Height-Weight Table for Persons Aged 65 Years and Older

| | Men | | | | | |
|---|---|---|---|---|---|---|
| | Weight (lb) | | | | | |
| Ht. (in) | 65–69 y | 70–74 y | 75–79 y | 80–84 y | 85–89 y | 90–94 y |
| 61 | 128–156 | 125–153 | 123–151 | | | |
| 62 | 130–158 | 127–155 | 125–153 | 122–148 | | |
| 63 | 131–161 | 129–157 | 127–155 | 122–150 | 120–146 | |
| 64 | 134–164 | 131–161 | 129–157 | 124–152 | 122–148 | |
| 65 | 136–166 | 134–164 | 130–160 | 127–155 | 125–153 | 117–143 |
| 66 | 139–169 | 137–167 | 133–163 | 130–158 | 128–156 | 120–146 |
| 67 | 140–172 | 140–170 | 136–166 | 132–162 | 130–160 | 122–150 |
| 68 | 143–175 | 142–174 | 139–169 | 135–165 | 133–163 | 126–154 |
| 69 | 147–179 | 146–178 | 142–174 | 139–169 | 137–167 | 130–158 |
| 70 | 150–184 | 148–182 | 146–178 | 143–175 | 140–172 | 134–164 |
| 71 | 155–189 | 152–186 | 149–183 | 148–180 | 144–176 | 139–169 |
| 72 | 159–195 | 156–190 | 154–188 | 153–187 | 148–182 | |
| 73 | 164–200 | 160–196 | 158–192 | | | |

| | Women | | | | | |
|---|---|---|---|---|---|---|
| | Weight (lb) | | | | | |
| Ht. (in) | 65–69 y | 70–74 y | 75–79 y | 80–84 y | 85–89 y | 90–94 y |
| 58 | 120–146 | 112–138 | 111–135 | | | |
| 59 | 121–147 | 114–140 | 112–136 | 100–122 | 99–121 | |
| 60 | 122–148 | 116–142 | 113–139 | 106–130 | 102–124 | |
| 61 | 123–151 | 118–144 | 115–144 | 109–133 | 104–128 | |
| 62 | 125–153 | 121–147 | 118–144 | 112–136 | 108–132 | 107–131 |
| 63 | 127–155 | 123–151 | 121–147 | 115–141 | 112–136 | 107–131 |
| 64 | 130–158 | 126–154 | 123–151 | 119–145 | 115–141 | 108–132 |
| 65 | 132–162 | 130–158 | 126–154 | 122–150 | 120–146 | 112–136 |
| 66 | 136–166 | 132–162 | 128–157 | 126–154 | 124–152 | 116–142 |
| 67 | 140–170 | 136–166 | 131–161 | 130–158 | 128–156 | |
| 68 | 143–175 | 140–170 | | | | |
| 69 | 148–180 | 144–176 | | | | |

*Source:* Reprinted with permission from A.M. Master et al. *Journal of the American Medical Association,* Vol 172, p. 659. Copyright © 1960, American Medical Association.

what can be accounted for as a mere function of the aging process.[101]

At present, the most clinically applicable procedure for evaluating the degree of muscle loss and adipose mass depletion is anthropometry, particularly skinfold and circumference measurements. These techniques have particular limitations in elderly subjects, due in part to the previously mentioned physical alterations in body composition associated with aging. In addition to the changes in lean muscle tissue and adipose tissue, other factors exist that make these measures more difficult to interpret in elderly subjects. With aging, there are changes in elasticity, hydration, and compressibility of the skin and in subcutaneous adipose and connective tissues that can alter the relationship of skinfold thickness measurements to body composition.[102] These changes may also affect both the accuracy and precision of the skinfold measurements. Additional problems relating to measuring technique become apparent when working with elderly subjects who have loose skin on the arms and upper body. Therefore, it is imperative that standardized techniques be used[83] and that any major abnormalities in skin and fat distribution be noted.

### Skinfold Measures

Skinfold measurements are relatively simple to obtain, are less affected by hydration status than is weight, and are independent of height. Skinfold measurements have been shown to correlate with body fat measured by more sophisticated techniques.[103–107] Formulas have been developed for predicting total body fat from one skinfold[108] and from multiple skinfold measurements.[103] Data from a large study of elderly subjects indicated that skinfold measurements on the trunk may be more reliable predictors of body fat in men, whereas skinfold measurements on the extremities seem to be more accurate in women.[104] In elderly people, the use of multiple skinfold measurements should add to the reliability of the predicted value of body fat. Numerous equations have been developed to determine body composition from skinfold measurements, all of which use various combinations of measurements from different sites.[109]

While there is no universal agreement about whether to use right-side or left-side body measures, it is very important that the same side of the body always be used for both skinfold and circumference measurements of a given subject. The most commonly used anatomic sites for skinfold measurements are triceps, biceps, subscapular, and suprailiac. The following methods for identifying these sites and performing the measurements are taken from the *Anthropometric Standardization Reference Manual*.[110]

Triceps skinfold is measured at a point midway between the lateral projection of the acromial process of the scapula and the inferior margin of the olecranon. This point is determined by using a tape measure, with the subject's elbow flexed to 90°. The midpoint is marked on the lateral side of the arm. Subjects are measured while standing, if possible; if not, they should be propped upright in a chair or bed. The skinfold is measured with the arm hanging loosely and comfortably at the subject's side. The triceps skinfold is picked up with the left thumb and index finger, approximately 1 cm proximal to the marked level, and the calipers are applied to the skinfold at the marked level. The skinfold should be held for the duration of the measurement. The measurement site must be in the midline posteriorly when the palm is directed anteriorly.

Biceps skinfold is measured by lifting the skin on the anterior aspect of the upper arm, directly above the center of the cubital fossa at the same level as the triceps skinfold. The crest of the fold should run parallel to the long axis of the arm. The subject stands, facing the measurer, with the arm relaxed at the side and the palm directed anteriorly.

Subscapular skinfold is measured by lifting the skin 1 cm under the inferior angle of the scapula with the shoulder and arm relaxed at the side of the body. To locate the site, the measurer palpates the scapula, running the fingers inferiorly and laterally along its vertebral border until the inferior angle is identified. For obese or elderly subjects, gentle placement of the subject's arm behind the back aids in identifying the site. The skinfold thickness is recorded to the nearest 0.1 cm.

Suprailiac skinfold is measured in the midaxillary line immediately superior to the iliac crest. The skinfold is grasped just posterior (about 2 cm) to the midaxillary line, following the natural cleavage lines of the skin. The crest of the fold should be horizontal. The caliper jaws are applied about 1 cm from the fingers holding the skinfold, and the thickness is recorded to the nearest 0.1 cm.

Equations for calculating total body fat and fat-free mass from the sum of the four skinfold measurements are given in Table 16–9. The most widely used data for evaluating skinfold and circumference measurements in elderly subjects are those from a cross-sectional sampling of American subjects aged 25 to 74 years from the NHANES I and II.[87] These data are presented in Tables 16–10 and 16–11. Available percentile norms for upper arm anthropometry in white men and women aged 60 to 89 years are presented in Table 16–12.[111]

---

**Table 16–9** Calculation of Fat and Fat-Free Mass

1. Determine the patient's age and weight in kilograms.
2. Measure the following skinfolds in millimeters: biceps, triceps, subscapular, suprailiac.
3. Compute $\Sigma$ by adding four skinfold values.
4. Compute the logarithm of $\Sigma$.
5. Apply one of the following age- and sex-adjusted equations to calculate body density ($D$) (in g/mL):

*Equations for men:*
Age Range (y)
17–19  $D = 1.1620 - 0.0630 \times (\log\Sigma)$
20–29  $D = 1.1631 - 0.0632 \times (\log\Sigma)$
30–39  $D = 1.1422 - 0.0544 \times (\log\Sigma)$
40–49  $D = 1.1620 - 0.0700 \times (\log\Sigma)$
50+    $D = 1.1715 - 0.0779 \times (\log\Sigma)$

*Equations for women:*
Age Range (y)
17–19  $D = 1.1549 - 0.0678 \times (\log\Sigma)$
20–29  $D = 1.1599 - 0.0717 \times (\log\Sigma)$
30–39  $D = 1.1423 - 0.0632 \times (\log\Sigma)$
40–49  $D = 1.1333 - 0.0612 \times (\log\Sigma)$
50+    $D = 1.1339 - 0.0645 \times (\log\Sigma)$

6. Fat mass is then calculated as: Fat mass (kg) = body weight (kg) $\times [(4.95/D) - 4.5]$
7. Fat-free mass is then calculated as: Fat-free mass (kg) = body weight (kg) – fat mass (kg)

*Source:* Reprinted with permission from J.V. Durnin and J. Womersley, "Body Fat Assessed from Total Body Density and Its Estimation from Skinfold Thickness" in *British Journal of Nutrition*, Vol. 32, p. 77, Copyright © 1974, Cambridge University Press.

**Table 16–10** Average Mid–Upper Arm Muscle Circumference in Adults

*Average Circumference (cm)*

| Age (y) | Men | Women |
|---------|------|-------|
| 45–54 | 28.2 | 22.7 |
| 55–64 | 27.8 | 22.8 |
| 65–74 | 26.8 | 22.8 |

*Source:* Reprinted with permission from *American Journal of Clinical Nutrition* (1981;34:2530), Copyright © 1981, American Society for Clinical Nutrition.

### Circumference Measurements

Circumferences are measurements that record the size of cross-sectional and circumferential dimensions of the body. They can be used alone, in combination with skinfold measurements, or in combination with other circumferences to help evaluate nutritional status. Specific techniques for measuring circumferences have been described.[112] These measurements require the use of a tape measure, which should be flexible but nonstretchable and should have markings on only one side, in either metric or English units. Circumferences should be recorded with the zero end of the tape held in the left

**Table 16–11** Average Triceps Skinfold Thickness in Adults

*Average Thickness (mm)*

| Age (y) | Men | Women |
|---------|------|-------|
| 35–44 | 12 | 23 |
| 45–54 | 11 | 25 |
| 55–64 | 11 | 25 |
| 65–74 | 11 | 23 |

*Source:* Reprinted from 1971-1975 National Health Survey, *Vital and Health Statistics Series No. 219*, U.S. Department of Health and Human Services, Public Health Service, 1981.

hand above the remaining part of the tape, which is held by the right hand. The tape should be maintained in a horizontal position, touching the skin and following the contours of the limb but not compressing underlying tissue. The tension applied to the tape by the evaluator affects the validity and reliability of the measurement. The mid–upper arm circumference is measured at the midpoint between the acromial process of the scapula and olecranon. This location is the same as that marked for the triceps and biceps skinfolds. The measurement is made with the elbow extended and the arm relaxed and hanging just away from the side of the trunk, with the palm facing the thigh.

The mid–upper arm circumference (MAC), in conjunction with the triceps skinfold (TSF) measurement, can be used to calculate the arm-muscle circumference (AMC) and the arm-muscle area (AMA), both of which are estimates of the amount of muscle or lean tissue in the body. Formulas that can be used for these calculations are as follows:

$$AMC \ (cm) = MAC \ (cm) - (3.14 \times TSF \ (mm))$$
$$AMA \ (cm^2) = AMC^2/12.56$$

Reference standards are given in Tables 16–10 and 16–11.

The use of calf circumference has been recommended as a more sensitive measure of the loss of total body muscle mass in the elderly than arm circumference and midarm muscle area.[113] The World Health Organization has recommended that calf circumference be included as a measure of nutritional status in the elderly.[91] Calf circumference is included as one of the anthropometric measures, in addition to MAC, BMI, and history of weight loss, in a Mini Nutritional Assessment form recently developed for assessing nutritional status as part of the geriatric evaluation.[114]

**Table 16–12** Percentile Norms for Measurements of Upper Arm Anthropometry

*Triceps Skinfold Thickness*

| Sex, Age (Y) Group | Sample | Mean | Percentile | | | | | | |
| | | | 5th | 10th | 25th | 50th | 75th | 90th | 95th |
| | | | MM | | | | | | |
| **Women** | | | | | | | | | |
| 60–89 | 496 | 25.2 | 12.5 | 14.4 | 18.5 | 24.0 | 30.8 | 38.1 | 43.6 |
| 60–69 | 146 | 27.2 ±10.2* | 13.0 | 14.7 | 20.7 | 26.2 | 33.0 | 40.3 | 47.2 |
| 70–79 | 239 | 25.1 ±9.3 | 13.0 | 15.0 | 18.0 | 23.7 | 31.0 | 38.3 | 41.5 |
| 80–89 | 111 | 23.3 ±9.7 | 10.9 | 12.9 | 16.7 | 21.8 | 27.5 | 34.6 | 43.4 |
| **Men** | | | | | | | | | |
| 60–89 | 250 | 22.5 | 5.7 | 7.6 | 11.5 | 20.4 | 31.8 | 42.1 | 45.8 |
| 60–69 | 86 | 21.9 ±13.6 | 4.9 | 6.9 | 10.8 | 18.0 | 31.9 | 45.1 | 49.3 |
| 70–79 | 115 | 23.5 ±13.3 | 6.3 | 7.9 | 12.0 | 22.0 | 32.7 | 41.8 | 45.4 |
| 80–89 | 49 | 21.6 ±11.0 | 5.8 | 8.0 | 11.5 | 21.0 | 29.6 | 37.5 | 40.5 |

*Mid–Upper Arm Circumference*

| Sex, Age (Y) Group | Sample | Mean | Percentile | | | | | | |
| | | | 5th | 10th | 25th | 50th | 75th | 90th | 95th |
| | | | MM | | | | | | |
| **Women** | | | | | | | | | |
| 60–89 | 496 | 30.0 | 23.3 | 25.1 | 27.0 | 29.7 | 32.7 | 35.9 | 38.1 |
| 60–69 | 146 | 31.1 ±4.8 | 23.5 | 25.6 | 27.7 | 30.6 | 33.7 | 37.5 | 39.9 |
| 70–79 | 239 | 30.0 ±4.1 | 23.5 | 25.5 | 27.1 | 29.5 | 32.5 | 35.5 | 37.8 |
| 80–89 | 111 | 28.8 ±4.6 | 22.5 | 23.5 | 26.0 | 28.8 | 31.6 | 34.5 | 36.4 |
| **Men** | | | | | | | | | |
| 60–89 | 250 | 30.4 | 24.9 | 26.6 | 28.7 | 30.4 | 32.2 | 34.6 | 36.3 |
| 60–69 | 86 | 30.5 ±3.0 | 25.1 | 27.3 | 29.0 | 30.5 | 32.4 | 34.2 | 35.7 |
| 70–79 | 115 | 30.7 ±3.1 | 25.3 | 26.8 | 29.0 | 30.7 | 32.4 | 34.6 | 36.6 |
| 80–89 | 49 | 29.6 ±3.5 | 23.4 | 24.9 | 27.6 | 29.6 | 31.5 | 35.3 | 36.5 |

*continues*

**Table 16–12** continued

### Mid–Upper Arm Muscle Circumference

| Sex, Age (Y) Group | Sample | Mean | Percentile (MM) | | | | | | |
|---|---|---|---|---|---|---|---|---|---|
| | | | 5th | 10th | 25th | 50th | 75th | 90th | 95th |
| **Women** | | | | | | | | | |
| 60–89 | 496 | 22.0 | 16.7 | 17.7 | 19.8 | 21.9 | 24.3 | 26.9 | 28.3 |
| 60–69 | 146 | 22.6 ±3.6 | 17.8 | 18.4 | 20.2 | 22.3 | 24.6 | 27.5 | 29.2 |
| 70–79 | 239 | 22.1 ±3.5 | 16.7 | 17.8 | 19.8 | 21.9 | 24.2 | 26.7 | 28.2 |
| 80–89 | 111 | 21.4 ±4.1 | 15.2 | 16.7 | 19.1 | 21.3 | 24.2 | 26.7 | 27.5 |
| **Men** | | | | | | | | | |
| 60–89 | 250 | 23.3 | 16.6 | 18.1 | 20.5 | 23.4 | 26.2 | 28.4 | 29.7 |
| 60–69 | 86 | 23.7 ±4.4 | 16.1 | 18.0 | 20.5 | 23.7 | 26.7 | 28.9 | 31.7 |
| 70–79 | 115 | 23.3 ±4.1 | 17.0 | 18.2 | 20.4 | 23.4 | 26.3 | 28.4 | 28.7 |
| 80–89 | 49 | 22.8 ±3.3 | 16.6 | 18.2 | 20.7 | 22.8 | 24.9 | 27.3 | 28.6 |

### Mid–Upper Arm Muscle Area

| Sex, Age (Y) Group | Sample | Mean | Percentile (MM) | | | | | | |
|---|---|---|---|---|---|---|---|---|---|
| | | | 5th | 10th | 25th | 50th | 75th | 90th | 95th |
| **Women** | | | | | | | | | |
| 60–89 | 496 | 39.9 | 22.2 | 25.0 | 31.1 | 38.0 | 47.1 | 57.7 | 63.8 |
| 60–69 | 146 | 41.6 ±13.5 | 25.1 | 27.0 | 32.6 | 39.6 | 48.3 | 60.3 | 67.6 |
| 70–79 | 239 | 39.8 ±12.7 | 22.1 | 25.1 | 31.2 | 38.0 | 46.7 | 56.6 | 63.2 |
| 80–89 | 111 | 37.9 ±13.3 | 18.4 | 22.3 | 29.0 | 36.1 | 46.5 | 56.8 | 60.2 |
| **Men** | | | | | | | | | |
| 60–89 | 250 | 44.6 | 22.0 | 26.2 | 33.5 | 43.6 | 54.4 | 64.1 | 70.4 |
| 60–69 | 86 | 46.0 ±16.5 | 20.7 | 25.8 | 33.4 | 44.8 | 56.8 | 66.7 | 79.7 |
| 70–79 | 115 | 44.6 ±14.6 | 23.0 | 26.4 | 33.3 | 43.7 | 54.8 | 64.3 | 65.7 |
| 80–89 | 49 | 42.3 ±11.8 | 21.9 | 26.5 | 34.2 | 41.5 | 49.4 | 59.1 | 64.9 |

*Mean ±standard deviation.

*Source:* Adapted from G. Falciglia, Upper Arm Anthropometric Norms in Elderly White Subjects. Copyright The American Dietetic Association. Adapted by permission from *The American Dietetic Association*, Vol. 85, p. 1296, © 1985.

Another measure of lean body mass (LBM) is the creatinine height index (CHI), which has been used to assess nutritional status in the elderly.[115] Creatinine is formed irreversibly from the metabolism of creatine and creatine phosphate found primarily in muscle tissue. The daily production of creatinine is related to the total LBM content of the body and has been shown to be remarkably consistent from day to day.[116] The CHI has been adopted for evaluation of LBM in young, healthy adults and in hospitalized patients who may be protein-energy malnourished.

Several problems are associated with this measurement as a clinical tool in elderly individuals. The measurement requires an accurately timed, 24-hour urine collection, which is very difficult (and often impossible) to obtain from elderly patients. In addition, creatinine excretion must be related to an individual's measured height, which sometimes is difficult to obtain in elderly subjects, as discussed previously. Another problem relates to the fact that LBM decreases with age, and with this decrease there will be a decrease in creatinine excretion unrelated to nutritional status. Many elderly individuals have compromised renal function; if this is the case, urinary creatinine excretion may not be a reliable measure.[117] The usefulness of the CHI as a tool with which to predict PEM in an elderly population has been evaluated.[69] This research indicated that CHI was a more accurate predictor of PEM in elderly men than in elderly women. In a recent study to determine whether aging alters the usefulness of creatinine excretion as an index of LBM or muscle mass in healthy men and women,[118] total LBM was determined by total-body potassium counting, and cross-sectional areas of upper arm and thigh muscle were determined by magnetic resonance imaging. This study indicated that creatine excretion is useful for evaluating body composition in both young and old subjects.

## BIOCHEMICAL MEASURES

A number of biochemical measures are available for use in the assessment of nutritional status. They can be categorized into two groups on the basis of the diagnostic ability of the results.[116] The first group relies on nonspecific indices of nutritional status, and the second group uses nutrient-specific indices of nutritional status. The first group includes determinations of the plasma proteins, which are usually easier to obtain than the nutrient-specific analyses that can detect subclinical micronutrient deficiencies.

As with anthropometric measures, problems exist with the use of biochemical indices in the assessment of elderly people. Factors other than nutrient intake are known to influence biochemical marker levels in the body. General state of health, past and present history of diseases, and use and abuse of alcohol, tobacco, medications, and over-the-counter drugs can produce alterations in biochemical data. These factors are of particular concern in elderly individuals. There is also a lack of age-adjusted reference data for appropriate interpretation of available results.

### Protein Assessment

Several biochemical measurements are available that reflect dietary protein intake as well as body protein stores. Among these, analyses of serum albumin, transferrin, and total iron-binding capacity (TIBC) are the most readily available and least expensive. Transport proteins with more rapid turnover (eg, prealbumin and retinol-binding protein) may be more sensitive to changes in protein nutriture, but tests for these are less readily available. The level of circulating serum albumin is the most consistently used measure of visceral protein status because of its high reliability as a prognostic marker of PEM.

Albumin is the major visceral protein produced by the liver, and its synthesis is dependent on an adequate supply of protein and, to a lesser degree, total energy intake.[119] It has been used extensively as a marker of the degree of PEM, has been shown to correlate positively with postsurgical outcome,[120] and has been reported to be a good prognostic indicator of hospital survival in elderly patients.[121] Albumin has also been found to be a strong predictor of clinical outcomes of hospitalized elderly nursing home residents.[122]

Serum albumin levels appear to be only minimally affected by aging.[123,124] However, some studies indicate a slight reduction in the rate of albumin synthesis in aged subjects.[125] A recent study found hypoalbuminemia to be associated with several sociodemographic, lifestyle, and disease-related factors in community-dwelling older persons.[126] Others have reported lower serum albumin levels in the elderly to be associated with losses in muscle mass.[127] Functional impairment and disability have also been associated with low serum albumin in the elderly.[123,128]

Hypoalbuminemia has been shown to be a reliable predictor of protein malnutrition in elderly people.[69,129] In a study evaluating several nutritional indices for their predictive ability of mortality in elderly hospitalized patients, a serum albumin level of less than 3 g/dL was found to be the best single predictor of mortality; it has been suggested that this value could provide early identification of elderly people who are at increased risk of death.[121] Another more recent study evaluating predictors of early nonelective hospital readmissions in nutritionally compromised Medicare patients found low albumin levels along with any amount of weight loss to be the most predictive of readmissions.[130]

Even though decreased albumin levels are almost always present in malnourished individuals, caution, along with astute clinical judgment, must be exercised in their interpretation. Many of the concurrent diseases that are common in elderly people are known to alter plasma protein concentrations. Therefore, depressed serum albumin levels due to diminished production in liver diseases, and excess losses as a consequence of renal or gastrointestinal disease or protein-losing enteropathy, must be ruled out before this measure can be used as a reliable indicator of nutritional status. In addition, plasma albumin concentrations are directly influenced by hydration status. Any situation that results in a decrease in plasma volume will cause an artificially high serum albumin level unrelated to protein intake or albumin synthesis. Depressed levels of serum albumin are seen when plasma volume is expanded, as would occur in a patient with congestive heart failure or renal disease. Albumin values in these individuals might appear to be deceptively low and unrelated to nutritional status. Very old and acutely ill elderly patients are often confined to bed for extended periods of time, and this can contribute to depressed albumin levels.[131]

After the clinical findings described above are taken into account, a serum albumin level of less than 3.5 g/dL is suggestive of chronic PEM and warrants further evaluation. Albumin's relatively long half-life (approximately 14 to 20 days), explains its slow response to nutritional therapy. A refeeding period of at least 2 weeks usually is required before consistent improvement in serum albumin levels can be noted. Aggressive refeeding in a severely malnourished elderly patient often will result in a further decrease in serum albumin level before an increase is seen. This phenomenon is attributed to the redistribution of extracellular and intracellular fluids.

Another major visceral protein often used for monitoring nutrition status is serum transferrin. It is usually considered a more sensitive marker of protein nutriture than albumin because its half-life is approximately 9 days. However, its usefulness in an aged population is complicated by the fact that there is a strong negative correlation between circulating transferrin and tissue iron stores.[132,133] With advancing age, tissue iron stores increase, and as a result, serum transferrin levels are reduced.[134,135] Thus, some healthy elderly individuals may have transferrin values in the range commonly associated with nutritional deficiency.[136] This fact should always be considered before assuming that reductions in transferrin levels are due to protein malnutrition. Conversely, in individuals who have decreased iron stores, serum transferrin may be within the normal range, even in the presence of PEM.[136]

Often direct measures of serum transferrin are not available, necessitating the estimation of transferrin from TIBC.[135] This is usually accomplished by using the following formula:

$$[TIBC \ (mg/dL) \times 0.8] - 43$$

This may not be the best formula to use in all circumstances, however, and it has been suggested that each laboratory run its own regression analysis to determine a laboratory-specific formula for the estimation of transferrin levels from TIBC.[117]

Thyroxine-binding prealbumin (PA) and retinol-binding protein (RBP) are two serum proteins synthesized in the liver that have very rapid turnover rates and small body pool sizes; they are therefore sensitive to any changes affecting their synthesis and catabolism.[137] Because of these properties, they may be excellent indicators of subclinical malnutrition and may aid in the long-term management and monitoring of high-risk elderly patients.[138]

RBP is a glycoprotein with a half-life of approximately 12 hours; it is involved in the transport of retinol from the liver to peripheral tissues. Its synthesis is responsive to the need for retinol transport; therefore, circulating serum levels may reflect vitamin A status, not just protein nutriture. In addition, inflated levels of RBP can be seen in patients with renal failure, and the levels may be depressed in patients with liver disease. RBP circulates while bound to PA as a PA-RBP complex. PA has a half-life of 2 days and is responsible for the transport of thyroxine. Its synthesis is not dependent on vitamin A status.

The concentration of PA-RBP complex is decreased in the presence of protein-energy metabolism, responds positively to nutritional therapy, and has been shown to be useful as a prognostic indicator of nutritional status.[139-142] However, like albumin, both RBP and PA are acute-phase reactants and therefore are directly affected by infections and inflammatory states. PA is considered a negative acute-phase reactant because levels decrease after acute stress. This decrease is due to an interruption of hepatic synthesis rather than to increased catabolism or urinary excretion[143] and is influenced by hormonal changes rather than lack of available nutritional substrate. Discretion should be used before ascribing any change in these proteins to nutritional circumstances if either of these conditions exists. There are no data to indicate that RBP and PA are altered in elderly people. However, more research is needed to determine the effect of aging on the synthesis and catabolism of these visceral proteins.

## Cholesterol

There is some evidence, corroborated by serum protein levels, that serum cholesterol levels in elderly people are associated with poor health status.[144] Cholesterol levels as a disease predictor is different in older adults than it is in younger adults. There is a decreased association between serum cholesterol and coronary heart disease with advancing age,[145-149] and a link between serum cholesterol and mortality has been demonstrated.[150,151] This suggests that further investigation of biochemical measures and nutritional status of the elderly should be pursued.

## IMMUNOLOGIC MEASURES

The association between nutritional status and immunocompetence is complex and multifactorial.[152-155] However, one of the strong associations noted is that PEM is accompanied by a reduction in host defense, demonstrated by anergy measured by delayed cutaneous hypersensitivity and lymphocytopenia. Immunologic dysfunction is associated with infections, cancer, and autoimmune diseases and may be a serious problem in elderly adults.

The immune system does not function as efficiently in older individuals as it does in younger individuals. The cell-mediated immune system is related to the T cell system, which is responsible for the delayed cutaneous hypersensitivity response; responses to certain autoimmune diseases; responses to some bacteria, viruses, and fungi; and responses to cancers. An absolute decrease in the number of T cells with a relative increase in the number of T suppressor cells has been described in elderly subjects.[136,156] One explanation is a progressive decline in thymic function and the production of thymic hormone with advanced age. These factors contribute to the increase in immature lymphocytes and the related decrease in helper/inducer T lymphocytes.[156] These and other changes that occur in immune function are very similar to the changes that are often seen with PEM.[157,158]

The most commonly used assay for immunocompetence is antigen-recall skin testing. The ability to demonstrate a response to recall antigens diminishes with age.[159,160] This same effect has been demonstrated in PEM.[153,159,160] The similarity of the effects of the aging process and those of PEM on immune function makes the usefulness of routine immunologic testing in elderly subjects difficult to interpret. A relationship between anergy and mortality in a nursing home population has been shown,[161] and there appears to be evidence that restoration of some immune function in malnourished elderly patients can be induced by nutritional repletion.[156] The contribution of measures of immune function to the assessment of nutritional status in elderly people is difficult to isolate and therefore must be evaluated within the context of all the previously identified parameters.

## HEMATOLOGIC MEASURES

Epidemiologic evidence indicates that anemia is fairly common among elderly subjects[162,163] (Chapter 11). Whether the anemia is related to the aging process or to nutritional factors is difficult to determine. There is a strong similarity between the alterations in hematologic function seen with advancing age and those seen with PEM. In a study that examined multiple indicators of nutritional status in malnourished, elderly subjects, refeeding corrected most nutritional indicators (weight, serum albumin level, vitamin and mineral levels) but did not correct immunologic and hematologic indices (eg, hemoglobin level).[136]

Hematologic indices such as hematocrit, hemoglobin level, and total lymphocyte count are often available in the medical record since they are routinely obtained on admission to the hospital; they should be followed and changes noted. In a free-living or long-term care environment where complete blood counts are not obtained on a regular basis, it is probably more valuable to follow other nutritional indicators that will provide more reliable nutritional data, such as weight, serum albumin level, and dietary intake.

## DIETARY ASSESSMENT

Dietary assessment of elderly subjects should provide insight into both present and past nutrient consumption habits. Finding the methods that can best accomplish this task is complicated by the physical and psychologic impairments often seen in this group. While quantitative methods often may be impossible, a qualitative assessment can be used to reveal those individuals who are at risk for nutrient deficiencies. These methods should be able to identify those who are having problems consuming an adequate diet, those who limit their intake to one or two foods or categories of food, those who follow unusual dietary patterns, or those who exclude an important food or food group.[164] Methods available for collecting dietary intake data include diet histories with food frequency checks, food records kept over a specific time period, and 24-hour dietary recalls. All of these methods rely on the operation of the elderly subject and the knowledge and skills of the interviewer. Many hospitalized and institutionalized elderly patients are not competent enough to provide accurate self-reported dietary intake information. When this is encountered, the use of a surrogate source is advocated; surrogates include the spouse, child, or close relative or friend of the patient. For a very old individual, it may be difficult to find a person who can provide data adequate to reflect an accurate description of eating habits. In a review of the use of surrogate measures of dietary intake in elderly subjects, it was concluded that surrogate dietary data may introduce misclassification in analytic investigations but may be useful in descriptive studies.[165]

Dietary histories elicit information regarding what subjects generally eat and are based on food frequency checklists. Checklists should be constructed so that food intake over time can be estimated and should minimize the variation of day-to-day intake. Additional data should be gathered concerning food likes and dislikes; socioeconomic factors, such as transportation availability, cooking facilities, and income status; information on health-related special dietary requirements; and use of alcohol and over-the-counter drugs.

In a review by Hankin,[166] the following recommendations were made regarding the development of a diet history questionnaire for studies of older persons:

1. The questionnaire should include items that are representative of the population's usual diet to permit valid associations with biochemical and clinical findings. Both regional and ethnic foods should be included.
2. The questionnaire should provide both qualitative and quantitative information on the usual intake of foods, nutrients, and other dietary components. This can best be accomplished through the use of visual prompts: food models, common household measuring equipment, or actual photographs of serving sizes of different foods.
3. The questionnaire should be objective. Food items and groups should be clearly defined, the range of serving sizes specified, and the method of recording frequencies clearly presented. This will help to reduce variations among interviewers and will increase clarity and comprehension among the older subjects.
4. The validity of the questionnaire must be determined as accurately as possible.
5. The reproducibility of the questionnaire should be assessed by pretesting

on a random sample of the study population on two different occasions and assessing agreement of the two sets of data. This will also help identify potential problems that may occur in the administration of the instrument.

A simplified diet history questionnaire may be adequate for use in an elderly population because the diets of these individuals are usually less varied than those of younger subjects. This is a result of the physiologic, sociologic, and economic changes that are often encountered in this group.[166] Dietary history and food frequency questionnaires, if administered properly, are very time consuming and require a well-trained, experienced professional interviewer. The subjectivity involved in describing a usual eating pattern makes this method vulnerable to memory lapses and psychologic tendencies to exaggerate or minimize self-described behavior.[167]

Another method often used to assess the nutrient intake of free-living elderly persons is the self-written dietary food record. A 7-day record is considered to be of an optimal length to obtain a more representative sample of usual intake. The food record technique places most of the responsibility on the subject and is therefore less time consuming for the interviewer. However, this method can be used reliably only for individuals who are well motivated and who can read and write. Level of education is often a factor in determining who will complete a 7-day record[168]; the length of the food record is often a factor relating to compliance. The accuracy of record keeping has been shown to decline before the end of 7 days[168]; therefore, for an older person a 3-day record may be adequate, but it should include one weekend day. Physical abnormalities, such as arthritis or uncontrollable tremors as a result of neurologic damage, may make it very difficult for some elderly people to write. Alterations in eating patterns are often noted by individuals who record their intakes.

The 24-hour recall is used more often than any other technique for assessing dietary intake and the subsequent nutrient status of free-living as well as institutionalized or hospitalized elderly people. The reliability of this method has been questioned for use in this group.[169] Factors that may interfere with the reliability of the method relate to dependence on memory; short-term memory is one of the first physiologic functions to show changes with advancing age.

## SCREENING VERSUS ASSESSMENT

A thorough, comprehensive nutrition assessment is the approach of choice in determining the nutritional status of an individual and in promoting appropriate therapeutic interventions when necessary. During the past years, there has been much discussion about nutritional screening for the elderly, and screening has been incorporated into many community and institution-based programs. A screening tool should be easy to administer, easy to score, reliable, and valid. One such instrument is the DETERMINE Your Nutritional Health checklist, developed by the Nutritional Screening Initiative (NSI), a collaborative effort of the American Dietetic Association, the American Academy of Family Physicians, and the National Council on the Aging.[170] This one-page instrument poses 10 questions designed to identify eating, economic, and lifestyle behaviors that may contribute to the development of nutritional problems. This tool does not evaluate nutritional status, but it does help to alert service providers and individuals to potentially correctable habits that are associated with poor nutritional status. The DETERMINE checklist has been widely used and validated.[171-173]

Screening should not be confused with assessment but can be very helpful when it is properly used.

## CONCLUSION

Assessing nutritional status in elderly individuals is a challenging task for nutrition professionals because of the age- and disease-related alterations of parameters commonly used to evaluate nutritional condition. To assess nutritional status properly, a multifaceted evaluation of the individual is necessary to develop a comprehensive picture of nutritional state. A thorough evaluation should include a physical assessment, including an examination of skin, hair, nails, eyes, oral mucosa, and musculature; fluid balance; physical disability; sensory losses; medical, cognitive, and psychologic problems; and socioeconomic conditions. Measures of body composition, such as anthropometric measures including height, weight, skinfold thicknesses, and muscle circumferences, can

be used to estimate protein and energy stores. Biochemical, immunologic, and hematologic assessments contribute to a more comprehensive evaluation of nutritional status and provide some valuable biomarkers by which to track changes in nutritional status over time. A dietary history will contribute to a more complete profile of an individual's nutritional state and may serve to identify potential nutritional problems that are not obvious to the observer.

An evaluation of nutritional status will help to detect individuals who are at risk for malnutrition before the overt presentation of such a condition. Malnutrition may interfere with the successful treatment of acute medical conditions, with the ability of an individual to recover from an insult or injury, or with an adequate response by the immune system to fight infection. Nutrition assessment will help to identify patients who may benefit from successful nutritional intervention before heroic measures are needed to restore nutritional integrity.

## REFERENCES

1. Buzina R, Bates CJ, van der Beek J, et al. Workshop on functional significance of mild-to-moderate malnutrition. *Am J Clin Nutr*. 1989;50:172–176.

2. McLaren DS. Clinical manifestations of human vitamin and mineral disorders: a resume. In: Shils ME, Olson JA, Shike M, Ross, CA, eds. *Modern Nutrition in Health and Disease*. 9th ed. Philadelphia, Pa: Lea & Febiger; 1999.

3. Hammond K. Nutrition focused physical assessment. *Supp Line*. 1996;18:41–44.

4. Lavizzo-Mourey R, Johnson J, Stolley P. Risk factors for dehydration among elderly nursing home residents. *J Am Geriatr Soc*. 1988;36:213–218.

5. Ausman LM, Russell RM. Nutrition in the elderly. In: Shils ME, Young VR, eds. *Modern Nutrition in Health and Disease*. 9th ed. Philadelphia, Pa: Lea & Febiger; 1999.

6. Rowe J. Renal system. In: Rowe JW, Besdine RW, eds. *Health and Disease in Old Age*. Boston, Mass: Little Brown & Co; 1982.

7. Food and Nutrition Board. *Recommended Dietary Allowances*. 10th ed. Washington, DC: National Academy Press; 1989.

8. Chernoff R. Meeting the nutritional needs of the elderly in the institutional setting. *Nutr Rev*. 1994;52:132–136.

9. Chidester JC, Spangler AA. Fluid intake in the institutionalized elderly. *J Am Diet Assoc*. 1997;97:123–128.

10. Chernoff R. Thirst and fluid requirements. *Nutr Rev*. 1994; 52: 53–55.

11. Knapp A. Nutrition and oral health in the elderly. *Dent Clin North Am*. 1989;33:109–125.

12. Sullivan DH, Martin W, Flaxman N, Hagen JE. Oral health problems and involuntary weight loss in

a population of frail elderly. *J Am Geriatr Soc.* 1993;41:725–731

13. Pla GW. Oral health and nutrition. *Nutr Old Age.* 1994;21(1):121–133.

14. Jurdi-Haldeman D, Napier AK. Perceived relationships between taste and smell acuity and food intake in the elderly. *Top Clin Nutr.* 1988;3(4):4–8.

15. Rosenberg IH, Russell RM, Bowman BB. Aging and the digestive system. In: Munro HN, Danford DE, eds. *Nutrition, Aging, and the Elderly.* New York, NY: Plenum Publishing Corp; 1989.

16. Grzegorczyk PB, Jones SW, Mistretta CM. Age related differences in salt taste acuity. *J Gerontol.* 1979;34:834–840.

17. Miller IJ. Human taste bud density across adult age groups. *J Gerontol.* 1988;43:B26–B30.

18. Chauhan J, Hawrysh ZJ, Gee M, et al. Age-related olfactory and taste changes and interrelationships between change and nutrition. *J Am Diet Assoc.* 1987;87:1543–1550.

19. Langan MJ, Yearick ES. The effects of improved oral hygiene in taste perception and nutrition of the elderly. *J Gerontol.* 1976;31:413–418.

20. Doty RL, Shaman P, Applebaum SL, Rosenberg L. Smell identification ability: change with age. *Science.* 1984;1441–1443.

21. Duffy VB, Backstrand JR, Ferris AM. Olfactory dysfunction and related nutritional risk in free-living, elderly women. *J Am Diet Assoc.* 1995;95:879–884.

22. Chernoff R. Aging and nutrition. *Nutr Today.* 1987;22(2):4–11.

23. Chernoff R. Nutrition and chronic conditions. *Top Geriatr Rehabil.* 1989;5(1):69–78.

24. Kohrs MB, Czajka-Narins DM, Nordstrom IW. Factors affecting nutritional status of the elderly. In: Munro HN, Danford DE, eds. *Nutrition, Aging, and the Elderly.* New York, NY: Plenum Publishing Corp; 1989.

25. Sullivan DH, Patch GA, Walls RC, Lipschitz DA. Impact of nutrition status on morbidity and mortality in a select population of geriatric rehabilitation patients. *Am J Clin Nutr.* 1990;51:749–758.

26. Dwyer JT, Gallo JJ, Reichel W. Assessing nutritional status in elderly patients. *Am Fam Physician.* 1993;47:613–620.

27. Guigoz Y, Vellas B, Garry P. Assessing the nutritional status of the elderly: the mini nutritional assessment as part of the geriatric evaluation. *Nutr Rev.* 1996;54:S59–S65.

28. Posner BM, Jette A, Smigelski C, Miller D, Mitchell P. Nutritional risk in New England elders. *J Gerontol.* 1994;49:M123–M132.

29. Sullivan DH, Martin WE, Flaxman N, Hagen JE. Oral health problems and involuntary weight loss in a population of frail elderly. *J Am Geriatr Soc.* 1993;41:725–731.

30. Dargent-Molina P, Hays M, Breart G. Sensory impairments and physical disability in aged women living at home. *Int J Epidemiol.* 1996;25:621–629.

31. Ostwald SK, Snowdon DA, Keenan NL, et al. Manual dexterity as a correlate of dependency in the elderly. *J Am Geriatr Soc.* 1989;37:963–969.

32. Siebens H, Trupa E, Siebens A, et al. Correlates and consequences of eating dependency in institutionalized elderly. *J Am Geriatr Soc.* 1986;34:192–198.

33. Katz S, Ford AB, Moskowitz RW, et al. Studies of illness in the aged: the index of ADL; a standardized measure of biological and psychosocial function. *JAMA.* 1963;185:914–919.

34. Lawton MP, Brody EM. Assessment of elderly people: self-maintaining and instrumental activities of daily living. *Gerontologist.* 1969;9:179–186.

35. Fleming KC, Evans JM, Weber DC, Chutka DS. Practical functional assessment of elderly persons: a primary-care approach. *Mayo Clin Proc.* 1995;70:890–910.

36. Goodwin JS, Goodwin JM, Garry PJ. Association between nutritional status and cognitive functioning in a healthy elderly population. *JAMA.* 1983;249:2917–2921.

37. Marcus DL, Freedman ML. The role of vitamin and mineral metabolism in cognition. *Clin Appl Nutr.* 1991;1(2):71–80.

38. Franklin CA, Karkeck J. Weight loss and senile dementia in an institutionalized elderly population. *J Am Diet Assoc.* 1989;89:790–792.

39. Sandeman P, Adolfsson R, Nygren C, et al. Nutritional status and dietary intake in institutionalized patients with Alzheimer's disease and multiinfarct dementia. *J Am Geriatr Soc.* 1987;35:31.

40. Wright BA. Weight loss and weight gain in a nursing home: a prospective study. *Geriatr Nurs.* 1993;14:156–159.

41. Morley JE. Death by starvation: a modern American problem? *J Am Geriatr Soc.* 1989;37:184–185. Editorial.

42. Gray GE, Paganini-Hill A, Ross RK. Dietary intake and nutrient supplement use in a Southern California retirement community. *Am J Clin Nutr.* 1983;38:122–128.

43. Adams TL, Chernoff R, McCabe BM et al. *The Effect of Home-Delivered Meals on Length of Hospitalization for Elderly Patients.* 1991. Unpublished master's thesis.

44. O'Hanlon P, Kohrs MB, Hilderbrand E, et al. Socioeconomic factors and dietary intake of elderly Missourians. *J Am Diet Assoc.* 1983;82:646–653.

45. Baker H, Frank O, Thind IS, et al. Vitamin profiles in elderly persons living at home or in nursing homes, versus profile in healthy young subjects. *J Am Geriatr Soc.* 1979;27:444–450.

46. Singer JD, Granahan P, Goodrich NN, et al. Diet and iron status, a study of relationships: United States, 1971-1974. *Vital Health Stat.* 1982;229(11).

47. McGandy RB, Russell RM, Hartz SC, et al. Nutritional status survey of healthy noninstitutionalized elderly: energy and nutrient intakes from three day records and nutrient supplements. *Nutr Res.* 1986;6:785–798.

48. McIntosh WA, Shifflet PA. Influence of social support systems on dietary intake of the elderly. J Nutr Elderly. Fall 1984;4:5.

49. Blackburn GL, Bistrian BR, Maini BS. Nutritional and metabolic assessment of the hospitalized patient. *J Parenter Enter Nutr.* 1977;1:11–22.

50. Mitchell CO, Lipschitz DA. Detection of protein-calorie malnutrition in the elderly. *Am J Clin Nutr.* 1982;35:398–406.

51. Rossman J. The anatomy of aging. In: Rossman J, ed. *Clinical Geriatrics.* Philadelphia, Pa: JB Lippincott Co; 1979.

52. Dequeker JV, Baeyens JP, Classens J. The significance of stature as a clinical measurement of aging. *J Am Geriatr Soc.* 1969;17:169–179.

53. Miall WE, Ashcroft MT, Lovell HG, et al. A longitudinal study of the decline of adult height with age in two Welsh communities. *Hum Biol.* 1967;39:445–454.

54. Trotter M, Bleser G. The effect of aging on stature. *Am J Phys Anthropol.* 1951;9:311–324.

55. McPherson JR, Lancaster DR, Carroll JC. Stature changes with aging in black Americans. *J Gerontol.* 1978;33:2–25.

56. Young CM, Blondin J, Tensuan R, et al. Body composition studies of "older" women, thirty to seventy years of age. *Ann NY Acad Sci.* 1963;110:598–607.

57. Norris AH, Lundy T, Shock NW. Trends in selected indices of body composition in men between the ages of 30 and 80 years. *Ann NY Acad Sci.* 1963;110:623–639.

58. Hertzog KP, Garn SM, Hempy HO. Partitioning the effects of secular trend and aging on adult stature. *Am J Phys Anthropol.* 1969;31:111–116.

59. Chumlea WC, Garry PJ, Hunt WC, et al. Serial changes in stature and weight in a healthy elderly population. *Hum Biol.* 1988;60:918–925.

60. Abraham S, Lowenstein FW, Johnson CL. *Preliminary Findings of the First Health and Nutrition Examination Survey, United States, 1971-72: Dietary Intake and Biochemical Findings.* Washington, DC: US Government Printing Office; 1974. National Center for Health Statistics; US Dept of Health, Education, and Welfare publication HRA 74-1219-21.

61. Elahi VK, Elahi P, Andres R. A longitudinal study of nutritional intake in men. *J Gerontol.* 1983;38:162–180.

62. Forbes GB. The adult decline in lean body mass. *Hum Biol.* 1976;48:161–166.

63. Garth S, Young R. Concurrent fat loss and fat gain. *Am J Phys Anthropol.* 1956;14:497–504.

64. Hejda S. Skinfold in old and long-lived individuals. *Gerontology.* 1563;8:201–297.

65. Stoudt HW, Damon A, McFarland R, et al. Weight, height and selected body dimensions of adults, United States, 1960–1962. *Vital Health Stat.* 1963;35(11).

66. Enzi G, Gasparo M, Biondetti PR, et al. Subcutaneous and visceral fat distribution according to sex, age, and overweight, evaluated by computed tomography. *Am J Clin Nutr.* 1987;45:7–13.

67. Borkan GA, Hults DE, Gerzof SG, et al. Comparison of body composition in middle-aged and elderly males using computed tomography. *Am J Phys Anthropol.* 1985;66:289–295.

68. Baumgartner RN, Heymsfield SB, Roche AF, et al. Quantification of abdominal composition by computed tomography. *Am J Clin Nutr.* 1989;50:221–226.

69. Mitchell CO, Lipschitz DA. The effect of age and sex on the routinely employed measurements used to assess the nutritional status of hospitalized patients. *Am J Clin Nutr.* 1982;36:340–349.

70. Heymsfield SB, Tighe A, Wang Z-M. Nutritional assessment by anthropometric and biochemical

methods. In: Shils ME, Olson JA, Shike M, eds. 8th ed. *Modern Nutrition in Health and Disease.* Philadelphia, Pa: Lea & Febiger, 1994.

71. Lipschitz DA, Mitchell CO. Nutritional assessment of the elderly: special considerations. In: Wright RA, Heymsfield S, eds. *Nutritional Assessment.* Boston, Mass: Blackwell Scientific Publications Inc; 1984.

72. Gordon CC, Chumlea WC, Roche AF. Stature, recumbent length, and weight. In: Lohman TG, Roche AF, Martorell R, eds. *Anthropometric Standardization Reference Manual.* Champaign, Ill: Human Kinetics Publishers Inc; 1988.

73. Chumlea WC, Roche AF, Mukherjee D. *Nutritional Assessment in the Elderly Through Anthropometry.* 2nd ed. Columbus, Ohio: Ross Laboratories; 1987.

74. Mitchell CO, Lipschitz DA. Arm length measurement as an alternative to height in nutritional assessment of the elderly. *J Parenter Enter Nutr.* 1982;6:226–229.

75. Chumlea WC, Roche AF, Steinbaugh ML. Estimating stature from knee height for persons 60 to 90 years of age. *J Am Geriatr Soc.* 1985;33:116–120.

76. Harris JA, Jackson CM, Patterson DG, et al. *The Measurement of Man.* Minneapolis, Minn: University of Minnesota Press; 1930.

77. Chumlea WC, Guo S, Roche AF, et al. Prediction of body weight for the non-ambulatory elderly from anthropometry. *J Am Diet Assoc.* 1984;88:564–568.

78. Martin AD, Carter JEL, Hendy KC, et al. Segment lengths. In: Lohman TG, Roche AF, Martorell R, eds. *Anthropometric Standardization Reference Manual.* Champaign, Ill: Human Kinetics Publishers Inc; 1988.

79. Dwyer JT, Coleman A, Krall E, et al. Changes in relative weight among institutionalized elderly adults. *J Gerontol.* 1987;42:246–251.

80. Roche AF. Anthropometric variables: effectiveness and limitations. In: *Assessing the Nutritional Status of the Elderly: State of the Art. Report of the Third Ross Roundtable on Medical Issues.* Columbus, Ohio: Ross Laboratories; 1982.

81. Sullivan DH, Patch GA, Baden AL, et al. An approach to assessing the reliability of anthropometrics in elderly patients. *J Am Geriatr Soc.* 1989;37:607–613.

82. Metropolitan Life Insurance Company. New weight standards for men and women. *Stat Bull Metrop Insur Co.* 1959;40:1–4.

83. Metropolitan Life Insurance Company. Metropolitan height and weight tables. *Stat Bull Metrop Insur Co.* 1989;64:2–9.

84. Russell RM. Evaluating the nutritional status of the elderly. *Clin Nutr.* 1983;2:4–8.

85. Frisancho AR, Flegel PN. Elbow breadth as a measure of frame size for U.S. males and females. *Am J Clin Nutr.* 1983;73:311–314.

86. Novascone MA, Smith EP. Frame size estimation: a comparative analysis of methods based on height, wrist circumference, and elbow breadth. *J Am Diet Assoc.* 1989;89:964–966.

87. Frisancho AR. New standards of weight and body composition by frame size and height for assessment of nutritional status of adults and the elderly. *Am J Clin Nutr.* 1984;40:808–819.

88. Clark NG. Nutritional support of elderly patients, II: proposed answers. *Clin Consult.* 1982; 2:5–9.

89. Master AM, Lasser RP. Tables of average weight and height of Americans aged 65 to 94 years: relationship of weight and height to survival. *JAMA.* 1960;172:661.

90. Burt VL, Harris T. The third National Health and Nutrition Examination Survey: contributing data on aging and health. *Gerontologist.* 1994;34:486–490.

91. de Onis M, Habicht JP. Anthropometric reference data for international use: recommendations from a World Health Organization Expert Committee. *Am J Clin Nutr.* 1996;64:650–658.

92. Chernoff R, Mitchell CO, Lipschitz DA. Assessment of the nutritional status of the geriatric patient. *Geriatr Med Today.* 1984;3:129–141.

93. Mooradian AD. Nutrition modulation of life span and gene expression. *Ann Intern Med.* 1988;109:890–904.

94. Galanos AN, Peiper CF, Cornoni-Huntley JC, Bales CW, Fillenbaum GG. Nutrition and function: is there a relationship between body mass index and the functional capabilities of community-dwelling elderly? *J Am Geriatr Soc.* 1994;42:368–377.

95. *Nutrition Interventions Manual for Professionals Caring for Older Americans.* Washington, DC: Nutrition Screening Initiative; 1992.

96. Obesity in America: an overview. In: Bray GA, ed. *Obesity in America.* Washington DC: US Dept of Health, Education, and Welfare; 1980.

97. Thommas AE, McKay DA, Cutlip MB. A nomograph method for assessing body weight. *Am J Clin Nutr.* 1976;29:302–304.

98. Potter JF, Schafer DF, Bohi RL. In-hospital mortality as a function of body mass index: an age-dependent variable. *J Gerontol*. 1988;43:M59–M63.

99. Rosenberg IH. Summary comments. *Am J Clin Nutr*. 1989;50:1231–1233.

100. Evans WJ. What is sarcopenia? *J Gerontol*. 1995;50A:5–10.

101. Chumlea WC, Guo SS, Glaser RM, Vellas BJ. Sarcopenia, function and health. *Nutr Health Aging*. 1997;1:7–12.

102. Chumlea WC, Baumgartner RN. Status of anthropometry and body composition data in elderly subjects. *Am J Clin Nutr*. 1989;50:1158–1166.

103. Durnin JV, Womersley S. Body fat assessed from total body density and its estimation from skinfold thickness: measurements of 481 men and women aged from 16 to 72 years. *Br J Nutr*. 1974;32:77–79.

104. Steen B, Bfroce A, Isaksson B, et al. Body composition in 70-year-old males and females in Gothenburg, Sweden: a population study. *Acta Med Scand Suppl*. 1977;611:87–112.

105. Wilmore JH, Behnke AR. Predictability of lean body weight through anthropometric assessment in college men. *J Appl Physiol*. 1968;25:349–355.

106. Watson PE, Watson JD, Batt RD. Total body water volumes for adult males and females estimated from simple anthropometric measurements. *Am J Clin Nutr*. 1980;33:27–39.

107. Latin RW, Johnson SC, Ruhling RO. An anthropometric estimation of body composition of older men. *J Gerontol*. 1987;42:24–28.

108. Butterworth CE, Blackburn GL. Hospital malnutrition and how to assess the nutritional status of a patient. *Nutr Today*. 1975;10:8–18.

109. Fox EA, Boylan ML, Johnson L. Clinically applicable methods for body fat determination. *Top Clin Nutr*. 1987;2:1–9.

110. Harrison GG, Buskirk ER, Carter JEL, et al. Skinfold thickness and measurement technique. In: Lohman TG, Roche AF, Martorell R, eds. *Anthropometric Standardization Reference Manual*. Champaign, Ill: Human Kinetics Publishers Inc; 1988.

111. Falciglia G, O'Connor J, Gedling E. Upper arm anthropometric norms in elderly white subjects. *J Am Diet Assoc*. 1988;88:569–574.

112. Callaway CW, Chumlea WC, Bouchard C, et al. Circumferences. In: Lohman TG, Roche AF, Martorell R, eds. *Anthropometric Standardization Reference Manual*. Champaign, Ill: Human Kinetics Publishers Inc; 1988.

113. Chumlea WC, Guo SS, Vellas B, Guigoz Y. Assessing body composition and sarcopenia with anthropometry. Proceedings: CERI Symposium, Nutrition et personnes agees au-dela des apports recommandes; 1997:161–169. Paris, France.

114. Guigoz Y, Bruno V, Garry PJ. Assessing the nutritional status of the elderly: the mini nutritional assessment as part of the geriatric evaluation. *Nutr Rev*. 1996;54:S59–S65.

115. Mitchell CO, Lipschitz DA. Creatinine height index in the elderly. In: *Assessing the Nutritional Status of the Elderly: State of the Art. Report of the Third Ross Roundtable on Medical Issues*. Columbus, Ohio: Ross Laboratories; 1982.

116. Bloch L, Schoenheimer R, Rittenberg D. Rate of formation and disappearance of body creatinine in normal animals. *J Biol Chem*. 1941;138:155–161.

117. Morrow FD. Assessment of nutritional status in the elderly: application and interpretation of nutritional biochemistries. *Clin Nutr*. 1986;5:112–120.

118. Welle S, Thornton C, Totterman S, Gilbert F. Utility of creatinine excretion in body-composition studies of healthy men and women older than 60 y. *Am J Clin Nutr*. 1996;63:151–156.

119. Mobarhan S. The role of albumin in nutritional support. *J Am Coll Nutr*. 1988;7:445–452.

120. Mullen JL, Buzby GP, Waldman MT, et al. Prediction of operative morbidity and mortality by preoperative nutritional assessment. *Surg Forum*. 1979;30:80–82.

121. Agarwal N, Acevedo F, Leighton LS, et al. Predictive ability of various nutritional variables for mortality in elderly people. *Am J Clin Nutr*. 1988;48:1173–1178.

122. Ferguson RP, O'Connor P, Crabtree B, Batchelor A, Mitchell J, Coppola D. Serum albumin and prealbumin as predictors of clinical outcomes of hospitalized elderly nursing home residents. *J Am Geriatr Soc*. 1993;41:545–549.

123. Salive ME, Cornoni-Huntley J, Phillips CL, et al. Serum albumin in older persons: relationship with age and health status. *J Clin Epidemiol*. 1992;45:213–221.

124. Campion EW, deLabry LO, Glynn RJ. The effect of age on serum albumin in healthy males: report from the normative aging study. *J Gerontol.* 1988;43:M18–M20.

125. Munro HN. Nutrition and ageing. *Br Med J.* 1981;37:83–88.

126. Reuben DB, Moore AA, Damesyn M, Keeler E, Harrison GG, Greendale GA. Correlates of hypoalbuminemia in community-dwelling older persons. *Am J Clin Nutr.* 1994;66:38–45.

127. Baumgartner RN, Doehler KM, Romero L, Garry PJ. Serum albumin is associated with skeletal muscle in elderly men and women. *Am J Clin Nutr.* 1996;64:552–558.

128. Corti MC, Guralnik JM, Salive ME, Sorkin JD. Serum albumin level and physical disability as predictors of mortality in older persons. *JAMA.* 1994;272:1036–1042.

129. Finucane P, Rudra T, Hsu R, et al. Markers of the nutritional status in acutely ill elderly patients. *Gerontology.* 1988;34:304.

130. Friedmann JM, Jensen GL, Smiciklas-Wright H, McCamish MA. Predicting early nonelective hospital readmission in nutritionally compromised older adults. *Am J Clin Nutr.* 1997;65:1714–1720.

131. Eisenberg S. Postural changes in plasma volume in hypoalbuminemia. *Arch Intern Med.* 1963;112:544–549.

132. Lipschitz DA, Cook JD, Finch CA. The clinical evaluation of serum ferritin as an index of iron stores. *N Engl J Med.* 1974;290:1213–1216.

133. Bothwell TH, Charlton R, Cook J, et al. *Iron Metabolism in Man.* Oxford, England: Blackwell Scientific Publishers Ltd; 1979:295–297.

134. Lipschitz DA, Mitchell CO, Thompson C. The anemia of senescence. *Am J Hematol.* 1981;11:47–54.

135. Awad MO, Barford AV, Grindulis KA, et al. Factors affecting the serum iron-binding capacity in the elderly. *Gerontology.* 1982;28:125–131.

136. Lipschitz DA, Mitchell CO. The correctability of nutritional, immune, and hematopoietic manifestations of protein-caloric malnutrition in the elderly. *J Am Coll Nutr.* 1982;1:16–23.

137. Winkler MF, Gerrior SA, Pomp A, et al. Use of retinol-binding protein and prealbumin as indicators of the response to nutrition therapy. *J Am Diet Assoc.* 1989;89:684–687.

138. Prendergast JM. Nutritional evaluation of the institutionalized elderly. In: Armbrecht HJ, Prendergast JM, Coe RM, eds. *Nutritional Intervention in the Aging Process.* New York, NY: Springer-Verlag; 1984.

139. Kergoat MJ, Leclerc BS, PettitClerc C, et al. Discriminant biochemical markers for evaluating the nutritional status of elderly patients in long-term care. *Am J Clin Nutr.* 1987;46:849–861.

140. Ingenbleek Y, DeVisscher M, DeNayer P. Measurements of prealbumin as an index of protein-calorie malnutrition. *Lancet.* 1972;2:106–108.

141. Carpentier YA, Barthel J, Bruyns J. Plasma protein concentration in nutritional assessment. *Proc Nutr Soc.* 1982;41:405–417.

142. Bourry J, Milano G, Caldani C, et al. Assessment of nutritional proteins during the parenteral nutrition of cancer patients. *Ann Clin Lab Sci.* 1982;12:158–162.

143. Ramsden D, Prince H, Burr A, et al. The interrelationship of thyroid hormones, vitamin A and their binding proteins following acute stress. *Clin Endocrinol (Oxf).* 1978;8:109–122.

144. Goichot B, Schlienger J-L, Gruenenberger F, et al. Low cholesterol concentrations in free-living elderly subjects: relations with dietary intake and nutritional intake, *Am J Clin Nutr.* 1995;62:547–553.

145. Kaiser FE. Cholesterol, heart disease, and the older adult. *Clin Appl Nutr.* 1992;2(1):35–43.

146. Harris T, Cook EF, Kannel WB, et al. Proportional hazards analysis of risk factors for coronary heart disease in individuals aged 65 or older. *J Am Geriatr Soc.* 1988;36:1023–1028.

147. Benfante R, Reed D. Is elevated serum cholesterol a risk factor for coronary heart disease in the elderly? 1990;263:393–396.

148. Corti M-C, Guralnick JM, Salive ME, et al. HDL cholesterol predicts coronary heart disease mortality in older persons. *JAMA.* 1995;274:539–544.

149. Wilson PWF, Anderson KM, Harris T, et al. Determinants of change in total cholesterol and HDL-C with age: the Framingham Study. *J Gerontol Med Sci.* 1994;49:M252–M257.

150. Oster P, Muchowski H, Heuck CC, et al. The prognostic significance of hypocholesterolemia in hospitalized patients. *Klin Wochenschr.* 1981;59:857–860.

151. Rudman D, Mattson DE, Nagraj HS, et al. Prognostic significance of serum cholesterol in nursing home men. *J Parenter Enter Nutr.* 1988;12:155–158.

152. Cunningham-Rundles S. Effects of nutritional status on immunological function. *Am J Clin Nutr.* 1982;35:1202–1210.

153. Bistrian BR, Blackburn GL, Scrimshaw N, et al. Cellular immunity in semistarved states in hospitalized adults. *Am J Clin Nutr.* 1975;28:1148–1155.

154. Meakins JL, Pietsch JB, Bubenick O, et al. Delayed hypersensitivity: indicator of acquired failure of host defenses in sepsis and trauma. Surgery. 1977;82:349–355.

155. Chandra RK, Scrimshaw NS. Immunocompetence in nutritional assessment. *Am J Clin Nutr.* 1980;33:2691–2697.

156. Thompson JS, Robbins J, Cooper JK. Nutrition and immune function in the geriatric population. *Clin Geriatr Med.* 1987;3:309–317.

157. Katz AE. Immunity and aging. *Otolaryngol Clin North Am.* 1982;15:287–291.

158. Delafuente JC, Meuleman JR, Nelson RC. Anergy testing in nursing home residents. *J Am Geriatr Soc.* 1988;36:733–735.

159. Chandra RK. Serum thymic hormone activity in protein energy malnutrition. *Clin Exp Immunol.* 1979;38:228.

160. Stiehm ER. Humoral immunity in malnutrition. *Fed Proc.* 1980;39:3093.

161. Cohn JR, Hohl CA, Buckley CE III. The relationship between cutaneous cellular immune responsiveness and mortality in a nursing home population. *J Am Geriatr Soc.* 1983;3:808–809.

162. Lipschitz DA. Nutrition, aging, and the immunohematopoietic system. *Clin Geriatr Med.* 1987;3:319–328.

163. Lipschitz DA. Nutrition and the aging hematopoietic system. In: Hutchinson ML, Munro HN, eds. *Nutrition and Aging.* New York, NY: Academic Press; 1986.

164. Caliendo MA. Validity of the 24-hour recall to determine dietary status of elderly in an extended care facility. *J Nutr Elderly.* 1981;1:57–66.

165. Samet JM. Surrogate measures of dietary intake. *Am J Clin Nutr.* 1989;50:1139–1144.

166. Hankin JH. Development of a diet history questionnaire for studies of older persons. *Am J Clin Nutr.* 1989;50:1121–1127.

167. Mahalko JR, Johnson LK, Ballagher SK, et al. Comparison of dietary histories and seven-day food records in a nutritional assessment of older adults. *Am J Clin Nutr.* 1985;42:542–553.

168. Gersovitz M, Madden JP, Smiciklas-Wright H. Validity of the 24-hr dietary recall and seven-day record for group comparisons. *J Am Diet Assoc.* 1978;73:48–55.

169. Bowman BB, Rosenberg IH. Assessment of the nutritional status of the elderly. *Am J Clin Nutr.* 1982;35:1142–1144.

170. *Report of Nutrition Screening I: Toward a Common View.* Washington DC: Nutrition Screening Initiative; 1991.

171. Posner BM, Jette AM, Smith MA, et al. Nutrition and health risks in the elderly: the Nutrition Screening Initiative. *Am J Public Health.* 1993;83:972–978.

172. *Nutrition Screening Initiative Project: Status Report.* Hillsborough County, Fla: Senior Citizens Nutrition Program, Nutrition Screening Initiative Project; 1994.

173. *Delaware Nutrition Screening Program.* New Castle, Del: Delaware Health and Social Services, Division of Aging; 1993.

# CHAPTER 17

# Nutritional Support for the Elderly

*Ronni Chernoff*

Nutrition is essential to sustain life and health and plays a key role in the recovery from acute and chronic illnesses. For those who are not healthy, who have chronic conditions or episodes of acute illness, who suffer trauma, or who undergo surgeries or other invasive medical procedures, providing nutritional therapies that are timely and appropriate for the patient and the patient's condition is essential to maximize recovery and rehabilitation potential.

Since older adults consume the greatest percentage of health care resources[1,2] and occupy many of acute and chronic care beds, it becomes essential that the provision of nutritional therapies, particularly as enteral or parenteral infusions, is done with special consideration to the unique needs of elderly individuals. Many of these specific needs have been addressed in the examination of macronutrient and micronutrient requirements (Chapters 2 through 5) and in the discussion of nutritional assessment in Chapter 16. However, it is important to review these particular requirements with consideration of the benefits and limitations of nutritional support methodologies. Appropriate selection of nutritional interventions may be key to successful nutritional rehabilitation, correction of nutritional deficits, restoration of nutritional

reserves, and avoidance of difficult ethical dilemmas.

## INDICATIONS FOR NUTRITIONAL SUPPORT

Gradual loss of weight is a common occurrence among elderly individuals, although the etiology of the weight loss may be undetermined. Involuntary weight loss may occur with a variety of acute and chronic illnesses, such as cancer[3]; sepsis, diabetes, renal disease, and dementia[4]; however, weight loss in elderly subjects may not have an obvious cause.[5-9] Anorexia or diminished nutrient intake usually is associated with the loss of weight. Morley and colleagues[10] describe this syndrome as the "anorexia of aging" and have suggested that the diminished nutrient intake is a consequence of decreased metabolic rate and reduced energy output. Inadequate food intake due to compromised socioeconomic circumstances, depression or dementia, and functional dependency may also contribute to slow, chronic weight loss. Sometimes weight is maintained because of lack of activity and reduced requirements for energy, but chronic malnutrition may occur because of a deficit of essential nutrients other than energy. Depletion of nutrient stores, particularly tissue stores of water-soluble vitamins, may not be apparent until a physiologic insult such as an illness, an accident, a trauma, or emotional stress occurs. When an individual who is chronically undernourished encounters physical stress, his or her physical condition may deteriorate rapidly, and unexpected complications may occur. Repletion of nutrient stores and restoration of nutritional and reserve capacity may require aggressive nutritional intervention—enteral or parenteral support.

Protein-energy malnutrition is often secondary to a primary disease process such as cancer, a chronic cardiac condition, a chronic pulmonary disease, a renal or hepatic disease, or a gastrointestinal disorder.[8] Many studies indicate that protein-energy malnutrition is prevalent among elderly hospitalized patients[10–16] and institutionalized individuals[17–19]. Many consequences of undernutrition may contribute to delayed recovery or rehabilitation, which, in older adults, may complicate an already complex health status.

One of the profound consequences of protein-energy malnutrition in elderly individuals is impairment of immune function.[8] Immune responses are affected by age (Chapter 16), independent of nutritional status; however, compromised nutritional status contributes to an additional depression of the immune system.[20] This situation may prove life threatening in seriously ill individuals because of the increased risk of infection and a decreased ability to mobilize host defenses.

If protein-energy malnutrition is suspected in seriously ill patients, it is important that practitioners use clinical judgment to set therapeutic priorities and to select and initiate nutritional interventions. Major medical problems take priority over nutritional deficits and must be corrected before nutritional intervention is considered. Priorities include the management of infection; the control of

blood pressure; and the restoration of metabolic, fluid, and electrolyte balances. It is important to monitor fluid and electrolyte equilibration during the acute phase of an illness, or at the time of admission to an acute care facility, to establish the validity of certain nutritional markers. Nutritional indicators may appear to change after fluid and electrolyte therapy is instituted because of serum dilution or rehydration effects. True serum values are necessary for an accurate assessment of nutritional condition and the need for nutritional support intervention.

Even in the absence of overt protein-energy malnutrition, there may be an indication for nutritional support. Medical condition, diagnosis, prognosis, and treatment plans are all factors in the decision to provide medical nutrition therapy. A patient who suffers from multiple chronic conditions is less likely to respond swiftly to an acute insult and may need support through the critical phase. Although oral nutrition is the preferred method of feeding, it may be unreasonable to expect adequate oral nutrient ingestion, particularly since some patients may not be able to eat for extended periods of time because of coma, stroke, head injuries, oral surgery, or gastrointestinal injuries or impairments. Patients who are chronically ill and cannot ingest adequate amounts of nutrients because of anorexia, side effects of drugs such as those used in chemotherapy, or severe limitations on nutrient or fluid intake for therapeutic purposes may be candidates for nutritional support. Having gastrointestinal disease (eg, malabsorption, maldigestion, or motility disorders), surgery, or obstruction may contribute to the need for nutritional support.[21] If the gastrointestinal tract cannot be used, parenteral nutrition is a viable option.

Even in stable long-term care patients, chronic undernutrition may be a problem, despite the lack of active disease processes. Patients who require long-term care may have inadequate dietary intakes because of dementia[4] or the need for help with feeding.[22,23] The need for help with feeding may be a significant factor for both dependent and apparently independent nursing home patients, not only for adequate energy intake but also for nutrient density.[22,23] For patients who have permanent disabilities that interfere with adequate nutrient ingestion, absorption, or utilization, nutritional support may become a necessity for continued life.

## ORAL SUPPLEMENTS

The optimal method for nutritionally supporting patients who are at risk for malnutrition is to feed them a nutritionally dense, well-balanced diet. Patients should be encouraged to eat as much as possible within the limits of their disabilities, oral health status, and medical conditions. If an adequate diet cannot be consumed through standard mealtimes and patterns, consideration should be given to offering multiple small meals or nontraditional meal patterns. If intake can be enhanced by serving breakfast foods for the dinner meal or desserts as between-meal snacks, the opportunity to enrich dietary intake ought to be pursued; there is a great deal to be gained from this approach, and the patient will be the beneficiary.

It has been reported that only 10% of elderly people who have protein-energy malnutrition can ingest nutrients adequate to overcome their nutritional deficits.[24] However, since food is such an important part of life, being the focus of social, cultural, religious, and family gatherings, it is important to encourage elderly individuals to maintain their normal diets as long as they are able.[21]

Unless there is a compelling need or a specific request from the patient, restricting certain nutrients in the diet may contribute to unforeseen problems.[25] Many older people have difficulty in discriminating between moderation in eating habits and the elimination of entire groups of food products. Limiting intake of many foods may lead to previously unseen nutritional deficiencies. Liberalizing diet restrictions may lead to a more palatable diet and more interest in food and may not have a negative impact on medical interventions for chronic disease; it is possible that the patient may enjoy food more and consume a diet that reduces the risk of nutritional problems.[25] A thorough dietary history is essential before changes in the diets of patients or clients are initiated.

### Dietary Supplements

Many options are available to supplement the diets of individuals who are at risk for malnutrition. Carbohydrate and protein powders are available that can be added to the patient's usual diet to increase the nutrient density without changing the flavor, texture, or color. Vitamin supplements are readily available to compensate for vitamins and minerals that may be lacking in an individual's diet. In a study conducted on elderly Australians, the use of dietary supplements (eg, bran or wheat germ) or vitamin and mineral supplements had no effect on incidence of illness or use of medical resources; however, individuals who used such supplements did have more favorable dietary habits and were more nutritionally aware than those who did not use supplements.[26] Data are inconclusive as to the contribution of supplements to the nutritional value of the diets of elderly Americans.[27–30]

For people who have unpredictable appetite levels, snacks can be prepared in advance to be available as desired. These might include crackers; cheese; hardcooked eggs; peanut butter; fresh or dried fruit; small meals, such as half a sandwich and a glass of milk or juice; soup; milkshakes or fruit frappes; nutrition bars; or oral liquid nutritional supplements. Commercially available supplements may be nutritionally complete or may provide only a portion of the recommended dietary allowances (RDAs) for adults. Elderly patients who have chewing, swallowing, or feeding problems or gastrointestinal impairments may require either liquid diets or supplemented diets for extended periods of time because of their inability to ingest adequate nutrients from regular food. Consideration of fluid, mineral, or macronutrient (eg, protein) restrictions is essential to selection of an appropriate supplement in long-term care patients. Many elderly individuals experience problems with chronic cardiac, renal, pulmonary, and hepatic diseases that contribute to fluid or protein limitations. Careful evaluation of the nutritional profile of supplements is necessary to meet therapeutic guidelines for individual patients.[31]

Many elderly patients, especially African Americans and Hispanics, are lactose deficient or have conditions that temporarily render them lactose deficient (severe malnutrition, sprue, bacterial overgrowth, chemotoxicity); these individuals may need lactose-free nutritional supplements in place of milkshakes, custards, or cream soups.[31]

## Commercial Liquid Supplements

Oral supplementation of patients' diets with commercially available liquid formulas has been shown to be efficacious in long-term care patients[32]; patients with bone fractures,[33] infections,[34] or cancer[3,35]; and homebound elderly people.[36,37] In a study by Ching and associates,[35] nutritional status was maintained in a group of elderly cancer patients undergoing various cancer treatment modalities through supplementation with commercially available nutritional supplements. Nine long-term care patients benefited from the addition of a nutritional supplement to their diets, in a study reported by Andersson and colleagues.[36] Although the volume of food consumed did not change appreciably in this group of patients, they achieved positive nitrogen balances as a result of increased protein, calorie, and fat intakes. In a study of long-term nursing home patients with a variety of diagnoses (including dementia, diabetes mellitus, pulmonary and urinary tract infections, stroke, and pressure ulcers), oral supplementation with commercial liquid diets contributed to weight gain and improvement in nutritional parameters.[32]

Volkert and colleagues[37] found that subjects who received oral supplementation in hospital and during a 6-month follow-up period post discharge recovered more effectively than a control group who were not supplemented. In another study of homebound elderly who were dependent on home-delivered meals, the impact of oral nutritional supplements, based on overall nutritional intake, was significant.[38] However, another study on free-living, frail elderly failed to show a significant improvement in functional status despite weight gain.[39] Although these investigators did not find a significant improvement in strength or perception of health, they did record a statistically significant difference in the incidence in falls. This may be a meaningful finding for those who care for these individuals.

The composition of oral liquid supplements changes regularly. It is important to obtain current information from industry representatives about available products.

Nutritional intervention can be accomplished successfully by use of oral supplements; however, there are patients who cannot ingest adequate nutrients because of oral and swallowing problems (eg, malignancies, obstructions, wired jaws, lesions associated with chemotherapy or radiation therapy, fungus infections, mucositis); cognitive problems (eg, dementia, coma); functional impairments (eg, due to stroke or head or spinal cord injury); or increased nutrient needs associated with hypermetabolic states, cancer, thermal injuries, malnutrition, or malabsorption. For these patients and others who cannot obtain sufficient nutrients via the oral route, there are alternative methods for providing nutrition to elderly individuals in need of nutritional support. Enteral feeding by tube is the next option to consider, especially if the patient has a functional gastrointestinal tract.

## ENTERAL FEEDING

Aggressive nutritional support via enteral feeding has been shown to be efficacious in restoring nutritional status in individuals who are unable to orally ingest adequate nutrients.[16,40,41] Enteral feeding by tube provides a reasonably safe, cost-effective method of providing protein, calories, vitamins, minerals, trace elements, and fluid while preserving or restoring a functional bowel surface.[42–44] Because most enteral solutions can be prepared in a nonsterile environment or are feeding ready, can be administered without special equipment, and are relatively inexpensive, the choice of enteral solutions for nutritional support of elderly patients is a reasonable one.

### Selection of Enteral Feeding Route

Selecting an enteral feeding route is sometimes a challenging decision for a team of health care professionals and the patient or patient representative such as a family member, an ombudsman, or an individual with power of attorney. Decisions should be made in the context of prognosis, patient au-

tonomy, mental competency, quality of life, and other factors unique to the patient.[45] When a clinician makes the decision to place a feeding tube in a patient, he or she must consider the option that the tube may, at some time in the future, have to be removed. However, those making the decisions have alternatives to consider; enteral feeding solutions can be effectively delivered to the stomach, duodenum, or jejunum, but relative benefits and risks must be carefully evaluated when selecting an enteral feeding route for a specific patient. Feeding into the stomach via either a nasogastric or a gastrostomy feeding tube takes advantage of the normal physiologic processes of digestion and absorption.

One method of assisted feeding that is somewhat controversial and generally out of practice is syringe feeding. This method, using a feeding syringe with a 30-mL bulb or a piston syringe, has been used with patients who are difficult to feed with standard utensils or who could drink from a cup. This method should only be tried in patients who have intact swallowing function, who are alert, and who can sit upright. This method can be time consuming, since food boluses should be given in small amounts (approximately 1 teaspoon to 1/2 tablespoon) to avoid aspiration.[46]

### Gastric Feeding

The stomach acts to digest food through secretion of acid and hormones, contributes to regulation of pH, and controls release of partially digested meals into the small intestine. Release of liquid food into the small intestine is affected by osmoreceptors in the jejunum that delay emptying of hyperosmolar or hypoosmolar solutions; by acid solutions; by solutions with a high level of fatty acids, with a high nutrient density, or with high or low temperature; and by drugs such as narcotic analgesics and anticholinergic agents.[47]

Although there are many advantages to feeding into the stomach, there are potential risks, primarily associated with aspiration. In elderly patients, the risk of aspiration may be associated with high levels of gastric residuals or an impaired or absent gag reflex.[41]

Nasogastric feeding has been the most commonly used method throughout the history of enteral feeding because of the near-normalcy that it evokes.[47] For centuries, the administration of liquid meals through a tube into the stomach provided nutrition to individuals who could not otherwise obtain adequate nutrients.[48] Until the development of the Dobbhoff feeding tube and others like it (all of which are made from new-technology compounds that allow for soft, nonirritating, flexible tubes), the hazards of nasogastric feeding included the development of otitis media and nasopharyngeal lesions, aspiration, and voluntary tube removal. Even with the new materials and advanced technology, risks are still encountered with nasogastric tube feeding. In one case report, difficulty with nasal breathing due to the presence of a nasogastric tube contributed to respiratory failure in an elderly woman who was tube-feeding dependent as a result of a stroke.[49] Evaluation of nasal patency is an important step before the insertion of a nasogastric feeding tube.

Placement of a nasogastric tube is the most easily achieved of all tube placements, since it can be accomplished at the bedside, needs a minimal amount of equipment, and can be performed by nurses or other allied health professionals. There are risks associated with the placement of nasogastric tubes that should be prepared for by the individual placing them. Placement of a tube by an inexperienced practitioner can lead to trauma associated with insertion of the tube (eg, esophageal perforation, pneumothorax, pulmonary hemorrhage, pleural effusion, bronchopleural fis-

tula formation, pneumonia) or with aspiration.[49-55] Placement of feeding tubes may lead to other complications that, although uncommon, are potentially dangerous. For example, Lipman and colleagues[54] reported cases of nasopulmonary tube placement that resulted in pneumothorax in one patient and pneumonia and hydrothorax in another.

Despite these potential problems with tube insertion, nasogastric feeding can be used in both acute and chronic care patient settings. Feeding solutions may be administered continuously by using a slow-drip gravity method or an enteral feeding pump that maintains a constant rate of flow. In the acute care setting, nasogastric feeding is a commonly used means of providing short-term enteral nutritional support.[56] However, increasing numbers of long-term care patients are being fed by the enteral tube route; nasogastric feeding can be provided safely for long periods of time[57,58] (Chernoff R, Lipschitz DA, Milton KY. 1988. Unpublished data).

If the indications are that tube feeding will be required for extended periods of time, or if the patient is confused, demented, or combative, leading to inadvertent dislodgment of the feeding tube and putting the patient at serious risk of aspiration or mechanical complications,[51,58,59] the establishment of a permanent gastrostomy should be considered.[45,60–64] Permanent gastrostomies avoid most of the complications associated with nasogastric tube feeding, but there are some problems that occur with indwelling gastric tubes. Because access is accomplished through an incision in the abdominal wall, complications include intra-abdominal leakage of gastric contents, potentially causing peritonitis; leakage around the catheter insertion site, causing skin excoriation; and migration of the catheter into the abdominal cavity or pylorus.[51,61]

Percutaneous endoscopic gastrostomy (PEG) is an alternate method that may be used with some success in long-term tube-fed patients.[45,61,64–66] Clinicians must carefully evaluate elderly patients for the suitability of this method as part of their care; older patients who are malnourished may have mucosal thinning and skin fragility, which should be considered when placing a gastrostomy tube endoscopically. An organized appraisal of the value of this tube-feeding method should be conducted in long-term tube-fed patients to ensure its safety. In most cases, gastrostomy feeding is an efficacious method to use in elderly patients.

### Jejunal Feeding

Jejunal feedings are usually used when there is an obstruction in the upper gastrointestinal tract or stomach; when there is potential for the exacerbation of gastric disease, such as ulcers; when gastric dysfunction, such as atrophic gastritis or achlorhydria, exists; or when an individual has had surgery that precludes esophageal or gastric feeding.[67] Jejunal access has distinct advantages for patients who cannot be fed via the upper gastrointestinal tract, but it also has some potential risks that must be considered when selecting an enteral feeding route. Jejunostomies reduce the risk of gastroesophageal reflux and aspiration, a major consideration in elderly patients; however, jejunostomy tube placement frequently requires surgical procedures, which have their own risks.[68] Jejunostomy feeding should be considered if enteral support will be required for an extended period of time and the upper gastrointestinal tract will not be viable for feeding. Caution must be exercised to avoid inadvertent or purposeful tube dislodgment. Partial extraction of a jejunostomy tube can cause leakage of formula or intestinal contents into the peritoneum, leading to peritonitis.[68,69] The use of an indwelling jejunostomy tube should be carefully considered for elderly patients who require nutritional support; placement of a jejunal catheter should be seen as a solution for a long-term problem that will necessitate extended enteral nutritional support.

### Selection of Enteral Formulas

Many factors must be considered when selecting an enteral feeding formula for an elderly patient.[41,70–72] Some of these factors include an estimation of the duration of tube-feeding dependency; the location of the feeding tube; the energy, protein, and micronutrient requirements of the patient; the ability of the patient to digest and absorb nutrients; the need for disease-specific formulas; and the expense and availability of the product to be infused.

In a limited, short-term situation that is characterized by an acute episode, patients probably will be fed nasogastrically, although if the illness required gastrointestinal surgery, an indwelling gastric or jejunal catheter may be in place. In either of these short-term, acute situations, a formula can be selected to meet specific short-term needs. High-protein, high-calorie, predigested, or specially designed nutritional products can be selected to meet unique needs related to the medical condition. Acutely ill individuals may require disease-specific formulas that are part of the treatment plan. Elderly patients who have been undernourished for an extended period may have the additional problem of compromised absorptive capacity, for which a dilute solution or a partially predigested formula may be needed. Whenever enteral feeding is considered for an elderly patient, early feeding protocols should be followed with some caution. It is wise to start with a dilute solution that is infused slowly, to ensure tolerance before moving to full-strength, full-volume feeding.

The vast majority of elderly patients who are sustained on tube-feeding formulas are chronically ill and will be tube-feeding dependent for extended periods of time. Selecting a formula for use with long-term tube-fed patients requires consideration of energy, protein, vitamin, mineral, and fluid needs. Although energy needs may be lower related to a decrease in energy output and a slower basal metabolic rate, requirements for other nutrients remain the same, with only small variations. The challenge this represents is that small volumes of formula often do not provide the levels of protein, vitamins, minerals, and trace elements that are needed to maintain nutritional status.

Recent evidence emphasizes the need for careful formula selection for patients who will be dependent on tube feedings for 6 months or longer. Chernoff and colleagues[73] examined serum levels of trace minerals (including zinc and selenium) and trace proteins (carnitine and taurine) in long-term tube-fed elderly patients. They found deficiencies of selenium and low levels of carnitine and taurine in all the subjects who had been maintained on tube feedings for 6 months or longer; these deficiencies were corrected with the substitution of an enteral formula that contained small amounts of these nutrients. These nutrients have important roles in immune function (selenium) and fat metabolism (carnitine and taurine) and are important in long-term nutrition status. These data suggest that use of supplemented formulas should be considered for individuals who will be tube-feeding dependent for extended periods of time.

Even with supplemented formulas, adequate volumes must be infused to achieve an adequate intake of all nutrients. Inadequate volumes of enteral solutions may also be a factor in inadequate hydration of chronically tube-fed individuals.

Nutrient levels for tube-fed patients should meet basic needs for protein (approximately 1 g/kg of body weight); the RDAs for vitamins, minerals, and trace elements for adults older than 50 years; and fluid requirements of approximately 1500 mL/d. Fluid requirements can be met by providing at least 1 mL/kcal ingested, 30 mL/kg of body weight, or 125% of the volume of the formula. Of particular importance is the fact that the vast majority of enteral formulas require more than 1500 mL or 1500 kcal to meet 100% of the RDAs. Underfeeding of essential nutrients can be a chronic problem in enteral feeding–dependent elderly individuals, as described above.

Consideration must be given to the patient's metabolic status, gastrointestinal function, and diagnosis. Most long-term tube-fed patients can be supported by using a standard, 1 kcal/mL formula that provides the RDA or greater for vitamins and minerals.[40,74] There is rarely a demand for disease-specific, predigested, or nutrient-dense formulation; however, there may be indications for high-nitrogen products, such as for pressure ulcer healing.[75,76] Unfortunately, the development of pressure ulcers may be related in part to chronic undernutrition.

## Delivery of Enteral Feeding

### Enteral Access

The safe and successful provision of enteral nutrition is related to where and in what manner tube feeding is administered. The placement of the feeding tube may be one of the most important factors in minimizing potential complications. For short-term, or initiation of, enteral feeding, nasogastric tubes are frequently used.[56] New generations of nasogastric tubes are comfortable and can remain in place for extended periods of time.

Nasogastric tubes are relatively easy to place, particularly since many tubes have markings that indicate the length for nasogastric or nasoenteric placement.[77]

Nasogastric tubes allow the clinician to monitor the viability of the gastrointestinal tract by measuring tube-feeding residuals. Although the stomach acts as a reservoir, controlling the release of feeding solutions into the small bowel, the risk of pulmonary aspiration is greater with feedings that remain in the stomach for a time after infusion.[51,78] Individuals who have gastroesophageal reflux, gastroparesis, absent gag reflex, or swallowing dysfunction or who are comatose will be at greater risk for aspiration.[51]

The risk for pulmonary aspiration can be decreased by using a longer tube that permits feeding directly into the small intestine.[51] Nasoenteric tubes that can be passed into the duodenum or jejunum can be used where the risk of aspiration is great. These tubes tend to be small-bored, soft, and weighted so that they remain in place; some come with stylets that act as guidewires to ensure appropriate placement. The small bores that make these tubes comfortable also contribute to the limitation of formula choices that will flow unimpeded through them and the potential collapse of the tube when formula is aspirated to check residuals.[79] Placement of the tube may require the feeding formula be administered in a continuous infusion over 12 to 24 hours, since the reservoir function of the stomach is bypassed by feeding into the proximal small intestine.

For long-term feeding, clinicians often recommend gastric access placement of feeding tubes, usually PEG. Many approaches to direct feeding into the stomach, bypassing the nasal access route, have been used with variable success. These include Janeway, Stamm, and Witzel procedures, all of which require surgery to create a serosal tunnel through which a tube can be inserted. These procedures have had a common problem of gastric acid reflux or leakage around the stoma.[77] Placing a PEG minimizes this complication, is more comfortable for the patient, reduces the problems associated with tube obstruction or blockage, enables feeding of individuals who are unable to voluntarily consume adequate nutrients, and is cosmetically more appealing for the patient and care providers.[45,51,61,80,81]

Patients can be given feedings into the jejunum using the PEG procedure and a gastric jejunal tube. There are both advantages and disadvantages of jejunal feedings that are related to bypassing the digestive processes of the stomach and duodenum.[51] Formulas need to be partially digested and of a thin viscosity to be administered and absorbed with minimal complications.

### Enteral Infusion Rate and Volume

The site of tube placement is a major consideration in determining what schedule to establish for enteral feeding. If the infusion site is the stomach, there may be more options because the stomach acts as a natural reservoir, controlling release of nutrient solution into the duodenum. Because the stomach regulates the flow of formula into the small bowel, enteral feedings can be administered by either intermittent or continuous flow without serious concern about osmolarity, nutrient concentration, or formula viscosity. However, if infusion occurs distal to the stomach, either pump-controlled intermittent or continuous feeding is a better choice. Since the reservoir function of the stomach is lost, solutions should not be infused more rapidly than the small bowel can safely absorb. Too rapid infusion or too large a volume may cause problems with poor absorption or diarrhea.[51]

There is considerable diversity of opinion among nutrition professionals about how to infuse tube-feeding solutions effectively. The route, formula concentration, and flow rate should be dictated by patient tolerance. In older patients, individual tolerance should be the guide for formula-feeding progression.[61,82] The primary goal should be to provide an adequate volume of formula to meet patient needs while maintaining a safe, tolerable method of infusion.

### Complications of Enteral Feeding

There are many risks associated with enteral feeding in elderly patients (Table 17–1); some of these have already been described, but some complications must be addressed more specifically.

It is not uncommon to encounter elderly patients who will not tolerate enteral feeding tubes. Even small-bore, flexible tubes may be uncomfortable; patients are resistant to tube placement and become agitated; and elderly, confused patients may partially dislodge tubes, which can contribute to more serious complications.[4,14,17,51,83–86] Small-bore tubes are susceptible to clogging, kinking, and migration. One of the most frequent causes of clogging is the use of enteral feeding tubes for administering crushed medications. The only medications that should be put into feeding tubes are those that are dissolved in a liquid or are in fluid form. The internal diameter of the tube should permit the tube-feeding formula of choice to flow easily; more viscous formulas should only be administered through a moderate-sized tube (eg, 12 French).

Some enteral formulas leave a precipitate on the interior walls of the tube, which eventually leads to clogging. Flushing the tube regularly with liquid, such as water, under pressure minimizes this problem. Since all tube-fed patients require additional free fluid, flushing the tube with water will help to meet this need. Tube-feeding formulas are made of nutrients suspended in a liquid medium (water). The volume of the tube feeding is the total water and the displacement of the nutrient sources when dissolved or dispersed in the water. Often the total displacement is close to 25% of the total volume; that amount of free fluid should be provided to the patient either orally, if the patient can swallow, or by tube, added to the nutrient solution or used as a tube flush.

Tube location should be monitored at periodic intervals, especially after an episode of vomiting or when there is evidence that the patient has pulled on the tube.[41] Migration of the feeding tube can contribute to complications of aspiration, pulmonary infections, and gastrointestinal dysfunction.[14] Pulmonary complications are frequently, but not always, related to aspiration. Risk of aspiration can be minimized by always elevating the patient's head or the head of the bed when tube formula is being infused; by using pump-administered feeding; and by using tubes that are placed in the duodenum or jejunum. Particular attention should be paid to patients who have had strokes or neurologic or esophageal diseases that contribute to an impaired gag reflex or swallowing difficulties.[78,85]

Gastrointestinal complications that may be encountered include bloating, nausea, vomiting, diarrhea, and constipation. Frequently these problems can be alleviated by slowing the rate of the enteral infusion; altering the feeding regimen to a slow, controlled, continuous drip; or changing the formula. Diarrhea is the most commonly experienced gastrointestinal problem associated with tube feeding and is most frequently reported in intensive care settings.[86,87] Among elderly persons, residents of nursing homes have the highest incidence of diarrhea. In frail, elderly persons, the consequences of diarrhea may contribute to an increased mortality.[88]

**Table 17–1** Potential Enteral Feeding Problems in Elderly Patients

| Risk Factor | Problem |
| --- | --- |
| Decreased gastric emptying | Gastric retention → aspiration |
| Hiatal hernia | Gastric reflux → aspiration |
| Tissue fragility | Esophageal bleeding |
| Dislocation of tube | Muscosal ulceration |
|  | Pulmonary aspiration and infusion |
|  | Peritonitis |
|  | Gastritis |
| Altered glucose tolerance | Hyperglycemia → dehydration → altered mental status |
| Inadequate water | Hypernatremia |
|  | Hyperchloremia |
|  | Azotemia |
|  | Altered mental status |
| Decreased energy needs | Inadequate intake of nutrients |
| Decreased bowel motility | Constipation → fecal impaction |
| Achlorhydria | Increased susceptibility to bacterial contamination |
| Polypharmacy | Changes in formula osmolarity |
|  | Interference with drug absorption |
|  | Diarrhea |
| Confusion | Tube dislocation → aspiration |

Source: Adapted with permission from J.L. Rombeau and M.D. Caldwell, eds., *Clinical Nutrition: Enteral and Tube Feeding,* p. 394, © 1990, W.B. Saunders Company.

Diarrhea may be related to a number of conditions that affect elderly, hospitalized, or institutionalized patients. In the past, the use of milk-based formulations caused diarrhea, bloating, and gastrointestinal discomfort in lactase-deficient patients. There is now a greater understanding of the extent of this problem, and since the mid-1970s there has been a vast array of lactose-free products from which to choose. Bacterial contamination of tube-feeding formulas appeared to be a cause of diarrhea[89]; this problem has also been minimized with the availability of commercially prepared, ready-to-feed products. Homemade formulas were made from blended meats, strained vegetables, cooked cereals, pureed fruit, milk powder, juices, and other ingredients that could be contaminated easily by skin-, air-, and waterborne bacteria.[90]

Diarrhea can be caused by many different kinds of medications; when diarrhea is encountered, it is wise to review the drug profile to identify any drug that might be causing the problem.[87] Diarrhea can also be the result of a too-rapid infusion or a hyperosmolar formulation. Feeding regimens should be slowed to allow the patient time to adapt to the formula. Individuals who have been chronically undernourished may have incompetent bowel surfaces that contribute to malabsorption.[87] Concentrated or hyperosmolar feeding will lead to a watery diarrhea that can be reduced or corrected by diluting the formula and feeding it slowly.

One solution to the problem of diarrhea in tube-fed patients has been the addition of soluble fiber to the enteral feeding products. There is some evidence that fiber may resolve the diarrhea in tube-fed patients.[87,91–93] There have also been investigations that discuss some of the potential problems associated with fiber-supplemented enteral feedings.[94,95] A conservative approach is most appropriate in elderly patients. If diarrhea is present and the cause is not apparent (eg, medications), adding one or two cans (feedings) of a fiber-containing product to the patient's feeding regimen may resolve the problem.

Many other problems unique to older patients require clinical considerations that may not be included in standard enteral feeding protocols. Some of these are itemized in Table 17–2.

### Other Issues in Enteral Feeding in the Elderly

Enteral feeding frequently raises some difficult ethical questions when elderly individuals are involved. There are emotional issues that relate to the individuals' medical condition, prognosis, cognitive status, nutritional condition, and patient preference.[96] There is some evidence that many elderly are not familiar with enteral feeding processes or principles and are confused by informed consent materials.[51,83,97,98]

Attention has been brought to the issues surrounding tube feeding and hydration in patients who are cognitively impaired or incompetent or are unable to express their wishes. Certain accepted principles have been decided by the U.S. Supreme Court and state supreme courts in well-known cases such as those of Karen Quinlan,[99] Claire Conroy, and Nancy Cruzan.[97] The major relevant principle is that nutrition and hydration are medical therapy. While the right to refuse or withhold medical therapy is a personal decision,[99–101] there are many people who categorize nutrition and hydration as symbols of love, caring, and nurturance.[102]

Discussions about advance directives or living wills and durable power of attorney should be held while individuals are still healthy and mentally competent. Every attempt should be made to explain the processes and possible outcomes of enteral nutrition support to ensure that each patient can make the best choices for him- or herself.[97–102] It is equally important that health professionals accept the wishes of the patient even though these may be contrary to the beliefs held by the practitioner.

### PARENTERAL NUTRITION

Although enteral nutritional support is the preferred method of nutritional intervention for patients who are unable to ingest adequate nutritional substrate orally, the parenteral route may be used. There are very few data, and a great many unanswered questions, about the efficacy and safety of intravenous feeding in elderly patients. A multitude of studies have examined the use of parenteral nutritional support in different populations with assorted diagnoses, but only a few of them have examined the tolerance for parenteral nutrition in elderly individuals.[103,104]

The customary source of calories in parenteral solutions is hypertonic glucose solutions. Standard formulas are often greater than 20% glucose. It is known that glucose tolerance deteriorates with advancing age,[105,106] but the threshold of glucose infu-

**Table 17–2** Considerations when Tube-Feeding Elderly People

| Clinical Condition | Therapeutic Consideration |
|---|---|
| Functionally dependent with inadequate nutrient intake | Dental status<br>Ability to feed without assistance<br>Therapeutic restrictions<br>Cost<br>*Consider oral supplements, puddings, snacks* |
| Protein-energy malnutrition treated by enteral nutrition | Calorie density<br>Protein level<br>Volume tolerance<br>Renal function<br>Cost<br>*Consider high-nitrogen, high-calorie formula until nutritional status is restored, then provide adequate calories, nitrogen* |
| Diarrhea | Rate/volume of feeding<br>Medication profile<br>Fat content of formula<br>Osmolarity of formula<br>*Consider decrease in rate/volume for brief period, use of fiber-containing formula* |
| Long-term tube-feeding dependency | Placement of tube<br>Adequate caloric intake<br>Availability of pump<br>Cost<br>*Consider gastrostomy feeding with a formula providing complete nutrition* |
| Pressure ulcers | Calorie level<br>Protein level<br>*Consider high-calorie, high-protein formula* |
| Constipation | Residue content of diet<br>Fluid intake<br>Medical profile<br>Ambulation<br>*Consider fiber-containing diet with extra free water; increase physical activity if possible* |
| Intolerance to nasogastric tube | Type of tube<br>Anticipated length of tube dependency<br>Gastrointestinal physiology<br>*Consider soft, pliable, small-bore tube; gastrostomy, jejunostomy* |

*Source:* Adapted with permission from J.L. Rombeau and M.D. Caldwell, eds., *Clinical Nutrition: Enteral and Tube Feeding*, p. 394, © 1990, W.B. Saunders Company.

sion that can be administered safely to elderly patients has not been thoroughly investigated; the simultaneous infusion of insulin to enhance the absorption of intravenous glucose also warrants more careful study.

The use of intravenous fat emulsions has become a routine part of parenteral nutritional support. Lipid systems may prove to be very effective in elderly patients who are fluid restricted or who have glucose intolerance; however, lipid clearance rates and efficiency are usually not investigated before their use. The ability of elderly patients to adequately tolerate lipid emulsions is an area for further investigation. If lipids are well tolerated and rapidly cleared by older patients, their use in lipid-based peripheral parenteral systems might be very valuable. A combination of peripheral intravenous infusion and oral or enteral feedings might serve to provide an excellent source of nutrition, encourage the patient to take food or fluids by mouth or tube, and preserve gut integrity and function.

Protein solutions should be tolerated equally as well by elderly patients as they are by younger individuals. Limitations of protein infusion in older patients parallel those in younger patients and are usually associated with organ system dysfunction. Since parenteral nutrition solutions are aqueous, patients are usually well hydrated unless there is an excess of electrolytes in the formulation. The maintenance of hydration status in parenteral feeding–dependent patients is essential to a successful course of therapy.

As with other forms of nutritional therapy, adequate vitamins, minerals, and trace elements must be provided in the basic formulation to meet unique nutrition needs. Older patients must be monitored very carefully to ensure adequate hydration; sufficient calories, protein, and micronutrients; mainte-

nance or correction of metabolic status; and positive therapeutic effects. There is some risk, particularly of air emboli, venous thrombosis, and sepsis, associated with parenteral feeding. Careful, close monitoring of the elderly, parenterally fed patient is the prudent course.[107]

## HOME NUTRITIONAL SUPPORT

It is conceivable that elderly patients may be sent home with nutritional support when their medical condition stabilizes. Because of the management problems associated with the complex administration of parenteral feedings, the most likely method for home nutritional support is enteral feeding. Age-related changes in elderly patients must be considered when deciding to send them home with nutritional support.[108]

Impairments that may have an impact on the success of home nutritional support include alterations of vision; compromised hearing; loss of fine motor skills, coordination, and strength; and cognitive dysfunction. All of these age-related changes limit the patient's ability to understand and follow directions, recognize and correct potential problems, and communicate with caregivers and medical personnel. Successful nutritional support is dependent on the capacity of the patient and caregiver to manage care and obtain advice and guidance when problems arise.

Another factor of major importance is a thorough evaluation of the social circumstances of the patient. The patient's financial situation, including access to private health insurance or Medicare or Medicaid, Social Security benefits, and other sources of support, should be assessed. The availability of other social service systems should be explored as well. The home environment should be surveyed to appraise the availability of space needed for storage and formula preparation. The motivation of both patient and caregiver to undertake the responsibilities associated with home nutritional support must also be evaluated by a professional.

One viable alternative, assuming that Medicare or other health insurance is available, is use of the services of a home nutritional support company. This type of service may be more efficient because it can provide regular formula delivery, minimize the need for storage space, respond rapidly to problems, offer a reliable product, and provide regular monitoring. With careful advance planning, nutritional support can be safely and effectively provided to elderly patients.

## CONCLUSION

Nutritional support, whether in the acute, chronic, or home care setting, can be safely and successfully used in elderly patients. Careful attention must be given to gastrointestinal function, unique nutrient needs, tube site location, feeding regimen, and disease-specific requirements. Parenteral, enteral, and oral nutritional support may be used singly or together, as needed. Some caution must be built into the protocols developed for elderly patients; metabolic changes can occur rapidly and must be addressed quickly to avoid serious problems. Nutritional support can be an important component of life-saving or life-sustaining treatments in elderly individuals.

## REFERENCES

1. *A Profile of Older Americans: 1997.* Washington, DC: Program Resources Dept, American Associated of Retired Persons and Administration on Aging, Dept of Health and Human Services; 1998.

2. Hanson MJ. How we treat the elderly, *Hastings Cent Rep.* 1994; 24(5):4–6.

3. Pironi L. Nutritional aspects of elderly cancer patients. *RAYS* 1997;22(1 suppl):42–46.

4. Sheiman SL. Tube feeding the demented nursing home resident. *J Am Geriatr Soc.* 1996;44:1268–1270.

5. Martin KI, Sox HC, Krupp JR. Involuntary weight loss: diagnostic and prognostic significance. *Ann Intern Med.* 1981;95:568.

6. Rabinovitz M, Pitlik SD, Leifer M, et al. Unintentional weight loss: a retrospective analysis of 154 cases. *Arch Intern Med.* 1986;146:186.

7. Olsen-Noll CG, Bosworth MF. Anorexia and weight loss in the elderly. *Postgrad Med.* 1989;85:140–144.

8. Sullivan DH. The role of nutrition in increased morbidity and mortality. *Clin Geriatr Med.* 1995;11:661–674.

9. Zawada ET. Malnutrition in the elderly. *Postgrad Med.* 1996;100:207–225.

10. Morley JE, Silver AJ, Fiatarone M, et al. Geriatric grand rounds: nutrition and the elderly. *J Am Geriatr Soc.* 1986;34:823–832.

11. Constans T, Bacq Y, Berchot J-F, et al. Protein-energy malnutrition in elderly medical patients. *J Am Geriatr Soc.* 1992;40:263–268.

12. Mowe M, Bohmer T. The prevalence of undiagnosed protein-calorie undernutrition in a population of hospitalized elderly patients. *J Am Geriatr Soc.* 1991;39:1089–1092.

13. Reilly JJ, Hull SF, Albert N, et al. Economic impact of malnutrition: a model system for hospitalized patients. *J Parenter Enter Nutr.* 1988;12:371–376.

14. Sullivan DH, Moriarty MS, Chernoff R, et al. Patterns of care: an analysis of the quality of nutritional care routinely provided to elderly hospitalized veterans. *J Parenter Enter Nutr.* 1989;13:249–254.

15. Lovat LB. Age related changes in gut physiology and nutritional status. *Gut.* 1996;38:306–309.

16. Tierney AJ. Undernutrition and elderly hospital patients: a review. *J Adv Nurs.* 1996;23:228–236.

17. Morley JE, Silver AJ. Nutritional issues in nursing home care. *Ann Intern Med.* 1995;123:850–859.

18. Posthauer ME, Russell C. Ensuring optimal nutrition in long-term care. *Nutr Clin Pract.* 1997;12:247–255.

19. Abassi AA, Rudman D. Observations on the prevalence of protein-calorie undernutrition in VA nursing homes. *J Am Geriatr Soc.* 1993;41:117–121.

20. Goodwin JS, Burns EL. Aging, nutrition, and immune function. *Clin Appl Nutr.* 1991;1:85–94.

21. Pories WJ. Feeding the elderly patient. *NC Med J.* 1988;49:632–635.

22. Nguyen NH, Flint DM, Prinsley DM, et al. Nutrient intakes of dependent and apparently independent nursing home patients. *Hum Nutr Appl Nutr.* 1985;39A:333–338.

23. Morley JE. Anorexia in older persons: epidemiology and optimal treatment. *Drugs Aging.* 1996;8:134–155.

24. Lipschitz DA, Mitchell CO. The correctability of the nutritional, immune, and hematopoietic manifestations of protein calorie malnutrition in the elderly. *J Am Coll Nutr.* 1982;1:17–25.

25. Position of the American Dietetic Association: liberalized diets for older adults in long-term care. *J Am Diet Assoc.* 1998:98:201–204.

26. Horwath CC, Worsley A. Dietary supplement use in a randomly selected group of elderly Australians. *J Am Geriatr Soc.* 1989;37:689–696.

27. Garry PJ, Goodwin JS, Hunt WC, et al. Nutritional status in a healthy elderly population: dietary and supplemental intakes. *Am J Clin Nutr.* 1982;36:319–331.

28. O'Hanlon P, Kohrs MB. Dietary studies of older Americans. *Am J Clin Nutr.* 1978;31:1257–1269.

29. Tripp F. The use of dietary supplements in the elderly: current issues and recommendations. *J Am Diet Assoc.* 1997;97(suppl 2):S181–S183.

30. Gray-Donald K. The frail elderly: meeting the nutritional challenges. *J Am Diet Assoc.* 1995;95:538–540.

31. Bernard MA, Rombeau JL. Nutritional support for the elderly patient. In: Young EA, ed. *Nutrition, Aging and Health.* New York, NY: Alan R Liss Inc; 1986.

32. Johnson LE, Dooley PA, Gleick JB. Oral nutritional supplement use in elderly nursing home patients. *J Am Geriatr Soc.* 1993;41:947–952.

33. Delmi M, Rapin CH, Bengoa JM, et al. Dietary supplementation in elderly patients with fractured neck of the femur. *Lancet.* 1990;1:1013–1016.

34. Woo J, Ho SC, Mak YT, et al. Nutritional status of elderly patients during recovery from chest infection and the role of nutritional supplementation assessed by a prospective randomized single-blind trial. *Age Ageing.* 1994;23:40–48.

35. Ching N, Grossi C, Zurawinsky H, et al. Nutritional deficiencies and nutritional support therapy in geriatric cancer patients. *J Am Geriatr Soc.* 1979;27:491–494.

36. Andersson H, Falkheden T, Petersson I. A study on liquid diet in geriatric patients. *Aktuel Gerontol.* 1979;9:417–421.

37. Volkert D, Hübsch S, Oster P, et al. Nutritional support and functional status in undernourished geriatric patients during hospitalization and 6-month follow-up. *Aging Clin Exp Res.* 1996;8:386–395.

38. Lipschitz DA, Mitchell CO, Steele RW, et al. Nutritional evaluation and supplementation of elderly subjects participating in a "Meals on Wheels" program. *J Parenter Enter Nutr.* 1985;9:343–347.

39. Gray-Donald K, Payette H, Boutier V. Randomized clinical trial of nutritional supplementation shows little effect on functional status among free-living frail elderly. *J Nutr* 1995;125:2965–2992.

40. Allison SP. Cost-effectiveness of nutritional support in the elderly. *Proc Nutr Soc.* 1995;54:693–699.

41. Sullivan DH. Nutritional support for elderly patients. In: Morley JE, Glick Z, Rubenstein LZ, eds. *Geriatric Nutrition: A Comprehensive Review.* New York, NY: Raven Press; 1990.

42. Chernoff R, Lipschitz DA. Enteral feeding and the geriatric patient. In: Rombeau JL, Caldwell MD, eds. *Clinical Nutrition: Enteral and Tube Feeding.* 2nd ed. Philadelphia, Pa: WB Saunders Co; 1990.

43. Levine GM, Deren JJ, Steiger E, et al. Role of oral intake in maintenance of gut mass and disaccharide activity. *Gastroenterology.* 1974;67:975–982.

44. Tilson MD. Pathophysiology and treatment of short bowel syndrome. *Surg Clin North Am.* 1980;60:1273–1284.

45. Hasan M, Meara RJ, Bhowmick BK, et al. Percutaneous endoscopic gastrostomy in geriatric patients: attitudes of health care professionals. *Gerontology.* 1995;41:326–331.

46. Soriano R. Syringe feeding: current clinical practice and recommendations. *Geriatr Nurs.* 1994;15:85–87.

47. Kelly DG, Fleming CR. Physiology of the gastrointestinal tract: as applied to patients receiving tube enteral nutrition. In: Rombeau JL, Rolandelli RH, eds. *Clinical Nutrition: Enteral and Tube Feeding.* 3rd ed. Philadelphia, Pa: WB Saunders Co; 1997.

48. McCamish MA, Bounous G, Geraghty ME. History of enteral feeding: past and present perspectives. In: Rombeau JL, Rolandelli RH, eds. *Clinical Nutrition: Enteral and Tube Feeding.* 3rd ed. Philadelphia, Pa: WB Saunders Co; 1997.

49. Hernandez OG, Nelson S, Haponik EF, et al. Obligate nasal breathing in an elderly woman: increased risk of nasogastric tube feeding. *J Parenter Enter Nutr.* 1988;12:531–532.

50. Galindo-Ciocon DJ. Tube feeding: complications among the elderly. *J Gerontol Nurs.* June 1993;17–22.

51. Drickamer MA, Cooney LM Jr. A geriatrician's guide to enteral feeding. *J Am Geriatr Soc.* 1993;41:272–279.

52. Miller KS, Tomlinson JR, Sahn SA. Pleural pulmonary complications of enteral tube feedings. *Chest.* 1985;88:230–233.

53. Woodall BH, Winfield DF, Bisset GS. Inadvertent tracheobronchial placement of feeding tubes. *Radiology.* 1987;165:727–729.

54. Lipman TO, Kessler T, Arabian A. Nasopulmonary intubation with feeding tubes: case reports and review of the literature. *J Parenter Enter Nutr.* 1985;9:618–620.

55. McWey RE, Curry NS, Schabel SI, et al. Complications of nasoenteric feeding tubes. *Am J Surg.* February 1988; 155:253–257.

56. Rolandelli RH, Ullrich JR. Nutritional support in the frail elderly surgical patient. *Surg Clin North Amer.* 1994;74:79–92.

57. Heitkemper MM, Williams S. Prevent problems caused by enteral feeding: know about complications before they arise. *J Gerontol Nurs.* 1985;11(7):25–30.

58. Meer JA. Inadvertent dislodgment of nasoenteral feeding tubes: incidence and prevention. *J Parenter Enter Nutr.* 1987;11:187–189.

59. Pick N, McDonald A, Bennett N, et al. Pulmonary aspiration in a long-term care setting: clinical and laboratory observations and an analysis of risk factors. *J Am Geriatr Soc.* 1996;44:763–768.

60. Daly MP, Richardson JP. Geriatrics for the clinician: nutrition in old age. *Md Med J.* 1995;44:377–381.

61. Tealey AR. Percutaneous endoscopic gastrostomy in the elderly. *Gastroenterol Nurs.* February 1994; 151–157.

62. Sriram K, Palac B. Nasogastric feeding in the elderly. *JAMA.* 1984;252:1682.

63. Ciocon JO, Silverstone FA, Graver LM, et al. Tube feedings in elderly patients: indications, benefits, and complications. *Arch Intern Med.* 1988;148:429–433.

64. Pomerantz MA, Salomon J, Dunn R. Permanent gastrostomy as a solution to some nutritional problems in the elderly. *J Am Geriatr Soc.* 1980;28:104–107.

65. Larson DE, Fleming CR, Ott BJ, et al. Percutaneous endoscopic gastrostomy: simplified access for enteral nutrition. *Mayo Clin Proc.* 1983;58:103–107.

66. Miller RE, Kummer BA, Tiszenkel Hl, et al. Percutaneous endoscopic gastrostomy: procedure of choice. *Ann Surg.* 1986;204:543–545.

67. DeChicco, RS, Matarese LE. Determining the nutrition support regimen. In: Matarese LE, Gottschlich MM, eds. *Contemporary Nutrition Support Practice.* Philadelphia, Pa: WB Saunders Company; 1998.

68. Gorman RC, Morris JB. Minimally invasive access to the gastrointestinal tract. In: Rombeau JL, Rolandelli RH, eds. *Clinical Nutrition: Enteral and Tube Feeding.* 3rd ed. Philadelphia, Pa: WB Saunders Co; 1997.

69. Lambaise RE, Dorfman GS, Cronan JJ, et al. Percutaneous alternatives in nutritional support: a radiologic perspective. *J Parenter Enter Nutr.* 1988;12:513–520.

70. Pasulka PS, Crockett C. Selecting enteral products. In: Borlase BC, Bell SJ, Blackburn GL, Forse RA, eds. *Enteral Nutrition.* New York, NY: Chapman & Hall; 1994.

71. Gottschlich MM, Shronts EP, Hutchins AM. Defined formula diets. In: Rombeau JL, Rolandelli RH, eds. *Clinical Nutrition: Enteral and Tube Feeding.* 3rd ed. Philadelphia, PA: WB Saunders Co; 1997.

72. Matarese LE. Rationale and efficacy of specialized enteral and parenteral formulas. In: Matarese LE, Gottschlich MM, ed. *Contemporary Nutrition Support Practice*. Philadelphia, PA: WB Saunders Co; 1998.

73. Chernoff R, Milton KY, Lipschitz DA. The effect of enteral formula supplementation on carnitine, taurine and selenium status in long-term tube fed patients. *J Parenter Enter Nutr*. 1991;15:365.

74. Berner Y, Morse R, Frank O, et al. Vitamin plasma levels in long-term enteral feeding patients. *J Parenter Enter Nutr*. 1989; 13:525–528.

75. Chernoff R, Milton KY, Lipschitz DA. The effect of a high protein formula (Replete) on decubitus ulcer healing in long term tube fed institutionalized patients. *J Am Diet Assoc*. 1990;90(suppl):A130.

76. Finucane TE. Malnutrition, tube feeding, and pressure sores: data are incomplete. *J Am Geriatr Soc*. 1995;43:447–451.

77. Lysen LK, Samour PQ. Enteral equipment. In: Matarese LE, Gottschlich MM, ed. *Contemporary Nutrition Support Practice*. Philadelphia, Pa: WB Saunders Co; 1998.

78. Pick N, McDonald A, Bennett N, et al. Pulmonary aspiration in a long-term care setting: clinical and laboratory observations and an analysis of risk factors. *J Am Geriatr Soc*. 1996;44:763–768.

79. Powell SK, Marcuard SP, Farrior ES, et al. Aspirating gastric residuals causes occlusion of small-bore feeding tubes. *J Parenter Enter Nutr*. 1993;17:243–246.

80. Rees RG, Payne-James JJ, King C, et al. Spontaneous transpyloric passage and performance of "fine bore" polyurethane feeding tubes: a controlled clinical trial. *J Parenter Enter Nutr*. 1988;12:469–472.

81. Sloane PD, Rizzolo P. Gastric tube feeding in elderly patients. *Arch Fam Med*. 1993;2:927–928.

82. Sullivan DH, Chernoff R, Lipschitz DA. Nutritional support in long-term care facilities. *Nutr Clin Pract*. 1987;2(1):6–13.

83. Leff B, Cheuvront N, Russell W. Discontinue feeding tubes in a community nursing home. *Gerontologist*. 1994;34(1):130–133.

84. Mitchell SL, Kiely DK, Lipsitz LA. Does artificial enteral nutrition prolong the survival of institutionalized elders with chewing and swallowing problems? *J Gerontol Med Sci*. 1998;53A:M207–M213.

85. O'Mahoney D, McIntyre AS. Artificial feeding for elderly patients after stroke. *Age Ageing*. 1995;24:533–535.

86. Guenter PA, Settle RG, Perlmutter SG, et al. Tube-feeding related diarrhea in acutely ill patients. *J Parenter Enter Nutr*. 1991;15:277–280.

87. Beyer PL. Complications of Enteral Nutrition. In: Matarese LE, Gottschlich MM, ed. *Contemporary Nutrition Support Practice*. Philadelphia, Pa: WB Saunders Co; 1998.

88. Bennett RG, Greenough WB III. Approach to acute diarrhea in the elderly. *Gastroenterol Clin North Amer*. 1993;22:517–533.

89. Yen PK. Tube feeding safety. *Geriatr Nurs*. 1997;18:40–41.

90. Chernoff R, Bloch AS. Liquid feedings: considerations and alternatives. *J Am Diet Assoc*. 1977;70:389–391.

91. Zimmaro DM, Rolandelli RH, Koruda MJ, et al. Isotonic tube feeding formula induces liquid stool in normal subjects: reversal by pectin. *J Parenter Enter Nutr*. 1989;13:117.

92. Slavin JL, Nelson NL, McNamara EA, et al. Bowel function of healthy men consuming liquid diets with and without dietary fiber. *J Parenter Enter Nutr*. 1985;9:317–321.

93. Scheppach W, Burghardt W, Bartrarn P, et al. Addition of dietary fiber to liquid formula diets: the pros and cons. *J Parenter Enter Nutr*. 1990; 14:204–209.

94. Hart GK, Dobb GJ. Effect of fecal bulking agent on diarrhea during enteral feeding in the critically ill. *J Parenter Enter Nutr*. 1988;12:465–468.

95. Heymsfield SB, Roongspisuthipong C, Evert M, et al. Fiber supplementation of enteral formulas: effects on the bioavailability of major nutrients and gastrointestinal tolerance. *J Parenter Enter Nutr*. 1988;12:265–273.

96. Hodges MO, Tolle SW. Tube-feeding decisions in the elderly. *Clin Geriatr Med*. 1994;10:475–487.

97. Krynski MD, Tymchuk AJ, Ouslander JG. How informed can consent be? New light on comprehension among elderly people making decisions about enteral feeding. *Gerontologist*. 1994;34(1):36–43.

98. Ouslander JG, Tymchuk AJ, Krynski MD. Decisions about enteral tube feeding among the elderly. *JAGS.* 1993;41:70–77.

99. Ahronheim JC. Nutrition and hydration in the terminal patient. *Clin Geriatr Med.* 1996;12:379–391.

100. Meisel A. Barriers to forgoing nutrition and hydration in nursing homes. *Am J Law Med.* 1995;21:335–382.

101. Ackerman TF. The moral implications of medical uncertainty: tube feeding demented patients. *J Am Geriatr Soc.* 1996;44:1265–1267.

102. Paine CJ. Nursing home patients: can feeding tubes be withheld? *J La State Med Soc.* 1996;148:284.

103. Ferry M, Leverve X, Constans T. Comparison of subcutaneous and intravenous administration of a solution of amino acids in older patients. *J Am Geriatr Soc.* 1997;45:857–860.

104. Lutz BH. Total parenteral nutrition in the older patient. *Home Healthcare Nurse.* 1996;14:123–125.

105. Andres R. Aging and diabetes. *Med Clin North Am.* 1971;55:835–846.

106. Hofeldt FD. Diabetes mellitus and dyslipidemia disorders in the elderly. In: Jahnigan DW, Schrier RW, eds. *Geriatric Medicine.* Cambridge, Mass: Blackwell Science; 1996.

107. Chernoff R, Lipschitz DA. Total parenteral nutrition: considerations in the elderly. In: Rombeau JL, Caldwell MD, eds. *Clinical Nutrition: Parenteral Nutrition.* Philadelphia, Pa: WB Saunders Co; 1986:2.

108. Chernoff R. Home nutrition support in elderly patients. *Clin Nutr.* 1987;6(1):36–39.

# CHAPTER 18

# A Continuum of Nutrition Services for Older Americans

*Barbara E. Millen and Elyse Levine*

The 20th century has witnessed an epidemiological transition that is characterized by the progressive aging of the U.S. population and improvements in the health status of older Americans.[1-3] Average life expectancy in the United States at birth is now about 76 years,[4] compared with 42 years in 1900, and the proportion of those aged 65 years and older, currently estimated at 12%, is expected to increase to 20% through the year 2030.[5] Men who reach age 65 years will live an additional 15.3 years on average; women another 19 years.[6] Despite advancing age, most older Americans consider their health to be good to excellent[7] and believe that they have reasonable access to health, supportive, social, and rehabilitative services.[7] Consistent with these views, the rates of undiagnosed health problems in older persons are estimated to be decreasing, and the proportion of those who are well managed medically appears to be increasing.[7] These trends enable about 95% of older persons to live independently in community-based, noninstitutional settings.

Population aging emerged for several key reasons. Advances within this century in the prevention and treatment of infectious disease during pregnancy, infancy, and childhood allow women of childbearing age and children to survive the previously ravaging health problems in far greater proportions.[1-3]

Enhanced public health measures, including improved food quality, safety, and sanitation, have improved the nutritional status of the population.[8] As well, technological and clinical advances in the management of chronic diseases, their medical complications, and associated disability allow many more to reach a healthier, older age.[1-3,8]

Increased population life expectancy is not unique to the United States; indeed, population aging is a global phenomenon.[1-3,8,9] Average life expectancy worldwide has increased from 46 years in the 1950s to 65 years in 1995, and the gap in life expectancy between all countries has narrowed from 25 years in 1955 to 13.3 years in 1995.[9] These directions in global population aging have brought about dramatic changes in the world's health needs. Murray and Lopez[10] recently emphasized that chronic diseases, such as heart disease, hypertension and stroke, diabetes, pulmonary disease, and certain cancers, are either rapidly emerging or already established at high rates globally. Chronic diseases of aging account for nearly half of population morbidity and mortality in the developing regions of the world and over 85% of deaths and disability in developed regions.[2,3,8-10] Of particular importance is that in the poor population, nutritional status is estimated to account for over twice the estimated "burden of disease" of any other modifiable risk factor.[10] Suboptimal nutritional status, such as nutrient deficiencies and excesses, accounts for about 12% of total deaths and 16% of disability in the world's population (in terms of what is called *disability-adjusted life years* [DALY]). The attributable deaths and DALY for tobacco are 6.0% and 2.6%, respectively; for physical inactivity, 3.9% and 1.0%; and for alcohol 1.5% and 3.5%.[10] Clearly, the identification and treatment of nutrition-related problems in the population, including older persons, has important implications in the United States as well as globally.

Further advances in life expectancy and the quality of life of older Americans will depend on continued improvements in health, the prevention and early treatment of diseases or their complications, and better understanding of the aging process. Nutritional interventions and related services will play a central role in the promotion of successful aging. As noted by the U.S. Surgeon General,[11(p18)] "Sound public education directed toward this group [the older population]—and professional education directed toward individuals who care for older Americans—should focus on dietary means to reduce risk factors for chronic disease, [and] to promote functional independence."

Consistent with these recommendations, the U.S. National Institute on Aging (National Institutes of Health) recently recognized the importance of nutrition in the promotion of elder health and declared nutritional well-being in older Americans a priority research area.[12] *Healthy People 2000*,[13] the nation's health policy directive, also emphasized the importance of sound nutrition in advancing age and defined key objectives for reducing nutritional risk in the older population. In addition, over 25 professional organizations in the United States

formed the Nutrition Screening Initiative (NSI) to urge the development of methods for assessing the prevalence and determinants of nutrition-related problems in elders and the formulation of improved health care delivery standards that will enhance the nutritional status of older persons.[14]

In a similar vein and in recognition of the serious tolls associated with the chronic diseases of aging, the World Health Organization introduced a collaboration of nations in all regions of the world called the InterHealth Programme.[2,3] The purpose of this global initiative is to reduce risks for chronic diseases at the population level through integrated behavioral and policy-level interventions. Among the major features of integrated behavioral risk factor intervention planning is the promotion of sound eating practices in the population. Central to the InterHealth integrated strategy is the understanding that poor nutrition is associated with increased risks for multiple chronic diseases, including coronary heart disease, hypertension, diabetes mellitus, certain forms of cancer, and osteoporosis. Countries participating in InterHealth have established national policy statements on nutrition for noncommunicable disease prevention and control. These countries have also mounted numerous nutrition interventions at the national, community, household, and individual levels. In addition, the InterHealth collaboration has provided a mechanism for the systematic evaluation of its community-based interventions and the global sharing of information on strategies for chronic disease risk reduction in populations throughout the developed and developing world.[15] The global perspective on nutrition and the chronic diseases of aging is beyond the scope of this chapter, but the InterHealth Nutrition Initiative has been recently reviewed.[2,3]

The purpose of this chapter is to examine the interrelationships among nutrition, physical function, and health with advancing age, including the determinants of nutritional risk in elders; to describe major U.S. policy recommendations and interventions for improving the nutritional status of and enhancing the delivery of nutrition services to older Americans; and to review the nutrition services payment systems, in particular Medicare and Medicaid. Major emphasis is also placed on the recent national evaluation of the Elder Nutrition Program (ENP), the largest federally funded mechanism for the delivery of a continuum of home- and community-based nutrition and related health and supportive social services to the older U.S. adult population.

## NUTRITION, PHYSICAL FUNCTION, AND HEALTH IN ADVANCING AGE

Nutritional well-being is an integral component of the health, independence, and quality of life of older individuals.[14–17] Proper nutrition appears to mitigate existing health problems, improves the management of many chronic diseases, and extends years of healthy living with advancing age.[18] Conversely, the presence of malnutrition increases risk for medical and surgical complications, delays recovery from physical traumas, and is a primary risk factor for recurrent hospitalizations and costly, extended institutionalization.[19] Although the majority of persons aged 65 years and older in the United States consider themselves to be in good to excellent health, [6,11,20–22] over 85% of noninstitutionalized older persons have one or more chronic health problems that could be improved with proper nutrition, and up to half may have clinical evidence of various forms of malnutrition.[16]

Myriad nutritional problems exist in the older population. They span a broad spectrum ranging from frank nutrient deficiencies,

such as protein-energy malnutrition, to evidence of nutritional excesses, including obesity, dyslipidemia, hypertension, and higher than recommended levels of dietary lipids and other nutrients.[16,23–28] It is estimated that up to 15% of the free-living older population have demonstrable nutrient deficiencies. Up to 40% of the frail, homebound elderly and a similar proportion of the institutionalized older population may also suffer from protein-energy malnutrition and frank nutrient deficiencies (such as folate or vitamin $B_{12}$ deficiency).[16] In national nutrition studies, low dietary intakes of energy, fiber, calcium, magnesium, antioxidants, certain B vitamins, and other micronutrients are common in older persons.[21,29–31] As many as one in four older people may consume low levels of nutrients, which result in increased risk for nutrient deficiencies. Micronutrient imbalances may also increase risks for certain nutrition-related chronic diseases, such as diabetes and heart disease, and their complications. [16,20,32]

Factors that increase risk for nutrient deficiencies in the older population are not fully understood. The characteristics that appear to be associated with low nutrient intake are acute and chronic medical problems, particularly the presence of multiple, coexisting health problems; polypharmacy; losses of functional capacity; advanced age; oral health problems; declines in appetite; reductions in taste and olfactory acuity; social isolation; depression and other psychological disturbances; poverty; lack of nutrition knowledge; and susceptibility to fraud.[31–38] Among the noninstitutionalized elderly, those who are homebound and frail appear to be particularly at risk for nutrient deficiencies.[32,39,40] In addition, there are racial and income disparities in levels of food insecurity and access to food and nutrition services that increase risks for malnutrition in the poor and minority elder populations.[41]

Health problems related to nutritional excesses, including obesity, are also estimated to be quite common in the older population. Up to half of the free-living population 60 years of age and older consume diets with higher than recommended levels of nutrients, such as fat and sodium, which may have detrimental impacts on health.[16,39–41] It is estimated that 40% of older persons are overweight or obese by accepted clinical standards.[38–40] Nutritional excesses impose increased risk not only for the development of chronic diseases such as hypertension, coronary heart disease, diabetes, and certain forms of cancer but also for their adverse complications and outcomes, including death and physical disabilities.[40,42]

Little research has characterized the determinants of dietary excesses and related health problems in the older population. One study in a population-based sample of free-living elders in New England[18] suggested that smoking and male gender were associated with nutritional excesses, such as higher than recommended levels of nutrients (particularly dietary lipids). Those elders who continued to smoke were more apt to have a high dietary lipid intake. Older women were more likely than older men to comply with recent recommendations for "heart-healthy" nutrient intake.[18]

The available literature emphasizes that significant gaps exist in our understanding of nutrition-related problems and their etiology in the elder population. Few studies provide population-based estimates of the prevalence or etiology of nutritional excesses and deficiencies in the elderly. While the presence of combined forms of malnutrition (such as obesity and protein deficiency) has been reported,[31,42] particularly in the older institutionalized population, their prevalence and health-related outcomes are underresearched. There is also little known concerning the variation in nutrient requirements with advancing age, particularly in the presence of chronic and acute medical problems and treatments that may alter nutritional status. Furthermore, the efficacy of nutritional interventions among older individuals in community, home, or institutional settings is poorly understood.

Previous national health surveys such as the National Health and Nutrition Examination Surveys (NHANES I and II) have not examined persons 75 years and older,[43] nor have they subsampled segments of the older population who may be at particular nutritional risk, such as the homebound, frail elderly. NHANES III (1988–1994) corrected this situation by oversampling black and Mexican American populations 60 years and older and white Americans 60 to 69, 70 to 79, and 80 years and older.[44] However, little has been published to date. Horwath[45] reviewed over 90 studies on diet and nutritional status of older individuals and concluded that the majority were conducted on small, highly selected samples with limited generalizability. Little, if anything, is known about the prevalence of nutritional problems in the oldest old (those 80 years and older); the impact of chronic diseases and their complications on nutritional status; the health outcomes associated with malnutrition, particularly in the very old population; the directionality of the relationships between nutritional status and health characteristics and outcomes; or optimal methods of nutritional intervention in advanced age.

Several recent reports have identified the following research areas concerning nutrition and aging as priorities for investigation: the prevalence of nutrition-related problems in the older population, particularly in high-risk older populations such as the frail, homebound elderly; the role of nutritional factors in the etiology and prevention of chronic diseases and age-related impairments in organ system function; the development of guidelines for nutrition interventions that are appropriate for common morbidity patterns among older adults; relationships between nutrition, physical functioning, and health; and the nutritional determinants of cognitive and physical functioning and quality of life in older adults.[11,20,22,38,46,47]

## PUBLIC NUTRITION POLICY STATEMENTS AND RECOMMENDATIONS

In the last several decades, growing concern over nutritional risk in the older population has led to the development of key public policy statements to improve the nutritional status of older Americans and to enhance the delivery of nutrition and related health services. Many statements have attempted to provide guidelines and recommendations for optimal food and nutrient intake in advancing age. In addition, both public and private initiatives and programs have emerged to implement these policy directives. Such activities provide elements of a framework for the comprehensive assessment and monitoring of nutrition-related problems in the older population as well as the delivery of rational and appropriate nutrition services to elders. The policy statements and dietary recommendations are summarized in Table 18–1 and are discussed below. The recommendations for developing effective nutrition services and interventions are summarized in Table 18–2 and are described in the next section of this chapter.

The nation's most recent health policy statement, *Healthy People 2000*,[13] outlines a set of specific objectives to improve the health status of older Americans. (*Healthy People 2010* is scheduled for publication in January 2000.) Major goals were set to target

health status concerns, the need for risk reduction activities, and the need to improve the availability of key health promotion and protection services. Among the major health-related goals were to reduce morbidity and mortality associated with suicides, motor vehicle accidents, falls, hip fractures, and pneumonia; increase years of healthy and independent living; decrease hearing and visual impairments; improve dental health status; increase abilities to perform activities of daily living; improve access to and use of supportive social and primary health care services; decrease alcohol and tobacco use; and increase physical activity. In addition, related health objectives were identified for reducing the morbidity and mortality associated with chronic diseases, including heart disease, hypertension and stroke, certain cancers, and diabetes. A series of Year 2000 nutrition-related objectives for older persons were also set forth. Primary attention was placed on improvements in dietary intake of older individuals, particularly reducing total and saturated fat and sodium intakes; ensuring adequate dietary levels of essential micronutrients; reducing the prevalence of obesity; improving access to food and nutrition services (particularly home-delivered meals and congregate feeding); and promoting the availability of nutrition services, particularly nutritional assessment, counseling, and education, provided by qualified nutrition professionals to older individuals.[14]

While these policy directives provide overall goals for nutrition and related health intervention, they do not establish detailed recommendations for dietary planning in individuals. Such standards for planning were compiled by the Food and Nutrition Board of the National Academy of Sciences.[46] These guidelines, termed the *dietary reference intakes* (DRIs), expand and replace the recommended dietary allowances

**Table 18–1** Diet-Related Health Recommendations for Healthy Aging

| Originating Source, Year | Nutrition and Diet | Health and Related Recommendations |
|---|---|---|
| *Healthy People 2000,* 1992[13] | Reduce overweight and increase adoption of sound dietary practices combined with regular physical activity to attain appropriate body weight. Reduce fat to an average of 30% of calories or less and saturated fat to less than 10%. Increase complex carbohydrate and fiber containing food to 5 or more daily servings for vegetables (including legumes) and fruits and to 6 or more servings for grain products. Reduce salt and sodium intake (prepare foods without salt, avoid salt use at the table, use salt/sodium-modified foods). Use food labels. | Reduce morbidity and mortality associated with suicides, motor vehicle accidents, falls, hip fractures, and pneumonia; increase years of healthy and independent living; decrease hearing and visual impairments; improve dental health status; increase abilities to perform activities of daily living; improve access to and use of supportive social and primary health care services; decrease alcohol and tobacco use; and increase physical activity. As well, reduce morbidity and mortality associated with chronic diseases, including heart disease, hypertension and stroke, certain cancers, and diabetes. |
| *DRIs,* 1998[46] | Levels of recommended nutrient intake (RDAs and AIs) for healthy persons aged 51 to 70 and older than 70 years for calcium, phosphorus, magnesium, vitamin D, fluoride, thiamin, riboflavin, niacin, vitamin B₆, folate, vitamin B₁₂, pantothenic acid, biotin, and choline. Tolerable upper limits and estimated average requirements are also set for certain nutrients. Reference weights are also provided. | |
| *Surgeon General's Report on Nutrition and Health,* 1988[11] | Reduce consumption of fat, saturated fat, and cholesterol. Achieve and maintain desirable body weight. Increase whole grains, cereals, vegetables, and fruits. Reduce sodium intake. Take alcohol only in moderation, if at all. Depending on the individual's cir- | Diseases of dietary excesses and imbalances rank as the leading causes of death and disability in the United States including heart disease, atherosclerosis, certain cancers, hypertension and |

| | | |
|---|---|---|
| | ...cumstances, consider fluoride, calcium, and iron needs and the risks associated with sugar intake. Recommend adoption of the *Dietary Guidelines*.[48] | stroke, diabetes mellitus, and cirrhosis. Integrate nutrition services into all health care programs, including assessment, nutrition counseling, and referral to community-based nutrition and food assistance programs. Increase the use of food labels and food products that promote healthy nutrition. |
| *Surgeon General's Workshop*, 1988[22] | Promote good nutritional status for a high-quality life through physical, psychological, and social mechanisms. In doing so, consider the varying sociodemographic, functional, and physical conditions of elders and their medical care. | Improve quality of life of older Americans and promote autonomy. Promote research on nutrition, chronic diseases, and aging as well as the efficacy of nutrition services in the management of health problems in older persons. |
| Committee on Diet and Health, 1989[47] | Reduce total fat intake to 30% of calories or less; saturated fat to less than 10%; and cholesterol to less than 300 mg. Eat 5 or more servings of fruits and vegetables per day. Maintain protein intake at moderate levels. Balance food intake and physical activity to maintain appropriate body weight. Alcohol consumption not recommended. Limit sodium chloride intake to 6 g or less. Maintain adequate calcium intake. Avoid supplements in excess of RDAs. Maintain optimal fluoride intake. | Integrate geriatric nutrition curriculum into all professional education. Expand research on nutrition and aging, including research on nutrient requirements and on interactions between diet, health, and elders' sociodemographic and functional profiles. |
| Institute of Medicine, 1992[20] | Promote Committee on Diet and Health guidelines (see above). | |

*continues*

**Table 18–1** continued

| Originating Source, Year | Nutrition and Diet | Health and Related Recommendations |
|---|---|---|
| *Food Guide Pyramid, 1992*[48] | Outlines recommended daily food intake that is consistent with the Dietary Guidelines (see below): use fats, oils, and sweets sparingly; consume 3 to 5 servings from the milk, yogurt, and cheese group; consume 2 to 3 servings from the meat, poultry, fish, dry beans, eggs, and nuts group; consume 3 to 5 servings from the vegetable group; consume 2 to 4 servings from the fruit group; consume 6 to 11 servings from the bread, cereal, rice, and pasta group. | |
| Dietary Guidelines, 1992[48] | Eat a variety of foods. Maintain desirable weight. Avoid too much fat, saturated fat, and cholesterol. Eat foods with adequate starch and fiber. Avoid too much sugar and sodium. If you drink alcohol, do so in moderation. | |
| NCEP, 1993[49] | Provides dietary guidance to lower plasma total and LDL cholesterol levels. Two diet levels are outlined (Step One and Step Two) which target total and saturated fat and dietary cholesterol intake. | |
| NCI, 1994[50] | Emphasize 5 servings from the fruits and vegetables groups for the promotion of reduced cancer risk. | |
| NSI, 1997[60] | Nutrition guidelines specific to the management and prevention of the following diseases and their consequences: cancer, chronic obstructive pulmonary disease, congestive heart failure, coronary heart disease, dementia, diabetes mellitus, failure to thrive, hypertension, osteoporosis, and pneumonia. | Provides guidelines for nutritional screening and assessment. Recommends professional education strategies and includes educational materials. |

**Table 18–2** Recommendations for Nutrition Services and Interventions in Older Populations

| Originating Source, Year | Clinical/Medical Nutrition Services | Public/Professional Nutrition Education | Food Services |
|---|---|---|---|
| White House Conference on Aging 1981[38] | Committee resolution recommended reimbursement of nutritional assessment or counseling of elders provided by RDs from Medicaid/ Medicare programs. | Called for a task force appointed by the president to devise and execute a program for nutrition education through the mass media. Recommended that laws be strengthened to require public service time on radio and television. Advocated use of mass media for training neighborhood leaders. | Recommended that all food delivery systems and programs contain some form of nutrition education insofar as possible without hampering the delivery of foods. |
| *Surgeon General's Report*, 1988[11] | Recommended nutrition services to be provided within institutional and community-based services for older adults, including homebound elderly. | Called for more research on the efficacy of nutrition interventions and techniques that promote adequate food consumption in elders. Recommended elimination of nutrition-related health fraud. | Recommended that those providing food services be required to meet energy and nutrient needs of older clients, including frail and homebound elderly. |

*continues*

**Table 18–2** continued

| Originating Source, Year | Clinical/Medical Nutrition Services | Public/Professional Nutrition Education | Food Services |
|---|---|---|---|
| *Surgeon General's Workshop,* 1988[22] | Recommended that nutritional assessment be done at admission or enrollment in all institutional or community-based health services for older adults. Recommended employment of RDs or credentialed nutrition professionals in policy, planning, administrative, and coordination of aging programs. Addressed needs for health professionals to coordinate community-based services and institutional care. Urged the reimbursement of nutrition services for elders within inpatient, outpatient, and community settings by third-party payers. | Recommended that health-related agencies and associations develop and coordinate messages to meet needs of elderly; use advanced communication techniques appropriate to older adults; and develop and disseminate successful public/private sector models for health promotion. Recommended the reversal of shortages of knowledgeable personnel in areas of nutrition education, research, and service and the training of health professionals in nutrition. | Recommended that institutional and community-based food services be evaluated against appropriate nutritional standards for older individuals (RDAs, etc). |
| American Dietetic Association, 1993[40] | Recommended that nutrition services for elders be integrated into institutionally based health care facilities; private or group medical practices; health maintenance organizations; preferred provider practice settings; and ambulatory, home health, and social service settings. | Recommended that nutrition education be part of the continuum of health care for older adults, to be incorporated into all ambulatory, home, and institutional health care service activities. | |

| | | | |
|---|---|---|---|
| Institute of Medicine, 1992[20] | Recommended that nutritional screening, assessment, intervention, and care plans be required in hospitals, nursing homes, and other health care settings that receive federal funding. Promotion of dietary intervention for elders with atherosclerosis, hypertension, diabetes, and osteoporosis. | Promote self-care. Regulate nutrition fraud. Minimize polypharmacy and adverse drug-nutrient interactions. | Encourage participation in congregate and home-delivered meal programs to support functional independence. Develop and maintain nutrition and food service standards for nursing homes, long-term care facilities, and facilities that receive Medicare and Medicaid reimbursement. |
| NSI, 1992[59] | Six areas of intervention were identified: (1) social services to assist older persons in obtaining an appropriate diet; (2) oral health to improve food intake, diet quality, and socialization; (3) mental health to improve motivation and ability to meet nutritional needs; (4) assurance of proper medication use; (5) nutrition education and counseling; and (6) nutritional support to, as needed, increase or decrease nutrition intake; change the timing, composition, or size of meals; modify food textures; and change the route of feeding administration. | Use dietitians and nutritionists in family, individual, and professional nutrition education and counseling. | Food services, such as congregate and home meals programs, and other social services (like food stamps) should address key determinants of appropriate nutrient intake, including poverty, poor functional status, and social isolation. |
| *Healthy People 2000*, 1993[13] | Increase nutrition assessment and counseling by qualified dietitians and nutritionists in primary care settings. | Increase involvement in organized health promotion programs in community and elder service settings. | Increase home food services to those with impairments and need. |

(RDAs). They are designed to provide quantitative estimates of nutrient intake for uses in many settings, including the assessment of diets and menu planning to ensure the adequacy of intakes for energy, macronutrients, and selected micronutrients. The DRIs include RDAs as goals for the intake of individuals; they represent the recommended average daily intake that is sufficient to meet the nutrient needs of nearly all (97–98%) healthy people in a particular age group. They also include three new types of reference values: adequate intake (AI), tolerable upper intake level (UL), and estimated average requirement (EAR). An improvement over the earlier RDAs is the inclusion of two older adult groups: one aged 51 to 70 years and the other older than 70 years. When an RDA cannot be determined, an AI is set as the recommended intake level, on the basis of observational or experimental data on approximated nutrient intake in a group (or groups) of healthy people. The UL is the highest level of daily nutrient intake that is likely to pose no health risk in the general population. The EAR is the level of nutrient intake estimated to meet the nutrient needs of half of the healthy people in a group. The EAR is used in determining the RDAs and in assessing the adequacy of population group intake.

Several other groups, including the Office of the Surgeon General,[11,22] the Institute of Medicine,[20] and the Committee on Diet and Health of the National Research Council[47] have also published recommendations for nutrition and healthy aging. They are consistent with the Year 2000 and RDA guidelines. These reports emphasize the importance of targeting public nutrition education at the older population; using dietary interventions to lower chronic disease risk, promoting of elder functional independence and preventing adverse consequences from the use of medications that may alter nutritional sta-

tus.[11,22,48,49] It has been suggested that population-based recommendations for older persons might include the adoption of dietary recommendations to lower total fat and saturated fat; increase complex carbohydrates, fiber, and nutrient-rich fruits and vegetables; and reduce sodium intake.[20,47] The development of nutrition interventions for individuals with cognitive and physical impairments has been recommended to ensure the consumption of the recommended levels of essential nutrients.[20] These reports point out that population-based dietary guidelines established for the general adult population are suitable for promoting health and nutritional well-being in the older population. Cited reports include the Food Guide Pyramid and its related dietary guidelines[48] and the general adult population recommendations set forth by the Committee on Diet and Health,[47] the National Cholesterol Education Program,[49] and the National Cancer Institute.[50]

Additional recommendations set by NSI deserve particular attention.[19,51–60] While not a governmental body, NSI is a collaboration of over 25 professional organizations in the United States that are interested in improving the nutrition and health status of the older population. The initiative is committed to increasing public awareness of the nutritional needs of the older population, promoting optimal nutrition in advancing age, and developing strategies for nutritional risk assessment and intervention planning. Through a consensus-building process and ongoing research, NSI has developed methods for increasing consumer awareness of nutrition problems and methods for the in-depth detection of nutritional risk among older people.[19,51–59]

NSI has published dietary management guidelines for chronic disease care in older individuals.[60] The publication relied on *evidence-based* information, where available, to develop specific recommended strategies for managing the clinical features of various health conditions, including cancer, chronic obstructive pulmonary disease, congestive heart failure, coronary heart disease, dementia, diabetes mellitus, hypertension, failure to thrive, osteoporosis, and pneumonia. *Consensus-based* information was used to develop recommendations for dietary intervention where research was more limited or unavailable. Information was also assessed and provided on the expected outcomes of nutrition intervention and the profile of suitable providers of professional nutrition care. The report highlights the results of several recent research investigations on the cost-effectiveness of nutrition care in older adults in hospital and community settings. It was estimated that the delivery of appropriate nutrition intervention to elders would save up to $1.3 billion in health-related costs by the year 2002.[60(p1)]

## PROVIDING NUTRITION SERVICES TO OLDER PERSONS

The major recommendations of national government agencies and professional organizations for nutrition services and intervention activities among elders are summarized in Table 18–2. These policy statements and guidelines generally consider that older individuals, particularly those of advanced age or with multiple medical problems, may require a complicated array of nutrition and health-related services from various providers to maintain their health and nutritional well-being. In these circumstances, there is an urgent need to integrate and coordinate the provision of care to older individuals. This theme was voiced in the Surgeon General's recommendations regarding public nutrition services for the aging population.[22] It was suggested that nutrition services, with particular emphasis

on nutritional assessment and "guidance," be offered in institutional health care settings (hospitals, nursing homes, etc) as well as in community-based health and social service delivery settings (senior centers, congregate nutrition programs, adult day care centers, etc). It was also recommended that the emerging networks of social and support service providers (home health care providers, managed care networks, etc) recognize the importance of nutrition in advancing age and arrange for appropriate types of nutrition services for their older clients.

These recommendations are similar to those proposed by Posner et al in the American Dietetic Association (ADA)'s position paper on nutrition and aging.[40] The ADA advocated that nutrition services be included throughout the emerging continuum of long-term health care services for the elderly. The recommended types of nutrition services involved clinical or medical nutrition care, such as nutritional screening, assessment, monitoring, and evaluation; individual or family education and counseling; and enteral or parenteral medical nutrition support. Other recommended nutrition service activities included the delivery of prepared meals in congregate, institutional, or home settings; the establishment of food pantries or other community resources; related activities that improve access to food (such as transportation and shopping assistance and food stamps); and meal preparation and eating assistance-related activities (such as those carried out by homemakers, home health aides, or occupational therapists).[61,62]

*Nutrition screening* was described as a focused activity that is designed to identify people who need a particular type of nutrition service or program.[17,27,40,41,55,63] Screening is usually conducted by community agencies, programs, or clinic personnel to identify those with elevated risk for nutritional problems or to determine special considerations in managing an individual's situation (eg, edentulousness, confinement to bed, food allergies or preferences, and therapeutic diet needs). *Nutritional assessment* determines the individual's nutritional status, identifies significant nutritional problems, and investigates the problems' etiologies and possible solutions. In conducting assessments, trained professionals use a relatively complex and comprehensive set of clinical and laboratory techniques. *Nutritional status monitoring* is a process whereby assessments are conducted at predetermined, regular intervals, allowing an assessment of the changes in an individual's or population's nutritional status over time. *Evaluation research*, particularly *outcomes research* provides a formal mechanism by which to assess the impact of nutrition services on the individual's nutritional status and health. These studies may also include estimates of the costs of providing care and the potential health care cost savings that result from nutritional interventions. *Nutrition education* and *counseling* may occur on an individual level or in groups with families or clients. They are ideally carried out by professionals who are trained in the needs and learning strategies of older people. Medical nutritional support is a specialized form of clinical nutritional care that involves the planning and management of parenteral and enteral feedings. These services are discussed further by the ADA in *Nutrition Services Payment Systems.*[63]

The concept of a health care continuum, as emphasized in the ADA recommendations described above,[40] was first defined in a 1982 California law. It was proposed that there be established "a coordinated continuum of diagnostic, therapeutic, rehabilitative, supportive and maintenance services that addresses the health, social, and personal needs of (older) persons."[64] Posner and Krachenfels[27] present a model for integrating a continuum of nutrition and health services for older persons within institutional and community-based settings (see Figure 18–1). Like the ADA, they recognize that older people may receive health care services and related benefits in a variety of settings (at home, in the community, or within institutions) and that providers of necessary services may have diverse backgrounds, resources, and orientations. For example, food stamps may be handled by community agencies and personnel whose expertise lies in income-related services and programs. Adult day care and home care may be handled by local community social service agencies that provide a number of benefits (shopping assistance, social services) and refer clients to other programs and services (eg, homemakers and home health aides). The diagnosis and treatment of chronic diseases and the management of terminal illness may be carried out by a network of community-based health and social service providers (eg, health centers, HMOs, ambulatory care centers, private practitioners' offices, or hospices). Institutions (eg, hospitals, rehabilitation centers, and skilled nursing facilities) may provide acute and chronic care. Increasingly, hospitals are providing short-term care, and other community-based and home care providers deliver follow-up care in potentially less costly, alternative care settings.[40,41,65–69] This complex matrix of services, often referred to as the *long-term care system*, presents considerable challenges to those who are attempting to coordinate and monitor service delivery to their older clients.

The integration of nutrition and health care activities for elders is consistent with the recommendations of the Surgeon General, the White House Conference on Aging, the Insti-

**Figure 18–1** Nutrition in the continuum of long-term care for elders.

| Long-Term Care Providers | Community-Based Care/Services | Institution-Based Care/Services |
|---|---|---|
| | • Private Practitioner Settings | • Hospitals |
| | • Health Centers | • Rehabilitation Centers |
| | • HMOs | • Extended/Skilled Care Facilities |
| | • PPOs | • Hospices |
| | • Ambulatory Care Settings | |
| | • Home Health Care Agencies | |
| | • Adult Day Care Centers | |
| | • Senior Centers | |
| **Optional Nutritional Services** | • Screening ———————————————————→ | |
| | • Assessment ———————————————————→ | |
| | • Monitoring & Evaluation —————————→ | |
| | • Education & Training ———————————→ | |
| | • Counseling ———————————————————→ | |
| | • Meals/Food Services/Food Access Initiative (Food Stamps, Shopping Assistance, etc.) ——→ | |
| | • Case Management ————————————→ | |
| | • Clinical Nutrition Care ————————→ | |

tute of Medicine, and *Healthy People 2000*.[13,23,38] These reports underscore the importance of considering and planning for the nutritional needs of elders, regardless of the setting in which health care services are provided. Several of the reports explicitly recommend that health care reimbursement guidelines cover nutrition services provided by credentialed professionals, particularly RDs, and related food services (congregate and home meals), enteral and parenteral nutrition products, and supplemental feedings.

NSI has also developed guidelines and recommended methods for screening and in-depth evaluation of nutritional risk in older populations and the designation of appropriate interventions.[57,58] The NSI-validated method for assessing warning signs of poor nutritional status in older adults is an easily self-administered 10-item checklist.[56,57] The technique is intended to guide individuals to social service and health care professionals with whom to discuss nutritional concerns and, as needed, to refer those with potential problems to professionals for further assessment and follow-up. At initial in-depth nutritional assessment of the older individuals, NSI recommends concentrating on changes in body weight, eating habits, living environment, and functional status that may reflect adverse changes in nutritional status. More specific diagnostic techniques, such as anthropometric measurements, physical observations, laboratory data, cognitive and emotional assessments, and detailed questions to evaluate medication use, eating habits, living environment and functional status, are considered in further stages of nutrition assessment. The methods are intended to identify those individuals with common nutritional problems, such as protein-calorie malnutrition, obesity, and medical conditions, including cognitive impairment or depression, that

can have a profound adverse impact on nutritional well-being.[55,56]

NSI has urged clinicians to incorporate nutritional screening as part of routine activities in free-living and institutionalized elderly populations in order to develop appropriate interventions. Several recent publications provide guidelines for professionals who are involved in nutritional care of older individuals.[19,57–59]

In summary, there is striking consensus in recent national policy statements and the recommendations of professional groups that nutritional risk assessment and interventions are important components of health care delivery to older persons. There is recognition that the nutritional problems of the elderly span a spectrum from frank nutrient deficiencies, like protein-energy malnutrition, to nutritional excesses, exhibited in obesity, hypercholesterolemia, hypertension, and diabetes. Attention is given to the importance of ensuring that an individual's dietary intake is adequate to meet nutrient requirements, particularly among those who may experience food insecurity for financial, cognitive, functional, or other reasons. The recommendations stress that preventive nutrition is as important among elders as in younger populations, and they outline dietary management for the prevention of the chronic diseases of aging and their adverse complications. Guidelines are provided that promote energy intake to maintain ideal body weight, lower total and saturated fat intake, reduce sodium and sugar intake, and increase fiber-, calcium- and fluoride-containing foods.

Despite the increasing recognition of the importance of nutrition in ensuring the health of elders and the emerging consensus on nutrition services and interventions, serious constraints exist on the availability and delivery of nutrition services to elders throughout the various health care and social service delivery settings. The existing national recommendations have often not been translated into regulations or policies at the programmatic level. To exacerbate the situation, nutrition services for elders are not coordinated. Relevant activities may be administered separately by a wide range of community-based organizations or professional groups or by institutions providing temporary or long-term care. As a consequence, services (where they exist) may be duplicative but more often miss key aspects of nutritional care. At present, there is at best a loosely integrated network of health care providers who may or may not consider the nutritional needs of their older clients. At the heart of the problem associated with providing a coordinated continuum of nutrition and health services to older persons is the lack of definition and consideration given to reimbursement of nutrition services by insurance programs, notably Medicare and Medicaid. Until these issues are resolved, the goals set in the national policy statements for providing frameworks that ensure the optimal nutritional status of older Americans will not be met.

## NUTRITION SERVICES FOR OLDER POPULATIONS

Table 18–3 summarizes the features of the major federally funded nutrition programs that are available to elders including ENP and food stamps. The table also summarizes the major elements of Medicare and Medicaid health care reimbursement system that can be utilized for providing nutrition services to older individuals. The following sections discuss these programs, their eligibility requirements and service definitions, and their strengths and limitations in ensuring a continuum of nutrition services for older people.

### Federally Funded Nutrition Programs

#### *Titles III and VI Community-Based Nutrition Program for Older Americans*

In 1972, Congress amended the Older Americans Act of 1965 (OAA) to establish a national nutrition program for the elderly (ENP). This initiative was established after 4 years of successful community-based demonstrations projects that provided congregate meals (and home meals for the homebound elders) in community-based settings that encouraged social activities and support of noninstitutionalized elders. In the ensuing three decades, ENP has become the largest publicly funded and longest standing program of coordinated community- and home-based preventive health-related and social services for the nation's elders.[17,40,41] The program responds to evidence of prevalent malnutrition in certain older population segments and emerging evidence of the importance of nutrition in maintaining health and managing medical problems in elders.

ENP distributes funding under Title III of the OAA to states (state units on aging [SUAs]) and U.S. territories and under Title VI to Indian tribal organizations (ITOs) for a national network of programs that provide congregate and home-delivered meals for elderly people. ENP funding helps maintain an elaborate infrastructure of area agencies on aging and nutrition projects at the regional and local levels, respectively, for the delivery of nutrition and related health and supportive social services to older clients (Figure 18–2).

Nutrition programs are required to provide at least one meal a day that meets one third of the RDAs and to operate 5 or more days a week.[41] Less well known but of great importance is the role of ENP in administering and/or delivering other health and supportive so-

**Table 18–3** Nutrition Programs and Services Payment Systems for Older Adults

| Program | Type of Intervention | Funding Source | Eligible/Available Services | Percentage of Older Population Served |
|---|---|---|---|---|
| **Federal Nutrition Programs** | | | | |
| Title III and VI Elder Nutrition Program | Nutrition and socialization intervention. Providing meals, therapeutic diets, access initiatives, and community-based and home health and related supportive social services | DHHS OHDS AoA | Congregate and home meals; transportation; shopping assistance; outreach; information and referral; nutrition education; case management; homemakers; home health aides; legal and financial counseling; personal care and chore services; fitness and rehabilitation programs; social and recreational activities | 10.8% of population aged 65+ years 17.29% of the eligible low-income elderly aged 65+ years[70] |
| Food Stamps [Inadequate] | Income subsidy | USDA SSA | Coupons for food purchases or cash equivalent | 20% to 35% of eligible elders aged 60+ years[70] 13% of eligible elders aged 65+ years[70] |
| **Nutrition Services Payment Systems:** Medicare/Medicaid | Third-party payment system: hospital insurance, medical insurance, and extended benefits | DHHS HCFA SSA | Covers medical and health-related services provided by participating hospitals, HMOs, private medical practices, ambulatory centers, rehabilitation and skilled nursing facilities, home health agencies, and hospice programs. Eligibility for nutrition services varies depending on the setting (reimbursement for care) and their deemed medical necessity. Home meals, enteral/parenteral nutrition, and weight reduction are particularly limited | 40 million beneficiaries 65 years and older |

*Note:* AoA, U.S. Department of Health and Human Services, Administration on Aging; DHHS, U.S. Department of Health and Human Services; HCFA, U.S. Department of Health and Human Services, Health Care Financing Administration; HMO, health maintenance organization; OHDS, U.S. Department of Health and Human Services, Office of Human Development Services; SSA, Social Security Administration; USDA, U.S. Department of Agriculture.

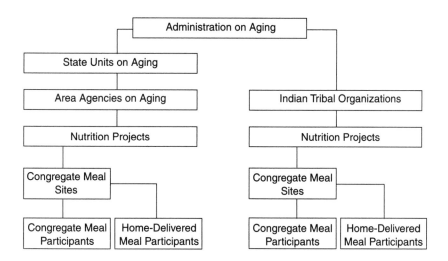

**Figure 18–2**  Title III and VI Elder Nutrition Program structure.

cial services including access initiatives (transportation, outreach, information and referral), in-home services (homemaker, home health aide, personal care, and chore assistance), and community-based health and supportive social activities (medical screening, case management, legal and financial assistance and counseling, physical fitness programs, rehabilitation services, and social and recreational activities).[42,72]

ENP maintains two major meal service delivery systems—one that provides community-based, congregate (group) and individual services to the ambulatory older population and one that delivers services to the frail, homebound elderly. ENP services emphasize preventive nutrition, particularly the provision of congregate and home-delivered meals (often called "Meals on Wheels"), as well as nutrition screening, education, and counseling.

Federal law mandates that ENP be available to all older Americans (those 60 years and older and their spouses, regardless of age) and that client contributions (payment) for services be strictly voluntary. Within fed-

eral funding limitations, ENP attempts to strategically place local projects in community facilities that serve those in greatest need—the poor, minority, and frail elderly. Older individuals voluntarily become ENP clients and are referred by health and medical providers (such as hospitals, private physicians, group medical practices, and social service agencies) as well as informal family and social networks.

The Administration on Aging currently distributes about $500 million annually in ENP federal funding to a national network of 57 state and territorial units on aging, 670 area agencies on aging, and over 200 ITOs. It is estimated that ENP provides services to 2.3 million elders through community sites and delivered meals and other in-home services to more than 877,000 frail elders.[41,67] In a 1987 report, the U.S. Department of Health and Human Services (DHHS) summarized federal expenditures for health promotion and disease prevention among all age groups and minority groups in the population. ENP, which was included in the Office of Human Development Service budget, accounted for over three fourths of expenditures by DHHS for health promotion and disease prevention.[68]

Title VI of the OAA establishes a separate grant program to tribal organizations to promote the delivery of social and nutritional services to older American Indians, Native Alaskans, and Native Hawaiians that are comparable to those provided under Title III. According to the most recent information from the Administration on Aging, about $17 million in Title VI are cited for nutrition and supportive services, including the provision of approximately 2.8 million meals to nearly 90,000 Native Americans and Native Hawaiians.

ENP gains additional spending power from a cash/commodity entitlement program supported by the USDA that expands the resources and meals available through the nutrition program. Federal legislation gives states the option to elect to receive food commodities, cash at a fixed amount per meal served to eligible participants per year, or a flexible combination of food and cash. In 1995 this support from the USDA exceeded $150 million.[69–71] Other ENP program revenues are realized from donations from older participants toward meal costs, private or public grant funding or donations, and the value of volunteerism in the program.

Many researchers have attempted to determine the impact of ENP on the nutritional well-being and health of older participants.[67,72–78] From these reports, it appears that ENP attracts "high-risk" elders, improves food and nutrient intake among participants, and provides beneficial socialization and recreation. Balsam and Rogers[61] found that many ENP sites were compelled to become innovative in meeting the nutritional needs of participants. These researchers found that many nutrition programs across the nation provide not only the congregate and home meals that are required by law but also therapeutic diets; food pantries; ethnic meals; luncheon clubs; breakfast, weekend, and evening meals; and meals for the homeless older population.

While evaluations of ENP have demonstrated its effectiveness, design issues limit their generalizability. Most have been conducted in selected local settings and have not provided a national perspective. Since the last comprehensive national program evaluation more than 10 years ago, ENP has undergone many changes. Since that time, there have been increased numbers of home-delivered meals, targeted services for older persons with the greatest economic or social needs, and the expansion of long-term care activities within the ENP infrastructure to support independent living and functional independence and to reduce risks for premature institutionalization in older clients.[32,72]

For these reasons, in 1992, Congress mandated a comprehensive evaluation of ENP to inform national health policy development, guided by a set of research questions, several of which are highlighted here: Are ENP services well targeted and reaching elders at greatest health risk? Does ENP favorably influence its major mandated health-related outcomes? What is the role of ENP in the provision of a continuum of long-term care health and supportive social services to elders?

The ENP evaluation study included a nationally representative sample of the program's ambulatory and homebound clients and a matched comparison sample of eligible elders who do not receive ENP services. Comparison sample elders were drawn from the Health Care Finance Administration (HCFA) Medicare beneficiary listings and were individuals in the same postal zip code areas as the ENP clients.[67]

Trained field staff conducted in-person interviews and elicited information on subjects' demographic profiles, health status indicators, nutrient intake, and levels of socialization. From a health status perspective, subjects were asked about their current medical conditions, recent hospitalizations and nursing home admissions, and level of physical functioning. Functional status was determined using standardized activities of daily living (ADLs) and independent activities of daily living (IADL) inventories.[79] Warning signs of poor nutrition were assessed using the NSI validated checklist and its criteria for interpretation.[19,54,55] Standardized protocols[67] were used to directly measure subjects' heights and weights for the purpose of calculating body mass index (BMI = weight (in kilograms)/height (in meters$^2$)). BMIs were compared against clinical standards for older persons to evaluate the prevalence of under- and overweight. Nutrient intake was estimated from 24-hour dietary recall interviews that were conducted with validated instruments[80] and standardized protocols. The University of Minnesota Nutrition Coordinating Center nutrient database (Data Collection NDS Version 2.6) was used to estimate nutrient intake of participants and nonparticipants.

The sociodemographic profiles of ambulatory and homebound ENP clients in the Title III and VI programs are compared with the overall U.S. population in Figure 18–3. Those served by Title III tend to be older by 4 to 6 years than U.S. elders overall and to include proportionately more women (69–70% of ENP participants are female, in contrast with 58% in the population 60 years and older overall). About twice the proportion of minority elders participate in the ENP than are in the older U.S. population; overall, 25% to 27% of clients (compared with 14%) are minority older individuals. Some 12% to 19% of Title III clients are black, and 5% to 12% are Hispanic minorities. The proportion of impoverished elders being served by Title III is more than twice that in the general population. Some 79% to 90% of ENP clients have incomes below 200% of the DHHS poverty level, in contrast to 38% nationally; the proportion of low-income minority elders that receive Title III services is about four times greater than their proportion in the overall older population. Title VI subjects are only slightly younger than U.S. elders overall (68 and 71 years in the congregate and home-delivered programs). As in Title III, women are more likely to participate in Title VI, and there are considerably more impoverished and minority participants than in the U.S. population overall.

The health characteristics of ambulatory and homebound Title III and VI clients are compared in Table 18–4. On average, ambulatory recipients of Title III services have 2.4 chronic health problems, compared with 3.0 in homebound clients; the proportions for Title VI subjects are 2.8 and 2.9, respectively. Some 26% to 43% of Title III and 30% to 37% of Title VI participants have been institutionalized (hospitalized or entered nursing homes) in the past year. About one quarter of ambulatory and 77% of homebound Title III clients and 23% and 44% of Title VI clients, respectively, have difficulty performing one or more activities of daily living, including shopping for food or preparing meals. About two thirds of both the ambulatory and homebound Title III and VI clients have a weight (as assessed by BMI) that is outside the healthy range for older persons; however, those who are ambulatory are more likely to be overweight, whereas homebound clients are more likely to be underweight.[67] From 64% to 88% of Title III and VI clients reported behaviors or profile characteristics that indicated moderate to high risk for potential nutritional problems by the NSI checklist criteria.

This study emphasized two priority outcomes of ENP that relate directly to overall

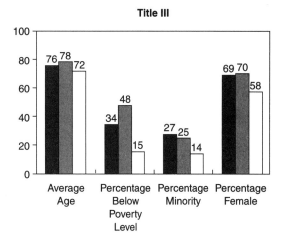

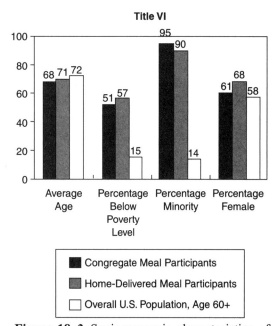

**Figure 18–3** Socioeconomic characteristics of ENP participants. *Source:* Reprinted from M. Ponza et al., *Serving Elders at Risk*, 1966, United States Department of Health and Human Services/Office of the Assistant Secretary for Aging/Office of the Assistant Secretary for Planning and Evaluation, 1996.

health and risk of institutionalization in the older population: improvements in participants' levels of nutrient intake and patterns of socialization. The mean daily nutrient intake

of ENP clients, expressed as a percentage of the RDAs[46] for persons 50 years of age and older, are compared with the matched research comparison group in Figure 18–4. ENP clients' mean daily nutrient intake approached or exceeded the RDAs for all nutrients except energy and zinc. For the entire range of essential nutrients studied, ENP clients had consistently higher levels of nutrient intake than matched-comparison elders. Intakes were significantly higher for all essential nutrients except vitamin $B_{12}$ and iron. In addition, mean intakes of dietary fat and cholesterol were not higher among ENP clients than among nonclients and approached or achieved recommended levels of intake (30% of total energy intake and under 300 mg/d, respectively; data not shown). The ENP meals were also found to contribute between 30% and 50% of total daily nutrient intake among congregate and homebound program participants.[67]

Socialization patterns of ENP clients were also compared with those of matched-comparison elders. Results of the ENP evaluation indicate that ENP clients experienced a 17% increase in monthly social contacts.[67]

Table 18–5 presents a summary of the long-term care health-related services that are currently offered by Title III and VI programs. Over half of the Title III and VI program sites currently offer their clients information and referral services, recreation and social activities, transportation services to a variety of settings (to meals, health care providers, etc), and counseling activities. About 7% to 14% of programs offer homemaker services; fewer provide personal care services and home health aides.

While service provision is relatively high in the ENP sites, the data in Table 18–5 underestimate the role of the ENP infrastructure in the delivery of long-term care services. As part of the ENP evaluation, various levels of the ENP program administrative structure

**Table 18–4** Health Characteristics of Ambulatory and Homebound Title III & VI Clients in Congregate and Home-Delivered Meal Programs[67]

| | Title III | | Title VI | |
| --- | --- | --- | --- | --- |
| | *Congregate* | *Home-Delivered* | *Congregate* | *Home-Delivered* |
| Average number of diagnosed chronic health conditions | 2.4 | 3.0 | 2.8 | 2.9 |
| Hospital/nursing home stay in previous year | 26 | 43 | 30 | 37 |
| Weight outside of health range | 61 | 64 | 65 | 69 |
| Difficulty doing one or more everyday tasks | 23 | 77 | 23 | 44 |
| Inability to prepare meals or much difficulty in preparing | 8 | 41 | 8 | 26 |
| Moderate to high nutritional risk | 64 | 88 | 80 | 78 |

were evaluated concerning their roles in long-term care. It is quite clear from comprehensive interviews conducted in the SUAs, the ITO administrative units, and the area agencies on aging that most are involved in the administration, coordination, and direct delivery of home- and community-based long-term care services.[67] This aspect of ENP activities is important to underscore, since ENP is often viewed strictly as a nutrition program. This evaluation documented the major role of these programs in attempting to provide a coordinated continuum of care for their elder clients.

The ENP evaluation demonstrates that the program is well targeted, efficient, and effective in providing health-related and supportive social services to the elders at greater health risk, particularly low-income and minority elders. The study underscores the emerging role of ENP in the coordination of long-term care activities for homebound and ambulatory elders in community settings. It is intriguing that the coordination of this care evolved from the long-standing activities of community providers in the delivery of meals to needy elders. Once again, this serves to emphasize the importance of nutrition and its central role in maintaining the health and independence of elders. ENP serves as a model framework for the coordination of a continuum of health and related supportive, social services to elders, particularly the low-income and minority elder populations.

### Food Stamps

The U.S. Department of Agriculture food stamp program, which was authorized by the 1964 Food Stamp Act, provides an income supplement to low-income households in the form of coupons used to purchase food. Recent studies estimate that between 13% and 35% of eligible elders[70] currently participate in the food stamp program. Reasons cited for nonparticipation by eligible older people include the "stigma of welfare" associated with the program's income means test, lack of information on program availability, and the perceived complexity of the application process.[81] To encourage participation by those residents aged 65 years and older, Wisconsin and California converted the food stamp benefit to a cash equivalent and added it to the individual's monthly supplemental security

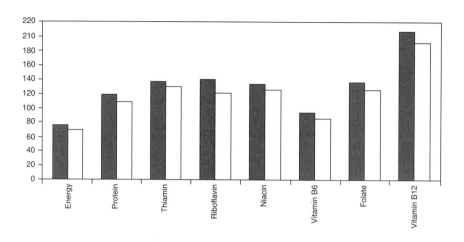

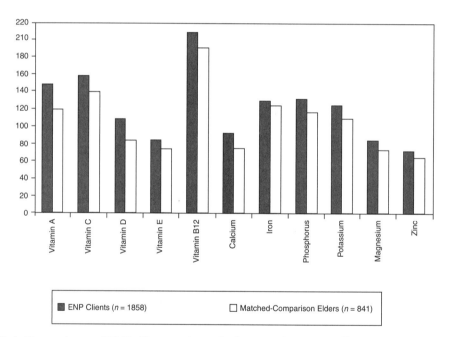

■ ENP Clients (*n* = 1858)        □ Matched-Comparison Elders (*n* = 841)

**Figure 18–4** Comparisons of ENP clients and matched-comparison elders.[67]

income (SSI) check. SSI provides a guaranteed minimal income to the nation's aged (those aged 65 years and older), blind, and disabled people.

Results concerning the impact of food stamps on the nutritional status of participating households have been inconclusive. Butler et al[82] concluded that elderly food stamp participants consumed levels of nutrients that were similar to those of nonparticipants who had otherwise similar characteristics. They suggested that food stamps act as an effective income supplement but may not be a mechanism to improve the nutrient intake of older

**Table 18–5** Nutrition Projects Offering Various Types of Non-Nutrition Services (%)[67]

| Services Provided | Congregate Meal Participants | Home-Delivered Meal Participants |
|---|---|---|
| Title III | | |
| Information and referral | 85 | 84 |
| Recreation and social activities | 69 | NA |
| Transportation to and from meal site | 68 | NA |
| Other assisted and nonassisted transportation | 57 | 58 |
| Other counseling | 53 | 55 |
| Home services | 12 | 14 |
| Personal care service | 4 | 5 |
| Home health aide services | 5 | 6 |
| Title VI | | |
| Information and referral | 89 | 86 |
| Recreation and social activities | 75 | NA |
| Transportation to and from meal site | 83 | NA |
| Other assisted and nonassisted transportation | 77 | 81 |
| Other counseling | 49 | 52 |
| Home services | 7 | 7 |
| Personal care service | 7 | 7 |
| Home health aide services | 4 | 4 |

*Note:* NA, Not applicable.

individuals. In contrast, Akin and colleagues[83] found that food stamp participants consumed higher levels of many nutrients than did members of nonparticipating households with similar incomes.

Further research is needed to resolve these conflicting findings. In particular, it is important to assess the specific role and impact of food stamps in the continuum of nutrition services and interventions involving older persons.

## NUTRITION SERVICES PAYMENT SYSTEMS

In addition to federally funded mechanisms for the provision of congregate and home meals and related services to elder populations (under ENP) and the provision of income subsidies in the form of food stamps to eligible elders, the major mechanism for providing nutrition services to elder clients is the third-party payment system, notably Medicare and Medicaid. These programs provide guidelines for the reimbursement of health-related services in institutional, community, and home settings. A summary of the general guidelines that determine the nature and extent of coverage for nutrition services within Medicare and Medicaid is found in Table 18–3. The following discussion provides an overview of general policies and procedures that affect reimbursement of nutrition services within Medicare and Medicaid. Further details are provided by the ADA on policies for nutrition care services coverage and reimbursement under Medicare and Medicaid[84]; and by the ADA's published procedures for implementing a nutrition services payment system,[63] including service definitions and documentation, fee setting, billing, and patient-monitoring procedures.

## Medicare

The Medicare program receives its statutory authority under Title XVIII of the 1965 Social Security Act and is administered by HCFA of DHHS. Medicare is a national health insurance program for persons 65 years and older, certain younger disabled persons, and those with kidney failure. HCFA forms partnerships with thousands of health care providers (hospitals, nursing homes, home health agencies, physicians, medical equipment suppliers, labs, and managed-care plans such as HMOs) to provide reimbursement for services to over 40 million Medicare beneficiaries (ie, eligible people aged 65 years and older and disabled people of all ages).[85] The Medicare program consists of three parts: part A (hospital insurance), part B (medical insurance), and part C (Medicare + choice). Part A covers inpatient hospital care, skilled nursing facility care, home health care, and hospice care. Part B provides reimbursement for "medical and other services" not covered by part A, including outpatient physicians' services and hospital services, laboratory services, durable medical equipment, and other clinical, therapeutic, or rehabilitative professional services deemed to be "incident to the provision of medical care." These include physical and speech therapy and nutrition services (as determined to be appropriate) and other items and services as specified by Medicare. Part C was established as part of the Balanced Budget Act of 1997 and is intended to enable Medicare enrollees to elect alternative health care (beyond the traditional fee-for-service plans) such as HMOs, preferred provider organizations, provider-sponsored organizations, and medical savings accounts. Medicare enrollees are required to pay deductible and coinsurance costs. They can also elect to purchase supplemental insurance, called Medigap insurance, a private insurance that is intended to help pay Medicare cost-sharing amounts.

### Part A: Medicare Hospital Insurance

Medicare part A provides reimbursement for all covered costs of care in hospitals and skilled nursing facilities during defined "benefit periods." Medicare beneficiaries are responsible for hospital deductibles and coinsurance costs during their stays. Part A pays for semiprivate room, meals, regular nursing services, drugs, medical supplies, lab tests, X-rays, and the use of operating and recovery rooms, intensive care and coronary care units, and other defined "medically necessary care." During hospital stays, Medicare does not pay for the use of phones, televisions, private-duty nurses, or extra charges unless they are medically necessary.

While Medicare patients are in skilled nursing facilities, Medicare Part A pays for semiprivate rooms, skilled nursing and rehabilitative services, and other defined services and supplies. Medicare provides full payment for skilled nursing facility care for up to 20 days, adjusted rates of payment from 21 to 100 days, and nothing after 100 days. Medicare Part A provides payments for unlimited home health care as long as the patient requirements for "defined need" are met. Part A home health care benefits include part-time or nursing care, home health aide services, durable medical equipment (some beneficiary copayment is required) and supplies, and other defined services. Hospice care is covered under Medicare Part A as long as a physician certifies a beneficiary's need. Reimbursed care includes pain relief, symptom management, support services for the terminally ill person, and respite services.

### Part B: Medicare Medical Insurance

Medicare Part B helps pay doctor bills and a wide range of medical services and supplies in both inpatient and outpatient settings. Reimbursed medical expenses include physician fees; surgical services and supplies; physical, occupational, and speech therapy (when provided by therapists of the approved Medicare facility); mental health services; clinical services of psychologists and social workers; clinical laboratory services; prosthetic devices; braces; diagnostic tests and durable medical equipment (wheelchairs, etc); and medical supplies (surgical dressings, ostomy bags, etc). Part B also helps pay for ambulance transportation and certain preventive services, such as flu shots, Pap smears, and mammography. Part B will also pay for home health care if beneficiaries do not have Medicare Part A coverage.

As with Part A, Medicare part B beneficiaries are responsible for certain copayments and deductibles. Many medical services and items are not covered by Medicare, including routine physical exams, most dental care and dentures, routine foot care, hearing aids, most prescription drugs, and eyeglasses, except if needed after cataract surgery.

### Nutrition Services Reimbursement Conditions of Participation

The rates of Medicare reimbursement to hospitals for costs incurred in patient care are fixed and are based on 470 diagnosis-related groups (DRG). There is a flat reimbursement rate for each DRG, regardless of the services that a patient receives. There is only limited flexibility within the Medicare reimburse-ment guidelines to adjust hospital reimbursement rates for patients who have unusually long hospital stays or multiple, complicated diagnoses. As a consequence, the DRG-based fixed payment system creates an incentive for hospitals that are able to limit patients' lengths of stay and encourage early patient discharge.

The Medicare program sets specific "conditions of participation" that must be met in order for the hospital to receive Medicare funding. Several of these conditions pertain to nutrition. A hospital that receives Medicare payments must have an organized dietary department. The guidelines, however, do not specify that it be headed by a registered dietitian. A consulting dietitian must be available to meet with medical and nursing staff and instruct patients on diet modifications, write diet histories, and participate in ward rounds and conferences. Diets must be recorded on patients' charts, and orders for therapeutic diets must appear there as well. Meals must be consistent with diet orders and must meet the National Research Council's RDAs.[46] While these guidelines provide general criteria for hospital nutrition services, they leave considerable latitude for determining the type and organization of these services and the availability of nutrition professionals for the provision of clinical nutrition care.

An additional factor that may determine the availability of nutrition services in the hospital setting is a voluntary hospital accreditation process that is carried out by the Joint Commission on Accreditation of Healthcare Organizations (Joint Commission). Hospitals that participate in this process, including about 5200 of the 6700 hospitals that participate in Medicare,[27] are required to maintain a set of basic nutrition care services, including routine dietary screening; nutritional assessment of individual patients; clinical nutrition care (including the availability of both enteral and parenteral nutrition); dietary counseling; and the administration of safe, appropriate, and sanitary food service operations. The Joint Commission guidelines add further emphasis on the availability of qualified nutrition professionals in the provision of both food service and clinical nutrition care activities.

Hospitals consider the services necessary for Medicare and Joint Commission participation and how to balance quality of care against cost efficiency. Under this system, the extent to which nutrition services are provided will, in part, depend on how they are perceived within the institutional framework. Nutrition services that are perceived as increasing the hospital's cost of providing care may be limited or not provided. Those nutrition services that are perceived as improving patients' rates of recovery or reducing hospital stays for a given diagnosis may be incorporated into the hospital's "core services."[68] This decision is made at the institutional level and is not regulated by the third-party payers. When provided, nutrition services are not reimbursed separately but are covered as part of the hospital's routine or administrative costs.

There appears to be specific wording in the Medicare policy that denies separate coverage for nutritional supplements such as enteral feedings in the hospital setting; supplements are considered to be "self-administered drugs" and ineligible for coverage.

### Special Considerations in Providing Nutrition Services under Medicare

*Ambulatory Settings.*    Medicare part B may cover nutrition services provided in hospital ambulatory centers or private physicians' offices if they are deemed "incident to medical care." Guidelines concerning nutrition services carried out in the hospital ambulatory center require that the nutrition profes-

sional be an employee of the hospital. Nutrition services provided in a private practice must be carried out by a professional who is an employee of the physician, rather than a private contractor; the physician must also be present to supervise the nutrition care. Nutrition services in hospital-based ambulatory centers and private practice settings are billed by the hospital or medical practice as a medical visit and are reimbursed as such.

*Health Maintenance Organizations.*    An HMO participating in the Medicare program must offer its Medicare beneficiaries the full range of services that are available to all HMO clients. The HMO legislation does include nutrition education and counseling as an allowable service but does not specify that these services be carried out by a professional with a specific background. Cost containment concerns guide the development of the available services of HMOs, much as they do in the hospital setting. For these reasons, the profiles of nutrition services paid for by HMOs differ considerably across the nation.

*Home Health Agencies.*    Home health agency services may be reimbursed under both Medicare parts A and B. To qualify, a patient or beneficiary must be homebound, under a physician's care, and in need of skilled nursing or speech or physical therapy. There are no limits to the number of home visits a person can receive, and, in home care, unlike institution-based skilled nursing or rehabilitative care, the beneficiary need not have been hospitalized before receiving the care. Home services that are considered appropriate for reimbursement are generally those that would be provided under hospital-based care. Home meals, however, are specifically excluded, since they are not viewed as a component of hospital care.

Home health agencies are reimbursed on a "reasonable cost" basis for visits; these rates include the administrative component of arranging care. In addition, the home health agency receives a negotiated overhead rate. Conditions for participation require that as part of administrative overhead the agency develop a treatment plan for each client, including his or her diet. Therefore, nutrition services are allowable under the agency's administrative costs. Home visits by nutrition professionals are generally not allowed as separate visits; rather, the nutrition professionals' time is likely to be reflected in administrative costs, and their level of effort is likely to be reflective of the agency's caseload. Parenteral and enteral nutrition products can be reimbursed under Medicare part B but must not be billed separately (ie, they are also included as an administrative cost).

*Hospice Care.* Medicare part A covers hospice care services, but guidelines specify limits on the length of allowable coverage and set ceilings on the total cost of service reimbursement per client. Many hospice programs across the country elect not to participate in the Medicare program because of these ceilings. Unlike other settings of care, dietary counseling is reimbursed directly. However, nutrition professionals are not designated as preferred providers of these services.

## Medicaid

Medicaid is a publicly funded health insurance program for persons who meet certain low- to moderate-income eligibility guidelines. Medicaid is funded under Title XIX of the Social Security Act. It is difficult to generalize about the Medicaid program, since each state determines the types of covered services on the basis of its resources and the needs of its population. However, Medicaid "conditions of participation" by settings of care are generally identical with those under

the Medicare program. Nutrition services may be covered if they are considered "incident to" ongoing medical care (as in hospital ambulatory care or private medical practice settings) or are part of service packages (as in the case of HMOs). Certain Medicaid programs may also specify guidelines for adult day care and personal care services provided to older people. These may exceed guidelines for services provided under Medicare. Despite similarities in participation guidelines, Medicaid coverage for services is generally considered more restricted than Medicare.

## Summary

In contrast with the emergence of public policy statements on nutrition and aging and the increasing recognition of the importance of nutrition in promoting the health of older populations, Medicare and Medicaid programs do not provide strong or comprehensive language concerning nutrition services provided by professionals. As the legislation and regulations for these programs are reviewed, it is important to advocate for the incorporation of definitions of appropriate nutrition services and their payment systems. No other set of activities could more effectively change the panorama of nutrition service options for elders, regardless of the settings in which health care is provided.

## CONCLUSION

The health and nutrition status of older people has improved in this century, but significant numbers continue to have unmet needs for nutritional services. The most prevalent nutritional problems of people aged 65 years and older are the nutrition-related chronic diseases of aging, including coronary heart disease, hypertension, diabetes, cancer, and osteoporosis. These affect many, if not most older people. There are also distinct groups of elders, notably those who are socially isolated, very old and frail, poor, or of minority populations, who are at greatest risk for nutrient deficiencies. The factors and personal characteristics that place the older population at risk of nutrition problems are poorly understood. Considerable research, both basic and applied, is needed to resolve these information deficits and to provide the critical basis for advocacy on behalf of elders and their nutritional needs.

ENP provides a framework for the delivery of nutrition and related health and supportive social services to elders. The recent national evaluation provides strong evidence of its success and favorable impacts on nutrition and socialization of elder participants. There is also emerging evidence that the agencies involved in the delivery of ENP have evolved into an infrastructure that is increasingly involved in case management and the delivery of a continuum of services, beyond simply meals, that support the independent living of

older clients. Funding limitations, however, restrict ENP to about 10% to 15% percent of eligible elders. These emerging roles of the ENP network are not well understood by other providers of health and related services to elders. As a consequence, there is only loose integration and communication between organizations in the provision of long-term care services. No single agency or entity has yet established responsibility for planning, coordinating, or providing nutrition services to older people in home, community, or institutional settings.

Medicare and Medicaid do not provide sufficiently explicit language to support the delivery of nutrition services by qualified professionals in the wide range of participating health care settings. Advocacy and research, particularly on the efficacy of nutrition services in advanced age, are needed to realize the goals set forth in the nation's public policy statements for a coordinated continuum of nutrition and health services for the older population.

## REFERENCES

1. Omran AR. A century of epidemiologic transition in the United States. *Prev Med.* 1977;6:30–51.

2. Posner BM, Quatromoni PA, Franz M. Nutrition policies and intervention for chronic disease risk reduction in international settings: The InterHealth Nutrition Initiative. *Nutr Rev.* 1994:52:179–187.

3. Posner BM, Franz M, Quatromoni P, InterHealth Steering Committee. Nutrition and the global risk for chronic diseases: the InterHealth nutrition initiative. *Nutr Rev.* 1994:52:201–207.

4. National Center for Health Statistics. *Vital Statistics of the United States, Table 118.* Hyattsville, MD: US Dept of Health and Human Services, Public Health Service; 1995.

5. US Bureau of Census. *Resident Population of the United States: Middle Series Projections, 2015–2030, by Age and Sex.* http://www.census.gov/

population/projections/nation/nas/npas1530.txt; 1996.

6. National Center for Health Statistics. *Vital Statistics of the United States, Table 119.* Hyattsville, MD: US Dept of Health and Human Services, Public Health Service; 1995.

7. *Aging in the Eighties: Preliminary Data from the Supplement on Aging to the National Health Interview Survey.* Hyattsville, Md: National Center for Health Statistics; 1986. Advance Data from Vital and Health Statistics, No. 115. US Dept of Health and Human Services publication PHS 86-1250.

8. *Diet, Nutrition and the Prevention of Chronic Disease.* Geneva, Switzerland: World Health Organization; 1990. Technical report series 797.

9. *Health for All in the 21st Century.* Geneva, Switzerland: World Health Organization; 1998.

10. Murray CJL, Lopez AD. *The Global Burden of Disease*. Geneva, Switzerland: World Health Organization; 1996.

11. US Dept of Health and Human Services, Public Health Service. Aging. In: *The Surgeon General's Report on Nutrition and Health*. Washington, DC: US Government Printing Office; 1988. DHHS (PHS) publication 88-50210.

12. National Institutes of Health, National Institutes on Aging. *Malnutrition in Older Persons*. 1994. PA-94-088.

13. US Dept of Health and Human Services, Public Health Service. *Healthy People 2000: National Health Promotion and Disease Prevention Objectives. Full Report, with Commentary*. Boston, Mass: Jones & Bartlett Publishers; 1992.

14. Dwyer, JT. *Screening Older Americans' Nutritional Health: Current Practices and Future Possibilities*. Washington, DC: Nutrition Screening Initiative; 1991.

15. *Guidelines for Protocols for Local Demonstration Projects*. Geneva, Switzerland: World Health Organization; 1990. Division of Noncommunicable Diseases and Health Technology. INTERHEALTH.

16. Posner BM, Fanelli MT, Krachenfels MM, Saffel-Schreier S. Position of the American Dietetic Association: nutrition, aging and the continuum of health care. *J Am Diet Assoc*. 1987;87:344–347.

17. Posner BM, Levine EL. Nutrition services for older Americans. In: *Geriatric Nutrition: A Health Professional's Handbook*. Gaithersburg, Md: Aspen Publishers; 1991.

18. Posner BM, Jette A, Smigelski C, Miller D, Mitchell P. Nutritional risk in New England elders. *J Gerontol Med Sci*. 1994;49:M123–132.

19. *Incorporating Nutrition Screening and Interventions into Medical Practice: A Monograph for Physicians*. Washington, DC: Nutrition Screening Initiative; 1994.

20. Institute of Medicine, Division of Health Promotion and Disease Prevention. *The Second Fifty Years: Promoting Health and Preventing Disability*. Washington, DC: National Academy Press; 1992.

21. Morley JE. Nutritional status of the elderly. *Am J Med*. 1986;81:679–695.

22. *Surgeon General's Workshop on Health Promotion and Aging*. Washington, DC: US Government Printing Office; 1988. Publication 1988-201-875/83669.

23. Dwyer JT, Coletti J, Campbell D. Maximizing nutrition in the second fifty. *Clin Appl Nutr*. 1991;4:19–31.

24. Dwyer JT. Nutrition concerns and problems of the aged. In: Satin D, ed. *Clinical Care of the Aged Person*. New York, NY: Oxford University Press; 1993.

25. Goodwin JS. Social, psychological and physical factors affecting the nutritional status of elderly subjects: separating cause and effect. *Am J Clin Nutr*. 1989;50:1201–1209.

26. Hutchinson M, Munro HN. *Nutrition and Aging*. New York, NY: Academic Press; 1986.

27. Posner BM, Krachenfels MM. Nutrition services in the continuum of care. *Clin Geriatr Med*. 1987;3:261–274.

28. Carroll MD, Abraham S, Dresser CM, eds. *Dietary Intake Source Data: U.S., 1976–80, NHANES I, II*. Hyattsville, Md: National Center for Health Statistics; 1983.

29. *A National Survey of Nutritional Risk among the Elderly*. Washington, DC: Food Research and Action Center; 1987.

30. Federation of American Societies for Experimental Biology, Life Sciences Research Office. Prepared for the Interagency Board for Nutrition Monitoring and Related Research. *Third Report on Nutrition Monitoring in the United States: Volumes 1 and 2*. Washington, DC: US Government Printing Office; 1995.

31. Ponza M, Ohls JC, Posner BM. *Elderly Nutrition Program Evaluation Literature Review*. Princeton, NJ: Mathematica Policy Research, Inc; 1994.

32. Posner BM, Smigelski CG, Krachenfels MM. Dietary characteristics and nutrient intake in an urban homebound population. *J Am Diet Assoc*. 1987;87:452–456.

33. Bailey LB. Vitamin B$_{12}$ status of elderly persons from urban low-income households. *J Am Geriatr Soc*. 1980;28:276–278.

34. Guthrie HA, Black K, Madden JP. Nutritional practices of elderly citizens in rural Pennsylvania. *Gerontologist*. 1972;12:330–335.

35. House Select Committee on Aging, Subcommittee on Health and Long-Term Care. *Quackery: A $10 Billion Scandal*. Washington, DC: US Government Printing Office; 1984. Publication 98-435.

36. US Dept of Health and Human Services. *Ten-State Nutrition Survey, V: Dietary*. Atlanta, Ga: Centers

for Disease Control; 1972: US Dept of Health and Human Services publication no. HSM 72-8133.

37. Vaughan LA, Manore MM. Dietary patterns and nutritional status of low income, free-living elderly. *Food Nutr News.* 1988;60:27–30.

38. White House Conference on Aging. *Final Report of the 1981 White House Conference on Aging: A National Policy on Aging.* Washington, DC: US Government Printing Office; 1981.

39. Assistant Secretary for Aging. *Food and Nutrition for Life: Malnutrition and Older Americans.* Washington, DC: Administration on Aging, Dept of Health and Human Services; 1994.

40. Posner BM, Saffel-Shrier S, Dwyer J, Franz MM. Position of the American Dietetic Association: Nutrition, aging, and the continuum of health care. *J Am Diet Assoc.* 1993;93:80–82.

41. Torres-Gil FM, Lloyd JL, Carlin J. Role of elderly nutrition in home and community-based care. *Perspect Appl Nutr.* 1995;2:9–15.

42. Posner BM. *Nutrition and the Elderly.* Lexington, Mass: Heath & Co; 1979.

43. US Dept of Health and Human Services. *Dietary Intake Source Data, United States, 1971–74.* Washington, DC: US Government Printing Office; 1979. DHEW publication (PHS) 79-1221.

44. Burt VL, Harris T. The Third National Health and Nutrition Examination Survey: contributing data on aging and health. *Gerontologist.* 1994;34:486–490.

45. Horwath CC. Dietary intake studies in elderly people. *World Rev Nutr Diet.* 1989;59:1–70.

46. Yates AA, Schlicker SA, Suiter CW. Dietary reference intakes: the new basis for recommendations for calcium and related nutrients, B vitamins, and choline. *J Am Dietet Assoc.* 1998;98:699–706.

47. National Research Council. (1989b). *Diet and Health: Implications for Reducing Chronic Disease Risk.* Washington, DC: National Academy Press; 1989.

48. US Dept of Agriculture. *The Food Guide Pyramid.* Hyattsville, Md: Human Nutrition Information Service; 1992. Home and Garden Bulletin No. 252.

49. Expert Panel on Detection, Evaluation and Treatment of High Blood Cholesterol in Adults. Summary of the second report of the National Cholesterol Education Program (NCEP) Expert Panel on Detection, Evaluation and Treatment of High Blood Cholesterol in Adults (Adult Treatment Panel II). *JAMA.* 1993;269:3015–3023.

50. Havas S, Heimendinger J, Reynolds K, et al. 5 a day for better health: a new research initiative. *J Am Diet Assoc.* 1994:94;32-36.

51. White JV. *Risk Factors Associated with Poor Nutritional Status in Older Americans.* Washington, DC: Nutrition Screening Initiative; 1991.

52. Ham RJ. *Indicators of Poor Nutritional Status in Older Americans.* Washington, DC: Nutrition Screening Initiative; 1991.

53. Lipschitz DA. *The Development of an Approach to Nutrition Screening for Older Americans.* Washington, DC: Nutrition Screening Initiative; 1991.

54. Posner BM, Jette AM, Smith KW, Miller DR. Nutrition and health risks in the elderly: the Nutrition Screening Initiative. *Am J Public Health.* 1993;83:972–978.

55. White JV, Dwyer JT, Posner BM, et al. Nutrition Screening Initiative: development and implementation of the Public Awareness Checklist and Screening Tools. *J Am Diet Assoc.* 1992;92:163–167.

56. White JV, Ham RJ, Lipschitz DA, Dwyer JT, Wellman NS. Consensus of the Nutrition Screening Initiative: risk factors and indicators of poor nutritional status in older Americans. *J Am Diet Assoc.* 1991;91:783–787.

57. *Report of Nutrition Screening 1: Toward a Common View.* Washington, DC: Nutrition Screening Initiative; 1991.

58. *Nutrition Screening Manual for Professionals Caring for Older Americans.* Washington, DC: Nutrition Screening Initiative; 1991.

59. *Nutrition Interventions Manual for Professionals Caring for Older Americans.* Washington, DC: Nutrition Screening Initiative; 1992.

60. White JV, ed. *The Role of Nutrition in Chronic Disease Care.* Washington DC: Nutrition Screening Initiative; 1997.

61. Balsam AL, Rogers BL. *Service Innovations in the Elderly Nutrition Program: Strategies for Meeting Unmet Needs.* Boston, Mass: Tufts University School of Nutrition; 1988.

62. Disbrow DD. The costs and benefits of nutrition services: a literature review. *J Am Diet Assoc.* 1989;89(4 suppl):53–66.

63. *Nutrition Services Payment Systems: Guidelines for Implementation.* Chicago, Ill: American Dietetic Association; 1985.

64. Monteith M. Role of nutritionists in community-based long term care. Presented at the Annual

Meeting of the American Dietetic Association; September 15, 1983; Anaheim, Calif.

65. Rubin DC. Waxing of the gray, waning of the green. In: Committee on an Aging Society, Institute of Medicine and the National Research Council, eds. *America's Aging: Health in an Older Society*. Washington, DC: National Academy Press; 1985.

66. Bezold C, Carlson RJ, Peck IC. *The Future of Work and Health*. Dover, Mass: Auburn House Publication Co; 1986.

67. Posza M, Ohls JC, Millen BE. *Serving Elders at Risk: The Older Americans Act Nutrition Programs. National Evaluation of the Elderly Nutrition Program, 1993-1995*. Washington, DC: US Dept of Health and Human Services, Office of the Assistant Secretary for Aging, Office of the Assistant Secretary for Planning and Evaluation; 1996.

68. US Dept of Health and Human Services, Public Health Service. *Prevention 86/87: Federal Programs and Progress*. Washington, DC: Public Health Service; 1987.

69. *The Aging Networks Guide to USDA*. Grand Rapids, Mich: National Association of Nutrition and Aging; 1988.

70. Subcommittee on Regulation, Business Opportunities, and Technology Committee on Small Business, US House of Representatives. *Hunger in America: public and private responses*. December 21, 1994.

71. Administration on Aging. *National Summary of Program Activities under Title III and Title VI of the Older Americans Act, Fiscal Year 1992*. Washington, DC: Office of State and Community Programs, Administration on Aging, US Dept of Health and Human Services; 1993.

72. Caliendo MA, Smith J. Factors influencing the nutrition knowledge and dietary intake of participants in the Title III-c meal program. *J Nutr Elderly*. 1981;1:65–77.

73. Kirschner Associates Inc, Opinion Research Corporation. *Longitudinal Evaluation of the National Nutrition Program for the Elderly* Washington, DC: Administration on Aging; 1980. US Dept of Health, Education, and Welfare publication 80-20249.

74. Kohrs MB, O'Hanlon P, Eklund D. Title VII nutrition program for the elderly, I: contribution to one day's dietary intake. *J Am Diet Assoc.* 1978;72:487–492.

75. Kohrs MB. Association of participation in a nutritional program for the elderly with nutritional status. *Am J Clin Nutr.* 1980;33:2643–2656.

76. LeClerc H, Thornbury ME. Dietary intakes of Title III meal program recipients and nonrecipients. *J Am Diet Assoc.* 1983;83:573–577.

77. Nestle M, Lee PR, Fullarton JE. *Nutrition and the Elderly: A Working Paper for the Administration on Aging*. San Francisco, Calif: Aging Health Policy Center, University of California; 1983. Policy Paper No. 2.

78. Zandt SV, Fox H. Nutritional impact of congregate meals programs. *J Nutr Elderly*. 1986;5:31–43.

79. Reuben DB, Siu AL. An objective measure of physical function of elderly outpatients: the physical performance test. *J Am Geriatr Soc.* 1990;38:1105–1112.

80. Posner BM, Smigelski C, Duggal A, et al. Validation of two-dimensional models for estimation of portion size in nutrition research. *J Am Dietet Assoc.* 1992;92:738–741.

81. US Senate Special Committee on Aging. *Developments in Aging: 1986. A Report of the Special Committee on Aging*. Washington DC: US Government Printing Office; 1987. ASI No. 25144.3.

82. Butler JS, Ohls JC, Posner BM. The effect of the food stamp program on the nutrient intake of the eligible elderly. *J Hum Resources*. 1985;20:405–419.

83. Akin JS, Guilkey DK, Popkin BM, et al. The impact of federal transfer programs on the nutrient intake of elderly individuals. *J Hum Resources*. 1985;20:382–404.

84. The Medicare program and nutrition Services. June 1997. http://www.eatright.org.med.html. American Dietetic Association; 1998.

85. US Dept of Health and Human Services. Health Care Financing Administration. *Your Medicare Handbook 1997*. Washington DC: US Government Printing Office. 1997. Publication 552-158.

# CHAPTER 19

# Health Promotion and Disease Prevention in the Elderly

*Beverly J. McCabe and Jessica L. Dorey*

In the decade since the 1988 Surgeon General's Workshop on Health Promotion and Disease Prevention and the 1989 US Preventive Services Task Force (USPSTF) report entitled *Guide to Preventive Services*, dramatic changes have occurred in the health care system in the United States.[1–6] Important scientific studies, lay interest, government policy, disease-related activities by private organizations, food industry advertising, and health professionals' practices all have added new luster to health promotion and disease prevention across the life span. The field of nutrition has moved from a focus on the prevention of nutrient deficiency diseases to a focus on the role of nutrition in the prevention of chronic diseases.[7–10] The value of exercise is no longer confined to children and young adults. Its value is being recognized among all geriatric populations including those with chronic diseases such as rheumatoid arthritis.[11–14] The importance of community-based, culturally sensitive interventions also has been recognized.[15–18] Strategies for health promotion and disease prevention have evolved from a single plan applied in many communities to use of focus groups to develop a local plan that directly involves the participants in decision making, implementation, and evaluation of the interventions.[15–19] Large intervention trials such as the Multiple Risk Factors Intervention Trial (MRFIT) program planned with the best of scientific methods have demonstrated only small changes.[17]

While scientific support for the benefits of health promotion has grown along with increased public awareness, the funding for intervention programs has not kept pace.[20] The lack of funding is due to several factors. In America, expensive health care for end-stage diseases consumes the bulk of resources (ie, hospital stays, nursing home care, physician services, nursing care, medications, and other services).[20,21] The last year, and especially the last months, of life cost nearly 30% of Medicare dollars compared with only 3% for prevention.[20,21] A consensus is building that more resources need to be spent on prevention if future health care costs are to be contained.

A major obstacle to funding decisions for prevention, especially among the elderly, is the lack of research to define the effectiveness of the prevention strategy.[22] Important questions include how, when, where, and by whom health promotion interventions are best provided.[22,23] Research is needed to determine if strategies and methods used successfully in the young apply to the old.[24]

## DEFINITIONS

Health promotion, wellness, and disease prevention may have different meanings. For some, wellness is defined as aerobic exercise while others see wellness and health promotion as smoking cessation, immunization, weight control, sanitation, and change in any number of other individual health behaviors. Several government reports use a working definition of health promotion originally coined by Green in 1979[25] as "any combination of educational, organization, economic, and environmental supports for behavior and conditions of living conducive to health."

Thus, health promotion focuses on personal health behavior while disease prevention is seen in the aggregate. Disease prevention is generally assigned to one of three levels: primary, secondary, or tertiary. Primary prevention interventions involve healthy people (eg, programs such as influenza vaccination or the Five-A-Day program), while secondary prevention measures involve individuals with a risk factor but whose disease is not apparent (eg, interventions such as a Pap smear or weight control efforts with a family history of type 2 diabetes mellitus). Tertiary prevention measures apply to individuals with an overt disease (eg, antibiotic therapy after injury or instruction on good food sources of potassium when diuretics are ordered).[3,5]

Aging has been described as a series of processes that increase vulnerability to challenges that can result in increased risk for disability and death.[26] Health promotion and disease prevention activities in the elderly aim to interrupt or slow the process of aging. Risk factors for the elderly may not be the same as those for the young or for a mature adult. For example, weight loss and low serum cholesterol may be greater risk factors than mild obesity and moderately high (greater than 250 mg/dL) serum cholesterol in the elderly.[27]

In the elderly, primary health prevention measures involve healthy lifestyle and good medical care with greater emphasis on eliminating or minimizing preexisting conditions (secondary prevention) or minimizing discomfort, disability, and dependency caused by established disease even if life cannot be saved (tertiary prevention). The goal of preventive medicine in older people should be not only the prevention of premature morbidity and mortality but also the preservation of function, independence (autonomy), and quality of life.[28] In general, the older the person, the less value primary prevention measures have.[22,29–31]

Quality of life has been characterized as an elusive phenomenon, encompassing biological, psychological, interpersonal, social, economic, and cultural dimensions.[31] The growth in life expectancy has greatly outpaced society's planning for the social economics and health care needs of older adults. The formulation of health care policy needs to encompass these multiple dimensions.[31] If prolonging life also prolongs disability at the end of life, then it is not optimizing the quality of life.[22]

Many of the determinants of health have little to do with medical care. Lifestyle, genetics, and environment contribute significantly to health and to quality of life. Lifestyle and behavior of individuals involve nutrition, substance abuse, use of protective devices, and physical activity. The environment includes education, literacy, income, housing, and exposure to toxins and pollutants.[31] Thus, effective health promotion must encompass individual behaviors, population-based initiatives, and physician actions. Decisions to include health promotion activities into clinical practice should be well grounded in scientific evidence.[30] A recent review of the literature by Patterson and Feightner[30] summarized recommendations that meet these criteria.

Two additional terms used in health promotion in the elderly have been recently defined by Hazzard:[32] preventive gerontology and preventive geriatrics. Hazzard distinguishes between the two by defining preventive gerontology as prevention occurring before old age and preventive geriatrics as prevention occurring in old age. Preventive gerontology is further defined as preventive measures taken before old age to retard processes that lead to premature morbidity and mortality. Interventions such as diet, exercise, controlled exposure to toxic substances, and limited adverse environmental exposure must be practiced on a long-term basis, requiring considerable personal choice and discipline. Should preventive gerontology be applied broadly, then Hazzard[32] sees geriatric medicine as becoming largely a field of caring for the frail elderly. Preventive geriatrics would focus on those interventions that are short term and yield a shorter return.[32]

While the benefits of health promotion are well documented in the general population, much less research has examined the benefits in the elderly population.[23] Early in the 21st century a fifth of the US population will be 65 years of age or older, and one third of the American life span will likely be spent in retirement.[33] Similarly, nearly 25% of the Canadian population will be over 65 years of age.[30]

Because of the increase in both absolute numbers and percentages of the population who will be classified as elderly, the importance of promoting "successful" and "healthy" aging becomes critical if health care costs are to be contained.[32] With few exceptions, Medicare, designed to cover the cost of acute illness, has not covered the cost of health promotion.[34] The Health Care Financing Administration (HCFA) funded a series of demonstration programs to evaluate the impact of providing health promotion and preventive services to Medicare recipients. Questions under consideration included whether health promotion would produce sig-

nificant improvements in the health of older Americans, whether money would be saved, and whether the elderly would participate in such services.[35–37] Other issues included whether such programs would simply delay the onset of disability or prolong the period of disability.

Currently, women live almost 7 years longer than men but they have almost twice as many years of disability prior to death.[38] The diseases in women that account for death and the consumption of health care resources are also diseases that are major contributors to disability. Interventions that affect heart disease, cancer, stroke, fracture, pneumonia, osteoarthritis, and cataracts would impact elderly women's health most.[38]

In a study in rural Pennsylvania, 41% of elderly participants were identified as eligible for a nutrition program, 11% for a smoking cessation program, 2% for alcohol counseling, and 7% for dementia and depression evaluations.[34,35] Participants not only varied across the type of program but also within programs by gender, education, and group assignment (hospital based versus physician based). Use of service was higher by participants with more education and by physician-based programs. Participant was greater in programs involving a single intervention (eg, immunization) than programs requiring more sessions and more participant action (eg, weight loss). Attendance was best in the five-session cholesterol-lowering program. Sixty-seven percent of the participants attended 75% or more of the sessions compared with 39% of participants attending at least 50% of the eight smoking cessation sessions and 40% attending at least 50% of the 16 weight loss sessions. Overall, at least one session was attended by 44.8% of those eligible for nutrition intervention, 17% for smoking cessation, and 57.5% for immunizations. Thus, rural Americans will use health promotion services if covered by Medicare.[34,35]

A small sample of Canadian elderly perceived differing benefits from individualized counseling and group wellness sessions.[36] Subjects described group sessions as a means to get general information about life and lifestyle choices but that some services are best provided to meet individualized needs.[36]

In California, 237 study participants over the age of 60 were randomly assigned to either a treatment or a control group after a standardized assessment.[39] The assessment included a health history, nutritional evaluation, and limited physical assessment by a nurse. The treatment group received a written personal health plan and counseling, while the control group received only the health assessment, risk identification, and limited verbal health plan counseling. The treatment group completed significantly ($p < .001$) more preventive referrals and health behavior changes upon reassessment 1 year later. The results support the conclusion that a client-centered process with supportive counseling by public health nurses combined with written health plans can significantly increase the prevention activities of older adults.[23]

These studies suggest that elderly Americans will participate in health promotion interventions if offered and that the referral of physicians will significantly improve participation. Guidelines for preventive services have been outlined by several expert panels.[3,10,25] The question is whether physicians and other health professionals will follow such guidelines to reduce morbidity and mortality.

Eleven urban hospitals and 46 primary care practitioners consented to a survey of 1,800 patients between the ages of 52 and 77 who had been followed by these physicians for at least 2 years.[39] Study physicians were primarily family or general practitioners (61%),

general internists (34%), and others (6%). Surveys were returned by 1,457 (81%) patients who were mostly female (59%), white (87%), with an income of $40,000 or less (75%), who possessed a high school education or more (78%), and who had health insurance (98%) with 51% Medicare and 20% health maintenance plan (HMP) coverage.

Of the 215 smokers, 93% had been told the health risks of smoking, 87% had been advised to stop smoking, 66% had been counseled, and 36% had been referred to a smoking cessation program. Physicians were least likely to discuss or ask about alcohol use (15%) or to advise the use of seat belts (17%).

Seventy-nine percent of the physicians recommended regular checkups, 73% asked about regular exercise, 72% discussed eating a healthy diet, 68% asked about smoking, and 67% recommended a flu shot. Physicians less frequently asked patients younger than age 60 about family history of early heart disease (56%), breast cancer (53%), or colon cancer (46%). At least 50% of the patients were offered and had a screening test within the past 2 years, regardless of the frequency of expert recommendations. When grouped, age trends were noted in increased likelihood of sigmoidoscopy ($p < .001$) and fecal occult blood tests ($p < .002$). While men were increasingly likely to be screened for prostate cancer ($p < .001$), women were decreasingly likely to receive most screening tests, particularly mammograms ($p < .001$) and Pap smear tests ($p < .02$). Patients with a positive family history were not more likely to receive screening than patients without.[39]

## COSTS VERSUS BENEFITS

If the benefits of health promotion in the elderly are demonstrated, if the elderly will participate in health promotion interventions, and if physicians appear to be using age more than risk to order screening tests, an important question is: At what age do the costs of intervention begin to outweigh the benefits? In 1980, a noted rheumatologist predicted that by the middle of the 21st century, the average human longevity would become stable at 85 years of age.[40] This prediction, coupled with limited data on benefits of preventive screening beyond the age of 85, has supported age 85 as a general cutoff range for conventional screening.[22,28,41] The risks, benefits, and costs of preventive gerontology with its long-term, low-cost, low-risk interventions partnered with individualized short-term, low-risk secondary prevention may yet demonstrate a maximal longevity of high quality for individuals and populations. That age has yet to be determined.[32]

The failure to use low-cost, low-risk screening tests such as mammograms in elderly women is disturbing in that breast cancer is among the leading causes of disability in the elderly.[39] As the benefits of exercise intervention (even in the frail elderly) and nutrition programs such as home-delivered meals in decreasing length of stay in hospitals become well documented, the assumption that health promotion interventions should cease at age 85 will likely be challenged.

## NUTRITION IN GENERAL HEALTH PROMOTION AND DISEASE PREVENTION

While interest in diet and nutrition as means of chronic disease prevention has grown steadily since the 1960s, it was not until three important reports were issued in 1988 and 1989 that a concerted effort began to help Americans translate dietary recommendations into a pattern that would emphasize chronic disease prevention over nutrient deficiency prevention.[42–45]

A number of other government agencies assisted in the process of revamping American eating patterns.[45,46] The US Congress established the National Nutrition Monitoring and Related Research (NNMRR) Act of 1990, which directed that the Department of Health and Human Services (DHHS) and the US Department of Agriculture (USDA) share responsibility for implementing the program and to contract with a scientific body such as the National Academy of Sciences (NAS) or the Federation of American Societies for Experimental Biology (FASEB) to interpret available data analyses and publish a report on the dietary, nutritional, and health-related status of the American people and the nutritional quality of food consumed in the United States at least once every 5 years.[44,45] The three reports issued under NNMRR provide five measurement components:

1. nutrition and related health measurements
2. food and nutrient consumption
3. knowledge, attitudes, and behaviors assessments
4. food composition and nutrient databases
5. food supply determinants[45]

Another important development was the 1990 Nutrition Labeling and Education Act (NLEA). It simplified the nutrition information provided on a label and required listing only those nutrients associated with chronic disease risks.[47,48]

This act also allowed food manufacturers to petition the Food and Drug Administration (FDA) for approval of health claims by providing data to demonstrate the validity of the claim. This significant change in food policy enabled food advertisements to provide messages about the role of nutrients and food constituents in health promotion and disease prevention.[47,48]

The USDA and DHHS released two important food guides for Americans in 1990.[49] The fourth edition of the USDA dietary guidelines assists in the selection of a diet that decreases dietary risks for chronic diseases while providing adequate nutrients and energy.[49] These seven revised guidelines are:

1. Eat a variety of foods.
2. Balance the food you eat with physical activity. Maintain or improve your weight.
3. Choose a diet low in fat, saturated fat, and cholesterol.
4. Choose a diet with plenty of vegetables, fruits, and grain products.
5. Choose a diet moderate in salt and sodium.
6. Choose a diet moderate in sugars.
7. Drink alcoholic beverages in moderation if you choose to drink.

In order to assist individuals in translating these dietary guidelines into appropriate food choices, the USDA replaced the Basic Four recommendations with the Food Guide Pyramid in 1990.[49,50] The pyramid recommends that the daily diet contain 6 to 11 portions of grain products, 2 to 4 servings of fruit, 3 to 5 servings of vegetables, 2 to 3 servings of meats or meat substitutes, and 2 to 3 servings of dairy products.

The National Cancer Institute developed the "5-A-Day" campaign to encourage the public to consume five servings of fruits and vegetables daily to promote diets that meet the Food Guide Pyramid guidelines.[10] More recently, the American Cancer Society convened an Advisory Committee on Diet, Nutrition, and Cancer Prevention to update the 1991 guidelines for cancer prevention.[10] These 1996 recommendations are to:

• Choose most of the foods you eat from plant sources. Eat five or more servings of fruits and vegetables each day. Choose green and dark yellow or cabbage-family vegetables. Use soy products and le-

gumes. Eat other plant source foods including breads, cereals, grain products, rice, pasta, and beans several times each day. Choose whole grains in preference to refined grains. Choose beans as a replacement for meats.

• Limit your intake of high-fat foods, particularly from animal sources. Choose foods low in fat. Prepare foods with little or no fat. Bake or broil meats and vegetables rather than fry foods. Choose nonfat and low-fat milk and dairy products. Eat smaller portions of high-fat dishes. Select low-fat food items when snacking or eating in restaurants. Limit meat intake, especially high-fat meats. Use lean meat more as a condiment and less as an entree. Choose seafood, poultry, or beans over beef, pork, and lamb.

• Be physically active. Achieve and maintain a healthy weight. Be active for at least 30 minutes several times a week. Control caloric intake. Be within your healthy weight range.

• Limit consumption of alcoholic beverages, if you drink at all. Limit alcoholic beverages to two or less drinks a day. Do not combine the use of tobacco and alcohol.

Table 19–1 lists the committee's best advice on how to reduce the risk of various types of cancer.[10]

The public's awareness of the role of diet and nutrition in the prevention of cancer continues to grow. So too is the scientific evidence of the importance of food and nutrients in cancer protection, and good news is coming from the American Cancer Society. In 1997, 1,382,400 new cases of cancer were projected for calendar year 1997.[51] A midyear adjustment reduced the estimate to 1,257,800, a decrease of 9%.[52] Landis and colleagues[53] predicted 1,228,600 new cases (an additional decrease of 2%) for the calen-

**Table 19–1** Advice on Risk Reduction for Various Types of Cancer

|  | Type of Cancer | | | | | | |
|---|---|---|---|---|---|---|---|
| Dietary Advice | Breast | Colorectal | Endometrial | Lung | Oral/Esophageal | Prostate | Stomach |
| Limit alcohol | X |  |  |  | XX |  |  |
| Eat vegetables/fruits |  | XX | X | XX | XX |  | XX |
| Be physically active | X | X | X |  |  |  |  |
| Avoid obesity | X | X | X |  |  |  |  |
| Consume less high-fat foods/saturated fats |  | X |  |  | X |  |  |
| Eat grains |  | X |  |  |  |  |  |
| Limit red meat |  | X |  |  |  | X |  |
| Avoid tobacco |  |  |  | XX | XX |  |  |
| Eat fresh foods |  |  |  |  | X |  | X |

Source: Data from American Cancer Society 1996, Advisory Committee on Diet, Nutrition, and Cancer Prevention, Reducing the Risk of Cancer with Healthy Food Choices and Physical Activities, CA: A Cancer Journal of Clinicians, Vol. 46, pp. 326–339, © 1996.

dar year 1998. Overall, this figure represents an 11% decrease over the original 1997 projection, largely due to fewer cases of prostate cancer. These figures reflect the first downward trend in cancer cases since recordkeeping began in the 1930s.[53,54]

In addition, 5-year relative survival rates also are improving but not equally well in all population groups and all specific cancer sites. Death rates in men have declined more than in women, largely due to increased death rates in women from lung cancer. Survival rates among African American men and women have improved, but to a lesser degree than those for whites.[54]

To better assess the overall diet quality and to monitor the compliance of Americans to the Food Guide Pyramid and the Dietary Guidelines, the Healthy Eating Index (HEI) was first computed using 1989 data from the Continuing Survey of Food Intakes by Individuals (CSFII).[55–57] The CSFII survey is a nationally representative survey containing information on people's consumption of foods and nutrients.[56] The HEI is the sum of 10 components, each representing different aspects of a healthful diet. Figure 19–1 illustrates the distribution of these components into a score of 100.[56]

The first five components measure the degree to which a person's diet complies with the recommendations for the five major food groups of the Food Guide Pyramid: grains, vegetables, fruits, meats, and milk. The percentage of total kilocalories from fat is the sixth component, while percentage from saturated fat is the seventh, total cholesterol intake is the eighth component, total sodium intake is the ninth component, and variety in the diet is the tenth component. An HEI score of over 80 is considered a "good" diet, an HEI score between 51 and 80 indicates a diet that needs improvement, and an HEI score below 51 is considered to be a "poor" diet.[56,57]

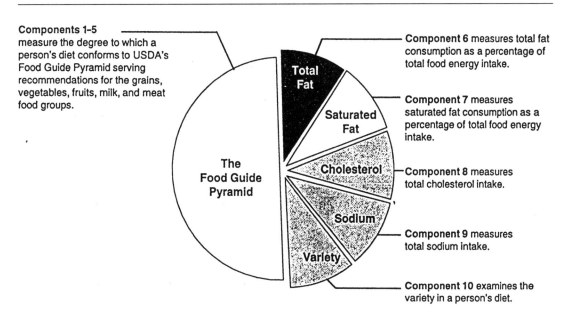

**Figure 19–1** Components of the Healthy Eating Index. *Source:* Reprinted from *Healthy Eating Index 1994–1996*, United States Department of Agriculture, Center for Nutrition Policy and Promotion, CNPP-5.

The Healthy Eating Index 1994–1996 provides a comparison of diet quality from 1989 to 1996.[57] Between 1989 and 1996 the overall HEI score improved from 61.5 to 63.8, a small but significant increase. In 1996 older females (51 years and above) had a better overall score than older men (67.5 and 65.2, respectively). Likewise women 19 to 50 scored higher than men in the same age group (62.7 and 60.6, respectively).[57]

The release of the first set of Dietary Reference Intakes (DRIs) in 1997 enlarged the concept of the single value Recommended Dietary Allowances (RDAs) to a range of values designed to go beyond the prevention of deficiency diseases and to include current concepts of the role of nutrients and food components in long-term health.[7–9,58–61] While the RDA is still included in this set, its purpose has been limited to that of being a goal for individuals.[7,8,58,61] For all other purposes, the three other reference values should be selected: the Adequate Intake (AI), the Tolerable Upper Limit (UL), and the Estimated Average Requirement (EAR).[61] Exhibit 19–1 presents the definitions of the DRIs.

The uses and preferred values to which the DRIs can be put include four primary areas:

1. assessing intakes of individuals for which the EAR would be used to examine potential for inadequacy and for which the UL would be used to examine for overconsumption;

2. assessing intakes of population groups for which the EAR would be used to examine prevalence of inadequate intakes within a group;

3. planning diets for individuals for which the RDA would be the target value if available, otherwise, the AI would be the target value (the UL would be used as a guide to limit intake of individuals on a chronic basis but not as a target intake); and

4. planning diets for groups for which the EAR would be used to set goals for the mean intake of a specified population.

An estimate of the variability of the group's intake would be required to set realistic goals. Thus, the appropriate use of the DRIs requires dietetic and other health professionals to invest time and effort in understanding how to use the DRIs and in collecting baseline data (eg, a group's intake of nutrients with which to use these tools most effectively).[7]

In addition, DRIs for many other nutrients and food components are not yet available. The DRI project has been divided into at least seven nutrient groups and two areas of general concern by the Food and Nutrition Board's Standing Committee on the Scientific Evaluation of Dietary Reference Intakes. The first two groups, calcium and related nutrients and folate and other B vitamins, have been released.[8,9] The third group, antioxidants (eg, vitamins C and E, selenium), is anticipated this year. No projected dates have been established for the remaining four groups: macronutrients (ie, protein, carbohydrates, and fats), trace elements (ie, iron, zinc), electrolytes and water, and other food components (eg, fiber and phytoestrogens).

The order and timelines for studying the nutrients are being determined by the interests of those funding the studies and by the availability of funds. If DRIs are not available for a nutrient, the 1989 RDAs remain the best available guidelines for assessing and planning diets.[58–61]

## NUTRITION IN GERIATRIC HEALTH PROMOTION AND DISEASE PREVENTION

### Nutrition Screening Initiative

The Nutrition Screening Initiative (NSI) began in early 1990 to promote nutrition

**Exhibit 19–1** Definitions of Terms Used in the 1997–1998 Dietary Reference Intakes

**Requirement.** The lowest continuing intake level of a nutrient that, for a specified indicator of adequacy, will maintain a defined level of nutriture in an individual.

**Basal Requirement.** The level of intake needed to prevent pathologically relevant and clinically detectable signs of a dietary inadequacy.

**Estimated Average Requirement (EAR).** The daily intake estimated to meet the requirement, as defined by the specific indicator of adequacy, in 50% of the individuals in a life-stage or gender group. The EAR is used to determine the RDA.

**Recommended Dietary Allowance (RDA).** The daily intake that is sufficient to meet the daily nutrient requirements of most individuals in a specific life-stage and gender group. If the variation in requirements is well defined, the RDA is set at 2 standard deviations (SDs) above the EAR.

$$RDA = EAR + 2\ SDs_{EAR}$$

If the variation is not well defined or available, a standard estimate of variance is applied. A coefficient of variation of 10% and equal to 1 SD is assumed for most nutrients.

$$RDA = 1.2 \times EAR$$

If the coefficient of variation is greater than 10% as it is with niacin (15%), then the RDA formula would be adjusted accordingly.

$$Niacin\ RDA = 1.3 \times EAR$$

**Adequate Intake (AI).** The recommended daily intake based on observed or experimentally determined approximations of the average nutrient intake by a defined population or subgroup that appears to sustain a defined nutritional state. The AI is used when scientific data are insufficient to determine an EAR and consequently the RDA.

**Tolerable Upper Intake Limit (UL).** The highest daily intake level that is unlikely to pose a risk of adverse health effects in almost all individuals in the specified life-stage and gender group. The UL is used to examine the potential fortification of foods and the use of dietary supplements. The UL is not intended as a recommended level of intake. The UL is based on a risk assessment model developed specifically for nutrients from careful literature review with systematic scientific considerations and judgments. The model is based on the lowest levels at which no observed adverse effects are found. Lack of data on adverse effects has limited the number of nutrients for which ULs have been set.

*Source:* Reprinted with permission from Institute of Medicine's Dietary Reference Intakes: Calcium, Phosphorus, Magnesium, Vitamin D, and Fluoride, pp. S1S7, © 1997, National Academy Press.

screening and better nutritional care for the elderly in the United States.[61] This multifaceted effort was a direct response to the 1988 Surgeon General's Workshop on Health Promotion and Aging and the DHHS call for nutrition screening. This project involved the American Academy of Family Physicians (AAFP), The American Dietetic Association (ADA), and the National Council on the Aging (NCOA) with advisors from medicine, health, nutrition, and aging.[62] The NSI Technical Review Committee provided the technical expertise and directions that produced the DETERMINE Your Nutritional Health Checklist and the Level I and Level II Nutrition Screening tools.[62–66]

More than 235,000 checklists and 22,500 screening manuals were distributed nationwide in the first 2 years.[67] These tools are being used in meal programs, senior citizen and adult day care centers, home services programs, physicians' offices, hospitals, and nursing homes to identify the nutrition needs of older Americans. The use of the checklist or Level I screen is usually the first step in screening individuals at high risk for poor nutrition states in order to identify who will benefit from nutrition interventions.[65] The Level II screen provides more specific diagnostic information. As more caregivers have recognized those at nutritional risk, interest in advice on nutrition has increased.[67]

**Nutrition Strategies**

The NSI Technical Review Committee identified specific strategies to improve the nutritional status of older Americans.[67] These strategies include:

- Place higher priority on nutrition screening and care in senior centers, congregate meal sites, physicians' offices, and hospitals.
- Establish interdisciplinary, community-based models for nutrition care.
- Integrate the use of foods and medical nutritionals for special dietary and medical purposes into nutrition counseling and support.
- Provide a range of practical therapeutic options.
- Develop highly structured practice protocols that measure outcomes in several ways.

- Reshape third-party reimbursement schedules to include nutrition screening and services.
- Offer continuing medical education with hands-on training to develop skills in nutrition diagnosis and treatment.
- Educate the public about the importance of nutrition status to overall health and quality of life and on ways to improve nutrition health.
- Stimulate partnerships and volunteer efforts in cooperation with a variety of lay people and professionals.[67]

In 1992 the Intervention Roundtable of the NSI involved 30 professionals who formed a consensus on recommendations in six areas of nutrition intervention: social services, oral health, mental health, medication use, nutrition education and counseling, and nutrition support.[67] In 1994 the NSI began to distribute a continuing education program for physicians, *Incorporating Nutrition Screening and Interventions into Medical Practices: A Monograph for Physicians*.[67] This monograph identifies ways to incorporate nutrition screening and intervention into quality preventive care for the geriatric patient.[67]

Nutrition screening differentiates individuals who are at high risk of nutritional problems and those who already have poor nutritional status. Screening begins with the DETERMINE Your Nutritional Health Checklist (Exhibit 19–2) of 10 items that if answered yes are scored as 0–2, good nutritional health; 3–5, moderate nutritional risk; or 6+, high nutritional risk.[62–67] The acronym DETERMINE outlines nine warning signs for nutritional risk (see Exhibit 19–3). The checklist was validated in both retrospective and prospective protocols to predict nutrition-related problems in the elderly. While it is not a diagnostic device, this instrument

**Exhibit 19–2** DETERMINE Your Nutritional Health Checklist

*The warning signs of poor nutritional health are often overlooked. Use this checklist to find out if you or someone you know is at nutritional risk. Read the statements below. Circle the number in the yes column for those that apply to you or someone you know. For each yes answer, score the number in the box. Total your nutritional score.*

|  | Yes |
|---|---|
| I have an illness or condition that made me change the kind and/or amount of food I eat. | 2 |
| I eat fewer than two meals per day. | 3 |
| I eat few fruits or vegetables or milk products. | 2 |
| I have three or more drinks of beer, liquor, or wine almost every day. | 2 |
| I have tooth or mouth problems that make it hard for me to eat. | 2 |
| I don't always have enough money to buy the food I need. | 4 |
| I eat alone most of the time. | 1 |
| I take three or more different prescribed or over-the-counter drugs a day. | 1 |
| Without wanting to, I have lost or gained 10 pounds in the last 6 months. | 2 |
| I am not always physically able to shop, cook, and/or feed myself. | 2 |
| **Total** |  |

**Total Your Nutritional Score. If It Is**

**0–2** **Good!** Recheck your nutritional score in 6 months.

**3–5** **You are at moderate nutritional risk.** See what can be done to improve your eating habits and lifestyle. Your office on aging, senior nutrition program, senior citizens center, or health department can help. Recheck your nutritional score in 3 months.

**6 or more** **You are at high nutritional risk.** Bring this checklist the next time you see your physician, dietitian, or other qualified health or social service professional. Talk with them about any problems you may have. Ask for help to improve your nutritional health.

*Source:* Reprinted with permission by the Nutrition Screening Initiative, a project of the American Academy of Family Physicians, the American Dietetic Association and the National Council on the Aging, Inc., and funded by a grant from Ross Products Division, Abbott Laboratories, Inc.

provides a valid measure of potential nutrition risks. It can be used by anyone, including the geriatric client or caregiver.[67]

The next step, the Level I Screen (Exhibit 19–4) differentiates those individuals who need further assessment and possibly nutrition intervention by calculation of body mass index (BMI) and change in body weight and evaluation of eating habits, living environment, and functional status. This tool can be used by a wide range of health care professionals. If an individual has a documented, significant, involuntary weight change or has a BMI above 27 or below 22, a referral to a

**Exhibit 19–3** Remembering the Warning Signs

*The nutrition checklist is based on the warning signs described below. Use the word* DETER-MINE *to remind you of the warning signs.*

- **Disease.** Any disease, illness, or chronic condition that causes you to change the way you eat, or makes it hard for you to eat, puts your nutritional health at risk. Four out of five adults have chronic diseases that are affected by diet. Confusion or memory loss that keeps getting worse is estimated to affect one out of five or more of older adults. This can make it hard to remember what, when, or if you've eaten. Feeling sad or depressed, which happens to about one in eight older adults, can cause big changes in appetite, digestion, energy level, weight, and well-being.

- **Eating poorly.** Eating too little and eating too much both lead to poor health. Eating the same foods day after day or not eating fruits, vegetables, and milk products daily also will cause poor nutritional health. One in five adults skip meals daily. Only 13% of adults eat the minimum amount of fruits and vegetables needed. One in four older adults drink too much alcohol. Many health problems become worse if you drink more than one or two alcoholic beverages per day.

- **Tooth loss/mouth pain.** A healthy mouth, teeth, and gums are needed to eat. Missing, loose, or rotten teeth or dentures that don't fit well or cause mouth sores make it hard to eat.

- **Economic hardship.** As many as 40% of older Americans have incomes of less than $6,000 per year. Having less—or choosing to spend less—than $25 to $30 per week for food makes it very hard to get the foods you need to stay healthy.

- **Reduced social contact.** One third of all older people live alone. Being with people daily has a positive effect on morale, well-being, and eating.

- **Multiple medicines.** Many older Americans must take medicines for health problems. Almost half of older Americans take multiple medicines daily. Growing old may change the way we respond to drugs. The more medicines you take, the greater the chance for side effects such as increased or decreased appetite, change in taste, constipation, weakness, drowsiness, diarrhea, nausea, and others. Vitamins or minerals taken in large doses can act like drugs and can cause harm. Alert your physician to everything you take.

- **Involuntary weight loss/gain.** Losing or gaining a lot of weight when you are not trying to do so is an important warning sign that must not be ignored. Being overweight or underweight also increases your chance of poor health.

- **Needs assistance in self care.** Although most older people are able to eat, one of every five have trouble walking, shopping, and buying and cooking food, especially as they get older.

- **Elder years above age 80.** Most older people lead full and productive lives. But as age increases, risk of frailty and health problems increases. Checking your nutritional health regularly makes good sense.

*Source:* Reprinted with permission by the Nutrition Screening Initiative, a project of the American Academy of Family Physicians, the American Dietetic Association and the National Council on the Aging, Inc., and funded by a grant from Ross Products Division, Abbott Laboratories, Inc.

**Exhibit 19–4** Level I Screen

### Body Weight

Measure height to the nearest inch and weight to the nearest pound. Record the values below and mark them on the body mass index (BMI) scale to the right. Then use a straight edge (ruler) to connect the two points and circle the spot where this straight line crosses the center line (body mass index). Record the number below. Healthy older adults should have a BMI between 24 and 27.

Height (in): _____

Weight (lbs): _____

Body mass index: _____
(number from center column)

Check any boxes that are true for the individual:

- ❏ Has lost or gained 10 pounds (or more) in the past 6 months
- ❏ Body mass index <24
- ❏ Body mass index >27

For the remaining sections, please ask the individual which of the statements (if any) is true for him or her and place a check by each that applies.

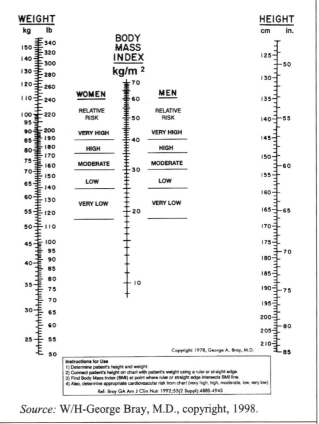

*Source:* W/H–George Bray, M.D., copyright, 1998.

### Eating Habits

- ❏ Does not have enough food to eat each day
- ❏ Usually eats alone
- ❏ Does not eat anything on one or more days each month
- ❏ Has poor appetite
- ❏ Is on a special diet
- ❏ Eats vegetables two or fewer times daily
- ❏ Eats milk or milk products once or not at all daily
- ❏ Eats fruit or drinks fruit juice once or not at all daily
- ❏ Eats breads, cereals, pasta, rice, or other grains five or fewer times daily
- ❏ Has difficulty chewing or swallowing
- ❏ Has more than one alcoholic drink per day (if woman); more than two drinks per day (if man)
- ❏ Has pain in mouth, teeth, or gums

### Living Environment

- ❏ Lives on an income of less than $6,000 per year (per individual in the household)
- ❏ Lives alone
- ❏ Is housebound
- ❏ Is concerned about home security
- ❏ Lives in a home with inadequate heating or cooling

*continues*

**Exhibit 19–4** continued

---

- ❏ Does not have a stove and/or refrigerator
- ❏ Is unable or prefers not to spend money on food (<$25–$30 per person spent on food each week)

**Functional Status**

Usually or always needs assistance with (check each that applies):
- ❏ Bathing

- ❏ Dressing
- ❏ Grooming
- ❏ Toileting
- ❏ Eating
- ❏ Walking or moving about
- ❏ Traveling (outside the home)
- ❏ Preparing food
- ❏ Shopping for food or other necessities

If you have checked one or more statements on this screen, the individual you have interviewed may be at risk for poor nutritional status. Please refer this individual to the appropriate health care or social service professional in your area. For example, a dietitian should be contacted for problems with selecting, preparing, or eating a healthy diet, or a dentist if the individual experiences pain or difficulty when chewing or swallowing. Those individuals whose income, lifestyle, or functional status may endanger their nutritional and overall health should be referred to available community services: home-delivered meals, congregate meal programs, transportation services, counseling services (alcohol abuse, depression, bereavement, etc), home health care agencies, day care programs, etc.

Please repeat this screen at least once each year—sooner if the individual has a major change in his or her health, income, immediate family (eg, spouse dies), or functional status.

*Source:* Reprinted with permission by the Nutrition Screening Initiative, a project of the American Academy of Family Physicians, the American Dietetic Association and the National Council on the Aging, Inc., and funded by a grant from Ross Products Division, Abbott Laboratories, Inc.

---

physician or nurse for further detailed screening is warranted. For those individuals who have other risk factors, referral for preventive interventions such as dietary counseling, shopping assistance, meal delivery, or nutrition support is appropriate.[65,66]

The Level II Screen (Exhibit 19–5) needs a more skilled administrator as this tool confirms the Level I Screen and expands to include more anthropometric measurements; laboratory tests; and evaluation of drug use, clinical features, eating habits, living environment, functional status, and mental/cognitive status. This tool also identifies major and minor indicators of poor nutritional status as shown in Exhibit 19–5.[64] Patients exhibiting one or more major indicators require immediate medical attention. Patients with less quan-

tifiable but multiple minor indicators should be referred to other health care or social service providers, as appropriate.[67]

Intervention-specific screening tools also are available for oral health, feeding difficulties, drug-nutrient interactions, and nutrition counseling. In addition, the NSI monograph also includes a social service intervention contact guide, an algorithm for nutrition support route selection, and a schematic diagram providing tips on how to incorporate nutrition screening and intervention into an office practice.[66,67]

Social service interventions can help improve the nutritional status of older Americans. Social isolation, poverty, and dependency and disability intervention programs include:

**Exhibit 19–5** Level II Screen

*Complete the following screen by interviewing the patient directly and/or by referring to the patient chart. If you do not routinely perform all of the described tests or ask all of the listed questions, please consider including them but do not be concerned if the entire screen is not completed. Please try to conduct a minimal screen on as many older patients as possible, and please try to collect serial measurements, which are extremely valuable in monitoring nutritional status.*

**Anthropometrics**

Measure height to the nearest inch and weight to the nearest pound. Record the values below and mark them on the body mass index (BMI) scale to the right. Then use a straight edge (paper, ruler) to connect the two points and circle the spot where this straight line crosses the center line (body mass index). Record the number below; healthy older adults should have a BMI between 24 and 27; check the appropriate box to flag an abnormally high or low value.

Height (in):_____
Weight (lbs):_____
Body mass index (weight/height$^2$):_____

Please place a check by any statement regarding BMI and recent weight loss that is true for the patient.

❑ Body mass index <24
❑ Body mass index >27
❑ Has lost or gained 10 pounds (or more) of body weight in the past 6 months

Record the measurement of mid-arm circumference to the nearest 0.1 centimeter and of

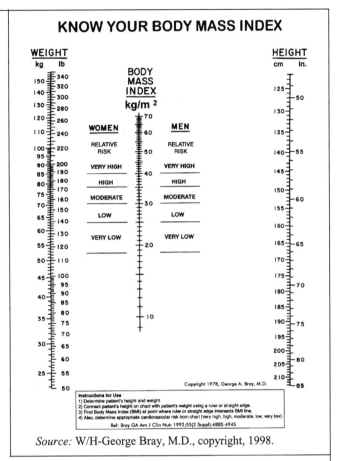

*Source:* W/H-George Bray, M.D., copyright, 1998.

triceps skinfold to the nearest 2 millimeters.

Mid-arm circumference (cm):_____
Triceps skinfold (mm):_____
Mid-arm muscle circumference (cm):_____

Refer to the table and check any abnormal values:

❑ Mid-arm muscle circumference <10th percentile
❑ Triceps skinfold <10th percentile
❑ Triceps skinfold >95th percentile

*Note:* Mid-arm circumference (cm) – [0.314 × triceps skinfold (mm)] = Mid-arm muscle circumference (cm)

For the remaining sections, please place a check by any statements that are true for the patient.

*continues*

**Exhibit 19–5** continued

### Laboratory Data

❑   Serum albumin below 3.5 g/dL
❑   Serum cholesterol below 160 mg/dL
❑   Serum cholesterol above 240 mg/dL

### Drug Use

❑   Three or more prescription drugs, over-the-counter medications, and/or vitamin/mineral supplements daily

### Clinical Features

Presence of (check each that applies):
❑   Problems with mouth, teeth, or gums
❑   Difficulty chewing
❑   Difficulty swallowing
❑   Angular stomatitis
❑   Glossitis
❑   History of bone pain
❑   History of bone fractures
❑   Skin changes (dry, loose, nonspecific lesions, edema)

### Eating Habits

❑   Does not have enough food to eat each day
❑   Usually eats alone
❑   Does not eat anything on one or more days each month
❑   Has poor appetite
❑   Is on a special diet
❑   Eats vegetables two or fewer times daily
❑   Eats milk or milk products once or not at all daily
❑   Eats fruit or drinks fruit juice once or not at all daily
❑   Eats breads, cereals, pasta, rice, or other grains five or fewer times daily

❑   Has more than one alcoholic drink per day (if a woman); more than two drinks per day (if a man)

### Living Environment

❑   Lives on an income of less than $6,000 per year (per individual in the household)
❑   Lives alone
❑   Is housebound
❑   Is concerned about home security
❑   Lives in a home with inadequate heating or cooling
❑   Does not have a stove and/or refrigerator
❑   Is unable or prefers not to spend money on food (<$25–$30 per person spent on food each week)

### Functional Status

Usually or always needs assistance with (check each that applies):
❑   Bathing
❑   Dressing
❑   Grooming
❑   Toileting
❑   Eating
❑   Walking or moving about
❑   Traveling (outside the home)
❑   Preparing food
❑   Shopping for food or other necessities

### Mental/Cognitive Status

❑   Clinical evidence of impairment (eg, Folstein < 26)
❑   Clinical evidence of depressive illness (eg, Beck Depression Inventory > 15, Geriatric Depression Scale > 5)

Patients in whom you have identified one or more major indicator of poor nutritional status require immediate medical attention; if minor indicators are found, ensure that they are known to a health professional or to the patient's own care or social service professional (dietitian, nurse, dentist, case manager, etc).

*Source:* Reprinted with permission by the Nutrition Screening Initiative, a project of the American Academy of Family Physicians, the American Dietetic Association and the National Council on the Aging, Inc., and funded by a grant from Ross Products Division, Abbott Laboratories, Inc.

- Food stamp program
- Congregate nutrition and home-delivered meal programs
- Social Security
- Supplemental Security Income
- Medicare/Medicaid
- Federally-assisted housing programs
- Employment training programs
- Adult day care services
- Transportation services
- Older Americans volunteer programs
- Case management services
- In-home health aide and personal care services
- Respite and caregiver support services[66]

A prospective study of newly hospitalized elderly patients found that 30 recipients of home-delivered meals had only half the length of stay of 30 nonrecipient controls matched by diagnosis, age, gender, and other factors.[68] In most states the cost of feeding one meal a day to an elderly person over a year's time was less than the price of one day's stay in a hospital. The relatively low cost of nutrition interventions that yield positive health costs savings is increasingly being documented.[69,70]

The NSI also has prepared two additional manuals to encourage health professionals in managed care practices and organizations and in home health agencies to incorporate nutrition screening and intervention processes.[69,70] These scientifically based manuals provide general guidelines on how to set up a nutrition screening and intervention program and how to incorporate the program into current services.[69,70] The manuals' algorithms provide visual summaries, while their graphs present data on the cost savings accrued through medical nutrition therapy.[69,70] Profiles and case studies provide materials for training staff. For example, one mnemonic device used is the NSI "Three Rs":

- **Remind.** Post charts to remind health care professionals and staff of the nutrition screening and intervention process.
- **Reach.** Keep references on procedures, risk factors, and interventions readily accessible.
- **Reinforce.** Communicate with all involved. Let them know what a valuable role they play. Keep them posted on the program's progress.[69]

In 1999 the NSI will release long-term care nutrition screening and intervention practice guidelines with five objectives:

1. Define the roles and responsibilities of the members of the interdisciplinary care team.
2. Provide guidance for the front-line care providers on how to conduct nutrition screening and assessment.
3. Distinguish different approaches to geriatric case management based on nutrition risk stratification of nursing facility residents.
4. Provide protocols for nutrition screening interventions to enhance nursing home staff who already use the HCFA Minimum Data Set and select resident assessment protocols to identify residents in need of medical nutrition therapies.
5. Advise on ways to develop and implement a nutrition care plan including follow-up nutrition assessment and interventions to maintain nutritional health.[71]

## NUTRITION AND HEALTH FOR OLDER AMERICANS

Analysis of the HEI results suggested some modification in the recommended number of servings in the Food Guide Pyramid for older adults due to the lowered energy requirements[55] (see Table 19–2).

**Table 19–2** Recommended Number of Food Guide Pyramid Servings Per Day for Older Adults

| Gender/ Age | Energy (k/cals) | Grain (servings) | Vegetables (servings) | Fruits (servings) | Milk (cups) | Meat (oz) |
|---|---|---|---|---|---|---|
| Females | | | | | | |
| 25–50 | 2,200 | 9 | 4 | 3 | 2 | 6.00 |
| Males | | | | | | |
| 25–50 | 2,900 | 11 | 5 | 4 | 2 | 7.00 |
| 51+ | 2,300 | 9.1 | 4.2 | 3.2 | 2 | 6.25 |

*Source:* Data from *The Healthy Eating Index 1994–96,* United States Department of Agriculture, Center for Nutrition Policy and Promotion.

The Expert Committee of Nutrition and Health for Older Americans recently developed a Food Guide Pyramid for older adults.[72] This pyramid focuses on the recommended food guides for older adults and features one unique feature. The base of this pyramid rests on water to emphasize the critical importance of fluid intake and the prevention of dehydration and its sequelae to the elderly with impaired thirst mechanisms and less reserve capacity for recovering from fluid deprivation.[72] This committee also has developed another important guide, the Exercise Guide for Older Adults.[72]

**Nutrition and Heart Disease**

Heart disease remains the leading cause of death in the United States, accounting for 32.8% of all deaths.[51] Among the elderly the number of deaths from circulatory diseases, ischemic heart disease, and cerebrovascular diseases has declined since their peak values in 1970.[51,73] The decline from the 1950 death rates has been the greatest for cerebrovascular diseases among those 70 to 74 years of age; the 1990 death rate was only 26.2% of the 1950 value, and only 44.3% among those 85 to 89 years of age. This change may be partially due to the implementation of Medi-care, but a similar value of 28.8% of the 1950 value also was noted among those 45 to 49 years of age, who are not recipients of Medicare benefits.[73] The availability of medical treatment has undoubtedly played a significant role in this decline in all age groups. For the other two categories, circulatory diseases and ischemic heart diseases, a much greater decline in death rates has occurred among those 45 to 49 years old than among those 70 to 74 and 85 to 89 years old. Among those 45 to 49 years old, the 1990 value was only one third of the 1950 rate while the decline was only about one half of the 1950 death rates in the two older age groups.[73]

Hypertension remains a substantial problem in elderly people. In the National Health and Nutrition Examination Survey (NHANES) III survey, prevalence was higher in females.[44] About 75% of females 80 years of age had elevated blood pressure compared with 60% of males in the same age group.[73] Table 19–3 presents data on the prevalence of hypertension by age, sex, and race/ethnicity as found in NHANES III, 1988–1991.[73]

High serum cholesterol is a major risk factor for coronary heart disease. Since 1970 public awareness of the relationship between diet and serum cholesterol has increased, but only 50% of US adults reported having had

**Table 19–3** Percentage of People 50 Years of Age and Older Who Have Hypertension Distributed by Sex, Age, and Race/Ethnicity

| Sex/Age (years) | All Groups | Non-Hispanic White | Non-Hispanic African American | Mexican American |
|---|---|---|---|---|
| **Males** | | | | |
| 50–59 | 42.2 | 41.8 | 55.9 | 36.0 |
| 60–69 | 52.1 | 51.3 | 63.6 | 53.8 |
| 70–79 | 60.7 | 60.3 | 68.0 | 52.1 |
| 80+ | 60.5 | 60.3 | 62.4 | 70.5 |
| **Females** | | | | |
| 50–59 | 38.8 | 36.8 | 47.9 | 33.5 |
| 60–69 | 53.5 | 50.9 | 77.8 | 59.3 |
| 70–79 | 67.6 | 66.9 | 72.6 | 67.0 |
| 80+ | 74.7 | 74.3 | 80.5 | 71.0 |

*Source:* Adapted from Third Report of NNMRRP, 1995.

their serum cholesterol checked in the NHANES III survey.[45] Of those who had had a serum cholesterol check, 85% reported being told by a physician or other health professional to change their diet, 54% were told to exercise, 47% were told to lose weight, and 20% were told to take medications; 89% reported they were currently following advice to change their diet compared with 70% who were trying to lose weight, exercise, and/or take medications.[45] Despite widespread education efforts by government and private agencies, only 60% of American adults were aware that "saturated fats" are more likely to raise "blood" cholesterol levels than "polyunsaturated fatty acids."[45] (*Note:* Quotation marks indicate specific terms used in survey items.) More people are aware of the relationship between dietary cholesterol and health than of the relationship between dietary "fat," "saturated fat," and health. People who were African American, over 60 years of age, less educated, and from lower income levels were less aware than white, middle aged, more educated people from higher income levels.[45] Only when nutrition policy changes allowed health claim advertisements and specially designed programs for minority populations did increases in diet knowledge begin to emerge among lower income, less educated, nonwhite populations.[47]

More recently, research interest has grown in potential risk factors other than serum cholesterol including the hypothesized relationship between vitamin intake and coronary heart disease secondary to hyperhomocysteine.[74,75] Subsequently 1,160 surviving elderly members of the Framingham Study cohorts were examined for their blood levels and dietary intakes of vitamin $B_{12}$, $B_6$, and folate compared with their serum homocysteine levels.[76] Homocysteine increased with both age and lower B vitamin intakes. Selhub and colleagues[76] suggest that a substantial majority of the cases of high homocysteine in the elderly may be due to vitamin status. In a later investigation of 70 participants between the ages of 54 and 81 years (the Boston Veterans Affairs Normative Aging Study), vitamin status and homocysteine levels were used to predict vascular disease status and cognitive performance.[77] Homocysteine levels did not appear to predict clinical diagnosis of vascular disease in this sample. No significant relationship was observed between plasma concentration of the B vitamins or homocysteine and age or years of education.[77] Plasma folate and vitamin $B_{12}$ concentrations were, however, negatively correlated with plasma homocysteine levels.[77]

In a review of over 75 studies involving more than 15,000 subjects, Parnetti and associates[78] concluded that homocysteine is an independent risk factor for cardiovascular diseases, especially for extracranial carotid atherosclerosis. They suggest that homocysteine may represent a metabolic link in the pathogenesis of atherosclerotic vascular disease and old-age dementias.[78] Ebly and colleagues[79] found low serum folate to be a significant explanatory variable for stroke and all types of dementias in 1,171 subjects in the Canadian Study of Health and Aging (CSHA). Several epidemiological and animal studies have suggested that vitamin E may play a significant role in the prevention of cardiovascular disease, but clinical trials now in progress will help shape any specific recommendations about the use of vitamin E in the prevention of cardiovascular disease.[80]

In a sample of 150 elderly people in Spain, the number of meals eaten was inversely related to serum cholesterol levels, very-low-density lipoprotein (VLDL) cholesterol and triacylglycerol levels.[81] As the number of meals increased, subjects came closer to meeting the recommended intake of energy and other nutrients (protein, fiber, vitamin C, thiamin, riboflavin, calcium, magnesium, and iodine).[81] Institutionalized subjects (n = 58) were less likely to eat four meals a day than noninstitutionalized subjects (n = 92).[81]

## Nutrition and Cancer

Cancer rates second among leading causes of all deaths in the United States, accounting for 23.4% of deaths in 1993.[52] Between 1950 and 1990, the death rate from all cancers rose among those over 70 years of age while falling nearly 20% among those 45 to 49 years old. Among those age 70 to 74, the 1990 death rate was 192.5% and for those age 85 to 89 the 1990 death rate was 172.8% of the 1950 death rates.[73] A new trend, however, is evident in the 1997 and 1998 cancer statistics, which show a decline in the number of new cases and death rates.[53–55] This trend may be due to prevention, early detection, or aggressive therapy.[55] Whatever the primary cause, efforts in all areas need to be encouraged.[55]

In a review of 206 human epidemiological studies and 22 animal studies on diet and cancer prevention, the consumption of vegetables and fruits was most favorable toward cancer prevention.[82] The evidence is particularly strong for cancers of the gastrointestinal and respiratory tracts; it is less strong for prevention of cancers related to hormones (eg, breast and prostate cancers).[10] The types of vegetables and fruits that are most often cited as protective include raw vegetables, allium vegetables (onion and garlic), carrots, green vegetables, cruciferous (cabbage family) vegetables, tomatoes, soy proteins, and legumes.[10,82] This protective effect is not limited to the value of vitamins such as beta carotene and minerals such as selenium but appears to include many other food constituents that are not classified as nutrients.[10,82] Examples of potential protective substances are fibers, phytochemicals such as flavonoids, terpenes, sterols, indoles, and phenols that are of plant origin.[10]

Elderly people tend to reduce their overall consumption of food due to multiple factors (eg, dental problems, limited access to shopping, loss of appetite, early satiety, indigestion, fatigue, and bone pain).[83–85] Many studies[10,43,51,85,86] document an intake of vegetables and fruits well below recommended levels. The NHANES III data reported older women averaged four servings of fruits and vegetables compared with the seven servings a day recommended by the Food Guide Pyramid and the Five-A-Day program advocated by the National Cancer Institute.[43,57] In addition, a pilot study of elderly women and men living in apartments in New York City found they consumed an average of 3.8 servings of fruits and 1.95 servings of vegetables.[85] Moreover, women living in rural east Tennessee public housing reported mean intakes for all vegetables as $15.1 \pm 9.7$ servings/week and for all fruit and juice as $9.9 \pm 9.8$ with a mean intake of $1,377 \pm 594$ kilocalories.[86] Even correcting for an underreporting of energy intake of 10% to 30% as reported in various studies comparing dietary intake data with energy expenditures as measured by doubly labeled water, these intakes would fall short of recommended intakes for many women, including the elderly.[87–89]

In a study of elderly Illinois women using a 7-day food record to estimate energy intake and doubly labeled water to estimate energy expenditure over a 6-day span, there was an underreporting of approximately 10% for a total energy intake of $1,599 \pm 126$ compared with a total energy expenditure of $1,782 \pm 253$.[89] Mares-Perlman and associates[90] estimated the dietary intake of middle-aged (43 to 64 years of age) men and women and of elderly (65 to 84 years of age) men and women in Wisconsin during the Beaver Dam Eye Study, using a modification of the Block Food Frequency Questionnaire. Older men and women consumed less protein, fat, cholesterol, niacin, riboflavin, calcium, iron, zinc, and lycopene.[90] Less energy came from protein and alcohol and more came from car-

bohydrates. The evaluation of the impact of dietary supplements on median intakes was greatest for vitamins A, C, and E; riboflavin; and calcium, but as previously noted, the use of supplements was less among those with a poor diet.[90]

## Nutrition and Osteoporosis

Osteoporosis affects more than 25 million Americans. It is the major underlying cause of bone fractures in elderly and postmenopausal women. (See Chapter X.) The 1.5 million fractures a year cost $10 billion in direct health care costs.[91]

The 1988–1994 NHANES III survey used dual-energy X-ray absorptiometry (DEXA) scanning of the proximal femur to assess the prevalence of bone mass density indicative of osteoporosis in 14,646 men and women aged 20 years or older who underwent direct standardized physical examinations and household interviews.[92] The prevalence of osteoporosis of the 1,249 women over 64 years of age was 29.3% by bone density findings, but only 6.3% of these women reported being told they had osteoporosis. These cross-sectional data suggest that over 90% of women with osteoporosis are unaware of their condition.[92] Women with higher education, living in urban areas, who had seen a physician in the last 6 months were more likely to self-report osteoporosis.[92]

Institutionalized elderly women are more likely to have lower bone density than noninstitutionalized controls.[93] Reduced peripheral fat was significantly associated with the lower bone density found in these institutionalized women.[93]

Bone health is dependent on many factors.[94] Thin, small, white or Asian women are at greater risk for the development of osteoporosis. African American women and men also may develop osteoporosis given long-term presence of lifestyle choices of a diet deficient in calcium, vitamin D, phosphorus, magnesium, or fluoride; lack of weight-bearing exercise; cigarette smoking; excessive alcohol intake; family history of osteoporosis; and use of some medications.[95] Long-term use of glucocorticoids, anticonvulsants, loop diuretics, anti-mitotics, cyclosporine, heparin, cholestyramine, thyroid hormones, and aluminum-containing antacids has been associated with osteoporosis.[91,95] The elderly may have limited sunlight exposure and may produce less cholecalciferol, have less renal ability to convert cholecalciferol to its active form, and may have a decreased ability to absorb calcium, thereby leading to a higher requirement for dietary vitamin D.[8]

A review paper recently summarized the evidence that vitamin K may play a role in bone metabolism as well as in coagulation synthesis.[96] Because the overall data for an association between diet and osteoporosis were so strong and the average intake of calcium by older women was less than 600 mg/day, nutrition policy about health claims was revised to allow claims to be made in food advertising.[47,48] The FDA began to approve the fortification of more foods with calcium and to allow claims on nutrition labels. For example, the fortification of orange juice, which was not previously considered a good source of calcium, has made it an important source of calcium for those individuals who cannot or will not consume dairy products.[46,90]

As noted in the 1994 National Institutes of Health (NIH) consensus conference, calcium intake in men and women older than 65 years is commonly less than 600 mg.[91] An analysis of calcium intake drawn from the 1994–1996 CSFII by McCabe and coworkers[97] yielded mean intakes and standard deviations of 578 ± 290 mg and 768 ± 397 mg for females and males 55 to 60 years of age, respectively. The mean intakes and standard deviations were 579 ± 290 mg and 720 ± 356 mg for females and males 75 to 80 years of age, respectively.[97]

The addition of three servings of a food fortified to become an excellent source of calcium would be needed to raise the mean intake to the AI of 1,000 to 1,500 mg recommended for older women.[8,97] (For a food to be labeled an excellent or high source of calcium, a serving must provide 200 mg.[46]) For older individuals at the 90th percentile of calcium intake, 955 mg for women and 1,240 mg for men ages 55 to 60, three calcium-fortified products a day would be well below the Tolerable Upper Limit of 2,500 mg calcium.[8,97] Thus, foods fortified with calcium could play a significant role in assisting elderly people attain these new recommended intakes of calcium.

Even with hormone replacement therapy (HRT), an adequate intake of calcium remains essential.[91] The use of HRT reduces the recommended daily calcium intake from 1,500 mg to 1,000 mg per day.[91] Moreover, the latest CSFII data suggest that the elderly are increasing their intakes of calcium and that many are using calcium supplements.[8,90,97] The average multiple vitamin and mineral supplement, however, does not provide sufficient calcium to move the current intake of elderly people to the recommended level of 1,000 to 1,500 mg per day.

## Nutrition, Hypertension, Obesity, and Diabetes

Hypertension, obesity, and diabetes share many common relationships and treatment strategies. They also are recognized as risk factors for the same diseases. Thus the literature becomes somewhat repetitious when viewed separately.

Hypertension remains a major health problem among the elderly, particularly in the southern United States and among African Americans.[98–101] The incidence of hypertension increases with age and is a major risk factor for both heart disease and stroke. Clinical trials of antihypertensive medication therapy have shown a reduction in these disease risks.[99,100] More recently, interest has grown in alternative approaches due to the potential for adverse effects of the drugs, drug-drug interactions, and the high cost of the drugs.[101] Obesity and dietary salt intake have been suggested as contributors to the development of hypertension. Weight loss and reduction of dietary sodium have been recommended for older persons based on clinical trials in middle-aged adults.[101,102]

A recent, randomized, controlled trial of nonpharmacological interventions in the elderly (TONE) in 875 men and women aged 60 to 80 years demonstrated that reduced sodium intake and weight loss are effective and safe therapies for hypertension in older persons upon withdrawal from antihypertensive drugs.[102] Obese subjects were randomized to weight loss, reduced sodium intake, both, or usual care. Antihypertensive drugs were withdrawn after 3 months of intervention. The combined weight loss–low-sodium intake regimen yielded the best outcome measures.[102] While this study did not offer other interventions such as increased physical activity, increased potassium intake, or other diet modifications, these approaches might offer additional benefits. This study did demonstrate that older subjects are both able to make and sustain lifestyle changes.[102]

Among the elderly, hypertension brings morbid effects such as cognitive impairment in the otherwise healthy individual and loss of mobility in community-dwelling persons.[99] The antihypertensive drug regimens and public education programs have proven effective overall, but less so in some populations.[44,47,98]

Older African Americans in the southeast United States present a stubborn public health problem.[98] In a study of 6,473 elderly South Carolinians, age was shown to be negatively related to lifestyle changes.[98] Social participation was identified as an important factor in willingness to change diet or exercise practices. The presence of comorbidities such as heart attack, stroke, kidney disease, atherosclerosis, and diabetes appears to be a relatively unimportant influence on lifestyle changes.[98] One possible explanation for this surprising finding is that the primary disease is being treated without providing health education for lifestyle change.[98]

Low-income, unmarried African American males were less likely to report changes; this group may need to be targeted differently than other groups of African American elderly. Extensive outreach initiatives, such as rides, meals, and fellowship, would appear to be justified for this hard-to-reach group.[98] In addition, socialization and feeding programs such as congregate meals and home-delivered meals can have positive impacts on health care costs.[68] A prospective observational study of newly hospitalized patients found that 30 recipients of home-delivered meals had only half the length of stay of 30 nonrecipients matched by diagnosis, age, gender, and other factors.[68] Outcomes studies are beginning to be documented more frequently.[103]

Obesity is widely accepted as a major risk factor for several diseases, particularly hypertension, heart disease, and type 2 diabetes mellitus, and as an aggravating problem for other chronic diseases such as osteoarthritis.[94] Obesity is a heterogeneous group of disorders characterized by an accumulation of excess body fat. The prevalence of overweight increases with age up to 50 years for men and up to 70 years for women.[94]

Clinical trials have established the benefits of weight loss and low-fat diets in obese middle-aged and older men in reducing the cardiovascular risk factors and in premenopausal women with diet or diet and exercise programs.[104] For older women, the benefits of weight loss in reducing the risks of cardiovascular disease have not been demonstrated. Weight loss through reduced daily energy intake and moderate endurance exercise has been the primary strategy in reducing cardiovascular risk factors in the obese based on clinical trials in younger adults. Fox and colleagues[105] demonstrated that weight loss in moderately obese older women was feasible but no effects on reducing common cardiovascular risk factors such as lipid lowering was observed with the weight loss.

A consensus exists about the health risks of overweight (BMI $\geq$ 25 kg/m$^2$) and obesity (BMI $\geq$ 30 kg/m$^2$).[106,107] No consensus exists, however, about the management of these conditions, especially in special groups such as the elderly. In order to evaluate published data and to determine the most appropriate treatment strategies, the National Heart, Lung, and Blood Institute and the Diabetes and Digestive and Kidney Diseases Institute joined in convening the Expert Panel on the Identification, Evaluation, and Treatment of Overweight in Adults. The panel recently released a set of clinical guidelines based on a systematic review of scientific literature from 1980 through 1997.[106,107] The guidelines present classifications of overweight and obesity by BMI, waist circumference, and associated disease risks. The general goals of weight loss and weight management are to prevent further weight gain, to reduce body weight, and to maintain a lower body weight. An algorithm summarizes the assessment and decision steps in the overall strategy for these goals.

The guidelines present the needs of special treatment groups including older adults.[106,107] They note that randomized clinical trials suggest that weight loss has a favorable effect on older adults in reducing heart disease risks. A caution is issued that food restrictions in the elderly can result in inadequate intake of some nutrients. Another risk is that involuntary weight loss due to occult disease might appear to be successful voluntary weight loss.[107] The summary statement offers the following guidance:

> A clinical decision to forego obesity treatment in older adults should be guided by an evaluation of the potential benefits of weight reduction for day-to-day functioning and reduction of the risk of future cardiovascular events, as well as the patient's motivation for weight reduction. Care must be taken to ensure that any weight reduction program minimizes the likelihood of adverse effects on bone health or other aspects of nutritional status.[107(p.913)]

The precautions above are well taken. The reduction of cardiovascular risk in middle-aged and older men is likely, but after menopause, cardiovascular disease is more common in women. This later onset in women and the finding of greater abdominal obesity in older women suggest that cardiovascular risk reduction should be gender and age specific. In a study of 41 healthy, moderately obese (120% to 140% of ideal body weight), postmenopausal women over the age of 60 years, the loss of body weight did not result in improved lipid levels.[105] Abdominal fat may be more of a risk than body fatness in other areas, and older women do not readily lose abdominal fat.

In other chronic diseases and disabilities, body fatness in elderly women may be protective or it may be predictive of increased risk. In a study of 22 institutionalized, but independent, Italian women (age range, 66 to 88 years), the experimental group was matched with 22 controls who were independent but not institutionalized. The institutionalized women had a lower bone density, and reduced peripheral body fat was found to be significantly associated with low bone mineral density.[93]

High body fat, however, is predictive of disability in older Americans.[108] In the Cardiovascular Health Study—an ongoing, population-based observational study of 5,201 older men and women (aged 65 to 100 years) in four states—a baseline prevalence for disability was 26.5% of the women and 16.98% of the men.[108] In a 3-year follow-up of those who had originally reported no disability, 20.3% of the women and 14.8% of the men reported onset of disability.[108] This increase in disability was not explained by age, physical activity, chronic disease, or other potential confounders. High body fatness, but not low fat-free mass, was predictive of disability.[108] This study used the simple, inexpensive and clinically feasible method of bioelectrical impedance to evaluate body composition.[108] While not considered the most rigorous method of estimating body composition, the results achieved with this approach equaled those obtained by the same investigators using the more sophisticated, expensive, and less clinically available DEXA method.[108,109]

Another chronic disease commonly found in the obese older adult is type 2 diabetes mellitus. Diabetes in the elderly is a major public health problem in the United States with a threefold or greater risk of hospitalization and institutionalization in nursing homes for people over the age of 65 who have diabetes compared with those who do not have the disease.[110] Estimates of the prevalence of dia-

betes in the elderly range from 18% at 65 years of age to 40% at 80 years of age.[110] Among African American women older than age 55, one in four is estimated to have diabetes.[111] African American women also have a higher prevalence of risk factors for diabetes and complications from diabetes.[111] Low-income African American women are less likely to have private health insurance and a regular source of medical care.[111]

Diabetes is an expensive and time-consuming disease to manage.[110–112] Acute and chronic stress have been found to affect insulin resistance and blood glucose control adversely.[110] Inexpensive, fat-filled, low-nutrient-density foods are common in African American communities with a high consumption of high-fat pork products such as sausage, luncheon meats, and bacon and a low consumption of fruits, vegetables, dietary fiber, and calcium.[111]

Other populations at high risk for diabetes are Hispanics and American Indians, who have not only a higher prevalence of type 2 diabetes but also poorer outcomes from treatment.[112,113] In a study of 51 Mexican Americans attending patient education trials, about half (n = 24) were judged in "good" glucose control and the other half (n = 26) were judged in "fair" or "poor" control.[112] None completely followed treatment plans.

Four key factors influenced the multiple treatment decisions they faced each day: (1) belief in the power of modern medicine, (2) desire to act and feel "normal," (3) desire to avoid physical symptoms, and (4) limited economic resources.[112] Patients preferred the quieter risk of hyperglycemia symptoms to the physical distress of hypoglycemic symptoms. Due to limited resources, the subjects were concerned about the greater costs of fresh fruits and vegetables not usually in the diets of their families. Some patients did eat correctly when they had the money but less appropriately when they were short on cash.[112]

Subjects reported taking medicine instead of making other behavioral changes. This overreliance on medications may partially result from physicians emphasizing medications during patient visits. The economic and social barriers are important factors in self-care by patients.[112,113] Care providers should avoid presuming that poor outcomes are due to ignorance or lack of motivation.[113]

The general nutrition guidelines for older adults with diabetes are no different than those for other type 2 diabetes patients.[110] Special problems may exist due to functional limitations that impact patient ability to shop for or prepare foods.[110] In a cross-sectional study of those over the age of 85 years, 26% were unable to prepare meals and 34% were unable to shop.[114] Older and obese diabetics are less likely to be able to shop and prepare foods than their nondiabetic cohorts.

Another hindrance to compliance with current recommendations is the ingrained belief that older diabetics simply need to avoid foods with sugar. Many elderly patients adhere to this belief and report that they cannot afford sugar-free foods.[109] Older, obese women were more likely to consume sugar-free foods such as sugar-free candies, cookies, and cakes and have lower quality diets than those who used both reduced-fat and reduced-sugar foods.[115]

The American Diabetes Association revised its recommendation that carbohydrates in the diabetic diet could be increased up to 60% of total kilocalories and lifted the prohibition against sucrose-containing foods.[110] Another important modification was the substitution of the goal of "reasonable" body weight for ideal body weight.[110] Improvement in diabetes control has been noted with a weight loss of 5 to 10 kg without achievement of "desirable" or ideal body weight.[116]

Very few studies have examined the effect of diet interventions in the elderly. Caloric restriction, while a cornerstone of weight loss in the obese, may result in malnutrition.[110] Only recently has the effect of nutritional risks on quality of life been reported.[117] A field-based, cross-sectional study of participants who received congregate meals or home-delivered meals assessed their quality of life. Quality of life was positively correlated with quality of health and negatively correlated with nutrition risk indicators, food insecurity, decreased enjoyment of food, depression, and impaired functional status.[117]

**Dietary Supplements**

While evidence of a relationship between diet and disease has grown steadily, largely from human epidemiological and animal studies, the use of dietary supplements has grown even more.[10,90,118–120] With the possible exception of folic acid supplementation, clinical trials of individual nutrients in prospective studies have not yet documented benefits unless dietary intakes were inadequate or specific diseases (eg, pernicious anemia) were present. Thus, The American Dietetic Association recommends that use of vitamin and mineral supplementation be based on individual assessment.[118,119] Over a 10-year period, the supplement use nearly doubled in a sample of older Wisconsin adults.[90] The increase was the greatest among individuals 65 to 84 years of age, with the major increase coming in regular use compared with occasional use. Approximately half of all females reported current use of supplements; 31% of males aged 43 to 64 years and 42% of males aged 65 to 84 years reported current use.[90]

In another study of supplement use among community-dwelling elderly aged 60 to 69 (n = 89), 80 to 89 (n = 90), and 100 and older (n = 76) in Georgia, usage was similar in all age groups.[120] Women were twice as likely to be current users. Subjects who were physically active, had stomach problems, used arthritis medications, and had healthier diets were more likely to use supplements. Healthier diets were defined as being lower in fat, higher in protein and fiber, and containing yogurt and whole-grain products.[120] Physically active elders were more likely to take calcium supplements and vitamin C than their sedentary counterparts.[90,120] Thus, supplement use does appear to be one among a cluster of health behaviors. Dietary intake studies of the elderly have shown both adequate and inadequate intakes.[90,116,120] In studying the effects of supplement use on disease, control for both dietary intakes and physical activity are essential.[120]

A number of studies have looked at the vitamin status and supplement use of one or more nutrients. Epidemiological, animal, and observational studies suggest that supplementing vitamin E beyond the amount normally consumed in a diet may be protective against cardiovascular diseases. Clinical trials are currently in progress that may demonstrate a reduction in cardiovascular events.[80]

While a high prevalence of vitamin $B_{12}$ deficiency in the older population has been established on the basis of low serum cobalamin concentrations, newer research[121,122] suggests this prevalence is underestimated. Anemia occurs in only the most severely $B_{12}$-depleted individuals.[121] In an examination of 548 Framingham subjects aged 67 to 96 years, the prevalence of cobalamin deficiency was established at 12% based on elevated serum concentrations of methylmalonic acid (MMA) and serum homocysteine (Hcys).[122] These two metabolites are considered highly sensitive indicators of tissue deficiency of cobalamin.[122] Thus, many elderly people are metabolically deficient in

cobalamin while appearing to have "normal" serum values.[122] More widespread use of MMA and Hcys tests could potentially prevent irreversible central nervous system damage and vitamin-dependency dementias.

In a placebo-controlled, double-blind trial of daily low-to-moderate micronutrient supplements, subjects aged 59 to 85 years showed significant increases in mean serum levels of ascorbate, beta carotene, folate, vitamin $B_6$, and alpha-tocopherol.[123] Improved delayed hypersensitivity skin test responses also were found in these healthy, independently living older adults.[123] Other studies in the elderly have suggested an association between enhanced immune responsiveness and vitamin E. Recommending vitamin E supplementation awaits further definition of the mechanisms between nutrition and immunity.[123]

Since the 1960s, folic acid deficiencies have been increasingly recognized in the presence of disease, polypharmacy, and poverty.[79,123–125] From 11% to 28% of the elderly have been estimated to have folic acid deficiency, largely from poor dietary intake.[124] A low red cell folate suggests a long-term dietary inadequacy.[125]

Dietary folate varies greatly in bioavailability and may also be destroyed in prolonged food preparation. When increased food folate intake did not lead to significant increases in folate status, attention turned to food fortification.[125] Ready-to-eat cereals were fortified with folate, and then flour was fortified with folate to provide additional folate to women of child-bearing age as a means to prevent neural tube defects.[125] Cereals and breads, however, are consumed in limited amounts by some elderly, who also are at increased risk of folate deficiency.

Institutionalized elderly are more likely to have low serum folate.[124] Milk was selected as a vehicle for folic acid supplementation in a prospective clinical trial. Forty-nine subjects received the fortified milk for at least 6 months and 40 controls received unfortified milk. The experimental group had a mean serum folate of 5.81 mcg/L compared with 2.16 mcg/L for the control ($p < .0001$); thus, fortified milk appears to be a feasible and effective vehicle for elderly subjects to receive folic acid supplementation.[124]

Three large trials of beta carotene, vitamin A, and alpha-tocopherol failed to duplicate the protection against cancer that had been associated with fruits and vegetables.[126] An increased risk for lung cancer occurred in smokers who received beta carotene supplements in the Alpha-Tocopherol–Beta-Carotene (ATBC) study.[127] Follow-up data on the ATBC subjects suggest that supplemental beta carotene is risky for smokers. Combined with the lack of benefits for nonsmokers in any of the other large trials, beta carotene supplementation is not recommended.[126]

Other supplements such as selenium, vitamin B$_6$, and iron also may have toxic or adverse effects in some individuals or in excess amounts.[128,129] The elderly are at special risk of iron overload because they have few mechanisms by which to excrete excess iron.[129] A number of clinical conditions that occur more frequently in the elderly promote blood loss such as gastrointestinal ulceration, aspirin-induced bleeding, ulcerative colitis, and colonic neoplasia.[129] Iron overload also can be iatrogenic. In infections, iron is bound to lactoferrin and transferrin to withhold iron from microorganisms. If the patient is mistakenly diagnosed as iron deficient and given iron supplements, the benefits of this natural defense mechanism of the immune system are lost.[129] To avoid iron overload, Mertz[130] proposes that nutritional supplements be made in two forms, one with and the other without iron.

Another potential cause of toxicity of dietary supplements in the elderly is chronic disease states.[131] Kidney and liver diseases raise the potential for nutrient toxicity such as for vitamin A.[131] Vitamin and mineral supplementation are not recommended for elderly patients with renal or liver disease.[131] The risk of nutrient toxicity reinforces the importance of individual assessment before recommending supplementation.[118]

Other "dietary" supplements include herbs, herbal medicines, and herbal teas. In 1996 herb sales were estimated to be in excess of $12 billion.[132] Americans are rapidly increasing their use of herbal remedies either in conjunction with, or as a substitute for, traditional medicine. Physicians and other health care providers need to ask direct questions about patient use of such products.

A major change in the marketing of herbs occurred when the Dietary Supplements Health and Education Act of 1994 allowed herbal manufacturers to make structure or function claims on their labels without approval from the FDA.[132] Four guidelines for claims are: (1) claims must be truthful and not misleading; (2) claims cannot be for cure, treatment, or prevention of disease; (3) a disclaimer must appear stating that the claim has not undergone FDA evaluation; and (4) claims must be based on scientific evidence that is kept in the manufacturer's files.[132] The manufacturer does not have to demonstrate compliance; the FDA must prove lack of compliance. The biggest problem with American herbal products is the lack of quality control. Products may be contaminated, may not contain the actual herbs listed, and may vary in strength.[132]

Outside the United States, careful evaluation and regulation of herbal medicine may be maintained. In Germany about 70% of primary care physicians prescribe herbal products.[133] In order to evaluate safety and efficacy of various herbs, the Federal Institute for Drugs and Medical Devices, commonly called Commission E, was established. The results of the first 300 evaluations have been translated and published in English.[133] Approximately 100 of the herbs were judged to lack safety, but the other 200 were seen to have some efficacy. This book provides additional information that can supplement previous American texts on pharmacognosy.[134] Herb-to-herb interactions can occur as with other medications and treatments; drug-herb interactions can happen as well.[133] No specific information has been published on food-herb interactions but the likelihood exists that they may occur.

## FOOD SAFETY

Increased incidence, severity, and risk of death from many foodborne illnesses occur in elderly people.[135] Susceptibility to foodborne infections appears to be age dependent.[135] Moreover, several clinical disease states appear to create these increased risks. As gastric acidity, intestinal microflora, intestinal mucus, mucosal epithelium, intestinal motility, and granulocyte function decline with age, the likelihood of serious infection increases.[135] Death rates for diarrheal diseases are five times greater in adults over the age of 74 years.[135] Part of this increased incidence and risk may be related to the previously unrecognized presence of other gastrointestinal diseases in the elderly.[136]

In the past, foodborne outbreaks occurred more frequently due to improperly cooked or stored chicken, eggs, milk, cheese products, and seafood. Increasingly, more fresh fruits and vegetables are being identified as the source of outbreaks, especially in the presence of inadequate washing and preparation.[137–140] In one case, imported raspberries were responsible for an outbreak of cyclosporiasis, a parasite.[137] In another case unwashed green onions were identified as the source of an outbreak of cryptosporidium, another parasite.[138]

The marketing of fresh, unprocessed fruit juices as healthier than conventionally processed juices also has contributed to the problem.[139,140] Unpasteurized, fresh-pressed apple juice was responsible for several outbreaks of *Escherichia coli* 0157.H7 and cryptosporidium.[139,140] The usual procedures for food sanitation become even more critical in group living situations for the elderly and in restaurants with a large elderly clientele.

An expert consortium has developed 18 recommendations that provide guidance on food safety policies and procedures. These recommendations may be readily accessed at www.cast-science.org.[141] The recommendations for education on food safety include:

- Educate the general public and food handlers relative to safe food preparation and handling.
- Identify high-risk populations and provide food safety education.
- Provide risk information relative to food choices to persons with enhanced disease susceptibility.
- Use and evaluate food labeling to communicate safe food preparation and storage practices to food preparers.[141]

## PREVENTION OF FRAILTY, DISABILITY, AND FALLS

Although no precise scientific definition of frailty exists, a practical definition is the diminished ability to carry out the important practical and social activities of daily living (ADLs) and little reserve capacity to tolerate stresses of life.[142–145] The Assessment of Frailty Scale measures 21 practical items, 9 social activities, and 5 reserve capacity items.[144] This model converges physical, social, and environmental factors and allows the dynamic state of frailty to be identified.[144]

The importance of preventing frailty is evident when its association with physical and cognitive impairment, falls, morbidity, institutionalization, and mortality is considered.[146] Frailty has been linked to physical inactivity, heavy alcohol intake, visual and hearing impairment, psychotropic drugs, depression, impaired strength in the extremities, and gait/balance disturbances.[142–144] Although a disabling disease may not be cured or prevented, many of the physiological decline factors can be overcome. For example, a recent study[143] found balance and strength to be the primary predictors between frail and nonfrail elderly. It is therefore important to maintain balance and strength during aging.

Several studies have investigated the most effective form of exercise for improving strength and balance in the elderly. Elderly involved in regular, high-intensity resistance training with weights appear to have the greatest increase in strength when compared with elderly subjects using low to moderate resistance training.[147] If weights and machinery are not available, other methods can be considered. One such method is Tai Chi. Small clinical trials have suggested that older people derive improved confidence in balance and movement along with a sense of well-being from Tai Chi.[148]

Only recently has exercise been advocated for elderly persons with diseases such as rheumatoid arthritis (RA).[149–151] The loss of lean body mass common to RA may be slowed by resistance training. Likewise, resistance training may reduce pain and improve function in people with RA, osteoarthritis, and fibromyalgia.[149]

To begin an exercise program, the patient with arthritis should first visit his or her physician. Selection of an exercise place with a warm indoor pool is ideal because water-based exercises strengthen muscles, tone the cardiovascular system, and put less stress on the joints. Resistance machines place less stress on hand joints than hand weights.[149]

Environmental hazards can be an aggravating factor for the frail elder. Because frailty is a primary cause of falls, removing environmental risks in the home can greatly benefit the individual. The following steps are recommended to reduce the risks of falls:

- Provide proper lighting.
- Install handrails on stairs and steps.
- Remove loose throw rugs or frayed carpeting.
- Install bars and/or adhesive strips in baths and showers.
- Eliminate trailing electrical cords, sharp corners, slippery floors, and storage locales that require a stool to access.
- Place the bed and other furniture at an easily accessible height.
- Choose footwear with appropriate traction (ie, thin soles allow a better feel of the floor surface than thick sports soles).[152]

Physiological loss can have many causes; therefore it is important to identify persons at risk. One important assessment tool may be the patient's self-report of health or perceived health or ADLs he or she can perform without assistance.[144,153] Regular clinical assessment of gait and balance, as well as eye tests, can identify risk factors before they contribute to a fall or a disability that may result from a fall.[142–145]

## AGING VERSUS PATHOLOGY

Differentiating age-related from age-dependent disorders challenges clinicians and researchers. Age-related diseases and disorders have specific temporal patterns. They display incidence peaks and then decline in frequency with advancing age. Ulcerative colitis, gout, peptic ulcers, and some cancers are age-related diseases. If the initiating factors can be determined and prevented or treated, the disease might never appear in the older person.[153] Evidence is growing that persons with lower health risk not only live longer, but also have a later onset and shorter period of disability.[154]

Age-dependent diseases are directly correlated with age and closely related to the usual aging processes. Coronary heart disease, adult-onset diabetes, and Alzheimer's disease are examples of age-dependent diseases. Most disability of old age is increasingly being associated with these age-dependent conditions, which ultimately are the primary causes of death and disability in persons over age 65.[38,52,73] Nonetheless, some diseases may be more or less dependent on age than previously thought. For example, an increase in type 2 diabetes mellitus is occurring more frequently in children and young adults. About one third of new cases of celiac disease (gluten enteropathy), once labeled a pediatric disease, are now being diagnosed in the seventh decade of life or above.[136] Adult celiac disease is associated with neurological complications and insulin-dependent diabetes mellitus and may be asymptomatic for years before diagnosis.[136]

### STRATEGIES FOR DISEASE PREVENTION AND HEALTH PROMOTION IN OLD AGE

Many studies[34-36,38,39] document the finding that the elderly will participate in health promotion programs if offered the opportunity. Most demonstrated improved attention to simple preventive measures such as having an annual checkup and obtaining immunizations.[34] Less success was noted in lifestyle changes that involve everyday activities such as weight control and smoking cessation.[23,34]

Nevertheless, elderly women are now eating more servings of vegetables a day than any other group of adults, and they score higher on the Healthy Eating Index than other adults.[45-47,85,89,90] Women in general are using more reduced-fat and reduced-sugar products and more supplements.[90,115]

Certain hard-to-reach groups need special targeting such as minorities who have been provided less health education and have less access to health care and who now experience much higher rates of chronic diseases such as hypertension and diabetes.[98,111-113] Community interventions require greater involvement of participants in planning and implementation if success is to be optimized. Moreover, a broader view of theoretical models needs to be considered in planning assessments and interventions.

Quality-of-life issues are likely to become even more important in obtaining resources, cooperation, and successful outcomes in health promotion intervention programs. Health professionals need to recognize the cohort of the clients in a program and the stresses that are present in order to interact more effectively.[153-155]

### TRAINING OF HEALTH PROFESSIONALS

Training of health professionals practicing in a wide variety of settings can be assisted by expert-compiled manuals published by the Nutrition Screening Initiative and by other practitioners with specialized interest and experience in gerontology.[69-72,156]

### CONCLUSION

Providing disease prevention and health promotion advice to older people presents a new challenge for health professionals. Recent research has begun to document the benefits of smoking cessation, diet modification, increased exercise, and limited intake of alcohol and drugs for older as well as younger adults. Health promotion strategies can improve function as well as reduce the risk of morbidity and premature death.

For those over age 50, health promotion is less about preventing the symptoms of disease and more about preserving function and maintaining independence, productivity, and personal fulfillment. Reasons for geriatric health promotion and disease prevention activities include the following:

• Aging is a lifelong phenomenon consisting of physiological, psychological, and behavioral processes.

• Aging occurs at different rates in different people; thus biological age may not be equal to chronological age.
• Most disabilities of old age are not inevitable, universal, or irreversible.[3]

Effective health promotion and disease prevention messages should be directed toward all older people when knowledge justifies such recommendations. Additional guidance and health interventions should be based on individual assessments of health status for those identified as being at high risk for disease or disability.

A geriatric assessment should be included as a regular part of health monitoring of older people, in addition to chronic disease screening. Nutrition screening and intervention can and should be a major part of any geriatric assessment.

## REFERENCES

1. *Healthy People: The Surgeon General's Workshop on Health Promotion and Disease Prevention.* Washington, DC: US Dept of Health, Education and Welfare; 1979. HEW publication 79-55071.

2. Koop CE. Keynote address, March 20–23, 1988. In: *Surgeon General's Workshop on Health Promotion and Aging.* Washington, DC: US Dept of Health and Human Services; 1988:1–4.

3. US Preventive Services Task Force. *Guide to Preventive Services.* Baltimore: Williams & Wilkins; 1989.

4. US Public Health Service. *Healthy People 2000: National Health Promotion and Disease Prevention Objectives.* Washington, DC: US Dept of Health and Human Services; 1991. DHHS publication (PHS) 91-50212.

5. Woolf SH, Jonas S, Lawrence RS, eds. *Health Promotion and Disease Prevention in Clinical Practice.* Baltimore: Williams & Wilkins; 1996.

6. Fishman P. Healthy people 2000: what progress toward better nutrition? *Geriatrics.* 1996;51:38–42.

7. Yates AA, Schlicker SA, Suitor CW. Dietary reference intakes: the new bases for recommendations for calcium and related nutrients, B vitamins, and choline. *J Am Diet Assoc.* 1998;98:699–707.

8. Institute of Medicine, Food and Nutrition Board. *Dietary Reference Intakes for Calcium, Phosphorus, Magnesium, Vitamin D, and Fluoride.* Washington, DC: National Academy Press; 1997.

9. Institute of Medicine, Food and Nutrition Board. *Dietary Reference Intakes for Thiamin, Riboflavin, Niacin, Vitamin B-6, Folate, Vitamin B-12, Pantothenic Acid, Biotin, and Choline.* Washington, DC: National Academy Press; 1998.

10. American Cancer Society 1996 Advisory Committee on Diet, Nutrition and Cancer Prevention. Reducing the risk of cancer with healthy food choices and physical activities. *CA Cancer J Clin.* 1996;46:325–341.

11. Lee I-M, Paffenbarger RS, Hennekens CH. Physical activity, physical fitness, and longevity. *Aging (Milano).* 1997;9:2–11.

12. Jones J, Jones KD. Promoting physical activity in the senior years. *Gerontol Nurs.* 1997;23:40–48.

13. Buchner DM. Preserving mobility in older adults. *West J Med.* 1997;167:258–264.

14. Rooks DS, Kiel DP, Parsons C, Hayes WC. Self-paced resistance training and walking exercise in community-dwelling older adults: effects on neuromotor performance. *J Gerontol A Biol Sci Med Sci.* 1997;52:M161–M168.

15. Powell RA, Single HM. Focus groups. *Int J Qual Health Care.* 1996;8:499–504.

16. Gulanick M, Keough V. Focus groups: an exciting approach to clinical nursing research. *Prog Cardiovasc Nurs.* 1997;12:24–29.

17. Hiatt RA. Where have we been? An overview. Paper presented at the American College of Epidemiology Annual Meeting; Sept 26–28, 1998; San Francisco, Calif.

18. Ockene JK. Community-based interventions. Smoking trials as an example. Paper presented at the American College of Epidemiology Annual Meeting; Sept 26–28, 1998; San Francisco, Calif.

19. Stevens PE. Focus groups: collecting aggregate-level data to understand community health phenomena. *Public Health Nurs.* 1996;13:170–176.

20. US Centers for Disease Control and Prevention. Estimated national spending on prevention—United States, 1988. *MMWR.* 1992;41:529–531.

21. Lubitz JD, Riley GF. Trends in Medicare payments in the last year of life. *N Engl J Med.* 1993;328:1092–1096.

22. Hickey T, Stilwell DL. Health promotion for older people. All is not well. *Gerontologist.* 1991;31:822–829.

23. Fox PJ, Breuner W, Wright JA. Effects of a health promotion program in sustaining health behaviors in older adults. *Am J Prev Med.* 1997;13:257–264.

24. Resnick B. Measurement tools: do they apply equally to older adults? *J Gerontol Nurs.* 1995;21:18–22.

25. Green LW. National policy in the promotion of health. *Int J Health Educ.* 1979;22:161–168.

26. Bogden JB, Louria DB. Micronutrients and immunity in older people. In: Bendich A, Deckelbaum RJ, eds. *Preventive Nutrition: The Comprehensive Guide for Health Professionals.* Totowa, NJ: Humana Press; 1998.

27. Chernoff R. Nutrition. In: Jahnigen D, Schrier R, eds. *Geriatric Medicine.* 2nd ed. Cambridge, Mass: Blackwell Scientific Publications; 1996:196–200.

28. Goldberg TH, Chavin SI. Preventive medicine and screening in older adults. *J Am Geriatr Soc.* 1997;45:344–354.

29. Pizzi ER, Wolf ZR. Health risks and health promotion of older women: utility of a health promotion diary. *Holist Nurs Pract.* 1998;12:62–72.

30. Patterson C, Feightner J. Promoting the health of senior citizens. *Can Med Assoc J.* 1997;157:1107–1113.

31. Keister KJ, Blixen CE. Quality of life and aging. *J Gerontol Nurs.* 1998;24:22–28.

32. Hazzard WR. Ways to make "usual" and "successful" aging synonymous: preventive gerontology. *West J Med.* 1997;167:206–215.

33. Fried LP, Freedman M, Endres TE, Wasik B. Building communities that promote successful aging. *West J Med.* 1997;167:216–219.

34. Lave JR, Ives DG, Traven ND, Kuller LH. Participation in health promotion programs by the rural elderly. *Am J Prev Med.* 1995;11:46–53.

35. Lave JR, Ives DG, Traven ND, Kuller LH. Evaluation of a health promotion demonstration program for the rural elderly. *Health Serv Res.* 1996;31:261–281.

36. Viverais-Dresler GA, Bakker DA, Vance RJ. Elderly clients perception: individual health counseling and group sessions. *Can J Public Health.* 1995;86:234–237.

37. US Preventive Services Task Force. *Guide to Clinical Preventive Services.* 2nd ed. Baltimore: Williams & Wilkins; 1997.

38. LaCroix AZ, Newton KM, Leveille SG, Wallace J. Healthy aging: a woman's issue. *West J Med.* 1997;167:220–232.

39. Love RR, Davis JE, Mundlt M, Clark C. Health promotion and screening services reported by older adult patients of urban primary care physicians. *J Fam Pract.* 1997;45:142–150.

40. Fries JF. Aging, natural death, and the compression of morbidity. *N Engl J Med.* 1980;3031:130–133.

41. Elder JP, Williams SJ, Drew JA, Wright BL, Boulan TE. Longitudinal effects of preventive services on health behaviors among the elderly cohort. *Am J Prev Med.* 1995;11:354–359.

42. *US Surgeon General's Report on Nutrition and Health.* Washington, DC: Government Printing Office; 1988. DHHS publication (PHS) 88-50210.

43. National Research Council, Food and Nutrition Board. *Diet and Health: Implications for Reducing Chronic Disease.* Washington, DC: National Academy Press; 1989.

44. Burt VL, Cutler JA, Higgings M, et al. Trends in prevalence, awareness, and treatment and control of hypertension in the adult US population: data from the heart examination surveys, 1960 to 1991. *Hypertension*. 1995;26:60–69.

45. Interagency Board for Nutrition Monitoring and Related Research, Life Sciences Research Office, FASEB. *Third Report on Nutrition Monitoring in the United States: Executive Summary*. Washington, DC: Government Printing Office; 1995.

46. Interagency Board for Nutrition Monitoring and Related Research. *Nutrition Monitoring in the United States: The Directory of Federal and State Nutrition Monitoring Activities, 1992*. Hyattsville, Md: Human Nutrition Information Services; 1992. DHHS publication (PHS) 92-1255-1.

47. Ippolito PM, Mathios AD. *Information and Advertising Policy: A Study of Fat and Cholesterol Consumption in the United States, 1977–1990*. Bureau of Economics Staff Report. Washington, DC: Federal Trade Commission; 1996.

48. Mackey MA, Hill BP. Health claims regulations and new food concepts. In: Kotsonis FN, Mackey MA, eds. *Nutrition in the 90's: Current Controversies and Analysis*. New York: Marcel Dekker; 1994;2.

49. USDA, USDHHS. *Nutrition and Your Health: Dietary Guidelines for Americans*. 4th ed. Washington, DC: Government Printing Office, 1995. Home and Garden Bulletin 232.

50 US Dept of Agriculture. *The Food Guide Pyramid*. Hyattsville, Md: Human Nutrition Information Services; 1992. Home and Garden Bulletin 252.

51. Parker SL, Tong T, Bolden S, et al. Cancer statistics, 1997. *CA Cancer J Clin*. 1997;47:5–27.

52. Wingo PA, Landis S, Ries LAG. An adjustment to the 1997 estimate for new prostate cancer cases. *CA Cancer J Clin*. 1997;47:239–242.

53. Landis SH, Murray T, Bolden S, et al. Cancer statistics, 1998. *CA Cancer J Clin*. 1998;48:6–29.

54. Rosenthal DS. Changing trends. *CA Cancer J Clin*. 1998;48:3–5.

55. Bowman SA, Lino M, Gerior SA, Basiotis PP. *The Healthy Eating Index 1994–96*. Hyattsville, Md: Human Nutrition Information Services; 1998. CNPP-5.

56. Kennedy ET, Ohls J, Carlson S, Feming K. The healthy eating index: design and applications. *J Am Diet Assoc*. 1995;95:1103–1108.

57. USDA Center for Nutrition Policy and Promotion. *The Healthy Eating Index*. Hyattsville, Md: Human Nutrition Information Services; 1995. CNPP-1.

58. Sims LS. Uses of the recommended dietary allowances: a commentary. *J Am Diet Assoc*. 1996;96:659–662.

59. Most frequently asked questions . . . about the 1997 dietary reference intakes (DRIs). *Nutr Today*. 1997;32:189–190.

60. National Research Council Subcommittee on the 10th Edition of the RDAs, Food and Nutrition Board, Commission on Life Sciences. *Recommended Dietary Allowances*. 10th ed. Washington, DC: National Academy Press; 1994.

61. Yates AA. Process and development of dietary reference intakes: basis, need, and application of recommended dietary allowances. *Nutr Rev*. 1998;56:S5–S9.

62. Shoaf LR, Wellman NS. The nutrition screening initiative: responsibilities, opportunities, and challenges for dietitians. *Top Clin Nutr*. 1991;7:71–76.

63. Nutrition Screening Initiative Technical Review Committee. *Report of Nutrition Screening I: Toward a Common View*. Washington, DC: Nutrition Screening Initiative; 1991.

64. Dwyer JT. *Screening Older Americans' Nutritional Health: Current Practices and Future Possibilities*. Washington, DC: Nutrition Screening Initiative; 1991.

65. White JV, Ham RJ, Lipschitz DA, Dwyer JT, Wellman NS. Consensus of the Nutrition Screening Initiative: risk factors and indicators of poor nutritional status in older Americans. *J Am Diet Assoc*. 1991;91:783–787.

66. Nutrition Screening Initiative Technical Review Committee. *Nutrition Interventions Manual for Professionals Caring for Older Americans*. Washington, DC: Nutrition Screening Initiative; 1992.

67. Nutrition Screening Initiative Technical Review Committee. *Incorporating Nutrition Screening and Interventions into Medical Practices: A Monograph for Physicians*. Washington, DC: Nutrition Screening Initiative; 1994.

68. Adams TL, Chernoff R, Winger RM, Hosig KW, McCabe BJ. The effect of home-delivered meals on length of hospital stay. *J Am Diet Assoc*. 1998;98:A12.

69. Nutrition Screening Initiative Technical Review Committee. *Keeping Older Americans Healthy at*

Home: *Guidelines for Nutrition Programs in Home Health Care.* Washington, DC: Nutrition Screening Initiative; 1996.

70. Nutrition Screening Initiative Technical Review Committee. *Managing Nutrition Care in Health Plans: A Guide to the Incorporation of Nutrition Screening Interventions in Managed Care.* Washington, DC: Nutrition Screening Initiative; 1996.

71. Nutrition Screening Initiative Technical Review Committee. NSI update. *Nutr Screening Initiative Newslett.* 1998;25:3–4.

72. Expert Committee of Nutrition and Health for Older Americans. *Nutrition and Health for Older Americans—A Campaign of The American Dietetic Association. Food Guide for Older Adults.* Chicago: The American Dietetic Association; 1998.

73. Smith DWE. Changing causes of death of elderly people in the United States, 1950–1990. *Gerontology.* 1998;44:331–335.

74. Clarke R, Daly L, Robinson K, et al. Hyperhomocysteinemia: an independent risk factor for vascular disease. *N Engl J Med.* 1991;324:1149–1155.

75. Stampfer MJ, Malinow MR, Willett WC, et al. A prospective study of plasma homocysteine and risk of myocardial infarction in US physicians. *JAMA.* 1992;268:877–881.

76. Selhub J, Facques PF, Wilson PFW, Rush D, Rosenberg IH. Vitamin status and intake as primary determinants of homocysteinemia in an elderly population. *JAMA.* 1993;270:2693–2698.

77. Riggs KM, Spiro A, Tucher K, Rush D. Relations of vitamin B-12, vitamin B-6, folate and homocysteine to cognitive performance in the Normative Aging Study. *Am J Clin Nutr.* 1996;63:306–314.

78. Parnetti L, Bottiglieri T, Lowenthal D. Role of homocysteine in age-related vascular and non-vascular diseases. *Aging (Milano).* 1997;9:241–257.

79. Ebly EM, Schaefer JP, Campbell NRC, Hogan DB. Folate status, vascular disease and cognition in elderly Canadians. *Age Aging.* 1998;27:485–491.

80. Tangney CC. Vitamin E and cardiovascular disease. *Nutr Today.* 1997;32:13–22.

81. Rodondo MR, Ortega RM, Zamora MJ, et al. Influence of the number of meals taken per day on cardiovascular risk factors and the energy and nutrient intakes of a group of elderly people. *Int J Vitam Nutr Res.* 1997;67:176–182.

82. Steinmetz KA, Potter JD. Vegetables, fruits and cancer prevention: a review. *J Am Diet Assoc.* 1996;96:1027–1039.

83. Morley JE. Anorexia in older persons: epidemiology and optimal treatment. *Drugs Aging.* 1996;8:134–155.

84. Morley JE, Flood HM, Perry HM, Kumar VB. Peptides, memory, food intake and aging. *Aging (Milano).* 1997;9:17–18.

85. Gilbride JA, Amella EJ, Breiner EB, Mariano C, Mezey M. Nutrition and health status of community dwelling elderly in New York City: a pilot study. *J Am Diet Assoc.* 1998;98:554–557.

86. Knol LL, Haughton B. Fruit and juice intake associated with higher dietary status index in rural East Tennessee women living in public housing. *J Am Diet Assoc.* 1998;98:576–579.

87. Johnson RK. In-person vs telephone collection of dietary intake data in children and women: validation with doubly labeled water. Paper presented at What We Eat in America: Research and Results Survey Conference; Sept 14–17, 1998; Rockville, Md.

88. Johnson RK, Soultanakis RP, Matthews DE. Literacy and body fatness are associated with underreporting of energy intake in U.S. low-income women using multiple-pass 24-hour recall: a doubly labeled water study. *J Am Diet Assoc.* 1998;98:1136–1140.

89. Gretebeck RJ, Boileau RA. Self-reported energy intake and energy expenditure in elderly women. *J Am Diet Assoc.* 1998;98:574–576.

90. Mares-Perlman JA, Klein BEK, Klein R, Ritter LL, Freudenhelm JL, Luby MH. Nutrient supplements contribute to the dietary intake of middle- and older-aged adult residents of Beaver Dam, Wisconsin. *J Nutr.* 1993;123:176–188.

91. NIH Consensus Development Panel on Optimal Intake. NIH Consensus. Optimal calcium intake. *JAMA.* 1994;272:1942–1948.

92. Division of Health Examination Statistics, National Center for Health Statistics, CDC, Osteoporosis among estrogen-deficient women—United States, 1988–1994. *MMWR.* 1998;47:969–973.

93. del Puente A, Postiglione A, Esposito-del Puenta A, Carpinelli A, Roman M, Oriente P. Peripheral body fat has a protective role in bone mineral density in elderly women. *Eur J Clin Nutr.* 1998;52:690–693.

94. Bidlack WR. Interrelationships of food, nutrition, diet and health: the National Association of State Universities and Land Grant Colleges white papers. *J Am Coll Nutr.* 1996;15:422–433.

95. Drugay M. Breaking the silence: a health promotion approach to osteoporosis. *J Gerontol Nurs.* 1999;23:36–43.

96. Weber P. Management of osteoporosis: is there a role for vitamin K? *Int J Vitam Nutr Res.* 1997;67:350–356.

97. McCabe BJ, Champagne CM, Allen HR. Calcium intake of selected age and gender groups from CSFII 1994–96. Unpublished data, 1998.

98. Ciesla JR, Piane G, Rubens AJ. Hypertension in community-dwelling elders from a statewide study: implications for nonpharmacological therapy. *J Health Care Poor Underserved.* 1998;9:62–75.

99. SHEP Cooperative Research Group. Prevention of stroke by antihypertensive drug treatment in older persons with isolated systolic hypertension: final results of the Systolic Hypertension in the Elderly Populations (SHEP). *JAMA.* 1991;265:3255–3264.

100. National High Blood Pressure Education Program Working Group. National high blood pressure education program working group report on hypertension in the elderly. *Hypertension.* 1994;23:275–285.

101. The Sixth Report of the Joint National Committee on Prevention, Detection, Evaluation and Treatment of High Blood Pressure. *Arch Intern Med.* 1997;157:2413–2446.

102. Whelton PK, Appel LJ, Espeland MA, et al. Sodium reduction and weight loss in the treatment of hypertension in older persons: a randomized controlled trial of nonpharmacologic interventions in the elderly (TONE). *JAMA.* 1998;299:839–846.

103. Barents Group of Peat Marwick. *The Clinical and Cost Effectiveness of Medical Nutritional Therapy: Evidence and Estimates of Potential Medicare Savings from the Use of Selected Nutrition Interventions.* Washington, DC: Nutrition Screening Initiative; 1996.

104. Dengel JL, Katzel LI, Goldberg AP. Effects of an American Heart Association diet with or without weight loss on lipids in obese middle-aged and older men. *Am J Clin Nutr.* 1995;62:715–721.

105. Fox AA, Thompson JL, Butterfield GE, Gylfadottir U, Moynihan S, Spiller G. Effects of diet and exercise on common cardiovascular disease risk factors in moderately obese older women. *Am J Clin Nutr.* 1996;63:225–233.

106. The National Heart, Lung, and Blood Institute Expert Panel on the Identification, Evaluation and Treatment of Overweight and Obesity. Clinical guidelines on the identification, evaluation, and treatment of obesity in adults: executive summary. *J Am Diet Assoc.* 1998;98:1178–1191.

107. Expert Panel on the Identification, Evaluation, and Treatment of Overweight in Adults. Clinical guidelines on the identification, evaluation and treatment of overweight in adults: executive summary. *Am J Clin Nutr.* 1998;68:899–917.

108. Visser M, Langlois J, Guralnik JM, et al. High body fatness but not low fat-free mass predicts disability in older men and women: the Cardiovascular Health Study. *Am J Clin Nutr.* 1998;68:584–590.

109. Visser M, Harris TB, Langlois J, et al. Body fat and skeletal muscle mass in relation to physical disability in very old men and women of the Framingham Heart Study. *J Gerontol A Biol Sci Med Sci.* 1998;53:M214–M221.

110. Fonseca V, Wall J. Diet and diabetes in the elderly. *Clin Geriatr Med.* 1995;11:613–624.

111. Rajaram SS, Vinson V. African American women and diabetes: a sociocultural context. *J Health Care Poor Underserved.* 1998;9:236–247.

112. Hunt LM, Pugh J, Valenzuela M. How patients adapt self-care recommendations in everyday life. *J Fam Pract.* 1998;46:207–215.

113. Carter JS, Pugh JA, Monterrosa A. Non-insulin dependent diabetes mellitus and ethnic minorities: the double jeopardy. *Ann Intern Med.* 1996;125:221–232.

114. Havlik RJ, Liu BM, Lovar MC. *Health Statistics on Older Persons.* US Vital and Health Statistics Services 3, No. 25. Washington, DC: Government Printing Office National Center for Health Statistics; 1987. DHSS publication (PHS) 87-1409.

115. Georgiou C, Goldman J, Anderson E. Reduced fat and reduced-sugar foods: Americans who use them and their diet quality. Paper presented at What We Eat in America: Research and Results Survey Conference; Sept 14–17, 1998; Rockville, Md.

116. Franz MJ, Horton ES, Bantle JP, et al. Nutrition principles for the management of diabetes and related complications. *Diabetes Care.* 1994;17:490–518.

117. Vailas LI, Nitze SA, Becker M, Gast J. Risk indicators for malnutrition are associated inversely with quality of life for participants in meal programs for older adults. *J Am Diet Assoc.* 1998;98:548–553.

118. Position of The American Dietetic Association. Vitamin and mineral supplementation. *J Am Diet Assoc.* 1996;96:73–77.

119. Tripp F. The use of dietary supplements in the elderly: current issues and recommendations. *J Am Diet Assoc.* 1997;97: S181–S183.

120. Houston DK, Johnson MA, Daniel TD, Poon LW. Health and dietary characteristics of supplement users in an elderly populations. *Int J Vitam Nutr Res.* 1997;67:183–191.

121. Allen LH, Casterline J. Vitamin B-12 deficiency in elderly individuals: diagnosis and requirements. *Am J Clin Nutr.* 1994;60:12–14.

122. Lindenbaum J, Rosenberg IH, Wilson PWF, Stabler SP, Allen RH. Prevalence of cobalamin deficiency in the Framingham elderly population. *Am J Clin Nutr.* 1994;60:2–11.

123. Bogden JD, Bendich A, Kemp FW, et al. Daily micronutrient supplements enhance delayed hypersensitivity skin test responses in older people. *Am J Clin Nutr.* 1994;60:437–447.

124. Keane EM, O'Broin S, Kelleher B, Coakley D, Walsh JB. Use of folic acid–fortified milk in the elderly population. *Gerontology.* 1998;44:336–339.

125. Cuskelly GJ, McNulty H, Scott JM. Effect of increasing dietary folate on red cell folate: implications for prevention of neural tube defects. *Lancet.* 1996;349:657–659.

126. Omenn GS. An assessment of the scientific basis for attempting to define the dietary reference intakes for beta carotene. *J Am Diet Assoc.* 1998;98:1406–1409.

127. Alpha-Tocopherol, Beta-Carotene Cancer Prevention Study Group. The effect of vitamin E and beta carotene in the incidence of lung cancer and other cancers in male smokers. *N Engl J Med.* 1994;330:1029–1035.

128. Nestle M. Nutrition. In: Wolfe SH, Jonas S, Lawrence RS, eds. *Health Promotion and Disease Prevention in Clinical Practice.* Baltimore: Williams & Wilkins; 1996.

129. Connor JR, Beard JL. Dietary iron supplements in the elderly: to use or not to use. *Nutr Today.* 1997;32:102–109.

130. Mertz W. Food fortification in the United States. *Nutr Rev.* 1997;55:44–49.

131. Russell RM. The impact of disease states as a modifying factor for nutrition toxicity. *Nutr Rev.* 1997;55:50–53.

132. Spaulding-Albright N. A review of some herbal and related products commonly used in cancer patients. *J Am Diet Assoc.* 1997;97:S208–S215.

133. Blumenthal M, Busse WH, Goldberg A, et al, eds. *The Complete German Commission E Monographs: Therapeutic Guide to Herbal Medicine.* Boston: Integrative Medicine Communications; 1998.

134. Tyler VE. *The Honest Herbal. A Sensible Guide to Use of Herbs.* 3rd ed. Binghamton, NY: Pharmaceutical Products Press Publishers; 1993.

135. Klontz KC, Adler WH, Potter M. Age-dependent resistance factors in the pathogenesis of foodborne infectious disease. *Aging (Milano).* 1997;9:320–326.

136. Beaumont DM, Mian MS. Celiac disease in old age: "a catch in the rye." *Age Ageing.* 1998;27:535–538.

137. Caceres VM, Ball RT, Somerfeldt SS, et al. A foodborne outbreak of cyclosporiasis caused by imported raspberries. *J Fam Pract.* 1998;47:231–234.

138. Quinn K, Baldwin G, Stepak P, et al. Foodborne outbreak of cryptosporidiosis—Spokane, WA, 1997. *MMWR.* 1998;47:565–567.

139. Millard PS, Gensheimer KF, Addiss DG, et al. An outbreak of cryptosporidiosis from fresh-pressed apple cider. *JAMA.* 1994;272:1592–1596.

140. Centers for Disease Control. Outbreaks of *Escherichia coli* 0157:H7 infection and cryptosporidiosis associated with drinking unpasteurized apple cider—Connecticut and New York, October 1996. *MMWR.* 1997;46:4–8.

141. Council for Agricultural Science and Technology (CAST). Foodborne pathogens: review of recommendations. www.cast-science.org (January 8, 1999).

142. Buchner DM, Wagner EH. Preventing frail health. *Clin Geriatr Med.* 1992;8:1–16.

143. Dayoff NE, Suhrheinrich J, Wigglesworth J, Topp R, Moore S. Balance and muscle strength as predictors of frailty among older adults. *J Gerontol Nurs.* 1998;24:18–27.

144. Raphael D, Cava M, Brown I, et al. Frailty: a public health perspective. *Can J Public Health.* 1995;86:224–227.

145. Brown I, Renwich R, Raphael D. Frailty: constructing a common meaning definition and conceptual framework. *Int J Rehabil Res.* 1995;18:93–102.

146. Guralnik JM, Simonsick EM. Physical disability in older Americans. *J Am Geriatr Soc.* 1993;48:3–10.

147. Sullivan D. Exercise in the frail elderly. Paper presented at Nutrition, Exercise and Aging. Nutrition and Aging XIII; Sept 16–17. 1998; Little Rock, Ark.

148. O'Grady M. Exercise and fall prevention. Paper presented at Nutrition, Exercise and Aging. Nutrition and Aging XIII; Sept 16–17, 1998; Little Rock, Ark.

149. Roubenoff R. Exercise for people with arthritis: can you and should you? Paper presented at Nutrition, Exercise and Aging. Nutrition and Aging XIII; Sept 16–17, 1998; Little Rock, Ark.

150. Borgenicht K, Carty E, Fergenbaum L. Community resources for frail older patients. *West J Med.* 1997;167:291–294.

151. Rall LC, Rosen CJ, Dolnikowski G, et al. Protein metabolism in rheumatoid arthritis and aging. *Arthritis Rheum.* 1996;39:1115–1124.

152. Haber D. *Health Promotion and Aging.* New York: Springer Publishing; 1994.

153. Wagner EH. Preventing decline in function: evidence from randomized trials around the world. *West J Med.* 1997;167:276–284.

154. Vita AJ, Terry RB, Hubert HB, Fries JF. Aging, health risks, and cumulative disability. *N Engl J Med.* 1998;338:1035–1041.

155. Wiliams SJ, Elder JP, Seidman RL, Mayer JA. Preventive services in a Medicare managed care environment. *J Community Health.* 1997;22:417–433.

156. Niedert KC, Dorner B, Gerwick C, Posthauer ME, Sichterman C, eds. *Nutritional Care for the Older Adult.* Chicago: The American Dietetic Association; 1998.

# Index